Fitness for Work
The Medical Aspects

FIFTH EDITION

Edited by

Keith T. Palmer
Professor of Occupational Medicine,
University of Southampton,
Southampton, UK

Ian Brown
Director and Head of Department,
Occupational Health Service,
University of Oxford;
Honorary Consultant Physician,
Occupational Health Medicine,
Oxfordshire Primary Care Trust,
Oxfordshire, UK

and

John Hobson
Consultant Occupational Physician,
Hobson Health Ltd,
Stoke-on-Trent, UK

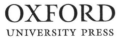

OXFORD
UNIVERSITY PRESS

OXFORD
UNIVERSITY PRESS

Great Clarendon Street, Oxford, OX2 6DP,
United Kingdom

Oxford University Press is a department of the University of Oxford.
It furthers the University's objective of excellence in research, scholarship,
and education by publishing worldwide. Oxford is a registered trade mark of
Oxford University Press in the UK and in certain other countries

© Oxford University Press 2013

Chapter 25 © Caroline L. Swales and Jeffrey A. Aronson 2013

The moral rights of the authors have been asserted

Fifth Edition published in 2013

Impression: 2

British Library Cataloguing in Publication Data
Data available

ISBN 978-0-19-964324-0

Printed in Great Britain by
Clays Ltd, St Ives plc

Foreword

By Dame Carol Black and Dr Bill Gunnyeon

The fifth edition of *Fitness for Work* is being published at a time of profound global economic challenge with its consequential impact on business growth and employment opportunity. At the same time the recognition and acceptance of the inextricable links between health and employment has never been greater, nor has the focus on supporting people with health conditions or disabilities to experience the benefits of work been sharper. Medical professional institutions in many countries have demonstrated their commitment to promoting the link between good work and good health by affirming that helping patients to remain in or return to work should be part of a healthcare professional's clinical function.

Safeguarding health at work, preventing loss of occupation as a result of ill health, and supporting prompt treatment and rehabilitation must be a joint enterprise. It must bring together the multiple aspects of a patient's concerns about their work in the face of health problems. It bridges the elements of clinical consultation and clinical management, functional assessment, and the workplace and welfare support agencies.

For some people an unavoidable consequence of illness and resulting disability is that they never work again. For many others this might result from failure to intervene sufficiently early when sickness threatens employment. There is consistent evidence in support of early intervention to help sick-certified people who do not have life-threatening or seriously disabling conditions to return to work. Such intervention should combine biopsychosocial and vocational rehabilitation, reaching beyond the usual limits of occupational health or of common clinical practice.

The needs of those who are not in productive employment—notably the young, the retired, and those unable to work—depend on the productive efforts of those who are working. With an ageing population the ratio is changing adversely and chronic disorders, common and rare, become more prevalent. This has obvious implications for attempts to extend working life. Besides underlining the importance of safeguarding and maintaining the health and well-being of people at all ages, it heightens attention to the preservation of function as an essential goal of clinical management, with a particular emphasis on capabilities that remain rather than those that have been diminished or lost.

The balance of this book is weighted towards clinical consultations and the functional consequences of health problems. Its chief concerns are the effects of medical conditions on employment and working capability, and the implications for the working life of patients with an illness or other disabling condition. This new edition builds on the foundations of the preceding edition, which reflected a growing understanding of the importance of appropriate 'good' work in maintaining health and well-being. The book provides an unrivalled source of information and guidance on the functional consequences of every significant health problem, their occupational impact, and how these can be minimized. Above all, it should help clinicians restore confidence to many people who—with a determination to meet the life challenges of less than perfect health and some impairment of function—can maintain a rewarding and fulfilling working life for as long as possible.

As we look to the future and to the growth in the economy required to support our increasingly elderly population, we will become more and more dependent on those with long-term health conditions and disabilities optimizing their participation in the world of work. Sound evidence-based decisions about fitness for work will be critical to achieving this. Like its predecessors, the new edition of *Fitness for Work: The Medical Aspects* should be accessible to all who have duties and responsibilities in this field.

Dame Carol Black
National Director for Health and Work (2006–2011)
Dr Bill Gunnyeon
Chief Medical Adviser
Department for Work and Pensions

Foreword

By Dr Olivia Carlton

The understanding of fitness for work underpins much of the practice of occupational medicine and occupational health. It is sometimes a complex matter, requiring knowledge of medicine and the related health disciplines. It also requires an understanding of individual psychology, the nature of work, the social milieu and social norms, cultural and gender differences, the barriers to work, and the incentives and disincentives which affect attitudes and behaviour.

The practitioner is not always a disinterested party, when advising on fitness to work. Part of their role may be to use their agency to help workers change their attitudes and behaviours towards their own fitness for work. This work on attitudes sometimes extends to employers and indirectly, or sometimes even directly, to families, work colleagues, and workplace employee advisers, including trade unions. The process of arriving at the point at which effective fitness for work advice can be given is a fascinating one. Working as I do in a safety critical industry, I am aware that some of the most interesting conversations I have had over a quarter of a century are about fitness for work decisions.

This outstanding textbook assists English-speaking people working in the occupational health arena all over the world to apply evidence-based knowledge in their decision-making. The first edition came out in 1987 and subsequent editions have reflected changes in knowledge, approach, and legislation, focused primarily on UK practice but with information that is useful worldwide. This fifth edition has new important and welcome chapters on cancer and on sickness absence. There has been a change of authorship in half of the chapters, which has brought a fresh approach to much of the subject matter. The underlying evidence for all chapters has been updated.

This is the Faculty of Occupational Medicine's flagship publication. I would like to thank all the contributors, and note my particular gratitude to the Editor in Chief, Keith Palmer, and his co-editors Ian Brown and John Hobson. I can attest to their tireless application in ensuring that the fifth edition builds on its predecessors and is of outstanding quality. All users of this book are in their debt.

Dr Olivia Carlton
President
Faculty of Occupational Medicine

Preface

Fitness for Work has become an established and essential source of guidance to all those involved in the practice of occupational medicine, including occupational physicians, occupational health nurses, general practitioners, and hospital doctors. It has also become an important point of reference for non-medical professionals such as personnel managers, safety officers, trade union officials, lawyers, and careers advisers amongst others. The requirement for sound, evidence-based advice on fitness decisions in workers with health complaints underpins the book's enduring popularity.

Since the last edition, awareness of the benefits of work has come to the forefront of public health and government thinking. The Black report, the Equality Act 2010, and the scrapping of compulsory retirement are all recent major developments with implications for assessing working-age health. The introduction of the 'fit note' may herald a sea change in thinking about return to work by both employers and general practitioners. Legislation to remove the 'default' retirement age provides a passport for people to work longer, but raises additional questions about fitness at older ages for suitable and, if necessary, appropriately tailored work.

Successive editions of this book have mentioned the fact that most employers and a large proportion of the workforce still do not have access to specialist occupational health advice. Occupational health is more important than ever and yet, paradoxically, there continues to be a decline in specialist training and established expertise, with little prospect of this trend being reversed in the near future. The existence of this book therefore remains an essential resource for non-specialist physicians to provide appropriate and accurate advice to employers.

The fifth edition follows the tried and trusted formula whereby most chapters are co-authored by a specialist occupational physician and a topic specialist. Every chapter has been updated and a number of other significant changes have been made. A new chapter has been added on managing and avoiding sickness absence, and a second on cancer survivorship and work; a former appendix on return to work after critical illness has been married with a chapter on fitness for work after surgery, to provide expert consensual guidance on expected return to work times; and, in all, some 29 new authors have contributed to this new edition. Most chapters have significant new content and there is increased emphasis on evidence, which has become easier to achieve with the further development of National Institute for Health and Clinical Excellence guidelines and the maturing of the Cochrane database. Where systematic off-the-peg evidence does not exist, *Fitness for Work* continues to provide a wealth of useful consensus guidance, codes of practice, and locally evolved standards with practical value to occupational health practitioners.

Although *Fitness for Work* is aimed at practice in the United Kingdom, we feel that most of the topics are universal and are covered in a sufficiently general way as to be of help wherever in the world there is a need to make informed decisions about the medical aspects of fitness for work. This book will be invaluable to anyone practising occupational medicine.

To an extent, occupational medicine, like medicine as a whole, is an art that tailors advice to individual patients under specific and unique circumstances. As with any clinical judgement, the medical advice that is given remains the responsibility of the doctor concerned and the general guidance contained in this book must always be interpreted in that light. Nonetheless, we believe this book will underwrite the considered opinions of clinicians and other professionals involved in the practice of occupational medicine.

Keith T. Palmer
Ian Brown
John Hobson

Acknowledgements

A book of this size, complexity, and significance would not be possible without tremendous effort on the part of many people and the support of several bodies. We would particularly like to acknowledge the 65 writers for this edition, who tread in the footsteps of previous authors making significant contributions to earlier editions of the work. These specialists have given freely of their time, shared their expertise and knowledge for the benefit of the health of working people, and have helped to create this much revised fifth edition of the Faculty's flagship publication. They have also borne patiently the enquiries of editors and publishers and can take credit for their individual chapters as we the editors take pride in the final book. We also wish to thank our many colleagues within the Faculty of Occupational Medicine of the Royal College of Physicians of London for providing both direct and indirect support throughout the book's gestation, and staff from Oxford University Press for their efforts in helping to coordinate this dauntingly large endeavour.

Keith T. Palmer
Ian Brown
John Hobson

Contents

Abbreviations

ABI	Association of British Insurers	BEA	British Epilepsy Association
ABR	auditory brainstem response	BHA	British Hyperbaric Association
ACC	American College of Cardiology	BM	bone marrow
ACE	angiotensin-converting enzyme	BMI	body mass index
ACJ	acromioclavicular joint	BMT	bone marrow transplant
ACL	anterior cruciate ligament	BNF	British National Formulary
ACOP	Approved Code of Practice	BP	blood pressure
ACP	American College of Physicians	BPH	benign prostatic hyperplasia
ACR	albumin:creatinine ratio	BPT	bronchial provocation challenge test
ADA	Americans with Disabilities Act	BSRM	British Society of Rehabilitation Medicine
ADL	activities of daily living		
AED	antiepileptic drug	BTS	British Thoracic Society
AHA	American Heart Association	CA	Court of Appeal
AIDS	acquired immune deficiency syndrome	CAA	Civil Aviation Authority
ALAMA	Association of Local Authority Medical Advisers	CABG	coronary artery bypass grafting
		CAPD	continuous ambulatory peritoneal dialysis
ALL	acute lymphoblastic leukaemia		
ALT	alanine transferase	CBI	Confederation of British Industry
AMAS	activity matching ability system	CBT	cognitive-behavioural therapy
AME	authorized medical examiner	CCDC	Consultant in Communicable Disease Control
AMED	Approved Medical Examiner of Divers		
AML	acute myeloid leukaemia	CD	Crohn's disease
AMRA	Access to Medical Reports Act 1988	CD4	cluster of differentiation 4 glycoprotein on T-helper lymphocytes
ANHOPS	Association of National Health Occupational Physicians		
		CEDP	Committee for the employment of disabled people
APD	automated peritoneal dialysis		
ARBs	angiotensin II receptor blockers	CEFEM	'Chance Encounter of Female Exceeding Male' strength
ARDS	acute respiratory distress syndrome		
ART	antiretroviral treatment	CEHR	Combined Equality and Human Rights Commission
AS	ankylosing spondylitis		
ATCO	air traffic control officer	CFC	chlorofluorocarbons
ATS-DLD	American Thoracic Society and the Division of Lung Disease	CFS	chronic fatigue syndrome
		CHD	coronary heart disease
AVC	additional voluntary contribution	CI	confidence interval
AWT	all work test	CIBSE	Chartered Institution of Building Services Engineers
BAC	blood alcohol concentration		
BBS	Behavioural Based Safety	CISD	Critical Incident Stress Debriefing
BCG	Bacillus of Calmette and Guérin	CJD	Creutzfeldt–Jakob disease
		CKD	chronic kidney disease
BCS	British Crime Survey	CLAW	The Control of Lead at Work Regulations

CLL	chronic lymphocytic leukaemia
CML	chronic myeloid leukaemia
CMP	Condition Management Programme
CMV	cytomegalovirus
CNS	central nervous system
COPD	chronic obstructive pulmonary disease
COSHH	Control of Substances Hazardous to Health
CPAP	continuous positive airways pressure
CPR	Civil Procedure Rules
CRE	Commission for Racial Equality
CSAG	Clinical Standards Advisory Group
CSF	cerebrospinal fluid
CSII	continuous subcutaneous insulin infusion
CT	computed tomography
CTS	carpal tunnel syndrome
CVD	cardiovascular disease
CVS	chorionic villus sampling
DAS	Disability Advisory Service
DAS28	Disease Activity Score-28
DB	defined benefit
DBCP	1,2-dibromochloropropane
dB	decibel
DC	defined contribution
DCU	Day Care Units
DDA	Disability Discrimination Act 1995
DDAVP	desmopressin
DDH	developmental dysplasia of the hip
DEA	Disability Employment Adviser
DHA	docosohexaenoic acid
DIP	distal interphalangeal joint
DIT	Disability Information Trust
DLA	Disability Living Allowance
DLF	Disabled Living Foundation
DMAC	Diving Medical Advisory Committee
DMARD	disease-modifying anti-rheumatic drug
DMPA	depot medroxyprogesterone contraception
DOTS	directly observed short-course treatment
DPA	Data Protection Act 1998
DSA	Disablement Services Authority
DSE	display screen equipment

DSM IV	*Diagnostic and statistical manual of mental disorders* (American Psychological Association)
DST	Disability Service Team
DVLA	Driving and Vehicle Licensing Agency
DVT	deep venous thrombosis
DWP	Department of Work and Pensions
DWR	Diving at Work Regulations 1997
EAA	extrinsic allergic alveolitis
EAGA	Expert Advisory Group on AIDS
EAP	Employee Assistance Programme
EASA	European Aviation Safety Authority
EAT	Employment Appeal Tribunal
EBMT	European Group for Blood and Marrow Transplantation
ECG	electrocardiogram
ECJ	European Court of Justice
EDH	extradural haematoma
EDTC	European Diving Technology Committee
EEG	electroencephalography
EFA	Epilepsy Foundation of America
ELISA	enzyme-linked immunosorbent assay
EMAS	Employment Medical Advisory Service
EMDR	eye movement desensitization and reprocessing
EMG	electromyogram
ENT	ear, nose, and throat
EOC	Equal Opportunities Commission
EPDS	Edinburgh Post Natal Depression Scale
ERC	Employment Rehabilitation Centres
ERS	European Respiratory Society
ERT	emergency response team
ESR	erythrocyte sedimentation rate
ESRD	end-stage renal disease
ET	Employment Tribunal
ETS	environmental tobacco smoke
EU	European Union
EWDTS	European Workplace Drug Testing Society
FCA	functional capacity assessment
FCE	functional capacity evaluation
FEFC	Further Education Funding Council
FEV_1	volume of gas expired in the first second
FIX	factor IX of the blood clotting cascade

FOM	Faculty of Occupational Medicine	HSW	Health and Safety at Work etc. Act 1974
FRC	functional residual capacity	HTL	hearing threshold level
FVC	forced vital capacity	HTLV1	human T-lymphotropic virus I
FVIII	clotting factor VIII of the blood clotting cascade	HTLVII	human T-lymphotropic virus II
		HTV	hand-transmitted vibration
FXI	factor XI of the blood clotting cascade	IAP	intra-abdominal pressure
G-CSF	granulocyte colony stimulating factor	IATA	International Air Transport Association
GCMS	gas chromatography–mass spectrometry	IB	Incapacity Benefit
		IBE	International Bureau for Epilepsy
GCS	Glasgow Coma Scale	IBS	irritable bowel syndrome
GFR	glomerular filtration rate	ICAO	International Civil Aviation Organization
GGT	gamma-glutamyl transferase		
GHJ	glenohumeral joint	ICD	implantable cardioverter defibrillator
GMC	General Medical Council	ICD-10	*International Statistical Classification of Diseases and Related Health Problems* (WHO)
GOLD	Global Initiative for Chronic Obstructive Lung Disease		
GORD	gastro-oesophageal reflux disease	ICFDH	International Classification of Functioning, Disability and Health
GP	general practitioner		
GvHD	graft versus host disease	ICOH	International Commission on Occupational Health
HAART	highly active antiretroviral therapy		
HAD	Hospital Anxiety and Depression Scale	IDDM	insulin-dependent diabetes mellitus
HAVS	hand–arm vibration syndrome	IDH	intradural haematoma
HbAS	heterozygous sickle cell disease	IDRP	internal dispute resolution procedure
HBcAB	hepatitis B core antibody	IHR	ill health retirement
HbeAG	hepatitis B e antigen	IIDB	Industrial Injury Disablement Benefit
HbIg	hepatitis B hyperimmune serum	IIDTW	Independent Inquiry into Drug Testing at Work
HbS	haemoglobin S (sickle haemoglobin)		
HBsAg	hepatitis B surface antigen	ILEA	International League Against Epilepsy
HbSC	sickle haemoglobin C disease	ILO	International Labour Organization
HbSS	homozygous sickle cell anaemia	IMiDs	immunomodulatory drugs
Hbsßthal	sickle beta thalassaemia disease	IMO	International Maritime Organization
HBV	DNA hepatitis B virus DNA	INR	international normalized ratio
hCG	human chorionic gonadotrophin	IOFB	intraocular foreign body
HCV	hepatitis C virus	IPSS	International Prostate Symptom Score
HD	haemodialysis; Hodgkin's disease	IPV	inactivated polio vaccine
HIV	human immunodeficiency virus	IRLR	Industrial Relations Law Report
HLA	human leucocyte antigen	IT	information technology
HNIG	human normal immunoglobulin	ITP	idiopathic thrombocytopenic purpura
HMFI	Her Majesty's Factory Inspectorate	IUCD	intrauterine contraceptive device
HMSO	Her Majesty's Stationery Office	IUD	intrauterine death
HPS	Heart Protection Study	IVF	*in vitro* fertilization
HRT	hormone replacement therapy	JAA	Joint Aviation Authorities
HSC	Health and Safety Commission	JCA	juvenile chronic arthritis
HSE	Health and Safety Executive	JRA	juvenile rheumatoid arthritis
HSL	Health and Safety Laboratory	KCO	carbon monoxide transfer coefficient

KS	Kaposi's sarcoma
KSHV	Kaposi's sarcoma associated herpes virus
L	litre
LACS	lacunar syndromes
LASIK	laser assisted *in situ* keratomilieusis
LBP	low back pain
LGV	large goods vehicle
LMWH	low-molecular-weight heparin
LTD	long-term disability
MAI	*Mycobacterium avium intracellulare*
MAOI	monoamine oxidase inhibitor
MCA	Maritime and Coastguard Agency
MCH	mean corpuscular haemoglobin
MCV	mean corpuscular volume
MDS	myelodysplastic syndrome
ME	myeloencephalitis
MED3	medical statements
METs	metabolic equivalents
MHSW	Management of Health and Safety at Work Regulations 1992
MI	myocardial infarction
MIT	multiple injection treatment
mL	millilitre
MND	motor neurone disease
mph	miles per hour
MRC	Medical Research Council
MRI	magnetic resonance imaging
MRO	Medical Review Officer
MRSA	methicillin-resistant *Staphylococcus aureus*
MS	multiple sclerosis
MTP	metatarsophalangeal joint
NA	nucleoside analogue reverse transcriptase inhibitor
NCYPE	National Centre for Young People with Epilepsy
NGO	non-governmental organization
NGPSE	National General Practice Study of Epilepsy
Nhanes III	Third National Health and Nutrition Survey
NHL	non-Hodgkin's lymphoma
NHS	National Health Service
NI	National Insurance
NICE	National Institute for Health and Clinical Excellence
NIDDM	non-insulin-dependent diabetes mellitus
NIOSH	National Institute of Occupational Safety and Health (US)
NMC	Nursing and Midwifery Council
NMR	nuclear magnetic resonance
NNRTI	non-nucleoside reverse transcriptase inhibitor
NPV	negative predictive value
NRR	noise reduction ratio
NRTI	nucleoside analogue reverse transcriptase inhibitor
NSAIDs	non-steroidal anti-inflammatory drugs
NSE	National Society for Epilepsy
NSH	National Study of Hearing
NTD	neural tube defects
nvCJD	new variant Creutzfeld–Jakob disease
OA	osteoarthritis
OH	occupational health
OHA	oral hypoglycaemic agent
OHS	occupational health services
OP	occupational physician
OPCS	Office of Population Censuses and Surveys
OPITO	Offshore Petroleum Industry Training Organization
OR	odds ratio
ORIF	open reduction and internal fixation
OTC	over the counter
PACS	partial anterior circulation syndromes
PBSC	peripheral blood stem cell
PCP	*Pneumocystis (carini) jiroveci* pneumonia
PCR	polymerase chain reaction; protein:creatinine ratio
PCT	Primary Care Trust
PCV	passenger carrying vehicle
PD	peritoneal dialysis; Parkinson's disease; Prescribed Disease
PE	pulmonary embolism
PEF	peak expiratory flow
PEFR	peak expiratory flow rate
PFEER	Prevention of Fire and Explosion, Emergency Response

PFO	patent foramen ovale	RTW	return to work
PGL	persistent generalized lymphadenopathy	RV	residual volume
PHI	permanent health insurance	SAMHSA	Substance Abuse and Mental Health Services Administration
PI	protease inhibitor	SARS	severe acute respiratory syndrome
PID	pelvic inflammatory disease	SCAT	standardized concussion assessment tool
PIP	proximal interphalangeal joint		
PMS	premenstrual syndrome	SCBA	self-contained breathing apparatus
PNH	paroxysmal nocturnal haemoglobinuria	SCD	sickle cell disease
		SCI	spinal cord injury
POAG	primary open-angle glaucoma	SCID	severe combined immune deficiency
POCS	posterior vertebrobasilar circulation syndromes	sCJD	sporadic Creutzfeldt–Jakob disease
		SCT	stem cell transplantation
PoM	prescription-only medicine	SDA	Severe Disablement Allowance
PPE	personal protective equipment	SEQOHS	Safe Effective Quality Occupational Health Service
PPI	proton pump inhibitors		
PPV	positive predictive value	SES	socio-economic status
PRK	photorefractive keratectomy	SLE	systemic lupus erythematosus
PRV	polycythaemia rubra vera	SMI	serious mental illness
PSA	prostate specific antigen	SPB	spontaneous preterm birth
PTA	post-traumatic amnesia	SPL	sound pressure level
PTCA	percutaneous transluminal coronary angioplasty	SSP	Statutory Sick Pay
		SSRI	serotonin selective re-uptake inhibitor
PTSD	post-traumatic stress disorder		
RA	rheumatoid arthritis	TB	tuberculosis
RADAR	The Royal Association for Disability and Rehabilitation	TED	thromboembolic deterrent
		TENS	transcutaneous electrical nerve stimulation
RADS	reactive airways dysfunction syndrome		
RAST	radioallergosorbent test	TfW	Training for Work programme
RCGP	Royal College of General Practitioners	THC	tetrahydrocannabinol
RCOG	Royal College of Obstetricians and Gynaecologists	TIA	transient ischaemic attack
		TLC	total lung capacity
RECs	research ethics committees	TLCO	carbon monoxide transfer factor
RF	rheumatoid factor	TPAS	The Pensions Advisory Service
RIDDOR	Reporting of Injuries, Diseases and Dangerous Occurrences Regulations 1995	TU	Trade Union
		TUC	Trades Union Congress
		UC	ulcerative colitis
RNIB	Royal National Institute for the Blind	UKPDS	UK Prospective Diabetes Study
RoC	receiver operating characteristic	UV	ultraviolet
RP	Raynaud's phenomenon	VA	visual activity
RPE	respiratory protective equipment; retinal pigment epithelium	vCJD	variant Creutzfeld–Jakob disease
		VCO$_2$	rate of elimination of carbon dioxide
RRT	renal replacement therapy	VDE	visual display equipment
RSD	reflex sympathetic dystrophy	VDU	visual display unit
RSI	repetitive strain injury	VR	vocational rehabilitation
RTI	reverse transcriptase inhibitor		

VTE	venous thromboembolic disease	VO_{2max}	maximum oxygen uptake
VZV	varicella zoster	WAI	work ability index
VWF	von Willebrand's factor; vibration-induced white finger	WHO	World Health Organization
		WRULD	work-related upper limb disorder
VO_2	oxygen consumption	ZDV	zidovudine

List of contributors

Jeffrey A. Aronson
Reader in Clinical Pharmacology
Green Templeton College
Oxford, UK;
Honorary Consultant in Clinical
Pharmacology and Honorary Consultant
Physician
Oxford Radcliffe Hospital NHS Trust
Oxford, UK

Tar-Ching Aw
Professor and Chair of Occupational Medicine
Department of Community Medicine
United Arab Emirates University
Al Ain, UAE

Mansel Aylward
Director
Centre for Psychosocial and Disability
Research;
Professor of Public Health Education
Cardiff University
Cardiff, UK

Ian Banks
President, European Men's Health Forum
Brussels, Belgium

Steve Boorman
Medical Director
UK Occupational Health Services
Abermed, London, UK

Henrietta Bowden-Jones
Consultant Psychiatrist
National Problem Gambling Clinic
London and Honorary Senior Lecturer
Department of Medicine
Imperial College
London, UK

David Brown
Consultant Occupational Physician
EDF Energy (Nuclear Generation)
Gloucester, UK

Edwina A. Brown
Consultant Nephrologist
Imperial College
Kidney and Transplant Centre
Hammersmith Hospital
London, UK

Ian Brown
Director and Head of Department
Occupational Health Service
University of Oxford;
Honorary Consultant Physician
Occupational Health Medicine
Oxfordshire Primary Care Trust
Oxfordshire, UK

Phil Bryson
Medical Director of Diving Services
Abermed Ltd
Aberdeen, UK

Tim Carter
Chief Medical Advisor
UK Maritime and Coastguard Agency
and Norwegian Centre for Maritime Medicine
Department of Occupational Medicine
University of Bergen, Norway

Deborah A. Cohen
Senior Medical Research Fellow
Centre for Psychosocial and Disability
Research
Cardiff University
Cardiff, UK

Andrew P. Colvin
Consultant Occupational Physician
Atos Healthcare for Scotland and Northern
Ireland
Glasgow, UK

Christopher Conlon
Consultant in Infectious Diseases
Nuffield Department of Medicine
John Radcliffe Hospital
Oxford, UK

Roger Cooke
Consultant in Occupational Medicine
Honorary Senior Lecturer
Institute of Occupational
and Environmental Medicine
University of Birmingham
Birmingham, UK

Sally E. L. Coomber
Clinical Lead
Safe Effective Quality Occupational Health
Service (SEQOHS)
Royal College of Physicians;
Consultant Occupational Physician
Suffolk Occupational Health
The Ipswich Hospital NHS Trust
Ipswich, UK

Paul Cullinan
Occupational and Environmental Medicine
Imperial College and Royal Brompton
Hospital
London, UK

Finlay Dick
Senior Occupational Physician
Capita Health and Wellbeing
Aberdeen, UK

Mike Doig
Regional Medical Manager
Health and Medical Services
Chevron Ltd
London, UK

Shirley D'Sa
Consultant Haemato-Oncologist
University London Hospitals
NHS Foundation Trust
London, UK

Sally A. Evans
Chief Medical Officer
UK Civil Aviation Authority
West Sussex, UK

Ursula T. Ferriday
Consultant in Occupational Medicine
Worcestershire Acute Hospitals
NHS Trust and Head
Working Well Centre
Worcester, UK

Iain S. Foulds
Consultant Dermatologist and
Senior Lecturer in Occupational Dermatology
Institute of Occupational and
Environmental Medicine
University of Birmingham
Birmingham, UK

Geoff Gill
Professor and Honorary
Consultant Physician
Department of Diabetes and Endocrinology
University of Liverpool
Clinical Sciences Centre
Aintree University Hospital
Liverpool, UK

Henry N. Goodall
Consultant Occupational Physician
Hampshire, UK

Neil Greenberg
Defence Professor of Mental Health
and Co-director of the Academic
Centre for Defence Mental Health
King's College London
London, UK

Charles Greenough
Clinical Director
The Golden Jubilee Spinal Cord
Injuries Centre
The James Cook University Hospital
University of Durham
Middlesbrough, UK

Paul Grime
Consultant Occupational Physician
Cambridge University Hospitals NHS
Foundation Trust
Cambridge, UK

John Grimley Evans
Professor Emeritus of Clinical Geratology
University of Oxford
Oxford, UK

Richard J. Hardie
Consultant Neurologist and Stroke Specialist
Department of Neurology
Frenchay Hospital
Bristol, UK

Peter A. Harris
Consultant Obstetrician and Gynaecologist
West Suffolk Hospital NHS Trust
Suffolk, UK

Simon Hellier
Consultant Gastroenterologist
Worcester Royal Hospital
Worcester, UK

Robbert Hermanns
Specialist Occupational Physician
Occupational Health Risk Management
Services Ltd, Milnathort
Scotland, UK

Richard Heron
President
Society of Occupational Medicine;
Vice President
BP PLC
London, UK

John Hobson
Consultant Occupational Physician
Hobson Health Ltd, UK

Gillian S. Howard
Employment Lawyer
London, UK

Richard S. Kaczmarski
Consultant Haematologist
Hillingdon and Ealing Hospitals
London, UK

David S. Q. Koh
Chair Professor of Occupational
Health and Medicine
PAPRSB Institute of Health Sciences
University Brunei Darussalam
Brunei Darussalam

Ian Lawson
Chief Medical Officer
Rolls-Royce PLC
Derby, UK

Paul Litchfield
Chief Medical Officer
BT Group PLC
London, UK

Chris Little
Consultant Orthopaedic Surgeon
Nuffield Orthopaedic Centre
Oxford, UK

Linda M. Luxon
Emeritus Professor of Audiovestibular
Medicine and Consultant Neuro-otologist
UCL Ear Institute/National Hospital for
Neurology and Neurosurgery
London, UK

Ira Madan
Consultant and Honorary Senior Lecturer
in Occupational Medicine
Guy's and St Thomas' NHS Foundation
Trust and King's College
London, UK

Heather G. Major
Senior Medical Adviser
Driver and Vehicle Licensing Agency (DVLA)
Swansea, UK

Stuart J. Mitchell
Head Aeromedical Centre and Occupational
Civil Aviation Authority
West Sussex, UK

Anne-Marie O'Donnell
Consultant Occupational Physician
Occupational Health Services
University of Oxford
Oxford, UK

Dipti Patel
Consultant Occupational Health Physician
Foreign and Commonwealth Office
London and Joint Director
National Travel Health Network and Centre
London, UK

Keith T. Palmer
Professor of Occupational Medicine
University of Southampton
Southampton, UK

Michael C. Petch
Consultant Cardiologist
The Queen Elizabeth Hospital
King Lynn's NHS Trust
Norfolk, UK

John Pitts
Consultant Ophthalmologist to the Civil
Aviation Authority
London, UK

Jon Poole
Consultant Occupational Physician
Dudley and Walsall NHS Trust
Health Centre
Dudley, UK

Richard Preece
Consultant in Occupational Medicine
Cheshire Occupational Health Service
Mid Cheshire Hospitals NHS Foundation Trust
Crewe, UK

Martin C. Prevett
Consultant in Neurology
Southampton University Hospitals NHS Trust
Southampton, UK

Anne E. Price
Consultant Occupational Physician
Hinchingbrooke NHS Trust
Huntingdon, UK

Dean Royles
Director
NHS Employers
Leeds, UK

Steve Ryder
Director of Occupational Health
Services NHS Highland
Inverness, UK

†Philip E. Sawney
Formerly of the Department for Work
and Pensions
Surrey, UK

Julia Smedley
Consultant Occupational Physician
and Head of Occupational Health
University Hospital Southampton NHS
Foundation Trust;
Honorary Senior Lecturer
University of Southampton
Southampton, UK

Caroline L. Swales
Consultant Occupational Physician
University Hospitals of Morecambe Bay
NHS Foundation Trust
North Cumbria University Hospitals Trust
Cumbria, UK

Bill Thomas
Consultant Surgeon and former
Clinical Director of Surgery
Sheffield Teaching Hospitals Trust
Sheffield, UK

Eugene R. Waclawski
Associate Professor
Division of Preventive Medicine
Faculty of Medicine and Dentistry
University of Alberta
Alberta, Canada

Karen Walker-Bone
Reader and Honorary Consultant in
Rheumatology
Brighton and Sussex Medical School
University of Sussex
Brighton, UK

Tony Williams
Medical Director of Working Fit
Kent, UK

Philip Wynn
Senior Occupational Health Physician
Durham County Council
Durham, UK

Chapter 1

A general framework for assessing fitness for work

Keith T. Palmer and Ian Brown

This book on fitness for work gathers together specialist advice on the medical aspects of employment and the majority of medical conditions likely to be encountered in the working population. Though personnel managers and others will find it of great help, it is primarily written for doctors so that family practitioners, hospital consultants, and occupational physicians, as well as other doctors and occupational health nurses, can best advise managers and others who may need to know how a patient's illness might affect their work. Although decisions on return to work or on placement must depend on many factors, it is hoped that this book, which combines best current clinical and occupational health practice, will be used by doctors and others as a source of reference and remind them about the occupational implications of illness.

It must be emphasized that, apart from relieving suffering and prolonging life, the objective of much medical treatment in working-aged adults is to return the patient to work. Much of the benefit of modern medical technology and the skills of physicians and surgeons will have been wasted if patients who have been successfully treated are denied work, through ignorance or prejudice, by employers or doctors acting on their behalf. A main aim of this book is to remove the excuse for denying work to those who have overcome injury and disease and deserve to be employed.

The book is arranged in chapters according to specialty or topic, most chapters having been written jointly by two specialists, one of whom is an occupational physician. For each specialty the chapter outlines the conditions covered; notes relevant statistics; discusses clinical aspects, including treatment, which affect work capacity; notes rehabilitation requirements or special needs at the workplace; discusses problems that may arise at work and necessary work restrictions; notes any current advisory or statutory medical standards; and makes recommendations on employment aspects of the conditions covered.

The first five chapters are applicable to any condition. This introductory chapter deals mainly with the principles underlying medical assessment of fitness for work, contacts between medical practitioners and the workplace, and confidentiality of medical information. Chapter 2 covers legal aspects, Chapter 3 focuses on the Equality Act, Chapter 4 outlines the current provision for support, rehabilitation, and restoring fitness for work, and important ethical principles of occupational health practice are elaborated in Chapter 5 (which is written by the Chair of the Faculty of Occupational Medicine's Ethics Committee).

A chapter on the possible effects of medication on work performance and additional chapters on the ageing worker, sickness absence, ill health retirement, health screening, health promotion in the workplace, return to work following critical illness, working with cancer, and fitness to drive are also included. Appendices on medical standards in various specific settings (civil aviation, merchant shipping, offshore work diving, work overseas) complete the book.

Health problems and employment

Workers with disabilities are commonly found to be highly motivated, often with excellent work and attendance records. When medical fitness for work is assessed, what matters is often not the medical condition itself, but the associated loss of function, and any resulting disability or handicap. It should be borne in mind that a disability seen in the consulting room may be irrelevant to the performance of a particular job. *The patient's condition should be interpreted in functional terms and in the context of the job requirements.*

Impairment, disability, and handicap

Handicap may result directly from an impairment (for instance, severe facial disfigurement), or more usually, from the resulting disability. To be consistent in the use of these terms, the simplified scheme of the *International classification of impairments, disabilities, and handicaps*[1,2] (now supplanted by the *International Classification of Functioning, Disability and Health*—see <http://www.who.int/classifications/icf/en/>) can be used as follows:

◆ A disease, disorder, or injury produces an *impairment* (change in normal structure or function).

◆ A *disability* is a resulting reduction or loss of an ability to perform an activity—for example, climbing stairs or using a keyboard.

◆ A *handicap* is a social disadvantage resulting from an impairment or disability, which limits or prevents the fulfilment of a normal role.

As examples:

◆ A relatively minor *impairment*, the loss of a finger, would be both a *disability* and a serious occupational *handicap* to a pianist, although not to a labourer.

◆ A relatively common *impairment*, defective colour vision, limits the ability to discriminate between certain hues. This may occasionally be a *handicap* at work, although there are in fact few occupations for which defective colour vision is a significant handicap.

Prevalence of disability and its impact on employment

Figures on the prevalence of disability and/or handicap in different populations vary according to the definitions and methods used and the groups sampled. There is no doubt that, however measured, disabling illness is common and an obstacle to gainful employment. One national population survey,[3] undertaken in the UK in 2001 by the Office of National Statistics, estimated that nearly one in five people of working age had a long-term disability (3.7 million men and 3.4 million women). Some 3.4 million disabled people were in employment, although at a rate significantly lower than that of those without disabilities (48 per cent vs. 81 per cent). Roughly half of the disabled population was economically inactive (44 per cent of men and 52 per cent of women) as compared with 15 per cent of the non-disabled population. The overall proportion of people reporting long-term illness or disability that restricted daily activities was 18 per cent, but the age-standardized rate was three times higher in the long-term unemployed than in managerial and professional occupations (Figure 1.1).

Many other statistics paint a similar picture, of common illnesses that commonly erode work capacity:

◆ Sickness absence cost the UK economy almost £17 billion in 2010, with 190 million working days lost.

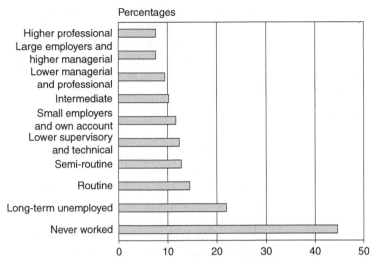

Figure 1.1 Age-standardized rates of long-term illness or disability restricting daily activities: by socioeconomic status, 2001, England & Wales (Office of National Statistics, reproduced with permission © Crown Copyright 2001).

◆ In the National Health Service (NHS) in England alone, the annual loss has been put at 10.3 million working days—the equivalent of being without 45 000 whole-time staff at an annual direct cost of £1.7 billion.[4]

◆ Some 9 per cent of adults in Britain suffered mixed anxiety and depression in 2007, 230 out of a thousand visited a general practitioner (GP) every year with mental health problems and a tenth of these were referred to specialist psychiatric services.[5]

◆ The Health and Safety Executive (HSE) estimated that in 2009/10 2.1 million working-aged adults in Britain were suffering from an illness which they believed was caused or made worse by work, contributing 28.5 million working days lost due to work-ascribed ill health or injury.[6]

◆ One in three men and one in four women suffer a critical illness between the ages of 40 and 70 years.[7]

◆ In England and Wales some 22 000 replacements of hip or knee joints are carried out annually on adults aged 15–59 years.[8]

◆ The European Community Respiratory Health Survey[9] estimated that 10 per cent of adults aged 20–44 years wheeze at work, while 4 per cent have work-related respiratory disability.

◆ A cohort study of 20 000 French electricity workers reported that diabetics were 1.6 times as likely as other workers to quit the labour force;[10] people with diabetes are also more likely to experience problems in obtaining employment.[11]

◆ In a community-based survey in the north east of England[12] the unemployment rate for economically active patients with epilepsy was 46 per cent, as compared with 19 per cent in age and sex-matched controls.

The experience in other countries is similar. Thus, according to the 2009 American Community Survey,[13] some 9.9 per cent of Americans aged 15–64 years (19.5 million people) had a disability and their employment rate was half that of people without a disability.

Is this experience justified and reasonable? We would argue not, in many instances. Self-evidently, serious illness can prevent a person working, but many people with major illness *do* work with proper treatment and workplace support. Thus the relation with unemployment is not as inevitable as these gloomy statistics suggest. Rather, the job prospects of people with common illnesses and disabilities can often be improved with thought, both about the work that *is* still possible and the reasonable changes that could be made to allow for their circumstances.

The Equality Act 2010

These ideas are captured in primary legislation. The Equality Act 2010 and its forerunner, the Disability Discrimination Act 1995, have major significance both for the disabled and for occupational physicians. In broad terms, and with certain important details of interpretation, the Act makes it unlawful for employers to discriminate against workers, including job applicants, on grounds of medical disability; rather, it requires that all reasonable steps be taken to accommodate their health problems. This is a form of positive discrimination in favour of preserving employment opportunities. It is also the legal embodiment of good occupational health values; long before the Act, occupational health professionals strove for the same outcome. However, employers are influenced strongly by legal mandate, so the Act is an instrument for good, as judged from the viewpoint of the disabled.

Occupational physicians need a good working knowledge of this legislation. Such is the Act's importance that a whole chapter (Chapter 3) is devoted to its application and the recent development of case law, while references to the effects of the Act in clinical situations are made throughout the book. Here, only a few essential points are made.

In the Act, 'disability' is not defined in terms of working ability or capacity but in terms of 'a substantial and long-term adverse effect on the ability to carry out normal day-to-day activities'. Work itself does not, therefore, have to be considered in deciding whether an individual is disabled or not, but of course it does have to be considered when a disabled person is in a work situation. It is in this circumstance that the opinion of the occupational physician will be required. The physician may be asked:

◆ Whether an individual's disability falls within the definition of the Act?

◆ If it does, what adjustments may be needed to accommodate the disabled individual in the workplace?

Adjustments may be to the physical and psychological nature of the work or to the methods by which the work is accomplished. It is for management, not the occupational physician, to decide in each individual case whether such adjustments are *reasonable*, although occupational health services may be well placed to *identify* potential adjustments. Before offering such opinions the occupational physician must make an accurate determination of the individual's disability, not in medical but in functional terms; this requires a detailed understanding of the work and the workplace in question—another abiding principle of good occupational health practice.

The 'fit note'

To raise awareness of the principle that many jobs can be performed adequately by people with health limitations, and to support its implementation, the UK Government introduced a redesigned Statement of Fitness for Work ('fit note') in 2010 to replace the old 'sick note'. The new form includes an option for the certifying doctor to indicate that, while not fit for normal work, the patient may be capable of working in a suitably modified job. In doing so it supports the right to work of those with short- and long-term health problems, and recognizes that suitable work can bring tangible health benefits.[14] Advice on completing a fit note is provided in Chapter 4 and elsewhere.[15,16]

At the time of writing, a report by Dame Carol Black to the government has recommended that a new independent assessment service be created to assist employees, their family doctors, and employers in functional assessment and advising those absent from work for 30 days or more. Whether this ambition is realized and if so, how much it facilitates earlier rehabilitation and return to work must await description in a new edition of this book; but sickness absence is an important practical topic, taken up in detail in a chapter new to this edition (Chapter 30).

The ageing worker

One circumstance in which reasonable accommodation may be required is the employment of older workers. With increasing longevity and a growing shortfall in pension resources the pension age is being extended and the default retirement age of 65 phased out. In future, people may well work significantly past the traditional retirement age. This may be beneficial to individuals' wealth and health, though some will need modifications to their work or working time to accommodate impairments of ageing. Age, per se, can no longer be a blanket bar to gainful employment, though the advice contained in this book and the advice of an occupational health professional may be needed to integrate the older worker into employment effectively.

Some major issues surrounding practice in this area are aired in Chapter 26. Here we stress the importance of the topic and its close relation to occupational medicine. As the 'demographic time bomb' looms large, the slack to discard valuable skills and experience will diminish. Avoidance of ageist judgements about work fitness and greater flexibility in job deployment will become commercially important; these are already basic values in occupational health practice, while the underpinning medical advice will come from health professionals with experience in the occupational setting.

Occupational health services

All employees should have access to occupational health advice, whether this is provided from within a company or by external consultants. Such advice may be provided by occupational health-trained nurses or by specialist occupational physicians, but for some problems advice from a specialist will be essential—e.g. in providing evidence for industrial tribunals or in other medico-legal cases. The nature and size of the occupational health service to which a company needs access depend on its size and the hazards of the activities in which it is engaged. Some companies find it advantageous to buy in or share occupational health services.

The local Employment Medical Advisory Service (EMAS) of the HSE can advise on the availability and sources of local occupational health services and occupational health practitioners. EMAS may give advice to individual employees, although the principal role their medical inspectors (doctors) and occupational health inspectors (nurses) fulfil is to support the HSE's general inspectorate.

In the main, occupational health services advise on fitness for work, vocational placement, return to work after illness, ill health retirement, work-related illness, and the control of occupational hazards. Some of these functions are statutory (e.g. certain health surveillance) or advisable in terms of meeting legal responsibilities (e.g. guidance on food safety, application of the Equality Act). Some employers regard the main function of occupational health services to be to control sickness absence. Although occupational health professionals can certainly help managers to understand and possibly reduce sickness absence, its control is ultimately a management responsibility.

Contacts between the patient's medical advisers and the workplace

The patient's own medical advisers have an important part to play. The importance of their contact with the workplace cannot be overemphasized. Consultants, as well as family practitioners, should ask the patient if there is an occupational health service at the workplace and obtain written consent to contact the occupational physician or nurse.

Where there is no occupational health service, early contact between the patient's doctor and management (usually the personnel manager) may be useful. It helps the employer to know when the patient is likely to return to work, and whether some work adjustment will be helpful, while family practitioners will be helped by having a better understanding of their patient's job and better equipped to complete a meaningful 'fit note'.

Confidentiality

Usually, any recommendations and advice on placement or return to work are based on the functional effects of the medical condition and its prognosis. Generally there is no requirement for an employer to know the diagnosis or receive clinical details. A simple statement that the patient is medically 'fit' or 'unfit' for a particular job often suffices, but occasionally further information may need to be disclosed using a fit note, particularly, if modifications to work are being proposed. The certificated reason for any sickness absence is usually known by personnel departments, which maintain their own confidential records.

The patient's consent must be obtained, preferably in writing, before disclosure of confidential health information to third parties, including other doctors, nurses, employers, and staff of career services. The purpose of this should be made clear to the patient, as it may help to identify suitable safe work. A patient who is deemed medically unfit for certain employment should be given a full explanation of why the disclosure of unfitness is necessary. Further advice may be found in the Faculty of Occupational Medicine's *Guidance on Ethics for Occupational Physicians*[17] (see also Chapter 5).

Medical reports

When a medical report on an individual is requested, the person should be informed of the purpose for which the report is being sought. If a medical report is being sought from an employee's GP or specialist, then the employer (or their medical advisers) should inform the employee of their rights under the Access to Medical Reports Act 1988 (which include the right to see the report before it is sent to the employer and the right to refuse to allow the report to be sent to the employer). Reports by occupational physicians will also come under the Access to Medical Reports Act if they have had clinical care of the patient. Even if the occupational physician has not cared for the patient, it is good practice to meet the same standard. Employees are also generally entitled to see their medical records, including their occupational health records, and any medical reports on them.

Any doctor being asked for a medical report should insist that the originator of the request writes a referral letter containing full details of the individual, a description of their job, an outline of the problem, and the matters on which opinion is sought.

At the outset the doctor should obtain the patient's consent, preferably in writing, to examine him and furnish the report. Even if the patient has given consent the report should not contain clinical information, unless it is pertinent and absolutely essential. The contents should be confined to addressing the questions posed in the letter of referral and advising on interpreting the person's medical condition in terms of functional capability and their ability to meet the requirements of their employment. The employer is entitled to be sufficiently informed to make a clear decision about the individual's work ability, both currently and in the future, and any modifications, restrictions, or prohibitions that may be required. The doctor should express a clear opinion and must offer the employee an opportunity to see the report before it is sent. The employee can then request correction of any factual errors but they cannot require the doctor to modify the opinion expressed, even if they strongly disagree with it. A patient's return to work or continuation in work may depend on the receipt of a medical report from his GP, consultant, or occupational physician. It is in the patient's interest that such reports are furnished expeditiously.

When writing a medical report the occupational physician should always remember that the document will be discoverable if litigation ensues. It should be clear from the report's content, letter heading, or the affiliation under the signature, why the doctor is qualified to address the subject in question.

Assessing fitness for work: general considerations

The primary purpose of a medical assessment of fitness for work is to make sure that an individual is fit to perform the task involved effectively and without risk to their own or others' health and safety. It is not the intention to exclude the applicant from the job if at all possible, but to modify or adjust it as necessary to allow them to work efficiently and safely.

Why an assessment may be needed

1 The patient's condition may limit or prevent them from performing the job effectively (e.g. musculoskeletal conditions limiting mobility).

2 The patient's condition may be made worse by the job (e.g. physical exertion in cardiorespiratory illness, exposure to allergens in asthma).

3 The patient's condition may make certain jobs and work environments unsafe to them personally (e.g. liability to sudden unconsciousness in a hazardous situation, risk of damage to the remaining eye in a patient with monocular vision).

4 The patient's condition may make it unsafe both for themselves *and for others* in some roles (e.g. road or railway driving in someone who is liable to sudden unconsciousness or to behave abnormally).

5 The patient's condition may pose a risk to the community (e.g. infection transmitted by a food handler).

A clear distinction can be drawn between the first-party risks of (2) and (3) and the third-party risks of (5). In (4), first- and third-party risks may both be present.

Thus, when assessing a patient's fitness for work, the doctor must consider:

◆ The level of skill, physical and mental capacity, sensory acuity, etc., needed for effective performance of the work.

◆ Any possible adverse effects of the work itself or of the work environment on the patient's health.

◆ The possible health and safety implications of the patient's medical condition when undertaking the work in question, for colleagues, and/or the community.

For some jobs there may be an emergency component in addition to the routine job structure, and higher standards of fitness may be needed.

When an assessment of medical fitness is needed

An assessment of medical fitness may be needed for those who are:

1 Being recruited for the first time.

2 Being considered for transfer to a new job. (Transfer or promotion may bring new responsibilities and different fitness requirements.)

3 Returning to work after significant or prolonged illness or injury.

4 Undergoing periodic review relating to specific requirements (e.g. regular assessment of visual acuity in some jobs, statutory health surveillance if working with respiratory sensitizers).

5 Being reviewed for possible retirement on grounds of ill health (see Chapter 27).

6 Unemployed and seeking work in training, but without a specific job in mind.

For (1)–(5) the assessment will be related to a particular job or a defined range of alternative work in a given workplace. The assessment is needed to help both employer and employee, and should be directed at the job in question. In all of these situations there is also a legal requirement to consider 'reasonable adjustment' if the individual has a disability within the definition of the Equality Act, and it is good practice to do so in any case.

After a pre-placement or pre-employment medical examination ((1) or (2)), employers need to know if there may be consequences from a medical condition that may curtail a potential employee's future working life.

For (6), where there may be no specific job in view and the assessment must be more open-ended. Health assessments may be required, for instance, by employment or careers services seeking suitable work for unemployed disabled people. It is important to avoid blanket medical restrictions and labels (such as 'epileptic') that tend to label individuals in their search for work and limit their future choice.

Recruitment medicals

Employers often use health questionnaires as part of their recruitment process. These should be marked 'medically confidential' and be read and interpreted only by a physician or nurse.

Some individuals may be reluctant to disclose a medical condition to a future employer (sometimes with their own doctor's support), for fear that this may lose them the job. However, dismissal on medical grounds may follow if work capability is impaired or an accident arises owing to the concealed condition. An industrial tribunal could well support the dismissal if the employee had failed to disclose the relevant condition. It is not in the patient's interest to conceal a medical condition that could adversely affect their work, but it would be reasonable for the applicant to request that the details be disclosed only to a health professional.

For some jobs (e.g. driving) there are statutory medical standards, and for others, employing organizations lay down their own advisory medical standards (e.g. food handling, work in the offshore oil and gas industry). For most jobs, however, no agreed advisory medical standards exist, and for many jobs there need be no special health requirements. Job application forms should be accompanied by a clear indication of any fitness standards that are required and of any medical conditions that would be a bar to particular jobs, but no questions about health should be included on job application forms themselves. If health information is necessary, applicants should complete a separate health declaration form, which should be inspected and interpreted only by health professionals and only after the candidate has been selected, subject to satisfactory health.

The reason for a pre-placement health assessment should be confined to fitness for the proposed job and only medical questions relevant to that employment should be asked (Box 1.1).

Box 1.1 The status of medical standards

Medical standards may be advisory or statutory. They may also be local and tailored to specific job circumstances. Standards are often laid down where work entails entering a new environment that may present a hazard to the individual, such as the increased or decreased atmospheric pressures encountered in compressed-air work, diving and flying, or work in the high temperatures of nuclear reactors. Standards are also laid down for work where there is a potential risk of a medical condition causing an accident, as in transport, or transmitting infection, as in food handling. For onerous or arduous work such as in mines rescue or in firefighting, very high standards of physical fitness are needed. Specific medical standards will need to be met in such types of work: where relevant, such advisory and/or statutory standards are noted in each speciality chapter.

Recruitment and the company pension scheme

Many doctors and managers in industry still believe that their company pension fund requires high standards of medical fitness for new entrants. Usually this is not so. Fortunately, most pension funds follow the principle recommended by the Occupational Pensions Board: 'Fit for employment—fit for the pension fund'.[18] The only modification may be in relation to death in service benefit, which can be many multiples of annual salary. If a person has a condition that may significantly shorten their working life, the death in service benefit may be negotiated at a lower multiple. In general, a disease/disability should not be a reason per se for exclusion from pension schemes, nor should it be used as an excuse to deny employment.[19] Where company schemes still operate against people with disabilities, attempts should be made to amend them. However, with recent changes in legislation pensions can now be personal, flexible, and mobile; anyone with a medical disability may be advised to negotiate a personal policy that they can retain permanently irrespective of their employer.

Special groups

Young people

Medical advice on training given to a young person with a disability who has not yet started a career often has a different slant from that given to an adult developing the same condition late in an established career. The later stages of a particular vocation may involve jobs incompatible with the young person's medical condition or its foreseeable development, and timely advice may avoid future disappointment. Conversely, a mature adult's work experience may enable them to overcome obstacles posed by a disease or disability in ways that a young worker could not manage; a young person who is well motivated though, can often overcome the most astonishing disabling handicap, especially with help and encouragement.

It is particularly important that young people entering employment are given appropriate medical advice when it is needed. For instance, although a school-leaver with epilepsy might be eligible for an ordinary driving licence at the time of recruitment, it would be inadvisable for them to take up a position where vocational driving would be an essential requirement for career progression. Similarly, a young person with atopic eczema may not wish to invest in training for hairdressing if advised that hairdressing typically aggravates hand eczema.

Severely disabled people

Where a medical condition has so reduced an individual's employment abilities or potential that they are incapable of continuing in their existing work or of working in open competitive employment, even with all appropriate adjustments, then sheltered work may be the only alternative to early medical retirement.

The assessment of medical fitness for work

A general framework

As previously emphasized, the clinician's assessment should always be reported in terms of *functional capacity*; the actual diagnosis need not be given. Even so, an opinion on the medical fitness of an individual is being conveyed to others and the patient's written consent is needed for the information to be passed on, in confidence.

Each of the specialty chapters that follow outlines the main points to be considered when faced with specific health conditions. In this section we summarize a general framework, although not all of the points raised will be relevant to all individuals. The key outcome measure is the *patient's residual abilities relative to the likely requirements at the workplace*, so a proper assessment weighs functional status against job demands.

Functional assessment

To estimate the individual's level of function, assessments of all systems should be made with special attention both to those that are disordered and relevant to the work. As well as physical systems, sensory and perceptual abilities should be noted, and psychological reactions such as responsiveness, alertness, and other features of the general mental state. The effects of different treatment regimens on work suitability should also be considered; the possible effects of medication on alertness, or the optimal care of an arthrodesis, are two of many examples.

Any general evaluation of health forms the background to more specific inquiry. Assessment should also consider the results of relevant tests. The following factors may be material:

- *General*: stamina; ability to cope with full working day, or shiftwork.
- *Mobility*: ability to get to work, and exit safety; to walk, climb, bend, stoop, crouch.
- *Locomotor*: joint function and range; reach; gait; back/spinal function.
- *Posture*: ability to stand/sit for certain periods; postural constraints; work in confined spaces.
- *Muscular*: specific palsies or weakness; tremor; ability to lift, push, or pull, with weight/time abilities if known; strength tests.
- *Manual skills*: defects in dexterity, ability to grip or grasp.
- *Coordination*: including hand–eye coordination.
- *Balance*: ability to work at heights; vertigo.
- *Cardiorespiratory limitations*: including exercise tolerance; respiratory function and reserve; submaximal exercise tests, aerobic work capacity, if relevant.
- *Liability to unconsciousness*: including nature of episodes, timing, warnings, precipitating factors.
- *Sensory aspects*: both for the work and in navigating a hazardous safety environment.

- *Vision*: capacity for fine/close work, distant vision, visual standards corrected or uncorrected, aids in use or needed; visual fields; colour vision defects. Is the eyesight good enough to cope with a difficult working environment with possible hazards?
- *Hearing*: level in each ear; can warning signals and instructions be heard?
- For both *vision and hearing* it is important that if only one eye or one ear is functioning, this is recognized and thought given to safeguarding the remaining organ from damage.

◆ *Communication/speech*: two-way communication; hearing or speech defects; reason for limitation.

◆ *Cerebral function*: will be relevant after head injury, cerebrovascular accident, some neurological conditions, and in those with some intellectual deficit: presence of confusion; disorientation; impairment of memory, intellect, verbal, or numerical aptitudes.

◆ *Mental state*: anxiety, relevant phobias, mood, withdrawal, etc.

◆ *Motivation*: may well be the most important determinant of work capacity. With it, impairments may be surmounted; without it, difficulties may not be overcome. It can be difficult to assess by a doctor who has not previously known the patient.

◆ *Treatment of the condition*: side effects of treatment may be relevant, e.g. drowsiness, inattention.

◆ *Further treatment*: if further treatment is planned, e.g. orthopaedic or surgical procedures, these may need to be considered.

◆ *Prognosis*: if the clinical prognosis is likely to affect work placement, e.g. likely improvements in muscle strength, or decline in exercise tolerance, these should be considered.

◆ *Special needs*: these may be various—dietary, need for a clean area for self-treatment (e.g. injection), frequent rest pauses, no paced or shiftwork, etc.

◆ *Aids or appliances* (in use or needed): implanted artificial aids may be relevant in the working environment (pacemakers and artificial joints). Prostheses/orthoses should be mentioned. Artificial aids or appliances that could help at the workplace (e.g. wheelchair) should be indicated.

◆ *Specific third-party risks*.

Requirements of the job

The requirements of work may relate not only to the individual's present job but also to their future career. Always considering the possibility of 'reasonable adjustment', some of the following aspects may be relevant:

◆ *Work demands*: physical (e.g. mobility needs; strength for certain activities; lifting/carrying; climbing/balancing; stooping/bending; postural constraints; reach requirements; dexterity/manipulative ability, etc.); intellectual/perceptual demands; types of skill involved in tasks.

◆ *Work environment*: physical aspects, risk factors (e.g. fumes/dust; chemical or biological hazards; working at heights).

◆ *Organizational/social aspects*: e.g. intermittent or regular pressure of work; public facing work.

◆ *Temporal aspects*: e.g. need for early start; type of shiftwork; day or night work; arrangements for rest pauses or breaks.

- *Ergonomic aspects*: workplace (e.g. need to climb stairs; distance from toilet facilities; access for wheelchairs); workstation (e.g. height of workbench; adequate lighting; type of equipment or controls used). Adaptations of equipment that could help at the workplace should be identified.
- *Travel*: e.g. need to work in areas remote from healthcare or where there are risks not found in the UK (see Appendix 5).

Too often, medical statements simply state 'fit for light work only'. The dogmatic separation of work into 'light', 'medium', and 'heavy' often results in individuals being unduly limited in their choice of work. A refinement of this broad grading is adopted by the US Department of Labor in its *Dictionary of Occupational Titles*.[20] Jobs are graded according to physical demands, environmental conditions, certain levels of skill and knowledge, and specific vocational preparation required, but occupational health practice requires more specific adjustment of the job to the individual. The physical demands listed in Table 1.1 express both the physical requirements of the job and capacities that a worker must have to meet those required by many jobs. The worker must possess a physical capacity that at least matches the physical demands made by the job. For example, if the energy or metabolic requirements of a particular task are known the individual's work capacity may be estimated and, if expressed in the same units, a comparison between the energy demands of the work and the physiological work capacity of the individual may be made. Energy requirements of various tasks can be estimated and expressed in metabolic equivalents, or METs. (The MET is the approximate energy expended while sitting at rest, defined as the rate of energy expenditure requiring an oxygen consumption of 3.5 mL per kilogram of body weight per minute.) The rough metabolic demands of many working activities have been published and the equivalents for the five grades of physical demands in terms of muscular strength adopted by the US Department of Labor are listed for information. Work physiology assessments in occupational medicine provide a semi-quantitative way of matching patients to their work, and are commonly used in Scandinavia and the US.

Factors influencing work performance

The ability to perform physical work, and even intellectual occupations involve some physical work, depends ultimately on the ability of muscle cells to transform chemically bound energy from food into mechanical energy. This in turn depends on the intake, storage, and mobilization of nutrient, and the uptake of oxygen and its delivery by the cardiovascular system to the muscles where it is oxidized to release energy. This chain of activities and processes is influenced at every juncture by other factors, both endogenous and external or environmental.

Factors which may influence work performance, directly or indirectly, include:

- Training or adaptation
- General state of health
- Gender (e.g. the maximal strength of women's leg muscles is 65–75 per cent of that of men)
- Body size
- Age (the maximal muscle strength of a 65-year-old man is about 75–80 per cent of that when he was 20 and at his peak)
- Nutritional state—particularly important when working in cold environments

Table 1.1 The typical physical demands of work

---

1. Strength

Expressed in terms of sedentary, light, medium, heavy, and very heavy

Measured by involvement of the worker with one or more of the following activities:

(a) Worker position(s):

(i) Standing: remaining on one's feet in an upright position at a workstation without moving about

(ii) Walking: moving about on foot

(iii) Sitting: remaining in the normal seated position

(b) Worker movement of objects (including extremities used):

(i) Lifting: raising or lowering an object from one level to another

(ii) Carrying: transporting an object, usually in the hands or arms or on the shoulder

(iii) Pushing: exerting force upon an object so that it moves away (includes slapping, striking, kicking, and treadle actions)

(iv) Pulling: exerting force upon an object so that it moves nearer (includes jerking)

The five degrees of physical demands are (estimated equivalents in METs):

S   Sedentary work (<2 METs): lifting 10 lbs (4.5 kg) maximum and occasionally lifting and/or carrying such articles as dockets, ledgers, and small tools. Although a sedentary job is defined as one that involves sitting, a certain amount of walking and standing is often needed as well. Jobs are sedentary if walking and standing are required only occasionally and other sedentary criteria are met

L   Light work (2–3 METs): lifting 20 lbs (9 kg) maximum with frequent lifting and/or carrying of objects weighing up to 10 lbs (4.5 kg). Even though the weight lifted may be only negligible, a job is in this category when it requires walking or standing to a significant degree, or sitting most of the time with some pushing and pulling of arm and/or leg controls

M   Medium work (4–5 METs): lifting 50 lbs (23 kg) maximum with frequent lifting and/or carrying of objects weighing up to 25 lbs (11.5 kg)

H   Heavy work (6–8 METs): lifting 100 lbs (45 kg) maximum with frequent lifting and/or carrying of objects weighing up to 50 lbs (23 kg)

V   Very heavy work (8 METs) lifting objects in excess of 100 lb (45 kg) with frequent lifting and/or carrying of objects weighing 50 lbs (23 kg) or more

2. Climbing and/or balancing

(a) Climbing: ascending/descending ladders, stairs, scaffolding, ramps, poles, ropes, etc., using the feet and legs and/or hands and arms

(b) Balancing: maintaining body equilibrium to prevent falling when walking, standing, crouching, or running on narrow, slippery, or erratically moving surfaces; or maintaining body equilibrium when performing gymnastic feats

3. Stooping, kneeling, crouching, and/or crawling

(a) Stooping: bending the body downwards and forwards by bending the spine at the waist

(b) Kneeling: bending the legs at the knees to come to rest on the knee or knees

(c) Crouching: bending the body downward and forward by bending the legs and the spine

(d) Crawling: moving about on the hands and knees or hands and feet

Table 1.1 (continued) The typical physical demands of work

---

4. Reaching, handling, fingering, and/or feeling

    (a) Reaching: extending the hands and arms in any direction

    (b) Handling: seizing, holding, grasping, turning, or otherwise working with the hand or hands (fingering not involved)

    (c) Fingering: picking, pinching, or otherwise working with the fingers primarily (rather than with the whole hand or arm as in handling)

    (d) Feeling: perceiving such attributes of objects/materials as size, shape, temperature, texture, by means of receptors in the skin, particularly those of the fingertips

5. Talking and/or hearing

    (a) Talking: expressing or exchanging ideas by means of the spoken word

    (b) Hearing: perceiving the nature of sounds by the ear

6. Seeing

Obtaining impressions through the eyes of the shape, size, distance, motion, colour, or other characteristics of objects. The major visual functions are defined as follows:

    (a) Acuity:

        Far—clarity of vision at 20 feet (6 m) or more

        Near—clarity of vision at 20 inches (50 cm) or less

    (b) Depth perception: three-dimensional vision: the ability to judge distance and space relationships so as to see objects where and as they actually are

    (c) Field of vision: the area that can be seen up and down or to the right or left while the eyes are fixed on a given point

    (d) Accommodation: adjustment of the lens of the eye to bring an object into sharp focus; especially important for doing near-point work at varying distances

    (e) Colour vision: the ability to identify and distinguish colours

---

Adapted from US Department of Labor. *Selected characteristics of occupations defined in the dictionary of occupational titles*. Washington, DC: US Government Printing Office, Copyright © 1981.

- Individual differences
- Attitude and motivation
- Sleep deprivation and fatigue
- Stress
- Nature of the work, workload, work schedules, work environment (heat, cold, humidity, air velocity, altitude, hyperbaric pressure, noise, vibration).

These factors are well summarized in *The Physiology of Work* by Rodahl.[21]

Objective tests

The result of any objective tests of function relevant to the working situation should be noted. For instance, the physical work capacity of an individual may be estimated using standard exercise tests, step tests, or different task simulations. Muscular strength and lifting ability can be assessed objectively by using either dynamic or static strength tests.

Matching the individual with the job

A functional assessment of the individual's capacities will be of most use when as much is known about the job as about the individual assessed. Sophisticated equipment is available to make a functional capacity assessment that will match an individual to a task. Less formally, the requirements of the task can be categorized, so that a match can be made with the individual's capacity.

There are wide variations in the practice of occupational medicine in different countries. In both France and Germany job matching is used formally in some work settings; and in Finland, the Work Ability Index (a short questionnaire-based self-assessment of work capacity) has been developed. But systematic job analysis and matching is rarely done at the workplace in the UK. Instead, a pragmatic solution often emerges when personnel staff and managers, company doctors, and supervisors discuss the placement needs of their disabled employees; as both worker abilities and task requirements are well known to them, a theoretical match is often superfluous. Outside the workplace itself, more formal assessments may be made in medical rehabilitation or occupational therapy departments (see Chapter 4).

A comprehensive review of current approaches to the analysis of both the physical demands of jobs and the physical abilities of individuals, job matching and functional capacity assessment has been published by Fraser.[22] Accommodation at the workplace is also discussed, and appendices include details of physiological and biomechanical techniques for work capacity measurement.

The occupational physician or nurse who is assessing medical suitability for employment must have an intimate understanding of the job in question.

Presentation of the assessment

If a written report is needed, it should be typewritten, clearly laid out, signed, and dated. The report should mention any functional limitations and outline activities that may, or may not, be undertaken. Any health or safety implications should be noted and the assessment should aim at a positive statement about the patient's abilities. Any adaptations, ergonomic alterations, or 'reasonable adjustments' to the work that would be helpful or required by the Equality Act should be indicated. Recommendations on restriction or limitation of employment, particularly for health and/or safety reasons, should be unambiguous and precise, and should be made only if definitely indicated.

Many standard functional profiles of individual abilities have been used in North America, Scandinavia, and the UK (mainly in the armed services). These profiles, which resemble each other, are known by acronyms of the initial letters of the parts of the body assessed, e.g. PULHEEMS (Physical capacity, Upper limb, Locomotion, Hearing, etc.), GULHEMP, PULSES. In the case of the GULHEMP profile each division is graded from 1 to 7. Other profiles have combined the evaluation of physical abilities with indications of the frequency with which certain activities may be undertaken. Although such profiles are relatively objective and systematic, and allow for consistent recordings on the same individual over a period of time, they take time to complete and much of the information may not be needed. Doctors in industry who have tried to introduce a PULHEEMS type of system have reported that it does not always help when dealing with the complex practical, problems affecting individual employees.

Other simple classifications are often used in clinical settings to monitor outcome after reha-bilitation or occupational therapy (e.g. the New York Heart Association functional classification of heart failure, the Barthel Index of stroke damage/recovery).

Recommendations following assessment

Recommendations following assessment depend on the circumstance of referral and the findings.

If the patient is employed, it should be possible to make a medical judgement on whether they are:

1 Capable of performing the work without any ill effects.

2 Capable of performing the work but with reduced efficiency or effectiveness.

3 Capable of performing the work, although this may adversely affect their medical condition.

4 Capable of performing the work but not without risks to the health and safety of themselves, other workers, or the community.

5 Physically or mentally incapable of performing the work in question.

For the employed patient, where the judgement is (2)–(5), the options of 'reasonable adjustment' may include work accommodation, alternative work on a temporary or permanent basis, shel-tered work, or, in the last resort, retirement on medical grounds.

If the patient is unemployed but is being given a pre-employment assessment for recruitment to *a particular job*, options (1)–(5) will still be appropriate.

Even if the patient is assessed as medically fit for a return to their previous job without modifi-cation, medical advice may still be needed on the timing of return to work. A clear indication to the patient or employer on when work may be resumed should be given wherever possible. Work should be resumed as soon as the individual is physically and mentally fit enough, having regard to their own and others' health and safety. Return to work at the right time can assist recovery, whereas undue delay can aggravate the sense of uselessness and isolation that so often accompa-nies incapacity due to illness, disability, or injury.

The contact between the patient's doctor and their employer or occupational physician, stressed earlier in this chapter, will ensure that preparations for the patient's return to work can be put in hand. Recommendations on when work may be resumed and on the patient's functional and work capacities should be clear and specific.

Patients who have been treated for cancer may have particular difficulties in integrating on their return to work, but, with modern treatment and suitable advice from an occupational physician, many cancer patients return to full and productive employment (see Chapter 32).

Work accommodation

The patient's condition, which may or may not come within the Equality Act, may be such that their previous work needs to be modified. Both physical and organizational aspects of the job must be considered. Simple features such as bench height, type of chair or stool, or lighting may need adjustment, or more sophisticated aids or adaptations may be required. The workplace environment may need to be adapted, for example, by building a ramp or widening a doorway to improve access for wheelchairs. Financial assistance may be available from the Employment Service. Further details are included in Chapter 4.

Information on equipment may be available from several voluntary organizations such as the Royal Association for Disability and Rehabilitation (RADAR), the Disabled Living Foundation

(DLF), and the Disabilities Trust (for a useful list of self-help and disease associations see <http://www.ukselfhelp.info/>), as well as the government website Directgov.

Certain organizational features of the work may need adjustment—for instance, adjustment of objectives, more flexible working hours, more frequent rest pauses, job sharing, alterations to shiftwork or arrangements to avoid rush-hour travel. A short period of unpaced work may be necessary before resuming paced work.

Alternative work

In some occupations, work accommodation or job restructuring is not possible and suitable alternative work, possibly only temporary, may have to be recommended. This is usually judged on an individual basis and is subject to periodic review. Where there are no occupational health services, the Employment Service's Disability Employment Advisers (DEAs) can visit the workplace to advise on work accommodation or alternative work (see Chapter 4). EMAS may be able to provide some advice to individual employees.

Early medical retirement

Medical retirement is a last resort, if further treatment is impossible or ineffective, if suitable alternative or sheltered work cannot be provided, or if the employee will not accept such initiatives. If the 'threshold of employability for a particular job' cannot be reached, either through recovery of fitness, or adjustment of work, retirement on medical grounds may have to be considered. *A management decision on early retirement on grounds of ill health should never be made without a supporting medical opinion that has taken the requirements of the job fully into account.* Medical retirement is discussed more fully in Chapter 27. Other aspects of early medical retirement in relation to the law are discussed in Chapter 2.

Recent developments and trends

Governmental initiatives

In recent times there has been great emphasis on maximizing fitness for work and job retention. Described in Chapter 4 are several flagship policy documents, including *Working for a Healthier Tomorrow* and *Improving Health and Work: Changing Lives*. Details are given also of recent initiatives and programmes such as the 'Pathways to Work' pilots, the fit note, the National Education Programme for Health and Work, and the Black review of sickness absence that complement long-standing arrangements (the Access to Work programme, residential training, Jobcentre Plus, the Job Introduction Scheme, etc.).

Another innovation has been the development of NHS Plus and the recent launch of the NHS Healthcare at Work Network, a network of over 150 NHS occupational health teams. Increasingly, NHS and independent occupational health services are participating in a quality assurance accreditation scheme developed by the Faculty of Occupational Medicine (Safe Effective Quality Occupational Health Service (SEQHS)).

Finally, the alignment of the HSE, within the Department of Work and Pensions, has encouraged a more holistic approach to health problems in employment. The important effort of controlling risks at work continues unchecked, but greater attention is being paid to rehabilitation and the common health problems that serve as barriers to job retention and job placement.

These initiatives are to be welcomed. At present between 2 per cent and 16 per cent of the annual UK salary bill is spent on sickness absence. Set against them, however, is a major retrenchment in Government spending on welfare from 2010, precipitated by European debt and banking crises. It is to be hoped that this does not derail the drive to improve employment for adults with health problems. The costs of making reasonable adjustments to retain an employee who develops a health condition or disability are likely to be far lower than the costs of recruiting and training anew. Moreover, work brings with it health benefits to the individual—it can be therapeutic, it is associated with lower morbidity and mortality, and it carries important social benefits and a sense of well-being and integration with society. Thus, in both financial and in human terms (as well as in terms of legal responsibilities), these efforts are important.

Maintaining fitness for work

From the occupational physician's viewpoint fitness for work does not end with medical assessment. An employee must remain fit, which means attention to those factors that will prevent the deterioration of health. These may include policies or advice on smoking, exercise, diet, and alcohol consumption. An educational leaflet from the Faculty of Occupational Medicine and the Faculty of Public Health has highlighted the importance of life-style factors in creating a healthy workplace and the costs to industry:

- An estimated 34 million days a year are lost in England and Wales through sickness absence resulting from smoking-related illness.
- Physical inactivity through its major health consequences (e.g. obesity, coronary heart disease, and cancer) is estimated to cost the wider English economy over £8 billion per year.
- Alcohol misuse among employees in England costs up to an estimated £6.4 billion pounds a year in lost productivity.

The subject of health promotion is covered in Chapter 31, and that of health screening in Chapter 29. These activities are important in terms of the well-being of working-aged people. The prevention of vascular disease is particularly important as this disease takes a high toll in the working population and simple initiatives can be effective. Doctors also have a duty to discourage smoking at work and support smoking bans and quit smoking initiatives. Finally, occupational physicians should encourage employers to provide facilities for employees to take regular exercise and be prepared to advise on sensible eating and the food available in eating places at work. Guidance from the National Institute for Health and Clinical Excellence (NICE) highlights workplace opportunities to combat physical inactivity, obesity and smoking.[23-25] The long-term prevention of ill health, by whatever means, is as important to the prudent employer as ensuring that a new employee is fit for work.

Conclusions

Medical fitness is relevant where illnesses or injuries reduce performance, or affect health and safety in the workplace. It may also be specifically relevant to certain onerous or hazardous tasks for which medical standards exist. Medical fitness should always be judged in relation to the work, and not simply the pension scheme. It has limited relevance in most employment situations: many medical conditions, and virtually all minor health problems, have minimal implications for work and should not debar from employment. Medical fitness for employment is not an end in itself. It must be maintained.

References

1 World Health Organization. *International classification of impairments, disabilities and handicaps.* Geneva: World Health Organization, 1980.

2 Wood PHN. The language of disablement: a glossary relating to disease and its consequences. *Int Rehabil Med* 1980; **2**: 86–92.

3 Smith A, Twomey B. Labour market experience of people with disabilities. Analysis from the LFS of the characteristics and labour market participation of people with long-term disabilities and health problems. *Labour Market Trends* 2002; **110**(8): 415–27.

4 Boorman S. *NHS health and well-being. Final report.* London: Department of Health, 2009. (<http://www.dh.gov.uk/prod_consum_dh/groups/dh_digitalassets/documents/digitalasset/dh_108907.pdf>)

5 McManus S, Meltzer H, Brugha T, *et al. Adult psychiatric morbidity in England, 2007: results of a household survey.* London: The Health & Social Care Information Centre, Social Care Statistics, 2009. (<http://www.ic.nhs.uk/webfiles/publications/mental%20health/other%20mental%20health%20publications/Adult%20psychiatric%20morbidity%202007/APMS%2007%20%28FINAL%29%20Standard.pdf>)

6 The Health and Safety Executive. *Statistics 2009/10.* London: HSE Books, 2010. (<http://www.hse.gov.uk/statistics/overall/hssh0910.pdf>)

7 Health Insurance. *The online guide to critical illness insurance. Vital statistics.* [Online] (<http://www.healthinsuranceguide.co.uk/statistics_mainbody.asp>)

8 Department of Health. *Hospital episode statistics: main procedures and interventions, 2009–10.* [Online] (<http://www.hesonline.nhs.uk/Ease/servlet/AttachmentRetriever?site_id=1937&file_name=d:\efmfiles\1937\Accessing\DataTables\Annual%20inpatient%20release%202010\MainOp3_0910.xls&short_name=MainOp3_0910.xls&u_id=8919>)

9 Blanc PD, Burney P, Janson C, *et al.* The prevalence and predictors of respiratory-related work limitation and occupational disability in an international study. *Chest* 2003; **124**: 1153–9.

10 Herquelot E, Guéguen A, Bonenfant S, *et al.* Impact of diabetes on work cessation: data from the GAZEL cohort study. *Diabetes Care* 2011; **34**: 1344–9.

11 Tunceli K, Bradley CJ, Nerenz D, *et al.* The impact of diabetes on employment and work productivity. *Diabetes Care* 2005; **28**: 2662–7.

12 Elwes RD, Marshall J, Beattie A, *et al.* Epilepsy and employment. A community based survey in an area of high unemployment. *J Neurol Neurosurg Psychiatry* 1991; **54**: 200–3.

13 Brault MW. US Census Bureau American Community Survey Briefs: Disability among the working age population: 2008 and 2009. Washington, DC: US Census Bureau, 2010. (<http://www.census.gov/prod/2010pubs/acsbr09-12.pdf>)

14 Waddell G, Burton AK. *Is work good for your health and well-being?* London: The Stationery Office, 2006.

15 Department for Work and Pensions. *Statement of fitness for work; a guide for general practitioners and other doctors.* London: Department for Work and Pensions, 2010. (<http://www.dwp.gov.uk/docs/fitnote-gp-guide.pdf>)

16 Coggon D, Palmer KT. Assessing fitness for work and writing a 'fit note'. *BMJ* 2010; **341**: c6305.

17 Faculty of Occupational Medicine, Royal College of Physicians. *Guidance on ethics for occupational physicians*, 6th edn. London: Faculty of Occupational Medicine, Royal College of Physicians, 2006.

18 Occupational Pensions Board. *Occupational pension scheme cover for disabled people.* Cmnd 6849. London: HMSO, 1977.

19 Brackenridge RDC, Elder WJ. *Medical selection of life risks*, 4th edn. London: Macmillan, 1998.

20 US Department of Labor Employment and Training Administration. *Dictionary of occupational titles*, 4th edn. Washington, DC: US Government Printing Office, 1991. (<http://www.oalj.dol.gov/libdot.htm>)

21 Rodahl K. *The physiology of work.* London: CRC Press, 1989.

22 Fraser TM. *Fitness for work: the role of physical demands analysis and physical capacity assessment.* London: Taylor & Francis, 1992.

23 National Institute for Health and Clinical Excellence. *PH13: Workplace health promotion: how to encourage employees to be physically active.* London: NICE, 2008. (<http://www.nice.org.uk/nicemedia/pdf/PH013Guidance.pdf>)

24 National Institute for Health and Clinical Excellence. *PH5: Workplace health promotion: how to help employees to stop smoking.* London: NICE, 2007. (<http://www.nice.org.uk/nicemedia/pdf/PHI005guidance.pdf>)

25 National Institute for Health and Clinical Excellence. *Obesity: the prevention, identification, assessment and management of overweight and obesity in adults and children (CG 43).* London: NICE, 2006. (<http://egap.evidence.nhs.uk/CG43/unknown_5>)

Chapter 2

Legal aspects of fitness for work

Gillian S. Howard

This chapter outlines some of the ways in which the law may affect the employment of people with health issues. There are three major legal sources relevant to employment in the UK—the common law, statute law, and European directives. Statutory employment protection in the form of unfair dismissal and protection from disability discrimination has transformed the rights and protection for employees who are injured or become ill at work and cannot work in the short or long term.

Common law

The English legal system is based on the common law. The common law system in England and Wales developed from the decisions of judges whose rulings over the centuries have created precedents for other courts to follow and these decisions were based on the 'custom and practice of the Realm'. The system of binding precedent means that any decision of the Supreme Court—the new name for the former House of Lords (the highest court in the UK)—will bind all the lower courts, unless the lower courts are able to distinguish the facts of the current case and argue that the previous binding decision cannot apply, because of differences in the facts of the two cases.

However, since the UK joined the European Union (EU), the decisions of the European Court of Justice (ECJ) now supersede any decisions of the domestic courts and require the English national courts to follow its decisions. (Scotland has a system based on Dutch Roman law, and some procedural differences although no fundamental differences in relation to employment law.) The Human Rights Act 1998 became law in England and Wales in 2000 (and in Scotland in 1998) in order to incorporate the provisions of the European Convention on Human Rights into UK law. The two most important Articles applicable to employment law are Article 8(1), the right to respect for privacy, family life, and correspondence, and Article 6, the right to a fair trial.

The common law covers both criminal and civil law. The law of negligence has grown out of the common law and forms part of the civil law of torts (civil wrongs). So, for example, a worker injured at work will sue in the civil courts, not in the employment tribunals, for damages for their injuries. For centuries, the common law courts have held employers liable for negligence if the injuries were reasonably foreseeable and the employer had not taken reasonable care for the health and safety of their workers. However, statute law since 1974 (the Health and Safety at Work etc. Act 1974 (HSW Act)) has developed to the point where there is a comprehensive regulatory framework of employment protection guaranteeing rights and freedoms of employees and imposing statutory duties on employers. This has been referred to by legal commentators as 'a floor of statutory rights'.

Common law duties of employers

At common law, employers have an obligation to take *reasonable care* of all their employees and to guard against the risk of injury to their workers only if the risks were *reasonably foreseeable*. These duties are judged in the light of the 'state of the art' of knowledge of the employer—what they either knew or ought to have known (see 'Standard of care of occupational physicians').

Standard of care of occupational physicians

The *standard of care* expected of a professional, such as an occupational health specialist, is set out in a case that established the so-called '*Bolam*' test.[1] This held that a doctor could not be held to be negligent where he had exercised the standard of care 'of the ordinary skilled man exercising and professing to have that special skill'. A 'doctor was not negligent if he acted in accordance with a practice accepted as proper by a responsible body of medical opinion'.

However, in *Bolitho*[2] the House of Lords held that *Bolam* would be followed only where that body of medical opinion had reached 'a defensible conclusion', i.e. where such a conclusion could be rationalized and justified. If the groundswell of medical opinion was outdated and clearly erroneous, the judges would not accept the opinion, even if it came from a respectable medical body.

The House of Lords held that if, in a rare case, it had been demonstrated that the professional opinion was incapable of withstanding logical analysis, the judge was entitled to hold that it could not provide the benchmark by reference to which the doctor's conduct fell to be assessed. In most cases the fact that distinguished experts in the field were of a particular opinion would be demonstration of the reasonableness of that opinion.

In the case of an accredited specialist in occupational medicine, the standard of care expected would be higher than for a general practitioner (GP) who works part-time in occupational medicine. Occupational physicians are deemed to exercise a standard of care that any reasonably competent occupational physician would exercise even if different occupational physicians might have come to very different conclusions.[3]

Duty to inform and warn of risks to health and safety

Employers are obliged to inform their workers, including prospective employees, of inherent risks of the job so that they can accept or decline employment having made an informed choice.[4] Any warning does not, of course, relieve the employer of the duty to take all reasonable care to guard against reasonably foreseeable risks of injury. What it does is to provide employees with information they would otherwise have lacked. Sometimes, and possibly most effectively, this information is imparted through the company's medical advisers.

The principle of *volenti non fit injuria*, i.e. that the individual knew about the risk, understood the exact nature of that risk, and accepted that risk, may conceivably be used by an employer in defence of a negligence claim. However, it has rarely proved to be a successful defence because the risk has to be accepted freely and without duress. If the only choice was dismissal or accepting a particular risk at the workplace, the courts would not be slow to disallow the defence of *volenti*.

In one of the several cases brought against Bernard Matthews for work-related upper limb disorders (WRULDs), it was successfully argued by Mrs Mountenay and others[5] that she had not been given sufficient warning of the inherent risk of WRULDs associated with eviscerating chickens on a paced production line. In the first case on 'stress' to reach the former House of Lords (*Barber* v. *Somerset County Council*[6]) the leading case of *Stokes* v. *Guest Keen and Nettlefold* was cited as still being good law.

In this case, the company had been found liable for the scrotal cancers that eventually killed several of its workers. It had employed a doctor who lectured in occupational medicine. This doctor had failed to warn the men of the dangers of cancer associated with the oils that contaminated their overalls, as he had not wanted to alarm them. He could, and should, have circulated a leaflet to the men warning of the dangers of scrotal warts, and should have instituted periodic medical examinations. The employer was held to be vicariously liable for this act of negligence on the doctor's part.

In summary, the employer's duties include obligations to:

◆ Take positive and practical steps to ensure the safety of their employees in the light of the knowledge that they have, or ought to have.

◆ Follow current recognized practice, unless in the light of common sense or new knowledge this is clearly unsound.

◆ Keep reasonably abreast of developing knowledge and not be too slow in applying it.

◆ Take greater than average precautions where the employer has greater than average knowledge of the risk.

◆ Weigh up the risk (in terms of likelihood of the injury and the possible consequences) against the effectiveness and the cost and inconvenience of the precautions to be taken to meet the risk.

Since *Barber* v. *Somerset County Council*, there has been further litigation in this area. In *Hartman* v. *South Essex Mental Health and Community Care NHS Trust*[6] the Court of Appeal held that the general principle remains that an employer is liable for psychiatric injury caused by stress at work where this is a foreseeable injury arising from the employer's breach of duty. As to whether psychiatric injury is to be regarded as reasonably foreseeable, the Court of Appeal reaffirmed the line taken by Lady Justice Hale in *Hatton*, widely regarded as comparatively favourable to employers.

In *Sutherland* v. *Hatton*,[7] the Court of Appeal held that to trigger the duty on an employer to take steps to safeguard an employee, the indications must be plain enough for any reasonable employer to realize that he should do something about it. The test is the same whatever the employment: 'there are no occupations which should be regarded as intrinsically dangerous to mental health' (see 'Balancing the risk').

Balancing the risk

In essence, a cost/benefit analysis must be done. In deciding what is 'reasonably practicable' to do in terms of eliminating risk and in determining what is reasonably foreseeable in terms of injury, the courts have determined a test that balances the quantum of risk against the time, trouble, and expense that the employer must go to, to avert that risk. The greater the risk to health or safety, the greater the time, trouble, and expense the law expects the employer to devote to mitigating that risk. In a leading case involving the National Coal Board,[8] the Court of Appeal held that the employer's obligation to discharge its duty of care would only be satisfied when the time, trouble, and expense required to avert the risk was grossly disproportionate to the risk involved. In other words, if the risk and gravity of harm is small or negligible, then the employer's duty to avert such risks would be considerably smaller.

Ignorance is no defence in law. Furthermore, if one member of the employer's staff knows about a risk or a health or safety problem, then (whether this is shared with the employer or not) the employer is deemed to know about it. This is called *constructive knowledge* (see Chapter 3 for further discussion on this point).

The state of the art

The courts will look at the state of knowledge at the time of the alleged act of negligence in judging whether the employer ought to have acted or not. Employers are not expected to be prophets, nor are they expected to remain ignorant of the growing knowledge of pertinent health and safety matters. Nor are they permitted to ignore advice and information given to them by their occupational health experts merely because other employers do not know about or concern themselves with these issues.

In cases concerning noise-induced hearing loss, the courts have investigated the state of knowledge among employers in the 1950s, even though the Ministry of Labour pamphlet *Noise and the worker* was not published until 1963. In *Baxter* v. *Harland and Wolff plc*,[9] the employer was held liable for noise-induced deafness as far back as 1953 because the employer failed to 'seek out knowledge of facts which are not in themselves obvious'. Harland and Wolff had not sought or heeded medical, scientific, and legal advice between 1953 and 1963, despite there being evidence of several incidents of noise-induced deafness problems in the naval shipyards in Devon before the Second World War and medical reports and papers on this in the early 1950s. Evidence was produced that an advertisement in *The Lancet* on 28 April 1951 had featured a protective earplug. The employer was held to be negligent because of its 'lack of interest and apathy . . . The defendants, knowing that noise was causing deafness among their workmen, should have applied their minds to removing the risk . . . (and) . . . sought advice'.

Greater duty of care: 'eggshell skull' principle

The employer owes a higher duty of care to any particularly vulnerable employee with a known, pre-existing medical condition. Those with an 'eggshell skull physique' are more vulnerable to serious injury than others of robust physical health. Those with a fragile personality may suffer far greater psychological damage than those with a robust personality. This is defined as the 'eggshell skull' principle, a classic example of which can be seen in the case of *Paris* v. *Stepney Council*.[10] Here the Council employed a labourer with only one eye. They failed to ensure that he was wearing eye goggles and as a result he suffered an injury to his other eye at work and was blinded. The courts held that his employers owed him a much higher duty of care as he was an individual with an extra risk of serious injury.

It is therefore important for employers to take informed advice from qualified occupational health professionals on fitness and placement decisions and the need for special arrangements or precautions. Failure to consider whether pre-employment medical checks are required and, if they are indicated, to arrange for them to be done by properly qualified and trained occupational health staff, may lead to a successful claim for negligence against the employer. This is all the more important today when disability discrimination claims may be brought and expert evidence required.

Duty owed in mental illness

In several cases the courts have extended the principle of the employer's common law duty to psychiatric injury. In a case that went to the House of Lords,[11] the negligent party was held liable for the onset of chronic fatigue syndrome precipitated by a car accident.

Although not the first case to establish an employer's duty of care to look after the mental wellbeing of employees, *Walker* v. *Northumberland County Council*[12] was the first successful claim for damages for not safeguarding the mental health of the employee once he had suffered his first nervous breakdown. The High Court held that it was reasonably foreseeable that in returning to his former post without adequate help and resources, Mr Walker would again become mentally ill—especially in the light of the medical experts' opinions that the nature and the volume of his work was the major contributory factor for his first nervous breakdown. In the *Barber* case in the Court of Appeal,[7] Lady Justice Hale laid down 15 useful propositions about an employer's duty of care in safeguarding its employees' mental health:

◆ There are no unique considerations applying to cases of psychiatric (or physical) illness or injury arising from the stress of doing the work the employee is required to do. The ordinary principles of employer's liability apply.

◆ The threshold question is whether this kind of harm to this particular employee was *reasonably foreseeable*. This has two components:
  • an injury to health (as distinct from occupational stress), which
  • is attributable to stress at work (as distinct from other factors).

◆ *Foreseeability* depends upon what the employer knows (or ought reasonably to know) about the individual employee. Because of the nature of mental disorder, it is harder to foresee than physical injury, but may be easier to foresee in a known individual than in the population at large. An employer is usually entitled to assume that the employee can withstand the normal pressures of the job unless he knows of some particular problem or vulnerability (staff who feel under stress at work should tell their employer and provide a chance to do something about it).

◆ The test is the same whatever the employment: there are no occupations that should be regarded as intrinsically dangerous to mental health.

◆ Factors likely to be relevant in answering the threshold question include:
  • *The nature and extent of the work done by the employee*:
  • Is the workload much more than is normal for the particular job?
  • Is the work particularly intellectually or emotionally demanding for this employee?
  • Are the demands being made of this employee unreasonable when compared with the demands made of others in the same or comparable jobs?
  • Are there signs that others doing this job are suffering harmful levels of stress?
  • Is there an abnormal level of sickness or absenteeism in the same job or the same department?

◆ *Signs from the employee of impending harm to health*:
  • Has he a particular problem or vulnerability?
  • Has he already suffered from illness attributable to stress at work?
  • Have there recently been frequent or prolonged absences that are uncharacteristic of him?
  • Is there reason to think that these are attributable to stress at work, for example, because of complaints or warnings from him or others?

◆ The employer is generally entitled to take what he is told by his employee at face value, unless he has good reason to think to the contrary. He does not generally have to make searching enquiries of the employee or seek permission to make further enquiries of his medical advisers.

◆ To trigger a duty to take steps, the indications of impending harm to health arising from stress at work must be plain enough for any reasonable employer to realize that he should do something about it.

- The employer is only in breach of his duty of care if he fails to take the steps that are reasonable in the circumstances, bearing in mind the magnitude of the risk of harm occurring, the gravity of the harm that may occur, the costs and practicability of preventing it, and the justifications for running the risk.

- The size and scope of the employer's operation, its resources, and the demands it faces are relevant in deciding what is reasonable; these include the interests of other employees and the need to treat them fairly, for example, in any redistribution of duties.

- An employer can only reasonably be expected to take steps that are likely to do some good; the court is likely to need expert evidence on this.

- An employer who offers a confidential advice service, with referral to appropriate counselling or treatment services, is unlikely to be found in breach of duty.

- If the only reasonable and effective step would have been to dismiss or demote the employee, the employer will not be in breach of duty in allowing a willing employee to continue in the job.

- In all cases, therefore, it is necessary to identify the steps that the employer both could and should have taken before finding him in breach of his duty of care.

- The claimant must show that that breach of duty has caused or materially contributed to the harm suffered. It is not enough to show that occupational stress has caused the harm.

- Where the harm suffered has more than one cause, the employer should only pay for that proportion of the harm suffered that is attributable to his wrongdoing, unless the harm is truly indivisible.

- The assessment of damages will take account of any pre-existing disorder or vulnerability and of the chance that the claimant would have succumbed to a stress-related disorder in any event.

In a more recent case—*Hartman* v. *South Essex Mental Health and Community Care NHS Trust* (and five other conjoined appeals)[13]—the Court of Appeal took extensive guidance laid down by that Court in the *Barber* case but it noted that the House of Lords had held that it was guidance only and that each case must be determined on its own facts. The overall test remains the conduct of the reasonable and prudent employer taking positive thought for his workers' safety in light of what he ought to know. In the *Hartman* case, liability for her stress-related illness was not made out even though the occupational physician was aware of her heightened susceptibility to stress, as this information remained confidential. The critical issue in this case was whether the Trust should have appreciated that Mrs Hartman was at risk of succumbing to psychiatric illness. The Court of Appeal held that the case was not reasonably foreseeable.

Finally, in *Intel Corporation (UK) Limited* v. *Daw*,[14] the Court of Appeal made it clear that liability for negligence was not avoided by offering counselling services (see the *Barber* case, discussed earlier in this section). It was not, according to the Court of Appeal, 'a panacea by which employers can discharge their duty of care in all cases'. Here Mrs Daw had made it clear at the time of her appraisal and thereafter that she was becoming ill due to her workload, but management failed to take appropriate action.

Employees' duties

In common law, employees have implied duties, including the duty to work with reasonable care and competence and to serve their employer loyally and faithfully. They are also under a duty to be reasonably competent, to co-operate with their employer, and to obey reasonable lawful instructions. So for example, an unreasonable refusal to submit to a medical examination by a doctor of the employer's choice and to consent to the disclosure of a medical report could constitute a breach of the duty to co-operate or to obey a reasonable instruction.[15]

Statute law

Health and Safety at Work etc. Act 1974

The HSW Act is superimposed on earlier Acts and the duties imposed by some of these (e.g. the Mines and Quarries Act 1954, the Factories Act 1961, and the Offices, Shops and Railway Premises Act 1963) must still be met, although most of their enforcement provisions have been replaced in the new legislation. The HSW Act imposes criminal liability, and the company, individual managers, and employees can be prosecuted for breaches of their statutory duties. Penalties for health and safety offences including failure to comply with an improvement or prohibition notice or for breaches of Sections 2–6 of the HSW Act are up to £20,000 and/or 12 months imprisonment in the lower (magistrates) courts and an unlimited fine and/or 2 years imprisonment if heard in the higher courts. There is provision in Section 47 of the HSW Act to permit employees injured at work to sue for their injuries in the civil courts under the Act, but this section has not been implemented to date. Employees who are injured at work as a result of a breach of any other statutory duties can sue in the civil courts, as the other statutory enactments impose both civil and criminal liability. The HSW Act covers everyone at work, including independent contractors and their employees, the self-employed, and visitors, but excludes domestic servants in private households.

Employers' statutory duties

The HSW Act imposes general duties on employers under Section 2 to ensure, so far as is reasonably practicable, the health, safety, and welfare at work of their employees. This specifically includes ensuring that:

- There is a safe system of work.
- There is a safe place of work.
- Staff are given information, instruction, and training on matters of health and safety, and are adequately supervised.
- There is a safe system for the handling, storage, and transport of substances and materials.
- There is a safe working environment.

Although there is no specific mention of a duty to conduct pre-employment medical examinations, part of a safe system of work could be interpreted as ensuring that the staff who have been recruited are fit to perform their duties where there is any question of medical fitness impinging on the work requirements. This can only be done after a job offer has been made (s.60 of the Equality Act 2010). Adequate medical data on new members of staff is essential. However, due care must be taken to observe the employer's duties under the Equality Act 2010 to not discriminate (see Chapter 3).

Employees' statutory duties

Employees have duties under Sections 7 and 8 of the HSW Act to 'take reasonable care' of their own health and safety, and the safety of others; to cooperate on any matter of health and safety; and to do nothing which could endanger their health and safety or that of others.

This duty could be taken to include the disclosure of a relevant medical condition once a job offer has been made. For example, an employee who failed to disclose that they had epilepsy, before starting work in a job where this could pose a hazard, might be in breach of their duty under Section 7 of the HSW Act. Failing to disclose material health information when requested to do so may also constitute grounds for lawful dismissal (see 'Unfair dismissal').

The institutions

The Health and Safety Executive (HSE) is an independent regulator with responsibility for enforcing health and safety legislation, including the HSW Act, in Great Britain. Formerly, the Health and Safety Commission (with its tripartite representation from government, industry, and the trade unions) was set up under the HSW Act to oversee national health and safety policy, but a merger of the two bodies in 2008 led to the HSE assuming both sets of powers. HSE has several divisions, the largest of which is Her Majesty's Factory Inspectorate. The Employment Medical Advisory Service is the field force of the medical division of HSE, and will be described in Chapter 4. Enforcement of the HSW Act in offices, shops, railway premises, and warehouses is carried out by environmental health officers, who are employed by the local authorities. Their powers are the same as those of factory inspectors.

Employment protection legislation

Employees have been given statutory protection from being unfairly dismissed; the relevant provisions can be found in the Employment Rights Act 1996. Several aspects of these measures are important for those who develop illnesses or injuries while at work. (Section 98(2)(a) defines 'capability' in Section 98(3)(a) in relation to an employee, meaning his capability assessed by reference to skill, aptitude, health, or any other physical or mental quality.) Employees have been given protection from unfair dismissal provided that they satisfy certain qualifying conditions, such as being ordinarily employed in Great Britain and 1 year's continuous service (other than for discriminatory dismissals).

Claims for unfair dismissal, discrimination, redundancy payments, certain breach of contract cases, and unlawful deductions from wages claims are heard by employment tribunals. These tribunals are chaired by a legally qualified solicitor or barrister of at least 15 years' standing, called an Employment Judge, and a panel of two lay members (one appointed by employers' organizations such as the Confederation of British Industry and one appointed by the Trades Union Congress or other trades union bodies). The lay members advise the Employment Judge as to good industrial practice. The Employment Judge directs the lay members as to points of law.

Appeals on points of law or a perverse decision lie with the Employment Appeal Tribunal (EAT), then with the Court of Appeal and the Supreme Court on points of law only and where leave has been given. Cases are only granted leave by petition to appeal to the Supreme Court on matters of public importance. In cases involving questions of European Community law, cases may be referred directly from employment tribunals to the ECJ. Many of these referrals concern questions arising from the UK's anti-discrimination legislation, which, has been alleged, fails properly to implement the EU directives.

Grounds for dismissal

Section 98 of the Employment Rights Act 1996 sets out five potentially fair grounds for dismissal. They are: conduct, capability, redundancy, illegality, and 'some other substantial reason'. In addition

to proving a fair reason for dismissal, there is a requirement for the employment tribunal to be satisfied that the employer followed a fair procedure and that the decision to dismiss fell within the band
of reasonable responses that any reasonable employer could have adopted. The words of Section
98(4) require an employment tribunal to be satisfied that in all the circumstances of the case, the
employer acted reasonably in treating 'that reason' as a sufficient reason for dismissal, taking into
account equity and the substantial merits of the case.

Employment tribunals are guided by the recommendations of the 'ACAS Code of Practice on
Disciplinary and Grievance Procedures' (2009). Breach of the ACAS code is not in itself unlawful
but employment tribunals are required to take its recommendations into account.

Right of representation

Employees are given the statutory right (s.10 of the Employment Relations Act 1999) to be accompanied by a fellow worker or trade union representative to any grievance meeting or disciplinary
meeting that could lead to a formal warning or other disciplinary action. However, in the public
sector it has been argued that if a professional, such as a doctor or teacher, could be struck off as a
result of a matter which led to their dismissal, Article 6 of the Human Rights Act 1998 (the right
to a fair trial) demands a right to be represented by a lawyer. This was recently tested by a doctor
(Court of Appeal in *Kulkarni* v. *Milton Keynes NHS Trust*) and a teacher, in the Supreme Court
(*R (on the application of G)* v. *The Governors of X School*[16]). Lord Dyson held in the latter case that
there was no requirement for the school's disciplinary proceedings to comply with Article 6; but
there may be circumstances in which legal representation could be a right under Article 6 where
the outcome of the dismissal would have a 'substantial influence or effect' on the regulatory proceedings (e.g. a process capable of barring an individual from a profession). Lord Dyson noted,
however, that where a decision in one set of proceedings determines the outcome in subsequent
proceedings that determine a person's civil rights, then the right to a fair hearing, and, by implication, legal representation, may be engaged at that first stage, which leaves the door open to legal
representation at disciplinary hearings in such circumstances.

'Capability': ill health cases

In order for an employer to justify the fairness of a dismissal on the grounds of ill health 'in all the
circumstances of the case' (Section 98(4) of the Employment Rights Act 1996), they must advance
factual evidence of the 'ill health' preventing the individual from performing the jobs that they
are employed to do, in order to justify the dismissal. In other words, the employer must obtain an
up-to-date medical report from the clinician in charge of the employee's treatment.[17]

Tribunals also have to be satisfied that the employer acted reasonably in all the circumstances
of the case, treating that reason as sufficient for dismissal, taking into account the size and administrative resources of the undertaking. In other words, large employers with human resources
experts and extensive resources are expected to adopt all the good practices of a model employer,
in contrast to a small employer who may be forgiven a failure to follow as thorough a dismissal
procedure. The tribunals have given guidance as to what constitutes reasonable conduct on the
part of the employer in this regard (see later in this section).

The mere fact that the individual is not prevented from performing all the duties that they
are required to perform under their contract, does not affect a decision to dismiss for ill health,
as long as the individual is unfit to perform some of the duties. This was stated in the case of
Shook v. *London Borough of Ealing*.[18] Miss Shook, who was employed as a trainee residential
care assistant, strained her back and was off work for some 9 months. She was declared unfit

to carry out her duties as a residential social worker because of the bending and lifting that was involved in her job and this was confirmed by both her GP and by the council's medical officer. She was eventually dismissed after having been offered alternative posts, which she had rejected. She argued that her employers did not have any fair reason to dismiss her because she was not disabled from all her contractual duties as her contract actually contained a very wide flexibility and mobility clause, and she worked in numerous posts within the Social Services Department of the council.

The Court of Appeal ruled that the dismissal was fair and rejected this argument: 'The Tribunal was entitled to reject the submission that an employee is not incapacitated from performing . . . the work which they are employed to do unless he is incapacitated from performing every task which the employers are entitled by law to call on him to discharge'. However widely that contract was construed, her disabilities related to her performance of her duties thereunder, even though her performance of all of them may not have been affected. In other words, a dismissal on grounds of ill health can still be fair even where an employee is not incapacitated from undertaking all their duties, if they cannot undertake an important and primary duty (such as, in this case, lifting residents).

Lying about previous health conditions

Lying has been accepted as being a potentially fair reason for dismissal under the Employment Rights Act 1996 (Section 98(1)(b)), being regarded as 'some other substantial reason for dismissal'. The tribunals have distinguished between lying on a pre-employment medical questionnaire and failing to volunteer the information. There is a subtle but important distinction. In some cases it has been held that there is no duty on employees to 'offer' voluntarily medical information about themselves. However, it is important to note that Section 60 of the Equality Act 2010 now prevents employers from asking about health conditions at the interview stage. Questions about medical or health conditions should only be asked after interview and an offer of employment (see later in this section). Nevertheless, if a direct question is not answered honestly and to the best of the individual's belief, then not only would a dismissal be potentially fair and non-discriminatory (if justified), but also the employer may be able to reclaim any sick pay. However, the question asked has to be clear, unambiguous, relevant, and job related, otherwise the employer will lose an unfair dismissal claim and possibly a discrimination claim, and will not succeed in reclaiming the sick pay paid.

In *Cheltenham Borough Council* v. *Laird*[19] the council learned a very expensive lesson, which was to ask the right questions. They asked Mrs Laird, their prospective new chief executive, whether she had 'any ongoing medical condition which would affect [her] employment?'. She replied 'no', although she mentioned that she occasionally had a migraine which did not affect her ability to work or usually require time off work. She did not mention any history of mental health problems. The form contained the following declaration: 'I declare that all the statements on the above answers are true and given to the fullest of my ability and acknowledge that if I have wilfully withheld any material fact(s), I am, if engaged, liable to the termination of my contract of service'.

She subsequently had significant time off for stress and was paid sick pay for a year before the council discovered that she had a history of depression and stress-related illnesses. The council sued her for misrepresentation to reclaim all her sick pay—and lost. The High Court held that as a lay person and not a medical person, Mrs Laird had given an honest answer. At the time of completing the questionnaire she had no ongoing medical condition. The occupational physician admitted that the questionnaire was 'very poorly drafted' and 'quite inadequate'.

According to the Judge:

> The question would reasonably be understood as relating to an ongoing condition that impaired her physical or mental abilities either generally or in January 2002. She was not depressed in January 2002 and had recovered from her previous illness. Similarly, her answer . . . was not false or misleading because although she had a vulnerability to depression, the vulnerability was ongoing but not the depression . . . From a lay person's perspective, I consider that the question would reasonably be understood as being directed at a condition that was continually suffered or at least regularly suffered and that her vulnerability was not such a condition.

The Judge suggested that a sweeping up question should have been asked, for example, 'Is there anything else in your history or circumstances which might affect our decision to offer you employment?'

Medical evidence and medical reports

In assessing fitness for work most employers rely on self-certificates for the first 7 days of absence and a Statement of Fitness ('Fit Notes') from the employee's GP thereafter. HM Revenue & Custom's *Employer Helpbook for Statutory Sick Pay*[20] suggests that employers may ask for any reasonable medical evidence of incapacity for work and this would include evidence from chiropractors, osteopaths, acupuncturists, and so on. If a Fit Note is provided, the helpbook suggests that this is strong evidence of incapacity and should usually be accepted as conclusive unless there is evidence to the contrary. Where there is evidence to the contrary, the employment tribunals have held that the employer is entitled to look behind the medical certificate, as happened in the case of *Hutchinson* v. *Enfield Rolling Mills Ltd*.[21] Mr Hutchinson was signed off for a week with sciatica but was seen marching in a trade union demonstration in Brighton. His employers took the view that this 'was not consistent with a person who was reputedly suffering from sciatica. In other words, if you were fit enough to travel to Brighton to take part in a demonstration, you were fit enough to report for work'. The EAT agreed with the employer.

However, contrast Hutchinson's case with that of *Scottish Courage Ltd* v. *Guthrie*[22] (unreported) where a warning shot was fired across the bows of employers deciding whether or not to pay sick pay in the face of an unchallenged medical certificate. Mr Guthrie's GP had given him a MED 3 (the forerunner of the Fit Note), but the employer's medical advisers said that he was fit to return to work. Neither medical adviser had suggested that Mr Guthrie's sickness was other than genuine. The employer's sickness absence policy provided that: 'Employees who are absent from work as a result of genuine illness and who fulfil all the requirements of the scheme rules will be eligible for [sick pay]' and 'Payment for sickness absence is conditional upon all appropriate procedures being followed and on management being satisfied that the sickness absence is genuine'. Mr Guthrie had followed the relevant procedures and in the past the company had always paid sick pay where employees produced medical certificates from their GPs. The company also agreed that Mr Guthrie did not have a poor sickness record. Mr Guthrie claimed that an unlawful deduction had been made from his wages. The EAT said that the tribunal was entitled to test whether the employer reached its decision in good faith. The decision to withhold sick pay was perverse, in that no reasonable employer could have reached it on the evidence gathered. Mr Guthrie was certified sick by his GP and, although the company's doctors differed as to when he could return to work, they had agreed that his illness was genuine. This case emphasizes the need for careful drafting of sick pay policies.

For a judicial definition of 'malingerer' see *Jeffries* v. *The Home Office* (unreported) in which the High Court held that: 'A malingerer is one who deliberately and consciously adopts the sick role, if necessary deceiving his medical advisers to persuade them that his complaints are true'.

Status of statements of fitness

If employers choose to rely upon statements of fitness (Fit Notes), then they are entitled to do so, although they are provided for 'Statutory Sick Pay (SSP) purposes only' and have no legal status in their advice to patients or employers. The Department for Work and Pensions[23] has published very useful advice to GPs, employers, and occupational physicians regarding the issuing of Fit Notes.

Not all duties are suspended when an employee is off sick

The definition of 'incapacity' for SSP purposes is inability to carry out *any* duties that it is reasonable to expect the employee to do under their contract. The definition requires consideration of the full range of the duties that it would be reasonable to expect the worker to conduct. Where, for example, an employee has his ankle in plaster 6 weeks after an operation, at a time when his consultant advises that he can weight bear and walk with crutches, that employee could carry out sedentary tasks, perhaps with adjustments to his working hours so that he can travel outside of the rush hour. If the GP continues to sign the employee off sick, careful discussions need to take place between the occupational physician and GP in order to resolve any concerns that the GP may have about his patient returning to work with his ankle in plaster. In *Marshall* v. *Alexander Sloan Ltd*[24] the EAT held that:

> The argument that all the appellant's obligations under the contract were suspended because she was off work ill so that her employers had no contractual authority to issue the order could not be accepted. Though a term has to be implied into a contract limiting the employee's obligation to perform all the terms of his contract when he is sick, such a term should be no wider than is necessary to give the contract business effect. Business commonsense requires only that when an employee is off sick, he is relieved of the obligation to perform such services as the sickness from which he is suffering prevents him from carrying out, not that all the employee's obligations are suspended.

In this case the tribunal found as a fact that the appellant could have complied with her employer's order and removed the stock from the car or got someone else to do so for her. Her sickness did not prevent her from carrying out her obligation to remove merchandise from the car. Therefore, she could be lawfully ordered to remove it.

Need for an up-to-date medical report

Employment tribunals have made it clear that employers should not rely on medical certificates alone. In *Crampton* v. *Decorum Motors Ltd* (unreported), the managing director received a MED 3 diagnosing Mr Crampton with angina pectoris. Believing that this was a serious heart condition, the director dismissed Mr Crampton on the basis of the MED 3 alone. This was held to be an unfair dismissal because a reasonable employer would have made further enquiries as to the seriousness of the condition before taking this drastic decision. In ill health cases, a full medical report should be sought from the occupational physician or nurse who should have obtained up-to-date medical reports from the treating doctors.

The employer is required to inform the doctor and the employee of the purpose for which the medical report is sought.[25] Typically, the employer will state that the report is needed to plan the work of the department, administer the sick pay scheme(s), and consider reasonable adjustments and alternative duties. A report could also be required for consideration for ill-health retirement or permanent health insurance.

Doctors should always ensure that every employee who attends for an assessment clearly understands its purpose and the intended use of the report. In case of doubt, the occupational physician should explain the situation to the patient prior to any examination. If necessary, the doctor should write to the originator of the request seeking clarification.

When employers without occupational health staff seek advice from an independent occupational physician, they should advise the doctor as to the purpose of their enquiry, the basic job functions of the individual, and length of absence to date. The employer should obtain prior, written informed consent to do this from the employee. Typically the report will be limited to non-clinical details and a functional assessment. If a medical report is sought from the employee's GP or specialist, then the employer is required under the Access to Medical Reports Act 1988 (see 'Access to Medical Reports Act 1988') to inform the employee of their rights under that Act (which include the right to see the report before it is sent to the employer and the right to withhold it from the employer). If a non-medically qualified person receives a medical report, they may not be able to understand it. Good practice dictates that they return it to the specialist seeking 'clarification and amplification'—*WM Computer Services* v. *Passmore* (unreported).

Data Protection Act 1998

Under Section 2 of the Data Protection Act 1998 (DPA), health data are designated as 'sensitive data' for which 'explicit consent' is required before an employer can process them. 'Processing' means obtaining, inputting, storing, using, disclosing, amending, deleting, erasing, etc. Part 4 of the Code of Practice published by the Information Commissioner[26] provides essential information on how employers must treat health data and the rights of data subjects to give or withhold their consent for data processing. If consent is obtained, employers (as opposed to occupational physicians or other treating doctors) may ask the specialist or GP a range of questions. If an occupational physician seeks the medical report, then the employer is entitled to the answers to the model questions listed by the British Medical Association (Box 2.1), although there must be no disclose of clinical or confidential information.

Box 2.1 Model letter to consultant or GP enquiring about an employee's return to work

1 When is the likely date of return to work?
2 Will there be any residual disability on return to work?
3 If so, will it be permanent or temporary?
4 Will the employee be able to render regular and efficient service?
5 If the answer is 'Yes' to question 2, what duties would you recommend that your patient does not do and for how long?
6 Will your patient require continued treatment or medication on return to work?

Under Section 7 of the DPA, data subjects (i.e. job applicants, employees, ex-employees, and other third parties) have a right of access to such personal data whether in electronic or paper form, subject to the restrictions and limitations placed on their rights in the Court of Appeal's judgment in *Durant* v. *Financial Services Authority (FSA)*.[27]

Mr Durant had been involved in litigation with Barclays Bank plc, which he lost. He then sought disclosure (under Section 7 of the DPA) of documents held by the FSA and related to the complaint against him. The FSA refused to provide certain documents on the grounds that they did not constitute personal data and/or were not part of a relevant filing system. Mr Durant brought a court action to seek disclosure which went to appeal. This examined:

+ The meaning of 'personal data'.

+ The meaning of 'relevant filing system'.

+ The withholding of personal data from a data subject on the grounds that third party personal data were also present.

+ The nature and extent of a court's discretion in deciding on disputes over subject access rights.

The court concluded that '*personal data*' does not necessarily mean every document that has the data subject's name on it. Rather, the over-riding test is whether the information (not the document) affects a person's privacy. Whether information can be classed as 'personal data' will depend on where it falls in the continuum of relevance or proximity to the data subject. There are two 'notions' that assist this task:

+ Is the information in itself significantly biographical?

+ Does it have the data subject as its focus?

A '*relevant filing system*' was held to be a record in which the information had a structure that allowed specific information about an individual to be identifiable with 'reasonable certainty and speed'. A paper file in which papers simply appear in date order, rather than by subject, is not a relevant filing system.

The court concluded that it is acceptable to blank out references to third parties where they have not given consent for their identity to be disclosed. But if the reference to the third party is a part of the personal data there is a tension between the duty of confidentiality to the third party and the duty to comply with the rights of the data subject. In those situations, the court must use its discretion based on the circumstances of the case.

The Information Commissioner stated that he supports the judgment of the court. His office has issued guidance to address the issues raised by this case.[26]

Access to Medical Reports Act 1988

Under the Access to Medical Reports Act 1988 (AMRA),[28] employees are entitled to see any medical report that relates to them, prepared by a medical practitioner responsible for their clinical care. Once an occupational physician (or a member of their staff) has treated an employee the Act will apply to all subsequent medical reports (in Section 2 'care' is defined as including examination, investigation, or diagnosis for the purposes of, or in connection with, any form of medical treatment); but it is less clear whether this may apply to other reports, such as a statement on fitness to work or job placement.

The court can order an individual to consent to the disclosure of clinical records and reports including correspondence between the occupational physician, the consultant, and managers of the company.[29] However, the courts and employment tribunals must first obtain the consent of the claimant, to avoid breaching the AMRA and the DPA[30] (see also Chapter 3).

Conflicting medical advice

In some cases, employers receive conflicting medical opinions—the employee's doctor stating the individual is unfit for work and the occupational health practitioner advising to the contrary. In this dilemma, tribunals have generally accepted that a reasonable employer would rely upon the view of its occupational physician[31] unless:

- The occupational physician has not personally examined the individual.
- The occupational physician's report is 'woolly' and indeterminate.
- The continued employment of the individual would pose a serious threat to health or safety of the individual or others.
- The individual is under a specialist and the occupational physician has not obtained a report from that specialist.
- The employee asks the employer to allow him to present another specialist opinion.

Tribunals have accepted that unreasonable refusal by an individual to return to work following the advice of the occupational physician constitutes misconduct on their part. The reason for dismissal is 'conduct'—refusing to obey a lawful and reasonable instruction. Employment tribunals have not been tolerant of employers who take decisions about the continued employment of an employee in haste, before the medical report is received.[32]

Consultation with the employee

The tribunals have ruled that in ill health dismissal, the employer should normally contact the employee by telephone or, ideally, by visiting them at home. The purpose is to consult the employee about their incapacity, to discuss any possible return date, the continuation or otherwise of company benefits and state benefits, the employment of a temporary or permanent replacement, and the future employment or termination of employment. Consultation like this replaces the warnings that employees are entitled to receive in poor performance or misconduct cases. This was stated in a number of leading cases.[33] Only in exceptional circumstances would an employer succeed in establishing that he had acted reasonably if he had failed to consult the employee prior to any decision.[34]

Seeking suitable alternative employment

The tribunals expect an employer to consider all alternatives other than dismissal. This includes looking for alternative employment within the organization or with any associated employers. The duty also includes considering whether any modification to the original job is possible. If the illness or injury is deemed to be a disability under the Equality Act 2010, there is a statutory duty to consider making reasonable adjustments to the workplace (see Chapter 3). Failure by the employer to seek alternative employment will normally render any dismissal for ill health unfair. This proposition received judicial approval in the House of Lords in *Archibald* v. *Fife Council*,[35] albeit in a case involving the former Disability Discrimination Act 1995.

Permanent health insurance benefits

Practitioners who advise employers offering long-term disability (LTD) or permanent health insurance (PHI) schemes ought to be aware that failure to consider offering such benefits in a particular case could be challenged in the common law courts as a breach of the employment contract.

The House of Lords ruled in *Scally* v. *Southern Health and Social Services Board*[36] that there was a positive duty on employers rather than their medical advisors to inform their staff of those benefits for which the employee must make an application. The same principle could apply to the claiming of sick pay or PHI or LTD and maternity rights. However, this implied duty on the employer does not extend to explaining to a sick employee the financial implications of resigning and taking an LTD scheme.[37] If an employer offers a PHI or LTD scheme it will be deemed to be a breach of contract to dismiss the employee before allowing them to become eligible for the scheme, as it is regarded as a contractual entitlement that cannot be frustrated by terminating the contract—*Aspden* v. *Webbs Poultry & Meat Group*.[38] If the employee commits gross misconduct, the employer has the right to dismiss them even if this deprives them of their right to PHI—*Briscoe* v. *Lubrizol Ltd*.[39]

In the context of PHI and LTD schemes, the duty may extend only to informing employees in the relevant circumstances that they may be eligible for participation. Consideration of eligibility for an LTD or PHI scheme, as an alternative to dismissal, may also be viewed by the tribunals as an important factor that could render the dismissal unfair. Company medical advisors should be familiar with the available benefits so that they can give appropriate advice. If such a scheme exists, the doctor ought to ask the employer whether the employee has been considered for it.

Early retirement on medical grounds

Some employees may be deemed permanently incapacitated for employment and dismissed and given an early retirement pension. The courts have indicated that the employer must act in good faith in such cases.[40] Medical practitioners must read the exact wording of any pension scheme in this regard, particularly if a medical examination is to be performed to assess eligibility. It would be wise for them to require a copy of the sick pay scheme, PHI scheme, and pension fund rules as they apply to early retirement pensions.

Management's role in sickness decisions

The tribunals have emphasized that the option to dismiss an employee who is off sick and unable to work is a management decision, not a medical one.[41] Doctors should not be pressured into making such decisions for managers. The doctor's role is to provide and interpret medical information so that employers are well placed to make proper decisions about the employee's position.

Pre-placement medical assessments

Pre-placement medical questionnaires should ask relevant questions and gather only information which is pertinent to assessing fitness for work; this should happen after and not before a job offer has been made (s.60 of the Equality Act 2010).

Duty of care in writing pre-employment reports

In *Kapfunde* v. *Abbey National plc*,[42] the Court of Appeal clarified to whom the occupational physician owes a duty of care when writing a report on the fitness for work of a job applicant. In this case, the court made it clear that the person commissioning the report (i.e. the potential employer) was the only person to whom the occupational physician owed a legal duty of care. However, the doctor still owes the patient the normal professional duty of care in clinical matters and must meet the standard expected by the General Medical Council (GMC) regarding 'Good

Medical Practice'. This includes ensuring that any assessment is conducted to the highest professional standards and that any significant abnormalities detected are notified to the patient and, with the subject's informed consent, to his GP.

Duty to be honest

In a case brought before the ECJ, *X* v. *Commission of the European Communities*,[43] it was ruled that prospective job candidates have the right to be informed of the exact nature of the tests to be carried out and to refuse to participate if they wish. In this case, Mr X complained that he had been screened for human immunodeficiency virus antibodies without his consent. The ECJ held that the manner in which the appellant had been medically assessed and declared unfit constituted an infringement of his right to respect for his private life as guaranteed by Article 8 of the European Convention on Human Rights. This right requires that a person's refusal to undergo a test be respected in its entirety; equally, however, the employer cannot be obliged to take the risk of recruitment.

Confidentiality

Ethical questions including the duty of confidentiality are covered in detail in Chapter 5. Apart from the Article 8(1) right to respect for private life, doctors and nurses are under strict ethical codes of conduct and can be struck off the medical register for serious breaches. The GMC periodically reviews and publishes guidance concerning confidentiality and the duties of a doctor, including an occupational physician. Recent guidance has been to offer to show or to give a copy of their report to the patient before it is supplied, as well as to the employer (paragraph 34 of the 2009 guidance).[44]

Employers are not entitled to require their staff to undergo medical examinations without obtaining their informed written consent on each occasion. This means ensuring that the employee understands the nature of the examination and tests, and the reasons for them. Medical staff should ensure that written consent forms are completed. On each occasion employers must also obtain the employee's written, informed consent to disclosure of the results or a more detailed medical report to a named individual in the company. In the absence of written consent no medical examination or disclosure should take place.

Expert evidence

Inevitably many occupational physicians will be asked at some time to give expert evidence, in employment tribunals in ill health dismissals, or disability discrimination cases, or in the High Court in personal injury claims. Expert witnesses give evidence of opinion as opposed to evidence of fact. Expert witnesses are governed by detailed rules and a Practice Direction in the Civil Procedure Rules (Part 1).

Pregnancy, discrimination, and the law

Any form of discrimination on the grounds of a woman's pregnancy is unlawful, constituting direct discrimination (Sections 13, 18, and 19 of the Equality Act 2010). All aspects of pregnancy, pregnancy-related illness, and maternity are covered, including the notification of intention to take maternity leave, the taking of maternity leave, and intention to return to work following maternity leave. Furthermore, pregnant women and breastfeeding mothers are given statutory protection at work as employers are under a duty to carry out risk assessments and to have adequate control measures where possible. Failing adequate control measures, the woman has a right to be transferred to another safer job, or, if this is not possible, a right to be suspended on normal pay (Section 64 of the Employment Rights Act 1996).[45]

European law

Directives which are adopted by the Council of Ministers are binding on member states and any emanations of the state, including former state bodies, such as nationalized industries, public utilities, and state schools, are bound by the directives. Their employees may sue for breach of an article of the directive directly in the UK tribunals. Employers in the private sector are not directly bound by a directive, but member states are required to adopt the directive into their national legislation within a defined timescale.

The Council of Ministers is represented by the appropriate minister from each member state. Each member state has a block vote, the number of votes depending on the size of its population. There are currently 25 member states. Except on matters of health and safety and product safety, voting must be unanimous for a directive to be adopted. The most important treaty is the Treaty of Maastricht, replacing the Treaty of Rome.

The Council of Ministers can also make recommendations. Recommendations are generally adopted by the institutions of the Community when they do not have the power to adopt binding acts or when they think that it is not appropriate to issue more constraining rules under the treaty. Although not legally binding, EU resolutions and recommendations have legal effect in particular when they clarify the interpretations of national provisions or supplement binding Community measures.

An important recommendation in the field of employment is the European Commission Recommendation and Code of Practice on the protection of the dignity of women and men at work (92/131). This contains recommendations to employers, trade unions, and employees on avoiding and dealing with sexual harassment.

Working Time Directive

The Working Time Directive, which was adopted under the qualified majority voting system, requires member states to legislate for a maximum of 48 working hours in any 7-day period, with rest breaks and restrictions on the number of hours of work that can be performed at night. Draft regulations were published in April 1998 and became law in the UK in October 1998.

The Working Time Regulations 1998 (SI 1998/1833) provided workers with an entitlement to:

- A rest break where the working day exceeds 6 hours.
- At least 1 whole hour off in each 24 hours.
- At least 24 hours off in every week.

Other provisions include at least 4 weeks of paid annual leave; restrictions on night work (including an average limit of 8 hours in 24); organization of work patterns to take account of health and safety requirements, and the adaptation of work to the worker; an average working limit of 48 hours over each 7-day period, calculated over a reference period of 17 weeks (Regulation 4(3) of the Working Time Regulations 1998).

A further statutory instrument, amending the first Working Time Regulations, became law in December 1999—The Working Time Regulations 1999. These regulations simplified the meaning of the unmeasured hours and those workers who work unmeasured hours are now exempt from the 48-hour week; it also amended the requirement for employers to keep records of the hours worked by workers who had opted out of the 48-hour maximum working week.

The directive is littered with derogations that exempt certain types of work. There are some general exceptions that exclude workers in air, sea, rail, and road, inland waterways and lake transport, sea fishing and other work at sea, as well as doctors in training. The major provisions for which there are no derogations are the 4 weeks of paid annual leave and the 48-hour working week.

Other exceptions may arise through national legislation or collective agreements for those whose working time is self-determined or flexible (e.g. senior managers or workers with autonomous decision-taking powers, family workers, and workers officiating at religious ceremonies). In addition, workers may agree voluntarily to work longer hours than those laid down in the directive. In other cases, the workers must be permitted compensatory rest breaks if they work for more than 48 hours in a week (e.g. those whose job involves a great deal of travelling, security and surveillance workers, those whose jobs involve a foreseeable surge in activity such as tourism and agriculture, and emergency rescue workers). In *Landeshauptstadt Kiel* v. *Jaege*[46] the ECJ ruled that being on call, even if not actually working, constituted working time under the directive. The ECJ held that:

> A period of duty spent by a hospital doctor on call, where the doctor's presence in the hospital is required, must be regarded as constituting in its entirety working time for the purposes of the Working Time Directive, even though the person concerned is permitted to rest at their place of work during periods when their services are not required . . . An employee available at the place determined by the employer cannot be regarded as being at rest during the periods of his on-call duty when he is not actually carrying on any professional activity.

Under the Working Time Regulations 1998 employers are required to give a minimum paid holiday of 20 days. In accordance with an important ECJ decision, holidays accrue during sick leave and the employee can opt to take this accrued leave when they return to work even if they have entered a new holiday year.[47]

Other health and safety directives

The 'Six Pack' regulations[48] made it mandatory for employers to carry out risk assessments in situations where there were 'significant and substantial' risks to health or safety and to appoint 'competent' people to assist them. Employers are required to maintain and update these risk assessments and to document them. Other regulations require regular health surveillance such as under the Control of Substances Hazardous to Health Regulations (Regulation 11).

The Health and Safety (Display Screen Equipment) Regulations 1992 ('DSE' Regulations), and Code of Practice and Guidance Notes sought to regulate the use of display screen equipment (visual display units (VDUs)). The regulations lay down ergonomic rules relating to the work station, and covering screens, keyboards, desks, chairs, the work environment, and software. In addition, the Code of Practice and Guidance Notes recommend rest breaks for habitual VDU users. The regulations also require employers to provide free eye sight tests and free spectacles if required for VDU use. Employers are also required to undertake regular risk assessments of the workstation and the work in order to highlight any particular or individual problems before they become more serious.

Acknowledgement

This chapter contains Parliamentary information and public sector information licensed under the Open Government Licence v1.0.

References

1 *Bolam v. Friern Hospital Management Committee* [1957] 1 WLR 582.

2 *Bolitho v. City and Hackney Health Authority* [1997] 4 All ER 771.

3 *Kapfunde v. Abbey National plc* [1998] IRLR 583 at paragraph 33.

4 *Stokes v. GKN* [1968] 1 WLR 1776.

5 *Mountenay v. Bernard Matthews PLC* [1994] 5 Med. LR 293.

6 *Barber v. Somerset County Council* [2004] IRLR 475.

7 *Sutherland v. Hatton* (the first of the four conjoined appeals) [2002] IRLR 263.

8 *Edwards v. NCB* [1949]1 ALL ER 743.

9 *Baxter v. Harland and Wolff plc* [1990] IRLR 516.

10 *Paris v. Stepney Council* [1951] 1 All ER 42.

11 *Page v. Smith* [1995] 2 WLR 644.

12 *Walker v. Northumberland County Council* [1995] IRLR 35.

13 *Hartman v. South Essex Mental Health and Community Care NHS Trust* [2005] IRLR 293.

14 *Intel Corporation (UK) Limited v. Daw* [2007] IRLR 355.

15 *Langston v. AUEW* [1973] IRLR 82 and *BT v. Ticehurst* [1992] IRLR 219.

16 *R (on the application of G) v. The Governors of X School* [2009] IRLR 829 and [2011] IRLR 756.

17 *East Lindsey District Council v. Daubney* [1977] IRLR 181 and *Rao v. CAA* [1994] IRLR 240.

18 *Shook v. London Borough of Ealing* [1986] IRLR 46.

19 *Cheltenham Borough Council v. Laird* [2009] IRLR 621 [1979] IRLR 140.

20 HM Revenue & HM Customs. *Employer helpbook for statutory sick pay* (Employer helpbook E14/2011). London: HMRC, 2012.

21 *Hutchinson v. Enfield Rolling Mills Ltd* [1981] IRLR 318.

22 *Scottish Courage Ltd v. Guthrie.* UKEAT/0788/03/MAA.

23 Department for Work and Pensions. Fit note. [Online] (<http://www.dwp.gov.uk/fitnote/>)

24 *Marshall v. Alexander Sloan Ltd* [1981] IRLR 264.

25 *Whitbread & Co plc v. Mills* [1988] IRLR 507.

26 Information Commissioner's Office. [Online] (<http://www.informationcommissioner.gov.uk>)

27 *Durant v. Financial Services Authority (FSA)* [2003] EWCA Civ 1746.

28 British Medical Association. *Access to medical reports—guidance from the BMA ethics department*, June 2009. [Online] (<http://www.bma.org.uk/images/accesstomedicalreportsjune2009_tcm41-186891.pdf>)

29 *Nawaz v. Ford Motor Company Ltd* [1987] IRLR 163.

30 *Hanlon v. Kirklees Borough Council.*

31 *Jones v. The Post Office* [2001] IRLR 381 and *British Gas Plc v. Breeze EAT 503/87 Evers v. Doncaster Monks Bridge* (unreported).

32 *Rao v. CAA* [1994] IRLR 248.

33 *East Lindsey District Council v. Daubney* [1977] IRLR 181; *Spencer v. Paragon Wallpapers Ltd* [1976] IRLR 373.

34 *Eclipse Blinds Ltd v. Wright* [1992] IRLR 133; *AK Links Ltd v. Rose* [1991] IRLR 353.

35 *Archibald v. Fife Council* [2004] IRLR 651.

36 *Scally v. Southern Health and Social Services Board* [1991] IRLR 522.

37 *Crossley v. Faithful and Gould Holdings Ltd* [2004] IRLR 377 (Court of Appeal).

38 *Aspden v. Webbs Poultry & Meat Group* [1996] IRLR 521.

39 *Briscoe v. Lubrizol Ltd* [2002] IRLR 607 Court of Appeal.

40 *Mihlenstedt v. Barclays Bank International Ltd and Barclays Bank plc* [1989] IRLR 522.

41 *The Board of Governors, The National Heart and Chest Hospitals* v. *Nambiar* [1981] IRLR 196.

42 *Kapfunde* v. *Abbey National plc* [1998] IRLR 583.

43 *X* v. *Commission of the European Communities* [1995] IRLR 320.

44 General Medical Council. *Confidentiality*, 2009. [Online] (<http://www.gmc-uk.org/guidance/ethical_guidance/confidentiality.asp>)

45 *Hardman* v. *Mallon t/a Orchard Lodge Nursing Home* [2002] IRLR 516.

46 *Landeshauptstadt Kiel* v. *Jaege* [2003] IRLR 804.

47 *Perada* v. *Madrid Molividad SA* [2009] IRLR 959.

48 The Management of Health and Safety at Work Regulations 1992 replaced by the 1999 Regulations; Health and Safety (Display Screen Equipment) Regulations; Personal Protective Equipment at Work Regulations 1992; Provision and Use of Work Equipment Regulations 1992; Manual Handling Operations Regulations 1992; Workplace (Health, Safety and Welfare) Regulations 1992.

Chapter 3

Disability and equality law

Gillian S. Howard and Tony Williams

Introduction

The Equality Act 2010 (EqA) (which applies in Great Britain and not in Northern Ireland) replaces the Disability Discrimination Act 1995 (DDA) and all the other antidiscrimination statutes and regulations (e.g. Sex Discrimination Act 1975; Race Relations Act 1976). The EqA has updated, added to, and consolidated the various definitions of discrimination that existed in the previous legislation.

It makes discrimination because of various 'protected characteristics' unlawful. Disability is one of the 'protected characteristics'. This chapter focuses on the disability discrimination provisions of the EqA but covers some of the other 'protected characteristics' in passing.

> Anyone who thinks that there is an easy way of achieving a sensible, workable and fair balance between the different interests of disabled persons, of employers and of able-bodied workers, in harmony with the wider public interests in an economically efficient workforce, in access to employment, in equal treatment of workers and in standards of fairness at work, has probably not given much serious thought to the problem.[1]

> It is a paradox, in no way unique to disabled people, that the anti-discrimination approach requires that in order to assert their right to full and equal participation in society, they must continue to assert their differences. The price of being heard, and achieving some control over the consequences of disability, is to accept the label.[2]

Originally, antidiscrimination legislation was piecemeal, inadequate, and disparate. The EqA has pulled together the various pieces of antidiscrimination legislation, added explicit detail in some areas (e.g. includes a new definition of indirect disability discrimination), new concepts (e.g. 'discrimination on the grounds of combined characteristics') and modified the former approach under the disability discrimination legislation concerning comparisons with an 'able-bodied' person. These issues are explained in the following sections.

'Medical' model of disability

The UK's disability legislation was and still is in large measure based on the 'medical model' of disability—i.e. disability is caused by a medical condition, which can be cured or treated or not as the case may be. Many disability discrimination experts reject this model, instead preferring the 'social model' which posits that functional disability is perpetuated by societal barriers. For example, someone who is wheelchair-bound will be disabled from enjoying theatre if there is no wheelchair access, but will not be disabled if such access is provided.

Court judgments

Court judgments are recorded in various ways, and most are also 'reported', with added legal commentary. References may either be the neutral citation, referring only to the court judgment, or may be the reported citation which may not include the level of court. Most references included here are to the reported citation.

The hierarchy of the Courts in England and Wales is:

(a) Employment Tribunal

(b) Employment Appeal Tribunal (except in Northern Ireland)

(c) High Court

(d) Court of Appeal (Court of Session in Scotland)

(e) Supreme Court (replacing the House of Lords)

(f) European Court of Justice

The Codes of Practice and Guidance

There are a number of Codes of Practice and Guidance issued on antidiscrimination matters. These include the Equality and Human Rights Commission's (EHRC's) Code of Practice on Employment (January 2011)[3] and the Guidance on matters to be taken into account in determining questions relating to the definition of disability (2010).[4]

Employment tribunals and the courts will expect occupational health practitioners and employers to be aware of the codes' recommendations and guidance in dealing with disability cases.

Equal treatment?

The concept of equality may seem a simple one but there is a problem. For treatment to be unequal, it must be unequal in relation to someone else—a comparator (save in cases of pregnancy discrimination and some forms of disability discrimination). This need for a comparator is obvious in the case of race. Pregnancy discrimination, which is gender-specific, can only adversely affect the female sex. In such cases there is no need for a male comparator: what the woman has to show is 'but for' her pregnancy or pregnancy-related condition, she would not have been so treated.

In disability discrimination cases, the only comparator can be an able-bodied person and some degree of inequality is inevitable. A damaging case in the House of Lords, *London Borough of Lewisham* v. *Malcolm [2008] IRLR 700*, led to provisions in the EqA that removed the need for someone with a disability to have to show comparable treatment of an able-bodied person. In claims of discrimination arising from disability, there is now no defence for an employer to show that an able-bodied person would have been treated in the same manner and therefore there has been no discrimination against the disabled person.

Positive discrimination for one person may appear to be negative discrimination for another. In contrast to the USA, positive discrimination is generally unlawful in UK (although the EqA allows very rare exceptions, which are discussed later in the chapter).

Disability law has to be different. In order somehow to redress the balance and give equality to an already disadvantaged disabled person, some positive treatment is necessary in the form of 'reasonable adjustments'. Providing a free disabled parking space for use for people with physical disabilities is a simple example of positive discrimination. These issues are discussed in the following sections.

Different forms of disability discrimination

There are now six different forms of disability discrimination:

1 Direct discrimination

2 Indirect discrimination

3 Discrimination arising from disability

4   Failure to make reasonable adjustments

5   Harassment

6   Victimization.

A new concept of 'combined' discrimination is covered later in the chapter.

Role of the occupational physician

Occupational physicians (OPs) have an important part to play in most areas of equality law and a critical role in the area of disability—in particular in advising on the need for 'reasonable adjustments' that may assist someone with a disability to secure work, stay in work, or return to work after a period of absence.

Antidiscrimination laws which protect individuals' rights need special care when OPs are giving advice. OPs may have to advise their client or employer on disability-related cases which may lead to claims for discrimination in an Employment Tribunal or for personal injuries in the High Court. In such cases employers will often seek their medical advisor's opinion and may require them to give evidence in Court. The Faculty of Occupational Medicine's guidance stresses that such advice must be *evidence-based*.

The OP's particular expertise lies in assessing the effects of work on health and the impact of the employee's health on his/her performance and that of others. In sickness absence cases a key role is to evaluate the functional capacity and limitation of the employee and to advise on reasonable adjustments that will help the employee back to work. Where necessary this advice may require additional information from other medical specialists. It will also help if the OP is prepared to learn about disability law so as to understand the issues that may arise.

Employment tribunals not uncommonly concur with the OP's opinion (in contrast to the evidence of a general practitioner (GP)), according to a review of tribunal judgments.[5]

The question of disability can *only* be determined finally by the court or tribunal. The role of the OP is *not* to advise an employment tribunal as to whether an individual is disabled for the purposes of the Act or what is or is not a normal day-to-day activity. It is reasonable for an OP to express an opinion of this kind when advising employers to assess job applicants and employees with health problems. The OP can advise as to the *likelihood* of the EqA applying and the adjustments the employer should consider making. Ultimately, whether adjustments seem 'reasonable' must be decided by the employer in light of their business operations and other constraints such as cost and efficacy.

In *Vicary* v. *British Telecommunications PLC [1999] IRLR 680* the Employment Appeal Tribunal (EAT) stated:

> It is not for a doctor to express an opinion (to an ET) as to what is a normal day-to-day activity. Nor is it for the medical expert to tell the tribunal whether the impairments which had been found proved were or were not substantial. Those are matters for the ET to arrive at its own assessment.

This point was reinforced in *Abadeh* v. *British Telecommunications PLC [2001] IRLR 23* which also stated (in relation to the same OP as in the *Vicary* case):

> The medical report should deal with the doctor's diagnosis of the impairment, the doctor's observation of the applicant carrying out day-to-day activities and the ease with which he was able to perform those functions, together with any relevant opinion as to prognosis and the effect of medication.

GP or specialist evidence?

Many employees with disabilities are not under consultant care. A question then arises from the viewpoint of tribunals as to the standing of generalist, as compared with specialist advice.

The evidence from a GP who has been treating the patient does carry weight. In *J* v. *DLA Piper LLP [2010] IRLR 936*, the EAT held that:

> A GP was fully qualified to express an opinion on whether a patient was suffering from depression, and on any associated questions arising under the DDA: depression was a condition very often encountered in general practice.

However, the EAT qualified this statement by adding that the evidence of a GP would 'have less weight than that of a specialist and in difficult cases the opinion of a specialist may be valuable; but that does not mean that a GP's evidence can be ignored if the evidence of a specialist is not available or is inconclusive'.

Equally in *Paul* v. *National Probation Service [2004] IRLR 190*, the EAT criticized the occupational health adviser (OHA) for only seeking an opinion from the GP and not from the specialist psychiatrist treating Mr Paul. The EAT held that in such cases employers are duty bound to seek 'competent and suitably qualified medical opinion'. (This last situation was complicated by the fact that the GP was not treating Mr Paul's illness.)

Where a 'difficult' medical condition is alleged, employers and OPs may elect to seek an additional specialist opinion. This can help in supporting assessment of the diagnosis, prognosis, and causation, as well as assisting the assessment of resulting disability.

Sometimes an OP may disagree with the employee's GP over assessment of fitness to work. In some cases sick pay has been denied by employers because of such a disagreement. The assumption that sickness absence is not genuine because two doctors disagree may, however, be successfully challenged in the Tribunals. In *Scottish Courage Ltd* v. *Guthrie [2004] UKEAT/0788/03/MAA* the employee was denied sick pay on the basis of an OP's assessment that the employee was fit for work. Guthrie's GP continued to sign him off sick. The sick pay scheme provided for 'Payment for sickness absence (being) conditional upon all appropriate procedures being followed and on management being satisfied that the sickness absence is genuine . . .'.

The OP believed that Mr Guthrie could return to full duties whilst the GP believed that he could do only 'light duties'. The EAT held, as the occupational physician had not found that the employee was '*malingering*', that the difference of opinion between the two doctors was in terms of what the employee could realistically do. His sickness absence was deemed 'genuine' and because of the wording of the contractual sick pay, the employer's denial of sick pay was ruled unlawful. (Notwithstanding the detail of this case, it should be noted that OPs rarely use the term 'malingering' in reports because of its pejorative overtone.)

Medical evidence may not only be conflicting, but unclear. The OP may be in a position to assist the court in distinguishing between evidence based on fact and evidence based on opinion. For example, a GP diagnoses post-traumatic stress disorder (PTSD) based on reported symptoms from their patient. However, PTSD as defined in ICD-10 and DSM IV has strict criteria that must be met before an expert psychiatrist can diagnose this condition, and the OP may assist the tribunal by commenting on this.

OPs must ensure that the advice given is full and appropriate, to ensure the employer is sufficiently informed to make reasonable adjustments. In *Secretary of State for DWP* v. *Alam [2009] UKEAT/0242/09/LA*, Mr Alam was depressed, partly because of financial problems. He wanted a second job and asked to leave work early for a job interview. This was denied but he left anyway and was disciplined. Smith J noted that if an employer did not know or could not be deemed to know of the disability and could not reasonably be expected to be aware of a relevant effect of the disability, no duty to make reasonable adjustments would arise. As Mr Alam's GP had not specifically stated that an effect of his depression might be difficulty in asking for permission when it was required, the employer had no duty to make an adjustment for this.

In *Project Management Institute* v. *Latif [2007] IRLR 579*, the EAT held that it is sometimes for the claimant to advise the employer about what adjustments they are seeking, so that the employer can consider whether these would be reasonable. The EAT stated that:

> That is not to say that in every case the claimant would have to provide the detailed adjustment that would need to be made before the burden would shift. It would, however, be necessary for the respondent to understand the broad nature of the adjustment proposed and to be given sufficient detail to enable him to engage with the question of whether it could reasonably be achieved or not.

Ethical considerations

> The occupational physician plays a different role from that of other specialists or general practitioners (Faculty of Occupational Medicine, 2009).

This arises because typically, the OP has a formal contractual relationship with the employer, an obligation to remain independent and an important duty to maintain the employee's confidentiality. This last duty overrides that of disclosure to an employer. Issues of confidentiality and informed consent are dealt with in the Faculty of Occupational Medicine's *Guidance on Ethics for Occupational Physicians*, publications from the General Medical Council and British Medical Association (including *Medical Ethics Today*, 2012), and in Chapter 5 of this book. 'The fact that a doctor is a salaried employee gives no other employee in the company any right of access to medical records or to the details of the examination findings. . . .' *(Medical Ethics Today)*.

With appropriate informed consent, however, the OP can enter into constructive dialogue with managers over reasonable adjustments and support for the employee and other issues such as fitness constraints.

Disability considerations

It will help employers to understand when specific and strict legal duties arise in relation to the need to make reasonable adjustments. However, employers who pay due regard to the needs of their staff when ill or injured will not distinguish between employees who are technically regarded as 'disabled' under the Act and those who are not. Good medical and employment practice dictate that, even where an employee's medical condition might not qualify as a disability under the exact terms of the Act, he/she should be treated in a similar manner to someone who is disabled, in terms of reasonable adjustments to encourage early return to work. Helping and supporting all employees with an illness or injury to return to work would seem good business sense.

Protected characteristics EqA S4

The EqA repealed all the existing antidiscrimination statutes and regulations and introduced nine characteristics protected in law from the various forms of discrimination. In additional to disability, they comprise: age, sex, race, religion or belief, sexual orientation, pregnancy and maternity, gender reassignment, marriage and civil partnership.

Much of the workload of OPs will involve cases of disability, although sometimes other protected characteristics, such as pregnancy, maternity, or gender reassignment, may also be cases which come under their care. This chapter focuses only on the key issues OPs are likely to face.

Definition of 'disability' EqA S6

> A person has a disability if they have a physical and mental impairment, and the impairment has a substantial and long-term adverse effect on their ability to carry out normal day-to-day activities.

The word 'substantial' has been held to mean 'more than minor or trivial' rather than 'very large' *Goodwin* v. *The Patent Office [1994] IRLR 4*.

The Courts and Employment Tribunals (ETs) have interpreted and defined variously 'disability', 'substantial adverse effects', 'effect of medical treatment', and 'likely to recur'. For example, dyslexia—a learning difficulty and not an illness or injury—can be held to be a disability (a mental impairment) under the Act where it has substantial adverse effects. In *Paterson* v. *MPC [2007] IRLR 763*, the EAT held that a person needing extra time in promotion examinations because of dyslexia was prejudiced in his 'normal' day-to-day activities (in a professional capacity) and so qualified as 'disabled'.

In addition the DRC's Code of Practice (paragraph 3.3) confirms that dyslexia may be covered under the Act as one of the '*hidden impairments*' (along with other learning difficulties). Whether the condition has a substantial adverse effect on the carrying out of a day-to-day activity or whether the employer has discriminated in some way against the employee (e.g. not making reasonable adjustments), will be determined by the tribunals and courts.

The focus in the legal definition of 'disability' is on how the condition impacts on ability to function rather than the condition itself.

Normal day-to-day activities

The EqA repealed a list of eight normal day-to-day activities previously in Schedule 1, para 1 of the DDA 1995, now leaving it to the ETs to make the determination.

However, the 2010 Guidance gives examples of 'normal' day-to-day activities. These are:

> Things people do on a regular or daily basis, and examples include shopping, reading and writing, having a conversation or using the telephone, watching television, getting washed and dressed, preparing and eating food, carrying out household tasks, walking and travelling by various forms of transport, and taking part in social activities. Normal day-to-day activities can include general work-related activities, and study and education-related activities, such as interacting with colleagues, following instructions, using a computer, driving, carrying out interviews, preparing written documents, and keeping to a timetable or a shift pattern.

In *Ekpe* v. *The Commissioner of Police of the Metropolis [2010 IRLR 605]*, the EAT held that:

> What is 'normal' for the purposes of the Act may be best understood by defining it as anything which is not abnormal or unusual (or, as in the Guidance issued by the Secretary of State, 'particular' to the individual applicant), just as what is 'substantial' may be best understood by defining it as anything which is more than insubstantial. What is normal cannot sensibly depend on whether the majority of people do it.

The tribunal decided that putting rollers in a claimant's hair was a normal day-to-day activity, even though carried out almost exclusively by women.

In *Goodwin* v. *The Patent Office [1998] EAT/57/98* it was held that tribunals and doctors should concentrate on what the individual *cannot* do, rather than what they can do, stressing that it was not the doing of particular acts that counted, but the ability to do them.

The guidance written for the EqA advises that any decision on terms such as 'normal day-to-day activities' and 'substantial' should be based on the ordinary meaning of the words and in most cases will be obvious in a commonsense way to most people.

Examples of what might be regarded as having a 'substantial adverse effect' are listed in the Appendix to the Guidance and include:

◆ Difficulty going out of doors unaccompanied—e.g. because the person has a phobia, physical restriction, or learning disability.

- Difficulty waiting or queuing—e.g. because of a lack of understanding of the concept, or because of pain or fatigue during prolonged standing.
- Difficulty on steps, stairs or gradients—e.g. because movements are painful, fatiguing, or restricted.
- Difficulty in environments that the person perceives as frightening.

Determination of disability

After receiving evidence on the impairment from a medical expert, the ET will seek evidence as to whether that impairment had a long-term, substantial adverse effect upon normal day-to-day activities in the individual.

In some cases of disability discrimination the issues before the ET are medical and the tribunal will need expert medical evidence in order to determine what, if any, impairment the claimant has. In other cases the ET will be able to make that assessment, based on the evidence of what effect the impairment has on normal day-to-day activities.

In *J* v. *DLA Piper LLP [2010] IRLR 936*, the EAT held that J's recurrent depressive illness was capable of falling within the Act as a disability and gave guidance as to the correct approach in determining disability. It acknowledged that:

> In some cases identifying the nature of the impairment from which a claimant may be suffering involves difficult medical questions. In many or most such cases it will be easier (and is entirely legitimate) for the tribunal to ask first whether the claimant's ability to carry out normal day-to-day activities has been adversely affected on a long-term basis. If it finds that it has been, it will in many or most cases follow as a matter of commonsense inference that the claimant is suffering from an impairment which has produced that adverse effect. If that inference can be drawn, it will be unnecessary for the tribunal to try to resolve the difficult medical issues.

Tribunal decisions are not binding on other tribunals, which limits their use as guidance. Decisions taken by higher courts where disability has been disputed are more useful as these are binding on future tribunals and lower courts. For disability to be determined there has to be an impairment, but a diagnosis or treatment does not necessarily signify this. Patients may take antihypertensive treatment to reduce a slightly raised risk of a future medical event but they have no impairment related to their high blood pressure, with or without treatment, and cannot be considered disabled.

However, disability can be determined where, if not for the treatment, the person would become disabled for normal day-to-day activities (e.g. the epileptic controlled by antiepileptic drugs or the arthritic patient rendered pain free by hip replacement).

Showing an impairment

The onus of proof rests with the claimant to provide clear medical evidence that they have an impairment. This normally requires the submission of a medical report from a GP or specialist, or in cases of dispute oral evidence from an expert.

In cases where there is overlay of psychological symptoms the burden of demonstrating physical or mental impairment remains, and can be difficult to establish.

Any decision on whether or not a claimant has a disability is ultimately for the ET to make. Where there is doubt, it is important that the OP presents the tribunal with clear factual and opinion evidence to help the tribunal decide whether the claimant has an impairment or not. This is particularly important when there are discrepancies between the stated impairment and observed impairment.

Covert surveillance

In disputed claims, covert surveillance has been used by insurers or employers to obtain evidence on the extent of a disability. Covert video footage is admissible in ETs, and may be admissible in the common law courts, although there may be issues of breach of the right to respect for privacy (Article 8 of the Human Rights Act 1998) and Courts have penalized employers for this breach by awarding costs against the employer, even when they have successfully defended the claim. Where an OP is asked to consider covert surveillance we suggest seeking legal advice and advice from the physician's medical insurer before agreeing to continue with the instruction.

What is an 'impairment'? EqA Sch1 S1 & 6

The DDA was amended in 2005 so that three conditions—cancer, HIV infection, and multiple sclerosis—were impairments automatically covered by the Act and these now appear in the EqA.[6] Someone registered blind or partially sighted is also automatically considered disabled if they can supply a certificate from an ophthalmologist. For these conditions, a doctor can state definitively that the person has a disability in accordance with the EqA, as the decision requires only a medical diagnosis. In all other situations, only a tribunal can decide (on the facts of the case) whether the person is disabled.

In *Kirton* v. *Tetrosyl Ltd [2003] IRLR 357*, Mr Kirton had incontinence following surgery for bladder cancer. His incontinence was considered to be a part of his disability from cancer as there was a causal link between the two. In the same way, it is important to consider whether symptoms or impairments such as hair loss following chemotherapy might be causally related to the cancer.

The Equality Act 2010 (Disability) Regulations 2010 include a list of conditions that are excluded from the definition of 'impairment'. These include addiction to alcohol, nicotine and other substances, tendency to set fires, tendency to steal, tendency to physical or sexual abuse of other persons, exhibitionism and voyeurism, piercings, tattoos, and seasonal allergic rhinitis.

However the ETs will determine whether any of these conditions is underpinned or caused by a medical condition covered by the Act (e.g. whether a tendency to physical abuse is caused by a mental illness) and could then rule that discrimination because of such a condition is unlawful under the Act.

In *Murray* v. *Newham Citizens Advice Bureau [2003] IRLR 340*, Mr Murray was imprisoned for stabbing someone (an excluded condition), but he had done so because of his schizophrenia. When Newham CAB found that he had been in prison for stabbing his neighbour, they rejected him as a volunteer worker. He complained that he had been unlawfully discriminated against because his mental illness rendered him liable to violent episodes. It was finally held that: '. . . . the applicant's tendency to violence was a consequence of paranoid schizophrenia and thus a manifestation of his disability', and that his claim for unlawful disability discrimination should succeed.

Long-term effects EqA Sch1 Part 1, S 2

The effect of an impairment is long-term if it has lasted for at least 12 months, it is likely to last for at least 12 months, or it is likely to last for the rest of the life of the person affected.

If an impairment ceases to have a substantial adverse effect, it is to be treated as continuing to have that effect if that effect is likely to recur.

If someone has had an impairment that met the criteria for a disability in the past, but has since recovered, they are still covered by the Act, provided that the effect upon normal day-to-day activities is '*likely to recur*'. This provision is designed to prevent discrimination on the grounds of a past impairment.

A distinction must be drawn between an impairment which 'recurs' over time and one which is 'repeated' over time. A rugby player may fracture an ankle aged 19, fully recover, and fracture an ankle again 10 years later. This is a new condition, not a recurrence of an underlying condition; he does not now have a 'disability' by virtue of an underlying condition lasting ten years.

By contrast, a woman with osteoporosis who fractures her wrist aged 50 and fractures the same wrist aged 60 years, would have an underlying condition linking the two recurrent events, and it would be appropriate to consider her disabled.

In many cases impairments do not last for 12 months or more, but are liable to recur. The words '*likely to recur*' have been the subject of litigation at the highest level. The House of Lords, in *SCA Packaging Ltd* v. *Boyle [2009] IRLR 746*, held that they meant '*could well happen*' rather than '*probable*' or '*more likely than not*'. This makes it easier for claimants to argue that their condition is likely to recur.

A case in point is depression. While a depressive episode may resolve within 6 months, 75–90 per cent of patients may have recurrent episodes.[6] Thus, once an individual has had one depressive episode which has a substantial effect upon normal day-to-day activity, they may be protected by the EqA. (This is not a hard and fast rule, as, for example, occurrence of a single severe depressive episode following bereavement would not ordinarily carry a high risk of recurrent depression.)

Sometimes the presenting condition is wrongly diagnosed, for example, as depression, when in fact it is not a depressive episode by the criteria of WHO ICD-10[7] or DSM IV.[8] This was noted in *J* v. *DLA Piper [2010] IRLR 936*, in which the EAT drew a distinction between 'clinical depression' and a reaction to 'adverse life events'. The EAT noted 'the looseness with which some medical professionals, and most lay people, use such terms as "depression", "anxiety", and "stress"'.

They considered that if someone had an episode of depression that lasted over 12 months, constituting a disability initially, and then a period of 30 years with no symptoms, followed by another episode of depression, that second episode would also need to meet the criteria for 'long term' rather than being linked to the first in order to constitute a disability. On the other hand, they considered someone who had a series of short episodes of depression over a 5-year period to have one single condition causing recurrent symptomatic episodes.

Anwar v. *Tower Hamlets College [2010] UKEAT/0091/RN* suggested the approach that should be taken when deciding whether a condition is likely to have a substantial adverse effect for more than 12 months when it has not yet lasted that long. Tribunals should consider the options for treatment (treatments already given, treatment it is reasonable to seek, and its availability and likely effects).

OPs will often see mental health issues in the context of workplace conflict, when advice in relation to the Act can be challenging. It may be safest to state that the EqA 'may apply', recommend appropriate adjustments, and leave it to managers to decide if these are reasonable or not. In such situations the OP can have a useful role in counselling the employee about the need to seek resolution and in exploring available options for mediation. They would be advised to do so at an early stage, as inertia and a consequent prolonged spell of absence can worsen the worker's prospects for eventual return to work and worsen the risk of legal dispute.

Severe disfigurement EqA Sch1 S3

> An impairment which consists of a severe disfigurement is to be treated as having a substantial adverse effect on the ability of the person concerned to carry out normal day-to-day activities.

A 'disfigurement' is the generic term for the aesthetic or visual impact of a scar, burn, mark, asymmetric, or unusually shaped feature or texture of skin on the face, hands or body. A '*severe disfigurement*' is to be treated as an impairment having a substantial adverse effect, whatever its actual effect may be. A mental impairment such as depression may occur as a direct result of the severe disfigurement, and in this case the person would be deemed to have a disability under the Act.

The term *'severe disfigurement'* is not further defined in the Act, so its determination will be a question of fact for an ET. However, certain deliberately acquired disfigurements, such as tattoos and body piercing, are excluded from coverage.

The *Guidance on matters to be taken into account in determining questions relating to the definition of disability (2010)* refers to examples of physical disfigurements such as 'scars, birthmarks, limb or postural deformation (including restricted bodily development) or diseases of the skin'.

'Substantial' EqA Sch1 S4

Impairment has to be 'substantial'. This has been defined by the *Guidance* to mean 'more than minor or trivial'. Account must be taken of the cumulative effect of several minor impairments. For example someone with obsessive–compulsive disorder might need to check switches, taps, and locks before leaving the house. The need to check one switch is a minor issue, but the cumulative effect of checking everything repeatedly before leaving the house may result in frequent and substantial lateness at work.

Certain conditions such as depression or arthritis may affect some patients substantially but have only a minor effect on others.

Effect of medical treatment EqA Sch1S5

An impairment is to be treated as having a substantial adverse effect on the ability of the person concerned to carry out normal day-to-day activities if measures are being taken to treat or correct it, and but for that, it would be likely to have that effect. 'Measures' includes, in particular, medical treatment and the use of a prosthesis or other aid.

This does not apply in relation to the impairment of a person's sight, to the extent that the impairment is, in the person's case, correctable by spectacles or contact lenses or in such other ways as may be prescribed.

This is an area where claimants need to provide sufficient medical evidence to establish that, without treatment, there would be a substantial adverse effect on a day-to-day activity.

In *Woodrup* v. *London Borough of Southwark [2003] IRLR 111*, the Court of Appeal had to establish whether there was a 'deduced effect' in relation to Ms Woodrup's anxiety neurosis (i.e. whether she would suffer symptoms with a substantial effect upon day-to-day activity if her treatment stopped). She alleged this, but offered only out-of-date medical statements from her GP and out-of-date letters from junior hospital doctors to support her case. The Court of Appeal held that an EAT had rightly judged this to be insufficient.

Progressive conditions EqA Sch1 S8

This applies to a person (P) if P has a progressive condition, as a result of that condition P has an impairment which has (or had) an effect on P's ability to carry out normal day-to-day activities, but the effect is not (or was not) a substantial adverse effect. P is to be taken to have an impairment which has a substantial adverse effect if the condition is likely to result in P having such an impairment.

The purpose of this provision is to provide support for individuals with progressive conditions such as motor neurone disease where the disabling effects may be slow to appear. In such cases the OP should consider what adjustments are necessary at each stage of the illness. ETs will consider whether at the time of dismissal the condition had manifested itself to the point of causing an effect which in future was liable to become substantial.

In *Richmond Adult Community College* v. *McDougall [2008] IRLR 227*, the Court of Appeal confirmed that the employer's knowledge of any disability, including a recurring condition, must be judged on the basis of the evidence available at the time of the employment decision, rather than the date of the ET hearing. In this case Ms McDougall's offer of appointment was withdrawn because she did not receive satisfactory medical clearance. The tribunal found that she had a mental illness but that there was no evidence at the time the decision was taken that the illness was likely to recur, and therefore no long-term effect. Subsequently, but prior to the tribunal hearing, she was admitted to hospital under the Mental Health Act. Lord Justice Pill held that:

> The central purpose of the Act is to prevent discriminatory decisions and to provide sanctions if such decisions are made. Whether an employer has committed a wrong must . . . be judged on the basis of the evidence available at the time of the decision complained of.

It was noted, however, that subsequent events should be taken into account in calculating damages.

Direct discrimination EqA S13

> A person (A) discriminates against another (B) if, because of a protected characteristic, A treats B less favourably than A treats or would treat others.

Direct discrimination—for example denying employment because someone has had a mental illness in the past or is a woman who may still bear children—is the crudest form of discrimination. It is unlawful and (apart from age discrimination) can never be justified.

The concept of 'less favourable treatment' requires a comparator; less favourable than someone else. Except in cases of pregnancy or maternity discrimination, a claimant needs an appropriate comparator to show different and less favourable treatment. We discuss next what comparator is required.

The wide definition of 'direct discrimination' includes 'perceived' and 'associative' discrimination. Perceived discrimination is discrimination because of a person's perceived characteristic (e.g. because a man is believed to be gay and harassed as a result).

In *English* v. *Thomas Sanderson Blinds Ltd [2009] IRLR 206*, Mr English, who was not gay, was nevertheless subjected to homophobic banter by his colleagues. The Court of Appeal held that:

> A person who is tormented by 'homophobic banter' is subject to harassment on the ground of sexual orientation within the meaning of (the former regulations) even though he is not gay, he is not perceived or assumed to be gay by his colleagues and he accepts they do not believe him to be gay. The conduct falls within both reg. 5 and the EC Equal Treatment Framework Directive.

'Associative discrimination' is discrimination because of an association with someone else (e.g. because of general prejudices over disability or race).

In *Coleman* v. *Attridge Law [2008] IRLR 722*. Ms Coleman was harassed, bullied, and finally forced to take voluntary redundancy because she claimed (successfully) she had to care for a severely disabled son. The ECJ held that this was disability discrimination by association and was unlawful.

Under the EqA, the perception that a person is disabled will be potential grounds for unlawful discrimination. The former Employment Equality (Age) Regulations already covered perceived (but not associative) discrimination.

There is no justification for direct disability discrimination—it is automatically unlawful if it is found to have occurred. If a case is made out, a finding of discrimination will be made with no cap on compensation (subject to the normal rules on compensation, relating to loss of future earnings, damages for injury to feelings, etc.).

Direct age discrimination is lawful, however, if it can be shown to be a proportionate means of achieving a legitimate aim. In *Wolf* v. *Stadt Frankfurt am Main ECJ C-229/08*, it was successfully argued that recruiting older firefighters was too expensive, given the limited period of service they could provide in a physically arduous job.

However the 'cost' argument is not an automatic justification. There has to be a cost plus justification. We refer to this later in the chapter.

Positive discrimination

Disabled employees and job applicants may receive 'positive discrimination', since the courts take regard of the inequality that may exist between an able-bodied and a disabled person. Making reasonable adjustments is seen as levelling the unequal playing field.

Positive discrimination may be lawful in the narrow area of 'training', where an employer can redress under-representation.

A major UK law firm fell foul of committing positive discrimination while selecting employees for redundancy. In *Eversheds Legal Services Ltd* v. *de Belin [2011] IRLR 448*, an employee absent on maternity leave was given a notional maximum score on a particular selection metric, and Mr De Belin was chosen instead for redundancy, despite consistently out-performing her before her leave. The case was declared to be unlawful discrimination on the grounds of sex. (However, a distinction exists between equal treatment for matters unrelated to pregnancy/childbirth and special treatment required in connection with it: allowing time off only to pregnant women to attend antenatal classes is lawful.)

It may be reasonable to consider the disabled person ahead of other candidates for a slightly higher graded job (if they cannot undertake their current job). The House of Lords in *Archibald* v. *Fife Council [2004] IRLR 651* held that:

> The Disability Discrimination Act is different from the Sex Discrimination and Race Relations Acts in that employers are required to take steps to help disabled people which they are not required to take for others. The duty to make adjustments may require the employer to treat a disabled person more favourably to remove the disadvantage which is attributable to the disability. This necessarily entails a measure of positive discrimination ... [This] ... could include transferring without competitive interview a disabled employee from a post she can no longer do to a post which she can do. The employer's duty may require moving the disabled person to a post at a slightly higher grade.

Combined discrimination EqA S14

The provisions on combined discrimination are still to be enacted at the time of writing. If it is not possible to demonstrate discrimination on the grounds of one characteristic it may be possible to argue that discrimination has taken place on the grounds of a combination of more than one protected characteristic. It is not possible, however, to combine direct discrimination for one characteristic with indirect discrimination for another, or indirect discrimination for both, or claim these combinations to be direct discrimination.

Discrimination 'arising from disability' EqA S15

Direct discrimination is rare nowadays. More common is discrimination 'arising from disability'— for example, using absence from work related to disability as a criterion for redundancy.

Such discriminatory treatment was defined under the DDA in terms of 'less favourable treatment' and automatically required a comparator. If the employer was able to show that an employee who had no disability with the same absence record would have been selected for redundancy, then the disability claim failed. The original legal argument defining the comparator occurred in *Clark* v. *TDG Ltd, t-a Novacold, [1999] IRLR 318*, using the example of a blind man needing to take a dog into a restaurant where dogs were banned. It was argued that the comparator was a sighted man without a dog, so preventing the blind man from entering with his dog was automatically discriminatory. It became more difficult with sickness absence. Should the comparator be someone without the condition who had not had sickness absence? That would imply that a disabled person could have unlimited sickness absence in relation to their disability.

However, in *London Borough of Lewisham v. Malcolm* [2008] IRLR 700, the House of Lords decided that the correct comparator for the purposes of the DDA was a person without a mental disability (a secure tenant in this case who had sublet his property) and not a secure tenant who has not sublet his property. Whilst this case related to the Local Authority's rights to evict a tenant, it was followed in later employment discrimination cases (e.g. *Aylott* v. *Stockton on Tees Borough Council, [2009] IRLR 994*).

The solution now enacted in the EqA was not to require a comparator:

> A person (A) discriminates against a disabled person (B) if A treats B unfavourably because of something arising in consequence of B's disability and A cannot show that the treatment is a proportionate means of achieving a legitimate aim.

The Act uses the word 'unfavourable' instead of 'less favourable'.

Other cases where disability is not the issue but, for example, the absence is due to pregnancy or gender reassignment treatment, may be regarded as discriminatory under the Act.

Justification

The employer will be left needing to show that such treatment is justified in terms of being 'a proportionate means of achieving a legitimate aim'.

In practice ETs will assess whether an objective balance had been struck between the discriminatory effect of the measure and the needs of the employer.

Indirect discrimination EqA S19

A person may seem to be fairly treated but still be placed at an unfair disadvantage by their disability. For example, a pub landlord may allow anyone to drink at the bar but the steps into the building prevent wheelchair access. Where there is indirect discrimination it is unlawful but can be justified. Not allowing a one-armed man to work as a scaffolder is discriminatory but if the job can only be done by someone with two arms that discrimination can be justified.

> A person (A) discriminates against another (B) if A applies to B a provision, criterion or practice (PCP) which is discriminatory in relation to a relevant protected characteristic of B's . . . A provision, criterion or practice is discriminatory in relation to a protected characteristic of B's if A applies, or would apply, it to persons with whom B does not share the characteristic, it puts, or would put, persons with whom B shares the characteristic at a particular disadvantage when compared with persons with whom B does not share it, it puts, or would put, B at that disadvantage and A cannot show it to be a proportionate means of achieving a legitimate aim.

This is perhaps the most important area of disability legislation, as indirect discrimination is more common than direct discrimination. It is inevitable that if someone has a disability it will put them at some form of disadvantage. A balance has to be struck, as in many cases discrimination is unavoidable. The law requires the employer to show that any disadvantage is a 'proportionate means of achieving a legitimate aim'.

The phrase 'provision, criterion or practice' (PCP) is not defined by the Act but it will be construed widely so as to include any formal or informal policies, rules, practices, arrangements, criteria, conditions, prerequisites, qualifications or provisions (including one-off decisions and decisions still to be applied).

This phrase, 'proportionate means of achieving a legitimate aim' is a significant departure from the DDA, which only required the employer to show that the reason was 'material and substantial'. A case demonstrating the change is *Jones* v. *The Post Office [2001] IRLR 384*. Mr Jones drove a postal van. Diabetes treated with insulin placed him at risk of hypoglycaemia and an OP advised that to lessen the risk he should drive his van for no more than 2 hours in any working day. This was discriminatory (as it would cost him valuable shift and overtime allowances), but his diabetes was a material fact in relation to the decision, and a hypoglycaemic event would be considered substantial, so the Court of Appeal allowed the employer's appeal of the original decision that the employer's conduct was discriminatory.

The EqA now required the employer to show that this was a 'proportionate means of achieving a legitimate aim'. If there were other ways of mitigating the risk of hypoglycaemia (e.g. periodic monitoring of blood glucose), then advice that the individual should not drive for more than two hours a day could be open to question.

Duty to make reasonable adjustments EqA S20

The first requirement is a requirement, where a provision, criterion or practice of A's puts a disabled person at a substantial disadvantage in relation to a relevant matter in comparison with persons who are not disabled, to take such steps as it is reasonable to have to take to avoid the disadvantage.

The second requirement is a requirement, where a physical feature puts a disabled person at a substantial disadvantage in relation to a relevant matter in comparison with persons who are not disabled, to take such steps as it is reasonable to have to take to avoid the disadvantage.

The third requirement is a requirement, where a disabled person would, but for the provision of an auxiliary aid, be put at a substantial disadvantage in relation to a relevant matter in comparison with persons who are not disabled, to take such steps as it is reasonable to have to take to provide the auxiliary aid.

Where reasonable adjustments are required, the employer is not entitled to require a disabled person to pay costs towards compliance with the duty. The disabled person may wish to provide their own auxiliary aid and should be allowed to do so if they wish, but they cannot be expected to provide or pay for it.

What is reasonable?

The Courts recognize 'reasonableness' in different ways. In unfair dismissal cases ETs use the measure of a 'band of reasonable responses' that different employers might adopt in order to assess the fairness of the particular employer's decision to dismiss. A tribunal cannot substitute its own views of what it would regard as a reasonable decision. Under the disability provisions of the EqA, however, it is for the tribunal to decide what is reasonable. This will depend on the circumstances for the employer. A large employer may be expected to spend substantial sums of money and resources on making physical adjustments to premises (e.g. installing lifts, enabling redeployment, offering retraining, or being more flexible with hours worked), but less may be expected of a small employer with fewer funds and less opportunity to make adjustments.

Sometimes employees with a disability expect adjustments that an OP considers unnecessary or (in the event of a progressive condition) premature. Sensitive handling is required if the OP's judgement is to be understood and accepted.

This is a complex area and the Code of Practice and Guidance are helpful in this regard.

The first step is for the employer to consider what adjustments might be made. In *Paul* v. *National Probation Service [2004] IRLR 190* cited earlier, where Mr Paul had a history of stress-related depression, an OHA recommended that it would be undesirable for him to work in a stressful role, and his application was rejected without any consideration of possible adjustments. The EAT held that this was disability discrimination because the employer had failed to consider reasonable adjustments, informed by specialist advice from the claimant's consultant on his fitness for the post in question, had not discussed this with the claimant, and had not entertained potential further dialogue with the OHA over measures to amend the job.

In *Yorkshire Housing Ltd* v. *Cuerden [2010] UKEAT/0397/09/SM*, Mrs Cuerden was off sick because of depression, panic disorder, and agoraphobia. Her employer refused to hold a meeting to discuss return to work arrangements with her (as recommended by her solicitor), until she was fit. This was found to be unreasonable.

What is unreasonable?

In *Kenny* v. *Hampshire Constabulary [1999] IRLR 76*, Mr Kenny, who had cerebral palsy, applied for the role of IT analyst/computer programmer. He stated that he needed help going to the toilet, with someone holding a bottle for him to urinate into and assistance to transfer to and from his wheelchair. Mr Kenny refused to allow his mother to assist as he did not want to place this burden on her. The EAT noted that 'a line has to be drawn on the extent of the employer's responsibilities in providing adjustments'. The requirement in question was not found to be reasonable.

In *Surrey Police* v. *Marshall [2002] IRLR 843*, Miss Marshall, who had a bipolar disorder with a history of hospital admissions and significant risk factors for a relapse, applied for a job as a fingerprint recognition officer. Her application was rejected. Given the need for first-time error-free processing of fingerprints, the EAT ruled that the adjustments suggested by the claimant would not have been reasonable.

In *Tameside Hospital NHS Foundation Trust* v. *Mylott [2011] UKEAT/0352/09 and UKEAT/0399/10/DM*, Mr Mylott was dismissed and claimed that as he was disabled there was a duty on the employer to facilitate his application for ill health retirement. The EAT determined that the duty to make reasonable adjustments applied only to employment, and not retirement from employment.

In *Burke* v. *The College of Law and Solicitors Regulation Authority [2010] EAT/0301/10/SM*, Mr Burke had multiple sclerosis and asked for additional time to sit his law examination. The EAT determined that the time requirement was a competency standard, and that it would be unreasonable to allow more time: 'the purpose of the examination as being to "assess the ability of the candidate to demonstrate their competence and capability in the subject matter under time pressure"'.

Sickness absence

Although many people with qualifying disabilities take little or no sickness absence, others do, with attendant costs to employers in sick pay and loss of productivity. Any action on the part of management to reduce sickness absence through disciplinary processes or capability action is likely to be discrimination arising from disability. Thus, to be defensible, it has to be shown to be proportionate and legitimate. Careful legal advice may be needed.

On the other hand, employees need to appreciate that very poor attendance can lead to a fair dismissal on grounds of capability. In *Royal Liverpool Children's NHS Trust* v. *Dunsby [2006] IRLR*

351, Mrs Dunsby had been absent for 38 per cent of her work time in a single year for various reasons (gynaecological problems, headaches and stress). The EAT accepted she was disabled but noted that the provisions of the DDA 'do not impose an absolute obligation on an employer to refrain from dismissing an employee who is absent wholly or in part on grounds of ill-health due to disability', and that it would be for a tribunal to determine if the employer is justified in such an action.

The key issue for most employers is to determine what is reasonable in the circumstances of the case. An OP may be asked to determine this, but should exercise due caution as the ultimate decision rests with the employer. In *The Board of Governors, The National Heart and Chest Hospitals v. Nambiar [1981] IRLR 196*, the EAT stated that any decision as to whether or not to dismiss was a management decision not a medical one. 'Seeking a report from a medical consultant did not carry with it the implication that the (employer) would be bound by any opinion that the consultant expressed.'

Advice from the doctor should be limited to views on what absence has been related to the disability, what would be expected in the circumstances, what future absence might be expected, and what reasonable adjustments could be made if any. A person with well-controlled diabetes would not be expected to have frequent sick leave from minor respiratory infections, but may need time off for treatment of recurrent leg ulcers arising from peripheral vascular disease. Any advice must be based on evidence and the facts known to the OP.

Employers should make adjustments to allow employees with a disabling condition to attend healthcare appointments and for treatment. This does not have to be counted as sickness absence or necessarily granted as paid leave. Many employers pay workers who are absent attending necessary healthcare appointments in work time. Agreeing to extended paid leave in respect of a disabled person (as defined under the Act) was rejected as a reasonable adjustment in the case of an employee who argued that cessation of sick pay would add to her stress (*O'Hanlon v. The Commissioners for HMRC [2007] IRLR 404*). However, paying sick pay beyond the contractually stated limit was considered a reasonable adjustment in *Meikle v. Nottinghamshire County Council [2004] IRLR 703* (Court of Appeal), because although there was no contractual duty to do so the employer had failed to make the 'reasonable' adjustments deemed necessary to hasten her return to work.

In *Stringer and Others v. HM Revenue and Customs [2009] IRLR 214*, the ECJ held that employees are entitled to accrue holiday entitlement during sickness absence, and in *Pereda v. Madrid Movilidad SA [2009] IRLR 959*, the ECJ held that accrued holiday in such cases could be carried over to a new holiday year:

> The purpose of the entitlement to paid annual leave is to enable the worker to rest and to enjoy a period of relaxation and leisure. He is entitled to actual rest, with a view to ensuring effective protection of his health and safety . . . It follows that a worker who is on sick leave during a period of previously scheduled annual leave has the right to take his annual leave during a period which does not coincide with sick leave . . . The employer is obliged to grant the worker a different period of annual leave, even if that period falls outside the reference period for the annual leave in question (ie the holiday year).

More difficult is the case where sickness or injury occurs at the start of, or during, a holiday. Employers should have a clear policy on whether that period can be treated as sick leave (instead of holiday) and if so what medical evidence is required.

The law defines a 'protected period' in relation to pregnancy, from the point where it begins (in practice when she informs her employer) normally to the end of her maternity leave. During this period, if, for example, she takes sickness absence for morning sickness this should not be included in any calculation of sickness absence for disciplinary purposes (although illness unrelated to pregnancy, such as a sore throat would count).

Redeployment and relocation

A person may no longer be fit for their current role and redeployment may be recommended. We have already referred to *Archibald* v. *Fife Council [2004] IRLR 651*. Mrs Archibald, a roadsweeper, could no longer work in that role because of severe nerve root pain following a minor operation. She was confined to a wheelchair and could only walk with the aid of two sticks. She applied for over one hundred other roles but was rejected for each. The House of Lords determined that she should have been offered an alternative role, even at a slightly higher grade without the need for competitive interview.

In *Beart* v. *HM Prison Service [2005] IRLR 568*, Mrs Beart had depression, and had a disagreement with her line manager. The OP recommended redeployment to a different work location (prison) but instead Mrs Beart was dismissed. The Court of Appeal determined that such redeployment would have been a reasonable adjustment.

In *Garrett* v. *Lidl Ltd [2008] UKEAT/0541/08/ZT*, Ms Garrett had fibromyalgia and was unable to carry out several of her duties as a store manager. The company was unable to make sufficient adjustments at her usual place of work, but could do so provided that she transferred to a nearby store. Her contract included a mobility clause, and Lidl offered her redeployment to this other store. The EAT found that this was a reasonable adjustment and she should be expected to move to take advantage of the offered adjustment.

In earlier interpretations of the Act, redeployment could only be required to a role that already existed, with no onus on employers to create a new role or transfer responsibilities from existing employees to accommodate the disabled employee. The case of *Chief Constable of South Yorkshire Police* v. *Jelic [2010] IRLR 744*, although fact-specific and not binding as a general rule, indicates how case law has developed. Mr Jelic, a police officer who developed chronic anxiety, was found no longer to be fit for front-line duties. He was assigned a desk job, but in due course it was decided to medically retire him. The EAT upheld the finding of an ET that it would have been a 'reasonable adjustment' for the police to have redeployed him into a job which did not involve facing the public. This could have been done by swapping his front-line post with that of a named police officer. The EAT rejected the argument that the most an employer is required to do in this context is to transfer the disabled employee to an existing vacancy.

That said, this case must come close to the edge of reasonableness. The tribunal said that because the police are a disciplined service the other police officer 'could simply be ordered to move, whether or not he liked it'. It is doubtful whether, in reality, it would be quite that simple.

Lifestyle reasons for disability

Perhaps the most contentious of all areas of disability legislation concern how the lifestyle choices of people with disabilities impact on their capability and the adjustments employers have to make.

The *Guidance* (paragraph B7) notes that:

> Account should be taken of how far a person can reasonably be expected to modify his or her behaviour to prevent or reduce the effects of an impairment . . . if a person can reasonably be expected to behave in such a way that the impairment ceases to have a substantial adverse effect . . . the person would no longer meet the definition of disability.

By way of example, the Guidance indicates that a person with back pain should be expected to give up parachuting, but not normal activities such as moderate gardening, shopping or using public transport.

Another issue is whether a disability is caused or aggravated by a failure to engage with treatment, and whether or not (with that treatment) the condition would not last or be likely to last for 12 months or more. This has been considered in *Anwar* v. *Tower Hamlets College [2010] UKEAT/0091/RN*, in which the EAT stated that it was relevant to consider the availability of potentially effective treatment and the claimant's failure to take this up. Tribunals are likely to expect the claimant to engage with medically appropriate treatment to mitigate their condition.

Irrelevance of alleged discriminator's characteristics EqA S24

It is irrelevant whether the employer or discriminator has the same protected characteristic. For example, if an employer is discriminating against someone with epilepsy, they cannot avoid the provisions of the EqA by claiming that they too have epilepsy.

Harassment EqA S26

> A person (A) harasses another (B) if A engages in unwanted conduct related to a relevant protected characteristic, and the conduct has the purpose or effect of violating B's dignity, or creating an intimidating, hostile, degrading, humiliating or offensive environment for B.

This includes unwanted conduct of a sexual nature which has the above purpose or effect, and where it has this effect, because of B's rejection or submission to the conduct, A treats B less favourably than A would treat B if B had not rejected or submitted to the conduct.

In deciding whether conduct has this effect, account must be taken of the perception of B, the other circumstances of the case, and whether it is reasonable for the conduct to have that effect.

In *Jenkins* v. *Legoland Windsor Park Ltd [2003] UKEAT/1155/02*, Mr Jenkins had a withered arm following a motorbike accident and had to wear a sling. Employees were given models to mark their service and his was the only model that showed him with his left arm in a sling. He went off sick with a depressive episode and did not return. The EAT held that the correct test was the perception that a reasonable employee would or might take of the treatment accorded to him. They held that a reasonable employee in Mr Jenkins' position might well take the view that he had been subjected to detriment by the way in which he was singled out from his colleagues at a substantial presentation ceremony to be identified by a (wrongly characterized) disability. His appeal against the dismissal of his discrimination claim succeeded and the EAT substituted a finding of unlawful discrimination.

Victimization EqA S 27

Victimization occurs where a person suffers a detriment upon bringing proceedings under various antidiscrimination statutes, or making allegations of discrimination, or offering to give evidence for someone in a discrimination claim. The conduct which resulted in an act of victimization is called a 'protected act'. In order to prevent people from being intimidated in this way or subjected to a detriment after doing so, victimization has been included in the EqA (as it was in earlier antidiscrimination laws):

> A person (A) victimises another person (B) if A subjects B to a detriment because B does a protected act, or A believes that B has done, or may do, a protected act.

Protected acts include bringing proceedings under the EqA, giving evidence or information in connection with proceedings under the EqA, and making an allegation that A or another person has contravened the EqA.

Giving false evidence or information, or making a false allegation, is not a protected act if done in 'bad faith'. 'Bad faith' is difficult to prove but would exist if a complaint was founded on malice.

Employees and job applicants EqA S39

An employer must not discriminate against a person in the 'arrangements' made for deciding to whom to offer employment, in the terms of employment, and in refusing employment. This applies both to direct discrimination against a protected characteristic and to indirect discrimination arising from policies and standards that define specific attributes or capabilities. The employer has a duty to make adjustments, and where a policy indirectly discriminates, the employer must demonstrate that the policy is a proportionate means of achieving a legitimate aim.

This is a particular issue for OPs advising on medical standards for employment. Blanket bans on certain conditions are only acceptable if (a) there is a statutory prohibition on employment; or (b) all those with the condition would be incapable or unsafe to work in that role; or (c) there is no proportionate way to distinguish between those who would be capable and safe, and those who would not.

There have been a number of successful challenges to policies that seemed completely reasonable at the time. As a result, for example, medical students with disabilities have increasingly been allowed to train, even though limited from some duties such as surgical procedures and resuscitation.

An employer must not discriminate against an employee in the terms of employment, in access to opportunities for promotion, transfer, training, or receiving any other benefit or service, or by dismissal.

There is a considerable body of case law in relation to promotion (referred to earlier), transfer and training. Where a person is unable to continue in their role because of disability, the employer has a duty to consider redeployment to another available role even if this might involve a promotion (*Archibald* v. *Fife*).

Employees and job applicants: harassment by a third party EqA S40

The employer is regarded as harassing an employee if he allows a third party (e.g. a work colleague) to harass that employee during their work. This has to have happened at least two other times (not by the same party) and with the employer's knowledge. The employer is only liable if he has failed to take reasonable steps to prevent harassment.

Enquiries about disability and health EqA S60

This new provision has caused concern for both occupational health practitioners and employers. It is headed 'Recruitment' and states that:

> A person (A) to whom an application for work is made must not ask about the health of the applicant (B) before offering work to B.

It is not unlawful per se to ask questions about health before making a job offer as s.60 goes on to state:

> A does not contravene a relevant disability provision merely by asking about B's health; but A's conduct in reliance on information given in response may be a contravention of a relevant disability provision.

This means that the use to which an employer puts an answer to a question about health may be unlawful if that answer is used to discriminate. The intention of the legislators was to stop employers asking health questions at interview and discriminating against job applicants ahead of a job offer.

However, there are important exceptions to the rule about not asking health questions at interview. For example, if the employer would need to make reasonable adjustments before asking the job applicant to undergo psychometric testing, or to establish whether the job applicant has a medical condition which would prevent him from working (e.g. vertigo if the job required working at heights).

> This section does not apply to a question that A asks in so far as asking the question is necessary for the purposes of:
> (a) Establishing whether B will be able to comply with a requirement to undergo an assessment or establishing whether a duty to make reasonable adjustments is or will be imposed on A in relation to B in connection with a requirement to undergo an assessment,
> (b) Establishing whether B will be able to carry out a function that is intrinsic to the work concerned,
> (c) Monitoring diversity in the range of persons applying to A for work,
> (d) Taking action to positively discriminate,
> (e) If A applies in relation to the work a requirement to have a particular disability, establishing whether B has that disability.

It is lawful to ask if someone is unable to climb stairs to attend an interview, or if they need information in a more accessible format, or to ask an applicant bus driver if they have any conditions that would prevent them meeting the DVLA Group 2 medical standards. Where the function is intrinsic to work (as in the case of the bus driver), it is only lawful to ask if it *remains* intrinsic to the work once the employer has complied with the duty to consider reasonable adjustments.

It is lawful to ask about disability if the purpose is to allow an organization to encourage sufficient numbers of disabled applicants or to monitor their health inequality policies and procedures.

It is also lawful if there is a requirement for the applicant to have a disability. For example, the RNIB may want a representative with a sight impairment, or a software company may have identified that people with autism spectrum disorder have particular skills they value.

It may still be necessary, however, for Occupational Health Advisers and OPs to acquire health information. Such questions must be 'a proportionate means of achieving a legitimate aim'. In most cases the time to ask is after the job offer has been made. If the person is clearly unable to perform effectively in the role despite reasonable adjustments it is lawful to terminate the application process after job offer and before employment, provided the job offer is clearly spelt out as conditional upon satisfactory medical assessment.

It is important in these circumstances to ensure that mechanisms are in place to complete the enquiries about disability and health in a timely manner and to ensure as far as possible that the job candidate does not start work until these enquiries are complete.

In the less than ideal situation where the person has already started the role, employment may still be terminated lawfully (either without notice in the first 4 weeks or with 1 week's notice or payment in lieu of notice thereafter), provided that the offer letter clearly identifies this as a possible outcome following receipt of the medical assessment. Good medical practice mandates that all pre-placement medical assessments relating to high risk and safety-critical posts should be completed before work is started.

Does s.60 apply to internal promotions?

It remains unclear at present whether section 60 applies in promotion interviews. The heading of s.60 is 'recruitment', and <http://Businessdictionary.com> defines 'recruitment' as 'the process of identifying and hiring the best-qualified candidate (from within or outside of an organization) for a job vacancy, in a most timely and cost effective manner'. Assuming this definition, s.60 would apply to internal promotions as well as to external recruitment. The Acas Guide to the Equality Act does not advise that s.60 is restricted to new external recruits.[9]

Positive action EqA SS158-9

If an employer considers that persons who share a protected characteristic suffer a disadvantage connected to that characteristic, and that participation by that group is disproportionately low, positive action may be taken (if a proportionate means of achieving a legitimate aim) to enable or encourage them to minimize the disadvantage or participate in activity.

In relation to recruitment and promotion positive action can only be taken to treat a person (A) more favourably than another person (B) if A is as qualified as B to be recruited or promoted.

The Acas Guide offers this advice:

> This does not mean they have to have exactly the same qualifications as each other, it means that your selection assessment on a range of criteria rates them as equally capable of doing the job.

> You would also need some evidence to show that people with that characteristic face particular difficulties in the workplace or are disproportionately under-represented in your workforce or in the particular job for which there is a vacancy. In these circumstances, you can choose to use the fact that a candidate has a protected characteristic as a 'tie-breaker' when determining which one to appoint.

> You must not have a policy of automatically treating job applicants who share a protected characteristic more favourably in recruitment and promotion. This means you must always consider the abilities, merits, and qualifications of all of the candidates in each recruitment or promotion exercise. Otherwise, your actions would be unlawful.

By way of example, Annexe 2 of the Acas Guide cites the appointment of a black head teacher ahead of a white one to reflect the ethnic mix in the population from which its pupils come (both candidates being equally qualified).

Lack of knowledge of disability EqA Sch 8 S20

> An employer is not subject to the duty to make reasonable adjustments if he does not know, and could not reasonably be expected to know that an applicant or potential applicant has a disability and is likely to be placed at a disadvantage.

An employer cannot make adjustments if he does not know or could not reasonably be expected to know that the employee has a disability. However ignorance is not a defence under all circumstances.

The ERHC Code (paragraphs 5.17 and 5.18) gives examples in which employers are deemed to know about a disability because their 'agent or employee' (e.g. OHA, OP, HR officer) knows about it. The code exhorts employers to ensure there 'is a means – suitably confidential and subject to the disabled person's consent – for bringing that information together to make it easier for the employer to fulfil their duties under the Act'.

Paragraph 5.15 of the code cites the example of a disabled man with a previously good attendance and performance record who develops depression and becomes emotional for no apparent reason, repeatedly late for work, and prone to make mistakes. In this example the worker is disciplined without being given the opportunity to explain that his difficulties at work arise from a disability and that the effects of his depression have recently worsened.

The sudden deterioration in the worker's time-keeping and performance and the change in his behaviour should have alerted the employer to the possibility that these were connected to a disability and it is likely to be reasonable to expect the employer to explore this further. Employers are expected to pay attention to the manifestations of both the employee's conduct and state of mind at work and the fact of their sickness absence.

In *H J Heinz & Co Ltd* v. *Kenrick [2000] IRLR 144*, an objective approach was taken to the issue of deemed or imputed knowledge of the employer. The EAT held that employers:

> through their medical adviser, had sufficient knowledge of the manifestations of the applicant's disability at the time they dismissed him for it to be held that they had treated him less favourably for a reason that related to his disability within the meaning of s.5(1)(a) of the Disability Discrimination Act, notwithstanding that his condition was not identified by name as chronic fatigue syndrome or medically confirmed until shortly after his dismissal.

This was reinforced by the EAT in *London Borough of Hammersmith and Fulham* v. *Farnsworth [2000] IRLR 691*. Here the council offered the job of residential social worker in an adolescence service unit to Ms F but then withdrew it. She was interviewed and given a provisional job offer but referred to the council's OP for medical clearance. The OP found that Ms F had a history of mental illness over a number of years:

> which at times has been severe and necessitated hospital admission . . . Although Ms Farnsworth's general practitioner reports that Ms Farnsworth's health has been good over the past year, in view of her medical history I am concerned that she may be liable to further recurrence in the future. If such a recurrence were to occur her performance and attendance at work could be affected.

As a result, the council withdrew its provisional offer of appointment. However, its argument that it did not routinely seek medical details of job applicants was held to be no excuse for ignorance of Ms F's disability. The fact that an employer does not know of a disability is not sufficient on its own—they must show that they could not reasonably be expected to know of it.

In *Wilcox* v. *Birmingham CAB Services Ltd UKEAT/0293/10*, the appellant had resigned following a requirement that she relocate to another office which would have meant further travelling from her home to the office. The EAT found, as the tribunal had done, that the CAB had neither actual nor constructive knowledge of Ms Wilcox's disability until after her resignation, when it had seen a full psychiatric report. Before the tribunal, Ms Wilcox had admitted that she had been embarrassed about the problem, that she had not wanted the CAB to make a decision based on her travel anxiety and that she had tried to delay the CAB's attempts to obtain a full medical report.

Since an employer cannot discriminate against a disabled person if it does not, and should not reasonably, know that the person has a disability, both Ms Wilcox's claims relating to her disability failed. The absence of disability discrimination also meant that she was not entitled to resign on that basis.

If an employer is contemplating terminating employment on grounds of capability because of sickness absence caused by an underlying medical condition, case law has established that the employer has a duty to: (a) obtain an up-to-date medical report on fitness for work and reasonable adjustments from either or both the treating physician and the occupational health service;

(b) consult the employee with the contents of that report; and (c) consider suitable alternative employment or reasonable adjustments to the original job.

There is a clear difference between the position of imputed or constructive knowledge at common law and under statute. In contrast to antidiscrimination legislation, the common law does not impute knowledge to an employer through its agent. Thus, job applicants and employees would need to inform their employer (rather than OHA or OP in confidence) about a relevant disability in order to pursue a later personal injury claim. Employers at common law are not deemed to know unless they actually know, and so they will not be held liable for personal injuries that could not be reasonably foreseen.

In *Hartman and ors v. South Essex Mental Health and Community Care NHS Trust and ors [2005] IRLR 293*, Mrs Hartman provided confidential information about her previous mental breakdowns to the occupational health department under the heading 'The following information is for use by the occupational health service only'.

The Court of Appeal held that despite knowledge of her previous mental health history being known to the employer's occupational health department:

> It was not right to attribute to the employers knowledge of confidential medical information disclosed by the employee to the occupational health department.

From a practical point of view, this means that disabled people seeking an adjustment, and those advising them, may have to reconsider the circumstances in which they will disclose their disability and waive their right to confidentiality.

Overall, therefore, there is a duty for an employer to make reasonable inquiries to determine whether the conduct, performance or sickness absence is underpinned by disability. If the employee insists on confidentiality and does not permit the employer to have any medical data, then the employer cannot be deemed to know about any disability and can take whatever reasonable steps that are necessary.

OPs should always be aware of their duty of confidentiality, even when asked a direct question in court. If they consider that the court does not need to know sensitive personal details they should ask the judge to make a ruling on the appropriateness of the question, explaining the issue and asking whether they need to give that evidence or not.

Health and Safety Law EqA Sch 22

There is an interesting relationship between health and safety legislation and equality legislation. An employer does not discriminate if their action is a requirement of an enactment or a relevant requirement or condition imposed by virtue of an enactment. Health and safety legislation and employers' duties therefore will 'trump' the EqA.

A rare example of this that came before an ET was that of *Lane Group PLC v. Farmiloe [2004] UKEAT 0352 03 2201*. Mr Farmiloe had psoriasis which prevented him from wearing safety boots. An environmental health inspector stated that failure to wear safety boots would contravene the PPE Regulations and would be unlawful. There were no other options available to the employer, so Mr Farmiloe was dismissed. The EAT held that dismissal was justified and that it triggered s.59 of the Disability Discrimination Act 1995 (which makes no act unlawful if it is done pursuant to a statute or regulation).

It is important, however, that the employer and the ET fully understand the requirements of the health and safety legislation. The cover of health and safety cannot be used as an excuse to discriminate. This is perhaps best expressed in a draft version of the Equality and Human Rights Commission Code of Practice on Employment (2009), which stated in paragraph 3.60:

> Disabled people are entitled to make the same choices and to take the same risks within the same limits as other people. Health and safety law does not require employers to remove all conceivable risk, but to ensure that risk is properly appreciated, understood and managed. Employers are advised to develop risk management policies which address the risks posed by or to all employees, rather than just focusing on the risks posed by or to disabled employees. If a disabled employee is singled out for a risk assessment, based on stereotypical assumptions, this may amount to direct discrimination or harassment.

A right to work?

Employees may believe that they have a right to work. Although there are exceptions, the general rule is that they do not. Their right is to be paid as long as they are ready, willing, and available to work, until dismissed. Employers may have to decide whether, although employees are ready willing and available, there is too great a risk to allow them to work. The employee's right not to be unfairly dismissed may have to be balanced against the employer's duty of care. The employer would be well advised to take specialist legal advice in such a case, with the benefit of OP advice as well.

Before the DDA, it was not unusual to see lists of automatically proscribed medical conditions throughout a profession or industry, to make it easier for employers and OPs to apply uniform fitness standards. The introduction of the DDA brought about substantial change, as it focussed on individual risk assessment and consideration of reasonable adjustments. There will always be some medical conditions that are incompatible with some roles on safety grounds (e.g. uncontrolled epilepsy in drivers or pilots). There will also be cases where a combination of conditions, poor symptom control, or a very specific safety role, will represent an unacceptable risk to health and safety. In most cases, however, it can be difficult to justify advising in a blanket way that a person cannot work on the grounds of diagnosis alone; each case must be weighed on its merits.

At common law employees are permitted to accept a higher risk to their health and safety if they are fully informed about that risk. In *Withers* v. *Perry Chain Co Ltd [1961] 1 WLR 1314*, Mrs Withers had dermatitis that was exacerbated by her work. Her employer tried her in various roles but all seemed to cause her some degree of dermatitis and she sued for damages. The Court of Appeal allowed the employer's appeal against this, arguing that:

> There is no duty at common law requiring an employer to dismiss an employee rather than retain him or her in employment and allowing him or her to earn wages, because there may be some risk.

Devlin LJ added:

> In my opinion there is no legal duty upon an employer to prevent an adult employee from doing work which he or she is willing to do. If there is a slight risk, as the judge has found, it is for the employee to weigh it against the desirability, or perhaps the necessity, of employment. It cannot be said than an employer is bound to dismiss an employee rather than allow her to run a small risk. The employee is free to decide for herself what risks she will run.

However as times changed and legislation was introduced, the courts took a different view. In *Coxall* v. *Goodyear Great Britain Ltd [2002] IRLR 742*, Mr Coxall had symptoms of asthma and was working as a paint sprayer. The OP recommended he should stop that work, but his employer failed to prevent him carrying on, and he subsequently developed occupational asthma and sued for damages. The employer cited *Withers* as a defence, but it was noted that the authority of *Withers* was 40 years old:

> ... and a lot has changed in the world of employment since 1961, not the least the COSHH regulations. Duties and obligations on employers are now much more stringent and it seems to me ... where a company doctor advises that an employee be moved, where a health and safety manager concurs with that suggestion and where the manager himself said that had he been aware of the advice he would have accepted that advice, failure to follow that advice ... does constitute a breach of the employer's duty.

The Court of Appeal in *Coxall* noted:

> The employer can only be reasonably expected to take steps which are likely to do some good. This is a matter on which the court is likely to require expert evidence. In many of these cases it will be very hard to know what would have done some let alone enough good. In some cases the only effective way of safeguarding the employee would be to dismiss or demote him. There may be no other work at the same level of pay which it is reasonable to expect the employer to offer him. In principle the law should not be saying to an employer that it is his duty to sack an employee who wants to go on working for him for the employee's own good.

The Court concluded that the *Withers* principle remained good law, but in some circumstances the employer's duty of care would overrule this where there was a 'very significant risk of being exposed to harm of a considerable magnitude'. In some circumstances, such as work-related stress, the risk to the health of the employee may possibly be greater if they lose their job than if they stay in work, with all its pressures. A difficult balance may need to be struck and the OP can be a helpful advisor in this situation.

Exemption certificates and 'disability clashes'

There may be cases where there is a 'disability clash'. For example, refusing to carry a disabled person in a taxi is unlawful, but if the taxi driver has a disability and cannot load a wheelchair into the vehicle, resolution is required. The answer in this case is an exemption certificate provided by the licensing authority.

Health practitioners may be asked to provide medical certificates but should not be required to provide exemption certificates, as this will require more than medical expertise. An appropriate balance must be struck between the two sides, which is a matter for the employer or licensing authority. The decision on what is proportionate is for the employer to take.

If an employer provides a minibus service for employees or members of the public it is likely that the duty to passengers would overrule the duty to make reasonable adjustments for the driver, so employing a driver who cannot assist passengers would not be reasonable if it meant that disabled passengers could not be carried.

Fitness standards

Certain occupations have standards of fitness for entry and continued employment which are laid down in statutes or regulations. Good physical and/or mental stamina may be an essential requirement and therefore people with certain disabilities may lawfully be denied employment. For example, airline pilots, air traffic controllers, police and the fire service and off-shore workers must undergo pre-employment and periodic fitness checks.

Old case law and standards have had to be revisited, however, and some of these fitness standards adapted to take account of disability discrimination provisions and issues of indirect discrimination.

Arguments of fitness in dismissal cases

In some cases employees have argued that their misconduct at work is caused or aggravated by their medical condition. Employers who discount such arguments without taking proper medical advice do so at their peril.

OPs should be prepared to give factual and impartial advice in such cases. Sometimes a medical condition can affect an employee's conduct at work or failure to attend work on time or at all, but not at others.

In *J* v. *DLA Piper LLP* cited earlier, J argued that her problems with lateness for work arose because she had difficulty sleeping and was on antidepressants and sleeping tablets which caused difficulty in waking. The EAT expressed concern at the respondent's expert psychiatrist statement that he was not aware 'of any mental illness which produces lateness as a specific symptom'.

The EAT stated that:

> We are bound to say that this comment has a snide tone which we hope was unintended. It appears from the material that depression can cause disturbance of sleep patterns, which may make it difficult for a patient to get up in the morning.

Similarly, in *The City of Edinburgh Council* v. *Dickson [200] UKEATS/0038/09/B1*, Mr Dickson had argued that his dismissal for viewing pornography on his work computer was unfair because he had hypoglycaemic attacks due to his poorly controlled diabetes which caused him to have no awareness of what he was doing. He provided his employer with literature which had references to the manifestations of hypoglycaemia as 'personality change, amnesia, cognitive impairment and automatism'. There was also an article about the phenomenon of 'hypoglycaemia unawareness' (in which a sufferer falls into a hypoglycaemic state without premonitory symptoms).

The employer ignored this literature and his arguments, and dismissed him. The dismissal was held to be unfair by both the ET and EAT because of the employer's failure to take expert medical advice about Mr Dickson's explanations.

Working abroad

Employees may be sent abroad to work on secondment or for longer periods of time. Careful attention has to be paid to remote deployment when employees have a medical condition or disability that may increase their risk of injury or ill-health. The employer's obligations to protect health and safety are greater in such cases, as there may be little or no supervision and working conditions may be more risky, with little or no access to sophisticated medical services.

For example, employees visiting certain parts of the world need vaccinations. Those using live viruses cannot be given to someone who is HIV positive. Careful and sensitive counselling of the individual and their employer will be needed, to safeguard the individual's confidentiality while protecting them from an employer's accusation that they are refusing to obey a lawful reasonable instruction to be vaccinated and travel.

Employers are advised to have up-to-date health and safety policies for employees working abroad with documentary evidence that those policies have been read by staff and any necessary vaccinations and medications administered. An individual risk assessment will be needed before sending an employee with a disability to work abroad. Further information on this appears in Appendix 5.

Policies

Finally, many employers have disability policies which set out their aims and goals and the measures that will be taken to assist staff with disabilities. There is a place within these policies for the role of occupational health practitioners to be spelt out.

Acknowledgement

This chapter contains Parliamentary information and public sector information licensed under the Open Government Licence v1.0.

References

1 Mummery LJ. *Clark* v. *TGC t/a Novacold* [1999] IRLR 318 CA p. 320.
2 Gooding C. *Disabling Laws, Enabling Acts*, p. 43. London: Pluto, 1994.
3 Equality and Human Rights Commission. *Equality Act 2010 Statutory Code of Practice: Employment.* London: The Stationery Office, 2011.
4 Office for Disability Issues. *Equality Act 2010 guidance: guidance on matters to be taken into account in determining questions relating to the definition of disability.* London: Department for Work and Pensions, 2010.
5 Williams AN. Are tribunals given appropriate and sufficient evidence for disability claims? *Occup Med* 2008; **58**: 35–40.
6 Grenden JF. The burden of recurrent depression: causes, consequences and future prospects. *J Clin Psychiatry* 2001; **62**(suppl 22): 5–9.
7 World Health Organization. *The ICD-10 classification of mental and behavioural disorders.* Geneva: WHO, 1993.
8 American Psychiatric Association. *Diagnostic and statistical manual of mental disorders, fourth edition (DSM-IV).* Washington, DC: American Psychiatric Association, 1994.
9 Acas. *The Equality Act – what's new for employers?* London: Acas, 2011.

Chapter 4

Support, rehabilitation, and interventions in restoring fitness for work

Mansel Aylward, Deborah A. Cohen, and †Philip E. Sawney

Introduction

Levels of disability and health-related work absence continue to increase and there is a pressing need to identify and address psychological and societal obstacles to recovery and a return to work. Moreover, the great majority of people in receipt of state incapacity benefits, and indeed very many patients who consult their general practitioners (GPs), report non-specific health complaints that have a high prevalence in the general population.[1,2] For these people sickness and incapacity for work are personal (psychological) and social problems rather than clearly medical ones.

Long-term sickness is a major problem in all industrialized countries. Paradoxically, despite improvements in healthcare and the population health in the UK,[3] people's sense of general health and well-being has not improved since the 1950s.[4] Indeed, we sometimes seem less able to cope with health problems and suffer more chronic disability than ever before. In the UK, the number of people on incapacity benefits increased from 700 000 in 1979 to 2.6 million in 1995.[5] Since then, it has plateaued, but has remained stubbornly high. An increasing proportion of state incapacity benefit is now related to 'common health problems' i.e. mild/moderate musculoskeletal and mental health conditions that consist mainly of symptoms rather than objective disease.[6] Ill health in people of working age is estimated to cost the UK £100 billion per annum.[7]

Addressing these trends depends on better understanding of sickness and disability.[8] 'Models'— which may be explicit or implicit—crystallize ideas and help to clarify thinking and communication with others, but they also channel and constrain our thinking. For example, if you consider that back pain is a sign of disease, you may seek medical investigation and treatment. If you think that it was caused by your work, you may stay off until it is better. But if you think that it is just your body's reaction to starting the sports season, you will deal with it very differently. So models matter: they determine not only how we think about our health, but also what we do about it and hence the ultimate outcome.

This shift from a traditional to a more flexible model of health and work and rehabilitation has now been accepted. Dame Carol Black in her 2008 report highlighted the need for a more proactive approach to rehabilitation.[7] The government response *Improving health and work: changing lives* (2008) recommended several initiatives to improve practice amongst GPs and other health professionals. One major outcome of the government's response was the introduction of the new Statement of Fitness for Work ('fit note'), introduced in April 2010.

The new note was designed to enable practitioners to have a more constructive conversation about work and health with their patients and consider what patients can do rather than what they cannot. The note also introduced changes to how the GP completed the statement.

Challenging conventional assumptions: health problems, sickness, and disability

The *sine qua non* of illness is that the individual has a health problem. Unfortunately, words such as 'ill', 'sick', and 'disabled' are often used as if they were interchangeable, which has caused confusion. Rational thinking depends on clear definitions and understanding of fundamental concepts.[9,10] The various concepts of ill health are summarized in Box 4.1.

These concepts are fundamental to defining entitlement and assessment of incapacity.[11] Diagnosis alone provides little information about incapacity for work.[8] Impairment is a bio-medical definition—it provides the most objective measure of a health condition, but does not give much information about the experience of the individual. Sickness and disability are social definitions, which focus on the individual's experience and functioning, and not just the health condition. 'Disability' is not synonymous with incapacity: about half of all 'disabled' people are working, including 25 per cent of those who say that their limitations are severe. Conversely, more than half those on incapacity benefits do not fit the traditional stereotype of 'disabled persons' and are better described as 'chronic sick' or prematurely retired. Indeed, the main problem today is with long-term sickness in people over the age of 50 years.[6] Most importantly, symptoms do not necessarily mean illness or incapacity for work. Symptoms, disability, and incapacity for work must therefore be distinguished—conceptually, in assessment, and as the basis for sick certification and incapacity benefits.

Many incapacity benefit recipients are not completely incapacitated but still retain some capacity for some work. Most benefit claimants have a genuine health condition, and many genuinely believe that they cannot or should not work. These beliefs are often reinforced by medical advice,[12,13] by employers who will not permit return to work until symptoms are 'cured',[14] and

Box 4.1 Concepts of ill health

- *Disease* is objective, medically diagnosed, pathology.
- *Impairment* is significant, demonstrable, deviation, or loss of body structure or function.
- *Symptoms* are bothersome bodily or mental sensations.
- *Illness* is the subjective feeling of being unwell.
- *Disability* is limitation of activities and restriction of participation.
- *Sickness* is a social status accorded to the ill person by society.
- *Incapacity* is inability to work because of sickness or disability.

Reproduced with permission from Gordon Waddell and Mansel Aylward, *Models of sickness and disability*, p. 3, Copyright © 2010 The Royal Society of Medicine Press, UK.

by the benefits system.[6] Virtually all claimants say that illness or disability affects their ability to work, and about three-quarters say that it is the main reason they are not working or seeking work. However, less than one-quarter say that they could not do any work at all. Ninety per cent of new incapacity benefit claimants initially expect to return to work eventually, and one-third to one-half of all recipients still want to work. All of these figures are based on the qualification of self-reporting.[15]

The relationship between work and health

Work forms a large part of most people's lives and allows full participation in our society, boosting confidence and self-esteem. The way we work has changed over the years. These days more women work outside the home, there is more shift work, and greater use of flexible hours. People may choose or need to work for longer. Jobs are no longer for life and during a working lifetime an individual is likely to do a variety of jobs and may work either full-time or part-time at different stages. In a broad sense, work need not necessarily be for financial gain: voluntary or charitable work brings many non-financial benefits of employment.

Just because someone has an illness, injury, or disability does not necessarily mean that they cannot work. There are many examples of people who work despite severe illness or disability. Work and health are intimately related. Health is not just a necessary condition for work, and work is not always a risk factor for health. There are more complex and positive interactions between individual health and the work environment. There is extensive evidence that work is generally good for health, and that the beneficial effects of work generally outweigh the risks of work and the harmful effects of worklessness.[7,16,17]

This reinforces economic, social, and moral arguments that work is an effective way to improve the well-being of individuals, their families, and their communities.

However, the pre-conditions are that: jobs are available; there is a realistic chance of obtaining work, preferably locally; allowance is made for age, gender, and (lack of) qualifications; and there are 'good' jobs from the perspective of promoting health and well-being.

The effects of unemployment and worklessness in terms of health are now recognized. Unemployment causes poor health and health inequalities, and this effect is still seen after adjustment for social class, poverty, age, and pre-existing morbidity. A person signed off-work sick for 6 months has only a 50 per cent chance of returning to work. By 1 year it is 25 per cent and by 2 years about 10 per cent. One study showed that after 6 months off work due to ill health the majority of people were suffering from depression, whatever the initial presenting problem. Most importantly regaining work may reverse these adverse health effects and re-entry into work leads to an improvement in health.[16] Worklessness and the problems it can bring is now recognized as important public health issues in the UK.[7,17]

While it is right to consider the health consequences of worklessness we also need to remember that despite comprehensive health and safety legislation, too many people are still injured or made ill as a result of their work. Unsafe working conditions may be a direct cause of illness and poor health; improvements in health and safety risk management could prevent much avoidable sickness and disability. This leads to a broader and more balanced view of the relationship between work and health. Safety will always be important, but a healthy working life is much more than this: it is 'one that continuously provides the opportunity, ability, support, and encouragement to work in ways and in an environment that allows workers to maintain and improve their health and well-being'[18]—a broader and more positive concept.[19]

There are, thus, implications for the provision of advice about work and for sick certification. Sick certification is a powerful therapeutic intervention, with potentially serious consequences if applied inappropriately, including in particular the slide into long-term incapacity.[12,13]

Common health problems

Workers' compensation and social security systems were originally designed for people with severe medical conditions and permanent impairment. These are still the stereotypes used in welfare debates. However, such conditions now account for less than a quarter of long-term sickness and their prevalence has been stable for many years.[6]

About two-thirds of long-term sickness absence, incapacity benefits, and ill health retirements are now due to common health problems—Table 4.1.[7,20,21]

Common health problems may be less severe in a medical sense, but that does not imply that they are minor or less important for those who experience them. These symptoms are very real, justify healthcare and may cause temporary limitations. Nevertheless, they are 'common health problems' in that they are similar in nature and sometimes even in degree to the bodily and mental symptoms experienced at times by most adults of working age.

When patients do seek healthcare for these symptoms, diagnosis is often non-specific—that is, the symptoms are not assignable to a particular cause, condition, or category. Such diagnoses are often nominal, they are simply labels, but the illusion that they are well understood can be misleading and cause iatrogenic harm.

These health problems are 'characterized more by symptoms and distress than by consistently demonstrable tissue abnormality'. They have been described as 'subjective health complaints'[24] or 'symptom-defined illness'.[25] They have also been described as 'medically unexplained symptoms' to emphasize the limited evidence of objective disease or impairment.[26] They usually are explicable in a clinical sense but only in terms of bodily or mental function and physiological disturbance, rather than disease or permanent impairment.[27] Comorbidity is common.[25] Between 60 per cent and 90 per cent of people with frequent back pain have other musculoskeletal pains. More than 50 per cent of people coming onto incapacity benefits have more than one long-term health problem, especially common mental health problems.[17]

Patients commonly seek and doctors regularly issue sick certificates for subjective health complaints. Family doctors and patients in the UK are well aware of these dilemmas and conflicting roles in the medical consultation.[28–30]

Table 4.1 Common health problems as causes of long-term sickness

	GP sick certificates[22]	Long-term sickness absence[23]	Incapacity benefits in payment	Ill health retirement
Mental health conditions	40%	Leading cause in non-manual workers	44%	20–50%
Musculoskeletal conditions	23%	Leading cause in manual workers	18%	15–50%
Cardiorespiratory conditions	10%	—	8%	c.10–15%

Reproduced with permission from Gordon Waddell and Mansel Aylward, *Models of sickness and disability*, p. 6, Copyright © 2010 The Royal Society of Medicine Press, UK.

Nevertheless, common health problems are insufficient *in themselves* to explain long-term incapacity:[20]

+ There is usually little objective evidence of disease or permanent impairment.
+ There is high prevalence in the general population.
+ Most acute episodes settle quickly—at least sufficiently to permit a return to most normal activities.
+ Most people with these conditions remain at work, and most of those who do take sickness absence return to work quickly.
+ Overall, only 3 per cent of episodes of sickness absence associated with common health problems go on to long-term incapacity.

These people have manageable health problems. Provided they are given proper advice and support, recovery is to be expected and *long-term incapacity is not inevitable*.

There is a conceptual distinction between these common subjective symptoms and objective disease or the severe medical conditions and permanent impairments for which sickness and disability benefit were originally defined.

Disability benefits and common health problems

Sissons et al.[21] examined the characteristics of Employment and Support Allowance (ESA) claimants in one-quarter of 2009 and explored their employment trajectories over 18 months. ESA claimants were slightly older than the general population of working age and were more likely to be male.

The prevalence of the two commonest health problems, musculoskeletal conditions (37 per cent) and mental health conditions (32 per cent), varied: mental health conditions were commoner among women and younger people whilst musculoskeletal conditions were commoner among men and older people. Multiple health problems and fluctuating conditions were reported by 66 per cent and 55 per cent respectively of the survey population. In those who were in work prior to claiming ESA, 72 per cent had a physical health condition dominated by musculoskeletal conditions; in 50 per cent the health condition was of recent origin and 27 per cent of conditions were attributed to work, mainly by men. In contrast, among those ESA claimants who were not working before their claim, mental health conditions (38 per cent) were most commonly reported and tended to be long-standing. Only a minority (11 per cent) considered their health condition to be work-related. Not unexpectedly, among those with non-work backgrounds 25 per cent had literacy difficulties and 28 per cent were in a disadvantaged group. Moreover the survey findings identified improvements or stability in health as pivotal to a return to work. Evidently, attitudes to work are important influences on return to work: encouraging people in the belief that work assists their health is more likely to achieve a successful return to work. Whilst health is a factor influencing return to work, other factors such as skills and qualifications, social disadvantage, beliefs in the benefits of working, and distance from the labour market are also important in explaining future employment trajectories.

Models of disability

Models are a practical approach to moving from theory to reality and a means of aiding understanding, research and management. There are strengths and limitations in adopting the traditional 'medical model'. Social models and the role of personal and psychological factors provide a better understanding of sickness and disability. They also impact on capacity for work and developing interventions aimed at facilitating return to optimal function and thus work. A *biopsychosocial model* of human illness that takes account of the person, their health problems and their social context has profound implications for healthcare, workplace management, and social policy.

The medical model

The medical model may be summarized as a mechanistic view of the body, in which illness is simply a fault in the machine that should be fixed.

This approach was originally, and is still primarily, a medical treatment model. Its focus on biological pathology and its treatment,[31] also leads it to be described as a *disease model* or *biomedical model*. Medical treatment is often regarded inappropriately as more or less synonymous with healthcare. This model has led to dramatic medical advances: it has worked well where it is possible to identify biological pathology for which there is effective treatment.[32] More generally, the medical model often leads to the assumption that all symptoms mean injury or disease, and that healthcare to 'cure' the symptoms is the (only) route to return to work.

The medical model underpinned modern workers' compensation and social security systems. Once treatment was complete, longer-term support would depend on the severity of permanent impairment, after allowance for rehabilitation and individual adaptation. The traditional occupational health paradigm viewed work as a potential hazard with the risk of occupational injury or disease.

Currently, the medical model remains deeply entrenched in the way that most people think about symptoms, disability, and healthcare. Common health problems are erroneously seen as medical problems that are a matter for healthcare, often caused by 'injury' and often work-related. Moreover symptoms are taken to imply incapacity, so sickness absence is considered necessary and justified until full recovery and complete relief of symptoms.

The weakness of the medical model is that it fails to take due account of the patient or their human qualities and subjective experiences.[33] The patient's accounts of illness are reduced to a set of simplistic symptoms and signs of disease.[34]

The problem is that focusing on disease and its *treatment* often leads to neglect of the person and the *management* of the health problem.

The social model of disability

Disability groups in the UK have rejected the medical model and proposed an alternative social model of disability.[35] It is argued that many of the restrictions experienced by disabled people do not lie in the individual's impairment but are imposed by the way society is organized for able-bodied living. Society fails to make due allowance and arrangements that would enable disabled people to fulfil their ability and potential.

The social model rests on the personal experience and views of disabled people and thereby has considerable social and political acceptance and reality.

The social model approach necessitates change in the work environment and thus in the attitudes and behaviour of employers, line managers, and other workers. Individuals may be empowered to adapt the work environment to meet their needs and other people also require education. The most powerful determinants of ill health are social gradients [36] and the linked problem of regional deprivation.[6]

The economic model

Financial benefits unquestionably affect illness behaviour. Work is fundamental to the family's socioeconomic situation, but in the circumstances brought by sickness or disability sick pay, social security and workers' compensation, benefits may assume greater importance.

Even more fundamentally, the economic model fails to recognize that some of the main drivers of sickness and disability are not financial but health-related and psychological.

Personal and psychological factors

None of the described models explain how people with similar health problems and healthcare behave so differently and in social or work contexts. They fail to allow adequately for personal and psychological factors.

Personal characteristics include gender, age, and genetic inheritance; family background and status; education, training, and skills; occupation and work history; and previous medical history. There may be little that can be done to modify these, at least in the short term, which reinforces the importance of development in early life.

Mental capital and mental well-being are critical to the healthy functioning of individuals, families, communities, and society.[37]

Psychologists study how people think and feel about their health condition, and how that affects their illness behaviour. There is extensive clinical evidence that psychological factors influence the course and outcome of human illness.[25,38,39] They are particularly important in chronic sickness and incapacity. Psychological factors influence when common bodily or mental symptoms become 'a health problem', and also influence sickness absence,[40] recovery, rehabilitation,[41] return to work,[42] and long-term incapacity.[6] Psychological factors colour all illness, including severe medical conditions, but are particularly important in common health problems: the more non-specific and subjective the health condition, the more important the role of personal and psychological factors.[43] Oversimplificating, capacity may be limited by a health condition but performance is limited by how the person thinks and feels about that health condition.[44]

Some of the most important psychological factors that influence sickness absence and return to work appear to be perceptions of health and its relationship to work. Although the focus is usually on the attitudes and beliefs of the individual, this is equally applicable to attitudes of health professionals and employers. These attitudes and beliefs reinforce behaviours (Box 4.2).

Box 4.2 Attitudes and beliefs about work and health

Individual perceptions

- Physical and mental demands of work.
- Low job satisfaction.
- Lack of social support at work (co-workers and employer).
- Attribution of health condition to work.
- Beliefs that work is harmful and that return to work will do further damage or be unsafe.
- Low expectations about return to work.

> **Box 4.2 Attitudes and beliefs about work and health** *(continued)*
>
> ## Organizational policy, process, and practice
>
> - Inappropriate medical information and advice about work; sick certification practice.
> - Lack of occupational health support.
> - Belief by employers that symptoms must be 'cured' before they can risk permitting return to work, for fear of re-injury and liability.
> - Lack of suitable policies/practice for sickness absence, return to work, modified work, etc.
> - Loss of contact and lack of communication between worker, employer, and health professionals.
>
> Reproduced with permission from Gordon Waddell and Mansel Aylward, *Models of sickness and disability*, p. 21, Copyright © 2010 The Royal Society of Medicine Press, UK.

For most people with common health problems, decisions about being unfit for work, taking sickness absence, or claiming benefits are conscious decisions, for which they must take responsibility.

The biopsychosocial model

Each of the earlier mentioned models reflects a particular perspective on sickness and disability: all have some validity, but each gives only a partial view of human illness. A complete model should include all of these perspectives.

From the time of Aristotle, the main determinants of health and sickness were considered to be lifestyle, healthy behaviour, and the social and physical environment, rather than biological status or healthcare. A public health perspective suggests that this is still true today.[45,46]

Engel[31] introduced the term 'biopsychosocial' and argued for a biopsychosocial model. The focus shifted from disease to illness, stressing that psychosocial factors influence the course of any illness and that healthcare must take account of the subjective experience of illness as well as objective biomedical data.

The contemporary biopsychosocial model

The biopsychosocial model can be defined as a model of human illness (rather than disease) that includes biological, psychological, and social dimensions, and the interactions between them:[15,18]

- Biological: illness originates from a health problem and always has a biological substrate in body or brain (whether or not a specific disease).
- Psychological: illness is by definition subjective and always has a personal/psychological dimension.
- Social: sickness and disability are social phenomenon, and illness is ultimately expressed in a social context.

Empirically, the biopsychosocial model is an interactive and individual-centred approach that considers the person, their health problem, *and* their social/occupational context.

The biopsychosocial model combines and balances the medical and social models, and introduces the personal/psychological dimension. It recognizes that some action must be at an individual level to deal with that person's health problem, but some must also be at a social level (as in the social model) to benefit all sick and disabled people (Table 4.2).

Table 4.2 Models of illness compared

Medical model	Biopsychosocial model	Social model
Sickness and disability are a direct consequence of impairment.	Sickness and disability originate from a health problem, but are also influenced by psychological and social factors, and the interactions between them.	Disabled people are disadvantaged by society's failure to accommodate everyone's abilities.
Sick and disabled people are pitied as the victims of personal tragedy.	Sick and disabled people suffer social disadvantage and exclusion, and society should make provision to accommodate them.	Disabled people are oppressed by current social and economic institutions.
Sickness and disability is best overcome through healthcare (and if necessary rehabilitation).		Disadvantage is best overcome by society removing social barriers.
Assumptions about work:		
Sick and disabled people can't work.	Sickness and disability are best overcome by an appropriate combination of healthcare, rehabilitation, personal effort and social/work adjustments.	Sick and disabled people are excluded from work.
	More could work if individual, psychosocial and system barriers were removed	

Reproduced with permission from Gordon Waddell and Mansel Aylward, *Models of sickness and disability*, p. 24, Copyright © 2010 The Royal Society of Medicine Press, UK, with data from Marilyn Howard, An Interactionist Perspective on Barriers and Bridges to Work for Disabled People, Institute for Public Policy Research, London, Copyright © 2003.

The factors that influence the process of disablement and recovery, and their relative importance, vary over time. Self-perceptions fluctuate, and individuals move between being disabled or not, and between working and varying degrees of incapacity.[47] Duration of sickness absence is fundamental to this process.[20]

The biopsychosocial model is not an aetiological model of disease, and arguments about whether the cause of a particular disease is biological or psychosocial obscure the main issue.[25] This model does not imply that psychosocial factors necessarily caused the underlying health problem. Overemphasis on psychosocial factors must not lead to neglect of the underlying health problem and its appropriate diagnosis and treatment.

Multiple interventions at several levels may be required. This is characteristic of many health and social policy interventions.

The major limitation of the biopsychosocial approach has been the lack of simple clinical tools to assess psychosocial issues and practical interventions to address them.[48,49] After more than 30 years, and despite agreement on the importance of psychosocial factors, there is relatively little empirical evidence for effective biopsychosocial interventions at an individual level. The challenge is to develop simple, practical, biopsychosocial tools for routine practice, and the evidence base that they are effective.

A biopsychosocial approach also demands a more egalitarian patient–doctor relationship. Patients want to be 'cured', but at the same time expect more human healthcare. This is not an impossible goal: it is a major part of modern medical training.[27]

The goal is to treat the person as well as their health condition: to strike the right balance between providing the most effective care and achieving the best social and occupational outcomes. Above all, patients need to be reassured that the biopsychosocial approach is an extension of standard healthcare and makes no assumptions about original causes.[25]

Workplace management

There is a strong business case for the effective management of health at work: simply, 'good health is good business'.[7,50–52]

Given the nature of common health problems, they cannot be left only to healthcare: they are equally matters of occupational management.[19,53,54] This moves the emphasis from traditional treatment (i.e. healthcare) to a more holistic approach of workers' health. As common health problems are an inevitable part of life, good workplace management is about preventing persistent and disabling consequences, which may include several overlapping strategies:[55]

+ Positive health at work strategies.

+ Early detection and treatment of mild to moderate symptoms.

+ Distinguishing temporary functional limitations from persistent or recurrent symptoms.

+ Interventions to minimize sickness absence and promote (early) return to (sustained) work.

Employers, unions, insurers, and government need to re-think workplace management of common health problems. The workplace, like healthcare, should tackle the entire health, personal, social, and occupational dimensions of health at work, identify barriers that prevent a return to work, and provide support to overcome them. Line managers play a key role in delivering this within the context of the employer's 'duty of care' to their employees.[56]

Sickness absence management, assisting return to work, and promoting rehabilitation are matters of good practice, good occupational management, and good business sense.[27,57,58]

Vocational rehabilitation

Concepts of rehabilitation

Vocational rehabilitation is *whatever helps someone with a health condition or disability to stay in, return to, or move into work*.[59] It is an idea and an approach, as much as an intervention or a service. Vocational rehabilitation is not a matter of healthcare alone: employers also have a key role.

The right balance must be struck between healthcare, the focus on work and all working together. That *is* a biopsychosocial approach.

The traditional approach to rehabilitation is a secondary intervention after medical treatment is complete but the patient is left with permanent impairment. It accepts that impairment is irremediable, and attempts to overcome, adapt, or compensate for it by developing to the maximum extent the patient's (residual) physical, mental, and social functioning. Where appropriate, patients may be helped to return to their previous or modified work. That approach remains valid for some severe medical conditions.

With common health problems, the approach to rehabilitation should be different. Recovery is generally to be expected, even if with some persisting or recurrent symptoms. Given the right opportunities, support, and encouragement, most people with these conditions have remaining capacity for some work. This reverses the question: it is no longer 'What makes some people develop long-term incapacity?', but rather 'Why do some people with common health problems not recover as expected?'.

Biopsychosocial factors aggravate and perpetuate sickness and disability; crucially, these factors can continue to act as obstacles to recovery and return to work. The logic of rehabilitation then shifts from dealing with residual impairment to *addressing the biopsychosocial obstacles that delay or prevent expected recovery and return to work.*[60]

The evidence for vocational rehabilitation

There is a strong evidence base for many aspects of vocational rehabilitation. There is also a good business case and more evidence on cost-benefits than for many health and social policy areas.[7]

The concept of early intervention is central: the longer anyone is off work, the greater are the obstacles to return to work and the more difficult vocational rehabilitation becomes. It is simpler, more effective, and cost-effective to prevent people going on to long-term sickness absence (Figure 4.1).

Return to work should be one of the key outcome measures for healthcare and workplace management. A stepped-care approach allocates finite resources most efficiently to meet individual needs.[61] This starts with simple, low-intensity, low-cost interventions that will be adequate for most sick or injured workers, and provides progressively more intensive and structured interventions for those who need additional help (Table 4.3).

Each stage involves a different set of expectations, behaviours, and social interactions. The outcome of any intervention may differ at different stages, so the timing of healthcare, rehabilitation, and social interventions is critical. The practical implication is that early intervention is generally simpler and more effective and cost-effective.

Given that vocational rehabilitation is about helping people with health problems stay at, return to, and remain in work, how can it be ensured that those of working age receive the help

Dimensions of disability	Obstacles to (return to) work	Corresponding rehabilitation intervention	Interactions Communication
Bio-	Health condition (+ health care) Capacity + activity level -v-job demands	Effective and timely health care Increasing activity levels & restoring function Modified work	
Psycho-	Personal / psychological factors Psychosocial aspects of work	Shift perceptions, attitudes & beliefs Change behaviour	
Social	Organisational + system obstacles Attitudes to health and disability Culture	Involvement of employer critical Social support Organisational policy, process & attitudes. Changing social attitudes	All players onside

Figure 4.1 Biopsychosocial obstacles to return to work with corresponding rehabilitation interventions. Reproduced with permission from Gordon Waddell G, Burton AK. *Concepts of rehabilitation for the management of common health problems.* London: The Stationery Office, 2004 © Crown Copyright 2004.

Table 4.3 Stages of sickness using low back pain as an example

Acute	Natural history benign and self-limiting.
0–4 weeks	Prognosis good, with or without healthcare.
(a health problem with social implications.)	90% of acute attacks settle within 6 weeks, at least sufficient to return to work, even if many people still have some persistent or recurrent symptoms.
	Minimize health care, avoid medicalization, avoid iatrogenic disability. Avoid 'labelling' and creating a 'culture' of disability and incapacity.
Subacute	Most people have returned to work, even if they still have some residual pain.
4–12 weeks	Those still off work now have significant risk of going on to chronic pain and incapacity.
	*Active interventions to control pain **and** improve activity levels are effective and cost-effective.*
	Window of opportunity for 'timely' health care, rehabilitation and administrative interventions.
Chronic	10% of patients account for 80% of healthcare use and 90% of social costs.
>12 weeks	Non-specific symptoms have now led to chronic incapacity.
(a disability problem with an underlying health problem)	Major impact on every aspect of their lives, their families, and their work.
	Poor prognosis and likelihood of return to work diminishes with time.
	Medical treatment and rehabilitation more difficult and lower success rate.
	Many people at this stage lose their jobs and attachment to the labour force. *Vocational rehabilitation becomes much more difficult.*

Reproduced with permission from Gordon Waddell and Mansel Aylward, *Models of sickness and disability*, p. 25, Copyright © 2010 The Royal Society of Medicine Press, UK, with data from Frank *et al.*, Disability resulting from occupational low back pain, Spine, Volume 21, Issue 24, pp. 2908–29, Copyright © 1996 and Krause and Ragland, Occupational disability due to low back pain: A new interdisciplinary classification based on a phase model of disability, Spine, Volume 19, Issue 9, pp. 1011–20, Copyright © 1994.

they need, when they need it? There are three broad types of clients, who are differentiated main-ly by duration out of work, and who have correspondingly different needs.[17] Each group requires a different management approach (Table 4.3). In the first 6 weeks or so, 90 per cent of people with common health problems can be helped to remain at or return to work by following a few basic management principles. Some 5–10 per cent of people with common health problems are still off work after about 6 weeks and need additional help to return to work, including timely identifica-tion, individual needs assessment, signposting to appropriate help, and interventions coordinated by a manager with assigned responsibility (Table 4.3). People who are out of work for more than about 6 months and on benefits need an intervention that can address the substantial personal and social barriers they face, including help with re-employment. In longer-term incapacity, the biological dimension and healthcare are only part, and often the lesser part, of the problem.

All successful rehabilitation programmes include some form of active exercise or graded activity component. The key element is activity per se, with the immediate goal of overcoming limitations and restoring activity levels: the ultimate goal is to increase participation and restore social functioning. These principles are equally applicable to mental health conditions, where increased physical activity has been shown to improve depression and general mental health.[17,62]

In principle, there should be steadily increasing increments of activity level, which are time-dependent rather than symptom-dependent. Properly implemented, a programme of increasing activity will increase a sense of well-being, confidence, and self-efficacy, which in turn will promote adherence.

Cognitive-behavioural and talking therapies

Attitudes, beliefs, and behaviour can aggravate and perpetuate symptoms and disability and addressing these issues is an essential part of management. This principle seems to apply generally across all rehabilitation for physical and mental symptoms, stress, distress, and disability.

Discussions about behaviour change with patients are integral to healthcare practice, e.g. smoking cessation, weight reduction, and diabetes management. Behaviour change methods are now also applied to managing rehabilitation and return to work. For GPs there are now specific training and e-learning programmes that address work and health and the management of the fitness for work consultation.[63]

Most psychological and behavioural approaches now combine *cognitive-behavioural* principles:[17]

- Cognitive approaches focus on changing how patients think about and deal with their symptoms; they teach patients to re-think their beliefs about their symptoms, and what they do about them, building confidence in their own abilities and skills.

- Behavioural approaches focus on changing patients' illness behaviour. they try to extinguish symptom-driven behaviours by withdrawal of reinforcements such as medication, sympathetic attention, rest, and release from duties and to encourage healthy behaviour by positive reinforcement.

- Cognitive-behavioural approaches try to address all psychological and behavioural aspects of the illness experience, in order to change beliefs, change behaviour, and improve functioning.

There is accumulating evidence for the applicability of the cognitive-behavioural approach across all the common health complaints.[64,65] For people experiencing common mental health problems at work brief (up to 8 weeks) individual therapy has been shown to be effective and cognitive-behavioural therapy (CBT) to be highly effective in retaining such people in the workplace.[66,67]

Engagement with therapies such as CBT is important. Ambivalence and motivation influence engagement. Understanding how motivation enhanced behaviour change within the alcohol and addiction field was the basis for the development of motivational interviewing (MI).[68] MI is now recognized as an important method for engagement and compliance across many areas of healthcare.[69]

Social and occupational interventions

Healthcare also has a key role in common health complaints but treatment by itself has little impact on work outcomes.[70] In fact healthcare interventions delivered in isolation can remove individuals from the workplace and act as a barrier to successful rehabilitation. (Employers also have a key role if rehabilitation is to be successful.)

There is strong evidence that a proactive approach from employers to attendance management that includes temporary provision of modified work and adjustments, are effective and cost-effective.[7] Modified work may take the form of temporary individual adaptations to reduce demand, or change to work organization, the primary goal being to facilitate a timely return to sustained regular work. A review of 29 empirical studies has demonstrated the success of modi-fied work as an intervention that halved the number of work days lost and the number of injured workers who went on to chronic disability.[42]

There is also strong evidence that for rehabilitation to be effective, both work-focused health-care *and* accommodating workplaces are required.[7]

Lower levels of organizational performance are associated with higher levels of sickness absence[71] and poor line manager support. The line manager can be thought of as 'the prism in which the organization is perceived'.[72] The line manager–employee relationship has a major impact on employee well-being[56] and therefore interventions must focus on both health profes-sionals and line managers if change is to be successful. Communication is an absolute prerequisite for a coordinated intervention.[73–75]

Training and organizational approaches that increased participation in decision-making and problem-solving, and improved communication have been found to be most effective at reducing work-related psychological ill health and sickness absence.[76]

Policies and procedures to improve line management have been developed.[56] However, the challenge required of line managers in undertaking the return to work conversation should not be underestimated. Being valued by the line manager and the organization are of great importance for employees and influences their attendance behaviours.

The 'fit note' introduced in April 2010 following Dame Carol Black's report (2008), provides a vehicle for communication with employers. It also tries to address an important misconception held by both healthcare workers and employers that an individual must be 100 per cent fit to return to work. This has been attempted by offering and option 'may be fit for work taking into account the following advice'. The note also allows doctors to recommend in the comments box that evaluation by occupational health specialists in complex cases should be sought.

A structured return-to-work programme provides a transparent pathway for employee and employer. It helps provide clarity, manage expectations, and integrate process with attendance management. Addressing psychosocial and inter-personal issues around return to work may be as important as modifying physical demands and should be central to any return-to-work pro-gramme. Such a programme should have the following features:

1 Communication between employee and employer soon after the onset of sickness absence.

2 Contact between the employee and line manager, continuing throughout the spell of absence.

3 The line manager should (with the employee's consent and where appropriate) inform co-workers of the absence and its likely duration.

4 The line manager should undertake a discussion with the employee on returning to work, to explore appropriate adjustments including modified work and psychosocial interventions.

5 Co-workers should be made fully aware of adjustments that are agreed (within the bounds of confidentiality and with the returning employees consent).

Educational interventions—the role of health services and healthcare professionals

Patients and some doctors fail to consider the likely implications of long-term certification. Fit notes, initially issued for acute illness or common health complaints, may then label people as sick and disabled, and thus unintentionally promote long-term incapacity. Many patients and doctors do not realize that a proportion of those who remain off work will lose their jobs and that a medi-cal certificate does not protect them.

GPs find certification and the work-related consultations challenging.[30] Many GPs also have strongly held beliefs that the management of certification, rehabilitation, and return to work lies outside their remit.

There is a pressing need to shift attitudes to health and work and in this context healthcare professionals should strongly challenge three incorrect assumptions:

♦ First, that work will be harmful—current evidence suggests that work is generally good for physical and mental health.[16,17]

♦ Second, that rest from work is part of treatment. On the contrary, modern approaches to clinical management stress the importance of continuing ordinary activities and early return to work as an essential ingredient of treatment.[7,17]

♦ Third, that patients should be 100 per cent fit before considering a return to work.

GPs as non-occupational health specialists nonetheless have a key role in relation to fitness for work advice. Most doctors who issue fit notes and advise about work and health have historically not been adequately trained in this area. For the majority of patients who return to work rapidly, this may not matter, but for those who receive repeated and long-term certification there is now compelling evidence that this may impact on their health and well-being.

Dame Carol Black's report (2008) led to the introduction of the new fit note and the development of a number of interventions to support a shift in attitude and improve training about health and work across all healthcare practitioners. For GPs this has included the National Education Programme for Health and Work, a collaborative project including a wide range of stakeholders. The programme has been now been evaluated and has shown to have increased GPs confidence in managing consultations about work and health. A review of the fit note 1 year on suggested that it has had some impact on the fitness for work consultation in general practice.[77] The Black report has also led to the development of e-learning modules for GPs and secondary care doctors, decision aids, as well as more easily accessible information, leaflets and guidance for all heath and work issues. These initiatives sit on a single website, Healthy Working UK (<http://www.healthyworking-uk.co.uk>), managed by the Royal College of General Practitioners. Other Royal Colleges and specialist societies have linked to this website prioritizing awareness of the importance of health and work in the patients they care for. Medical schools also have access to a wide range of resources to embed this training in their curricula via the Faculty of Occupational Medicine's website.

In November 2011 an independent review of the sickness absence system in Great Britain was published.[78] The review aimed to investigate sickness absence systems in the UK and understand the factors, which cause and prolong sickness absence. It investigated the impact of sickness absence on employers, the State and individuals. It recommended ways to improve the effectiveness of services and develop a more coherent service provision. The main recommendations included the funding of a new Independent Advisory Service (IAS), to be managed by approved health professionals and funded by Government. An IAS would provide an in-depth assessment of individuals' physical and/or mental function once they have been signed off work for a period of 4 weeks and would also be available to employers seeking advice about how an individual could be supported to return to work. The government response is still awaited at the time of writing.

'Pathways to Work' pilots

In studies, about three-quarters of those people in receipt of incapacity benefits say they would like to work.[17] Launched at the end of 2003 in UK pilot areas, the 'Pathways to Work' approach offered enhanced support to those who were in receipt of a state incapacity benefit including specialist personal advisers, a series of six work-focused interviews, and a £40 per week return to work credit and a 'Choices Package'. These voluntary components included a Condition Management Programme (CMP), delivered by the National Health Service, to help clients better manage their condition and to reduce the disability produced by chronic illness/injury. In 2006 the pilots were extended to cover the whole of Great Britain. This initiative doubled the number of benefit recipients re-entering work in some regions and was well received by the claimants and case managers.

Summary and conclusions

◆ Prolonged absence from normal activities, including work, is often detrimental to a person's mental, physical, and social well-being, whereas a timely return to appropriate work benefits the patient and his or her family by enhancing recovery and reducing disability.

◆ An approach to rehabilitation based upon a biopsychosocial model is necessary to identify and address the obstacles to recovery and barriers to return to work. It should also meet the needs of those with common health problems who do not recover in a timely fashion.

◆ Rehabilitation is dependent on labour market opportunities, and availability, as well as personal capabilities related to the physical and psychological demands of work.

◆ A patient's return to function and work as soon as possible after an illness or injury should be encouraged and supported by employers, health professionals, fellow employees, and rehabilitation service providers.

◆ A safe and timely return to work also preserves a skilled and stable workforce and reduces demands on health and social services.

Acknowledgements

This chapter is dedicated to our colleague and co-author Philip Sawney who sadly passed away after a long illness in September, 2012. We would like to acknowledge Gordon Waddell and Kim Burton whose concepts, work, and publications have been heavily drawn upon in preparing this chapter. We also thank Eleanor Higgins for administrative support. Text adapted with permission from Gordon Waddell and Mansel Aylward, *Models of sickness and disability*, Copyright © 2010 The Royal Society of Medicine Press, UK.

References

1 Wessely S. Mental health issues. In: Holland-Elliott K (ed), *What about the workers? Conference proceedings*, pp. 41–6. London: Royal Society of Medicine Press, 2004.

2 Aylward M. Needless unemployment: a public health crisis? In: Holland-Elliott K (ed), *What about the workers? Conference proceedings*, pp. 1–6. London: The Royal Society of Medicine Press, 2004.

3 Lopez AD, Mathers CD, Ezzati M, *et al.* Global and regional burden of disease and risk factors, 2001: systematic analysis of population health data. *Lancet* 2006; **367**: 1747–57.

4 Barsky AJ. The paradox of health. *New Engl J Med* 1988; **318**: 414–18.

5 Department of Health. *Choosing health: making healthier choices easier*. CM 6374. London: The Stationery Office, 2005.

6 Waddell G, Aylward M. *Scientific and conceptual basis of incapacity benefits*. London: The Stationery Office, 2005.

7 Black C. *Working for a healthier tomorrow: review of the health of Britain's working age population*, London: The Stationery Office, 2008.

8 Aylward M, Locascio JJ. Problems in the assessment of psychosomatic conditions in social security benefits and related commercial schemes. *J Psychosom Res* 1995; **39**: 755–65.

9 Boyd KM. Disease, illness, sickness, health, healing and wholeness: exploring some elusive concepts. *Med Humanit* 2000; **26**: 9–17.

10 Hofmann B. On the triad disease, illness and sickness. *J Med Philosophy* 2002; **27**: 651–73.

11 Aylward M, Sawney P. Disability assessment medicine. *BMJ* 1999; **318**: 2–3.

12 Anema JR, van der Giezen AM, Buijs PC, *et al*. Ineffective disability management by doctors is an obstacle for return-to-work: a cohort study on low back pain patients sicklisted for 3–4 months. *Occup Environ Med* 2002; **59**: 729–33.

13 Sawney P. Current issues in fitness for work certification. *Br J Gen Pract* 2002; **52**: 217–22.

14 James P, Cunningham I, Dibben P. Absence management and the issues of job retention and return to work. *Hum Res Manage J* 2002; **12**: 82–94.

15 Aylward M, Sawney P. Support and rehabilitation (restoring fitness for work). In: Palmer K, Brown I, Cox R (eds), *Fitness for work*, pp. 69–90. Oxford: Oxford University Press, 2006.

16 Waddell G, Burton AK. *Is work good for your health and well-being?* London: The Stationery Office, 2006.

17 Waddell G, Aylward M. *Models of sickness and disability: applied to common health problems*. London, Royal Society of Medicine Press, 2010.

18 Scottish Executive. *Healthy working lives: a plan for action*. Edinburgh: Scottish Executive, 2004. (<www.scotland.gov.uk/Resource/Doc/924/0034156.pdf>)

19 Lunt J, Fox D, Bowen J, *et al*. *Applying the biopsychosocial approach to managing risks of contemporary occupational health conditions: scoping review*. WPS/07/08. Buxton: Health & Safety Laboratory, 2007.

20 Waddell G, Burton AK. *Concepts of rehabilitation for the management of common health problems*. London: The Stationery Office, 2004.

21 Sissons P, Barnes H, Stevens H. *Research report: routes onto employment and support allowance*. London: DWP Research Report, 2011.

22 Shiels C, Gabbay MB, Ford FM. Patient factors associated with duration of certified sickness absence and transition to long-term incapacity. *Br J Gen Pract* 2004; **54**: 86–91.

23 Chartered Institute of Personnel and Development. *Absence management: annual survey report 2007*. London: Chartered Institute of Personnel and Development, 2007. (<http://www.cipd.co.uk>)

24 Ursin H. Sensitization, somatization, and subjective health complaints: a review. *Int J Behav Med* 1997; 4:105–16.

25 White P. *Biopsychosocial medicine: an integrated approach to understanding illness*. Oxford: Oxford University Press, 2005.

26 Page LA, Wessely S. Medically unexplained symptoms: exacerbating factors in the doctor-patient encounter. *J Royal Soc Med* 2003; **96**: 223–7.

27 Buck R, Barnes MC, Cohen D, *et al*. Common health problems, yellow flags and functioning in a community setting. *J Occup Rehab* 2010; **20**: 235–46.

28 Chew CA, May CR. The benefits of back pain. *Fam Pract* 1997; **14**: 461–5.

29 Cohen DA. *Inside the fitness for work consultation*. MD thesis, 2008.

30 Money A, Hussey L, Thorley K, *et al*. Work-related sickness absence negotiations: GPs' qualitative perspectives. *Br J Gen Pract* 2010; **60**: 721–8.

31 Virchow R. *Die cellular Pathologie in ihrer Begrundurg auf physiologische und pathologische*. Berlin: A Hirschwald, 1858.

32 Schultz IZ, Crook J, Fraser K, *et al*. Models of diagnosis and rehabilitation in musculoskeletal pain-related occupational disability. *J Occup Rehab* 2000; **10**: 271–93.

33 Engel GL. The clinical application of the biopsychosocial model. *Am J Psychiatry* 1980; **137**: 535–805.

34 Wade DT, Halligan PW. Do biomedical models of illness make for good healthcare systems? *BMJ* 2004; **329**: 1398–401.

35 Finkelstein V. *Attitudes and disabled people*. Geneva: World Rehabilitation Fund, 1980.

36 Marmot M. *Status syndrome*. London: Bloomsbury, 2004.

37 Foresight. *Foresight mental capital and wellbeing project. Final project report*. London: The Government Office for Science, 2008.

38 Halligan P, Aylward M (eds). *The power of belief: psychosocial influences on illness, disability and medicine*. Oxford: Oxford University Press, 2006.

39 Main CJ. Burton AK. Economic and occupational influences on pain and disability. In: Main CJ, Spanswick CC (eds), *Pain management. An interdisciplinary approach*, pp. 63–87. Edinburgh: Churchill Livingstone, 2000.

40 Alexanderson K, Norlund A (eds). Sickness absence—causes, consequences, and physicians' sickness certification practice. A systematic literature review by the Swedish Council on Technology Assessment in Health Care. *Scand J Public Health Suppl* 2004; **63**: 1–263.

41 British Society of Rehabilitation Medicine. *Vocational rehabilitation. The way forward*. London: British Society of Rehabilitation Medicine, 2000.

42 Krause N, Frank JW, Dasinger LK, *et al*. Determinants of duration of disability and return to work after work-related injury and illness: challenges for future research. *Am J Ind Med* 2001; **40**: 464–84.

43 Wormgoor MEA, Indahl A, van Tulder MW, *et al*. Functioning description according to the ICF model in chronic back pain: disablement appears even more complex with decreasing symptom-specificity. *J Rehabil Med* 2006; **38**: 93–9.

44 Nordenfelt L. Action theory, disability and ICF. *Disabil Rehabil* 2003; **25**: 1075–9.

45 Aylward M. Beliefs: clinical and vocational interventions—tackling psychological and social determinants of illness and disability. In: Halligan PW, Aylward M (eds), *The power of belief*, pp. xxvii–xxxvii. Oxford: Oxford University Press, 2006.

46 Marmot M. *Fair society, healthy lives: the marmot review*. London: UCL: 2010. (<http://www.instituteof-healthequity.org/projects/fair-society-healthy-lives-the-marmot-review/fair-society-healthy-lives-full-report>)

47 Burchardt T. The dynamics of being disabled. *J Social Policy* 2000; **29**: 645–68.

48 Kendall NAS, Linton SJ, Main CJ. *Guide to assessing psychosocial yellow flags in acute low back pain: Risk factors for long-term disability and work loss*. Wellington: Accident Rehabilitation & Compensation Insurance Corporation of New Zealand and the National Health Committee, 1997.

49 Kendall NAS, Burton AK. *Tackling musculoskeletal problems: the psychosocial flags framework—a guide for clinic and workplace*. London: The Stationery Office, 2009.

50 Hanson MA, Burton AK, Kendall NAS, *et al. The costs and benefits of active case management and rehabilitation for musculoskeletal disorders*. HSE Research Report 493. London: HSE Books, 2006.

51 PriceWaterhouseCoopers. *Building the case for wellness*. London: PricewaterhouseCoopers LLP, 2008. (<http://www.workingforhealth.gov.uk/Carol-Blacks-Review).

52 Burton AK, Kendall NAS, Pearce BG, *et al. Management of upper limb disorders and the biopsychosocial model*. HSE Research Report 596. London: Health and Safety Executive, 2008.

53 Health and Safety Executive. *HSE workshop on health models*, Manchester, 20 September 2005.

54 Hill D, Lucy D, Tyers C, *et al. What works at work? Evidence review by Institute for Employment Studies on behalf of the cross-government Health Work and Wellbeing Executive*. Leeds: Corporate Document Services, 2007.

55 Shaw W, Hong Q, Pransky G, *et al*. A literature review describing the role of return-to-work coordinators in trial programs and interventions designed to prevent workplace disability. *J Occup Rehab* 2008; **18**: 2–15.

56 Pransky G, Shaw WS, Loisel P, *et al*. Development and validation of competencies for return to work coordinators. *J Occup Rehab* 2009; **20**: 41–8.

57 Health and Safety Executive. *Managing sickness absence and return to work—an employers' and managers' guide*. London: HSE, 2004.

58 Buck R, Barnes MC, Cohen D, *et al.* Common health problems, yellow flags and functioning in a community setting. *J Occup Rehabil* 2010; **20**(2): 235–46.

59 Trades Union Congress. *Consultation document on rehabilitation. Getting better at getting back.* London: TUC, 2000.

60 Burton AK, Main CJ. Obstacles to recovery from work-related musculoskeletal disorders. In Karwowski W(ed), *International encyclopaedia of ergonomics and human factors*, pp. 1542–4. London: Taylor & Francis, 2000.

61 Freud D. *Reducing dependency, increasing opportunity: options for the future of welfare to work.* Leeds: Corporate Document Services, 2007.

62 Crowther RE, Marshall M, Bond GR, *et al.* Helping people with severe mental illness to obtain work: systematic review. *BMJ* 2001; **322**: 204–9.

63 Chang D, Irving A. *Evaluation of the GP education pilot: health and work in general practice.* London: Department for Work and Pensions, 2008.

64 Vlaeyen JW, Linton SJ. Fear-avoidance and its consequences in chronic musculoskeletal pain: a state of the art. *Pain* 2000; **85**: 317–32.

65 Von Korff M. Fear and depression as remediable causes of disability in common medical conditions in primary care. In: White P(ed), *Biopsychosocial medicine*, pp. 117–32. Oxford: Oxford University Press, 2005.

66 British Occupational Health Research Foundation. *Workplace interventions for people with common mental health problems: evidence review and recommendations.* London: British Occupational Health Research Foundation, Sainsbury Centre, 2005.

67 Secretaries of State of the Department for Work and Pensions and the Department of Health. *Improving health and work: changing lives: the government's response to Dame Carol Black's review of the health of Britain's working-age population.* London: The Stationery Office, 2008.

68 Miller W, Rollnick S. *Motivational interviewing: preparing people to change*, 2nd edn. New York: Guilford Press, 2002.

69 Rollnick S, Mason P, Butler C. *Health behavior change: a guide for practitioners.* Edinburgh: Churchill Livingstone,1999.

70 Waddell G, Burton K, Kendall N. *Vocational rehabilitation. What works, for whom, and when?* London: Vocational Rehabilitation Task Group, 2009.

71 Ashby K, Mahdon M. *Why do employees come to work when ill? An investigation into sickness presence in the workplace.* London: AXA PPP healthcare, 2010.

72 Aylward M. What are the outcomes of low back pain and how do they relate? Boston MA: Boston International Forum Primary Care Research on Low Back Pain, Harvard School of Public Health, 2009.

73 Sawney P, Challenor J. Poor communication between health professionals is a barrier to rehabilitation. *Occup Med* 2003; **53**: 246–8.

74 Beaumont DG. The interaction between general practitioners and occupational health professionals in relation to rehabilitation for work: a Delphi study. *Occup Med* 2003; **53**: 249–53.

75 Cohen D, Aylward M, Rollnick S. Inside the fitness for work consultation: a qualitative study. *Occup Med* 2009; **59**: 347–52.

76 Michie S, Williams S. Reducing work related psychological ill health and sickness absence: a systematic literature review. *Occup Environ Med* 2003; **60**: 3–9.

77 Fylan B, Fylan F, Caveney L. *An evaluation of the statement of fitness for work: qualitative research with general practitioners.* London: DWP, 2011.

78 Black C, Frost, D. *Health at work—an independent review of sickness absence.* London: DWP, 2011.

Chapter 5

Ethics in occupational health

Paul Litchfield

Introduction

Ethics, or moral philosophy, is an attempt to define principles that govern how people should behave in society. Healthcare is practised within communities and must reflect the cultural and ethical values of society as a whole. Professional codes of ethics are not unique to healthcare, but from as early as the 5th century BC ethical behaviour has been acknowledged as a cornerstone of good medical practice. The relationship between a health professional and a patient is one where power lies predominantly with the health professional and the various biomedical ethical codes seek, among other things, to redress that balance. Underpinning all of biomedical ethics are four main principles or shared moral beliefs first articulated by Beauchamp and Childress in the 1970s:[1]

+ Respect for autonomy of the individual.

+ Non-malfeasance (do no harm).

+ Beneficence (do good).

+ Justice (fairness and equality).

In some situations the principles can be opposing and each health professional must decide on the right course of action in those circumstances and be accountable for their decision. Material is available to help deal with such dilemmas and in the UK both the General Medical Council (GMC)[2] and the British Medical Association (BMA)[3] produce comprehensive guidance. Cultural and societal differences can lead to varied views on what is ethically acceptable and global guidance issued by bodies such as the World Medical Association[4] is particularly useful as people become more mobile internationally.

The issues in occupational health (OH) may differ from those in other branches of healthcare but the same four principles apply. A therapeutic relationship is uncommon in OH and blanket use of the term 'patient' in describing ethical duties may therefore be unhelpful since it may lead healthcare professionals and/or those to whom they are rendering services to believe that ethical guidance does not apply to much of their work. Internationally the term 'worker' is used much more widely in ethical guidance and this is the terminology that will be used throughout this chapter, whether or not a therapeutic relationship exists.

In practice, the ethical challenges and reasoning that should be applied are essentially the same, whether the relationship is a therapeutic one or not, since the power predominantly lies with the OH professional. A worker is far more likely to divulge confidential information to a member of the OH team than to a lay person and management is far more likely to accept guidance on health matters from an OH professional than from someone without a healthcare qualification. OH practitioners enjoy the authority and the status of their core professions—they must therefore apply the same ethical principles as their peers in other specialties.

Ethical guidance in OH has tended to be produced at national level, by and for individual professional groups within the discipline.[5,6] This has its benefits but does not reflect well the multidisciplinary nature of most OH teams or the increasing globalization of the workforce. The International Commission on Occupational Health (ICOH) has produced a code of ethics[7] that applies to all OH professionals and which is particularly helpful for those with international responsibilities.

There is sometimes confusion between acting ethically and acting lawfully. They are not the same. Laws sometimes allow health professionals to opt out on ethical or moral grounds (e.g. termination of pregnancy). Where that is not the case practitioners should reflect carefully, consult with appropriate colleagues and follow their conscience in full knowledge of any potential consequences for themselves of breaking the law. Simple legal compliance does not guarantee ethical behaviour and acting ethically may be unlawful. The hallmark of a professional is taking responsibility for one's own actions and acting with probity—that may be difficult but the application of sound ethical analysis can ease the process.

Governance

The concept of good clinical governance is understood and accepted by healthcare professionals. However, governance is a much wider concept which applies to the exercise of authority to manage activity and allocate resources in any organizational context. The principles focus on activities being undertaken in a way that promotes engagement, transparency, openness, due process, accountability, and clear communication. Good governance should also provide a sound audit trail in the event of adverse consequences that require examination or investigation. It therefore applies to all aspects of OH practice, not only clinical activity but also the organizational aspects of health and the commercial elements of providing a service. Many organizations have developed their own corporate values and ethical codes which OH staff will be expected to follow and they should satisfy themselves that there is no conflict with their professional ethics. However, OH professionals have a further duty over and above their business colleagues to promote the health and well-being of workers. This advocacy role may particularly be required when work is undertaken in a context where general healthcare is suboptimal.

Professional standards

OH professionals have a personal responsibility to continuously improve their own standard of practice and to promote the transfer of knowledge to others. Practice should be based upon the best evidence available and OH professionals should contribute to the knowledge base by disseminating findings from their own practice. They should develop protocols based on current evidence and undertake clinical audit to facilitate continuous improvement. Audit should be kept separate from any performance management system so that there is clarity of purpose for both activities. Lifelong learning for oneself and staff for whom one has leadership or managerial responsibility should be encouraged and issues such as budgetary constraints or service delivery requirements should be managed so as not to compromise essential education, training, or revalidation. OH professionals should contribute to the information, instruction, and training of workers in relation to occupational hazards and more generally to both clinical and non-clinical members of the team. Those providing or procuring services should give consideration to how they can help ensure the maintenance of professional expertise for the future. The Faculty of Occupational Medicine has published guidance[8] which is specifically for occupational physicians but which has wider applicability.

Commercial occupational health

Much OH provision is delivered on a commercial basis and the pressures inherent in this type of professional market can lead to ethical difficulties. OH professionals must abide by sound principles of business and biomedical ethics in their dealings with their client organizations and each other in order to safeguard their own reputations and that of the discipline as a whole. Potential areas of difficulty include advertising, competence, competitive tendering, transfer of services, resourcing, and contractual terms.

OH providers may wish to advertise their services but many OH professionals are subject to constraints imposed by their professional bodies[9] limiting them to the provision of factual information about professional qualifications and services. OH professionals should only accept or perform work which they are competent to undertake and recognize areas where specific expert knowledge is required. The terminology used to describe OH staff should be consistent with the definitions applied by relevant professional bodies.[10-12] Services themselves should work to appropriate standards and be subject to quality accreditation, such as SEQOHS.[13] Competitive tendering exercises should be conducted with integrity, which implies not only honesty but also fair dealing and truthfulness. Competitors should not be denigrated in any way and great care should be taken not to damage their professional reputations.

Clients change providers and the abiding principle in transferring OH services should be to safeguard the health, safety, and welfare of the workers. Early consideration should be given to issues such as the transfer of equipment, hazard information, and OH records with the interests of the affected workers, rather than commercial considerations, having primacy. Resources should be suitable and sufficient to meet the agreed needs of the client and, in particular, appropriate access to accredited specialist expertise must be ensured. It is important for OH staff to be aware of contractual service specifications since they could include provisions that are lawful but unethical, such as inappropriate access to clinical records. Where doubt exists it is prudent to seek advice from representative bodies or medical defence organizations.

Protecting health and promoting well-being

The scope of OH has broadened over time from simply addressing health issues of the workforce to considering the impact of work, its inputs, and its outputs on society as a whole. In parallel, the focus on only physical and mental ill health has shifted to include well-being, which incorporates the positive dimension of health in which citizens can realize their potential, work fruitfully, and contribute to society.[14] While the focus on the health of the individual worker remains undiminished, the levers to effect improvements are increasingly recognized as being work organization and health behaviours in the workplace. As the boundaries between OH and public health are eroded, the ethical issues faced by OH professionals broaden and can become more complex in balancing the needs of the individual with those of wider society.

It is the ethical duty of occupational physicians to do no harm (non-malfeasance) and this is consistent with the risk management hierarchy applied by businesses and the health and safety community. However, occupational physicians also have a duty to do good (beneficence) which does not necessarily translate into traditional management practice. In consequence, occupational physicians may find themselves acting as advocates for management action for which there is no legal requirement and commenting on areas of company activity (e.g. organizational design) which have not traditionally been viewed as health related.

Organizational health

The culture of an organization and the way that it conducts its activities can have a profound effect upon the health of the workforce. Management style is an important determinant of mental health and competencies[15] have been developed to help organizations train managers better. Workload, control, and change can also affect health and the perception of justice in the way the organization behaves is increasingly seen as being critical.[16] Some OH practitioners still focus only on the narrower issues of hazardous exposures and individual capability, thereby potentially neglecting their wider duty to protect health and promote the well-being of people of working age. Only a few will be in a position to influence behaviour directly at an organizational level but all should flag the issues on an opportunistic basis and link them, where valid, to individual cases on which they are advising.

Health promotion

The increasing prevalence of non-communicable diseases, including mental health problems, is a global issue[17] and lifestyle is critical. Promoting behavioural change in the work environment is particularly effective in public health terms and delivers benefits not only to the individual worker and society but also to the employing organization.[18] OH professionals are well placed to promote health and well-being in this way and respect for the autonomy of the individual should be paramount. The evidence should be presented in a balanced way that helps workers make their own decisions. Participation should be voluntary and OH practitioners should oppose, even well meaning, compulsion. A clear distinction should be drawn between fitness programmes designed to improve operational capability (e.g. service personnel, firefighters), which may well rightly be compulsory and those with more general aspirations to improve health status which should not. OH staff should disassociate themselves from spurious health arguments that others may seek to use in discriminating against workers who engage in habits of which they disapprove.

Pre-employment assessment

The rationale for having any pre-employment health assessment process should be established before it is implemented and the system should be reviewed periodically to ensure that it remains fit for purpose. Criteria to justify such a scheme might include statutory requirements, significant safety risks to the individual, the safety of others, or a material risk to the business by virtue of a critical position held or the associated financial exposure. A number of organizations, including the BMA,[19] recommend engagement at the pre-placement stage with a light touch process asking selected candidates if they have a health problem or disability for which they might need assistance. OH practitioners should reflect on whether activity in this area, which can constitute profitable business, is driven by benefit to their clients and workers rather than to themselves.

The content of the pre-placement assessment should reflect the nature of the work to be undertaken. There is rarely likely to be any justification for standardized general assessments of health, whether by physical examination or by completion of a health questionnaire. Invading the privacy of individuals by requiring them to disclose sensitive personal information which is not relevant to the assessment process is unethical and may well infringe their human rights. In the UK it also contravenes the principles enshrined in the Data Protection Act[20] which require that information sought is 'adequate, relevant and not excessive in relation to the purpose' and that it is only used for the declared purpose. Some jobs have health standards and OH professionals setting these should ensure that they are based on capability, rather than specific medical conditions, and that they are underpinned by robust evidence. Where health standards exist, they should be transparent and made available to applicants at an early stage in the recruitment process so that they do not have unrealistic expectations of a job offer.

Hazard control

Where an individual is at risk because of a particular vulnerability to a hazard at work there is a balance to be struck between all four ethical principles. The clinician may have to weigh the autonomy of the worker to decide the acceptability of a risk to their own health or safety against the clinician's duty to do no harm. A paternalistic approach, whereby the clinician makes the decision for the worker, is not acceptable in modern times but neither is an abrogation of responsibility to the individual. OH practitioners should take time to help the worker come to an informed decision about the level of risk that they find acceptable and then make their own decision on how to act. Every effort should be made to achieve a consensual decision but if the clinician feels that the risk of harm to the individual is too high, regardless of the worker's willingness to accept it, they should follow their conscience and refuse to provide health clearance for the activity. Where the risk of harm includes others, the ethical analysis is the same but the balance is shifted from autonomy towards non-malfeasance. Where the harm relates to matters such as legal liability, for which the OH practitioner lacks competence and authority, the consent of the worker should be obtained to pass on appropriate information to the relevant decision-maker.

Immunization

Immunization against occupational biohazards is another aspect of hazard control. The ethical issues again are influenced by whether the programme is primarily for the protection of the individual worker or for the protection of others. An ethical complication of immunization, unlike most health assessments, is that the procedure itself may cause harm to the individual worker and it may not always convey the desired protection. Immunization is also invasive and failure to obtain consent is therefore not just unethical but, potentially, an assault. Occupational physicians should ensure that policies are clear about how workers who fail to develop the anticipated immunity following vaccination will be managed, and that individuals have been apprised of this information before entering the programme. Similarly the approach to dealing with workers who decline immunization should be determined and promulgated in advance of implementing a programme. Some immunizations, notably against influenza, are offered partly for the protection of workers and those they come into contact with, but mainly to try and mitigate the operational disruption of sickness absence. OH staff should understand the reasons behind such programmes and must not misrepresent the benefits to workers. It is unethical for OH professionals to be party to the coercion of workers to undergo immunization based on operational or business benefits.

Health screening

Well-person health screening may be offered by employers for a variety of reasons but, once accepted, it is an activity for the sole benefit of the individual worker. It must be differentiated from health surveillance which is an activity undertaken as part of a hazard control programme or to ensure continuing fitness to work where there are specific health criteria. Health screening programmes should be evidence based and, to be ethically acceptable, should satisfy established criteria such as those published by the UK National Screening Committee.[21] Screening is a voluntary activity and while occupational physicians may encourage and promote participation they must avoid being complicit in programmes that use compulsion. Arrangements must be in place for the follow-up of abnormal results including referral with consent to the worker's own medical practitioners. If aggregated results of workforce screening are used it is essential that data are anonymized and presented so that linkage to identifiable individuals is prevented.

Health surveillance

While health screening is voluntary, health surveillance is not and is usually a condition of employ-ment in a given role. The ethical issues in ongoing health surveillance include those considered at pre-placement but the impact on the worker of the OH practitioner's decision is usually greater. Denying someone an opportunity to work is a major decision but taking their livelihood away is even more significant. Decisions must be based on sound evidence which should be confirmed if there is material doubt. Professional judgement must be objective and must not be swayed unduly by emotion, but compassion should be shown in communicating adverse results to the worker. Matters requiring medical intervention should be referred on appropriately and agree-ment should be sought from the worker to communicate the employment outcome (but not the health issues) to the employer. If the worker refuses consent for the outcome to be communicated, the OH practitioner must consider whether a public interest disclosure is indicated or whether it will suffice to advise the employer that health surveillance could not be completed because of withdrawal of consent.

Drug and alcohol testing

Trust is at the heart of a good relationship and instituting programmes to test that workers are complying with instructions, especially when these relate to personal behaviour rather than work activities, indicates a lack of trust. Programmes should therefore only be introduced after careful consideration of the full implications for the way an organization wishes to engage with its work-force. Clarity of purpose for any drug and alcohol testing programmes is essential and acceptance is more likely for those introduced for safety critical tasks than those put in place to enhance cor-porate image. The consumption of alcohol is lawful in most countries and the pharmacokinetics are relatively predictable, which allows workplace rules to be straightforward. The illegal nature of many other recreational drugs, the potential for confusion with prescribed medication, the lack of easily demonstrable dose–effect relationships, and the persistence of some substances create practical problems as well as potential civil liberties and human rights issues. No programme should be introduced without a detailed policy that sets out the reasons for testing, the procedures to be followed, and the role of OH staff. This issue is the subject of detailed guidance produced by the Faculty of Occupational Medicine.[22] Many organizations employ specialist contractors to conduct testing programmes which avoids potential conflict of interest for OH staff and removes confusion among workers about the role of the service.

Genetic testing and monitoring

Neither genetic testing nor monitoring is yet well developed, but knowledge is increasing rapidly and tests are becoming more widely available. Employers might feel that they want genetic information about their workers for a number of reasons including the following:

◆ To protect the public where employees with a genetic condition could represent a serious danger to others.
◆ To identify a worker's susceptibility to the effects of particular toxic or carcinogenic agents in an occupational environment.

- To detect damage caused by a workplace exposure to an agent in advance of physiological effects or disease.
- To assess a job applicant's long-term health prospects.

There are isolated instances of testing being used to discriminate against job applicants. This may well run counter to Article 6 of the Universal Declaration of the Human Genome and Human Rights; more information is available from the UK Human Genetics Commission.[23]

Criteria for voluntary genetic testing in the workplace[24] have been developed and may be helpful in advising employers in this complex area.

Health and work

OH professionals are often engaged to provide an impartial opinion on a worker's functional capacity and adjustments to overcome obstacles to effective working. Opinions may also be the gate to financial benefits for the worker from pension schemes, insurers, etc. There are therefore multiple stakeholders to satisfy and practitioners must resist inappropriate pressures to sway their objective and evidence-based judgement. Balancing these multiple responsibilities according to ethical principles is consistent with the injunction to 'make the care of your patient your first concern'.[25] That does not mean taking the side of the worker regardless of the circumstances but rather ensuring that clinical issues are given primacy.

Supporting the sick worker

OH practitioners may engage with sick workers while they are still working, but often OH input is only sought once they have commenced a spell of sickness absence. Such referrals may be part of an absence management process and OH practitioners should ensure that their prime focus remains the individual worker and not absence levels. There is often an emphasis on the report of a consultation but OH professionals must not neglect the advice they can give to the sick worker nor underestimate the impact that they can have in influencing the health and well-being of the person they are seeing. Workers must be treated with courtesy and respect recognizing that an OH assessment may well be a new experience which can feel threatening or intimidating. Clinical concerns should be explored and followed up without undermining the worker's confidence in the treatment they are receiving from their own practitioners.

Recommending adjustments

OH professionals should use their training and experience to define temporary adjustments that will help workers' rehabilitation. Recommendations must make sense and be practicable for the worker and the employer. It is for the employer to determine whether it is reasonable to make a specific adjustment but the OH practitioner who recommends totally unrealistic measures is behaving neither responsibly nor ethically. Permanent adjustments and alternative duties are usually more difficult to accommodate in the workplace than temporary measures. OH professionals should give very careful consideration before issuing advice that may render an individual unemployable. Many workers have a naïve view of the power of OH professionals and think that guidance they give must be followed by employers. They may therefore welcome OH statements which they perceive as making their working lives easier without realizing the longer-term implications. Recommendations that offer a desirable benefit to the worker at the expense of costing them their job do not represent sound ethical judgement.

Termination of employment

OH practitioners rarely have direct involvement in the termination of workers' employment but they do often provide information critical to the process. A key element is prognosis for recovery of capacity or return to work and OH professionals have a duty to provide realistic estimates based on sound evidence. It is not unusual for workers faced with performance or discipline cases to take extended certificated sick leave. OH professionals may be asked to determine whether a worker is fit to attend investigation and resolution meetings. The key issues are whether the worker is capable of understanding the case against them and of replying to the charges, either in person or by instructing a representative. Proceedings are invariably distressing for the worker but a prolonged delay is likely to be more damaging to their health. This is an issue poorly understood by many workers, their representatives, and their own healthcare practitioners. The OH professional should try to explain to all concerned the concept of doing least harm and supplement the advice with practical guidance on the mitigation of distress.

Health-related pension benefits

OH input is often sought in relation to enhanced benefits payable for medical retirement and in some cases for injury awards. Ethical responsibilities in this area are complex because stakeholders include the pension scheme trustee as well as the worker and the employer. OH professionals must be particularly clear about where their responsibilities lie, both in their own minds and in the way that they communicate with others. Assessments may be made on the basis of a physical consultation or as a 'papers only' process and neither is inherently superior from an ethical standpoint. The foremost responsibility in these cases is to the pension scheme and justice therefore has primacy among the four ethical principles.

Information

Confidentiality and the associated issues of disclosure and consent constitute the main area of ethical difficulty within OH. Data must be collected, stored, and processed ethically as well as to comply with legal requirements and professional standards. Respect for autonomy requires that the worker is given appropriate information to inform decision-making in the release of information. OH professionals must ensure that workers' personal information is kept confidential and that any disclosure is both appropriate and normally only made with consent. The duty of confidentiality is not an absolute one and it may be broken if required by the law or on the grounds of public interest.

Collection of information

OH professionals generally obtain personal information about workers either by conducting a clinical assessment of them or by communicating with third parties. Clinical assessments may be carried out on a face-to-face basis or undertaken remotely using electronic communications. Whatever the medium for the interaction, the ethical requirements are that the OH professional must aim to ensure that the worker understands from the outset the purpose, nature, and process of the consultation and, as far as possible, the potential outcomes. OH professionals have a similar duty when obtaining reports from third parties to explain why, what, and how information is to be sought and then how it is to be used. In both cases the consent of the worker is mandatory from an ethical standpoint and essential in practical terms. The primary purpose of a clinical record is to facilitate the OH care of the worker and it should therefore be contemporaneous, accurate, balanced, readily retrievable, and accessible to others who may need to use it in future.

Storage

Clinical records must be kept secure to minimize the risk of unintended disclosure and the arrangements are equivalent whether data is recorded on paper or electronically. Filing cabinets must be lockable with a secure key system and databases must be password protected. Access rights must be defined with suitable training on ethical issues for system administrators. Responsibility for administrative and IT systems may be delegated but accountability for the security of the clinical information rests with the OH professional. Good office housekeeping should be enforced rigorously so that documents are not left unattended. If it is necessary to transfer records between sites a secure system should be established with particular care paid to mobile equipment like laptops and memory sticks. A file tracking system should be in place along with a process for informing subjects if their information is lost.

Retention and transfer of records

It is good practice not to keep information for longer than is necessary and in the UK this is enshrined as one of the Data Protection Principles[20] in the Data Protection Act. Some retention periods are set by law but in general it is left to data controllers to define what is reasonable and to justify their decision if questioned. OH professionals are rarely data controllers in this context and should therefore work with their organizations to input appropriate advice. The range of retention periods for OH records is wide and can vary from 3 years to 30 years after the worker leaves that employment; 8–10 years is a common timeframe. Records must be destroyed appropriately so that, as far as possible, disclosure cannot occur. Shredding is the normal practice for paper records and specialist IT advice should be sought on the destruction of electronic files since simple deletion or overwriting is not sufficient. If OH records are transferred between providers, the responsible OH professional in the outgoing service has a duty to ensure that transfer is to an appropriate person for the new provider. Seeking individual worker consent to transfer records is usually impractical but the workforce should be advised of the change and be given the opportunity to opt out of any transfer.

Disclosure

Disclosure relates to personal information which the OH professional has acquired either directly from the worker or from a third party with the worker's consent. If an OH professional is asked by an employer or pension scheme to give a view on papers which are already in their possession that simply represents an interpretation of data, not a disclosure. A disclosure would only become relevant if the OH practitioner accessed additional personal information from records, from extra reports, or from assessing the worker.

Disclosures should normally only be made with the consent of the worker concerned. Disclosure can be made without consent if required by law but it is only ethical (as opposed to lawful) if the OH practitioner believes the law to be just. Disclosure without consent can also be made where circumstances dictate that it is in the public interest but the onus is on the OH practitioner to demonstrate that it is justified. Before making a disclosure without consent the OH practitioner should make all reasonable efforts to obtain consent from the worker and should only act against their wishes after due consideration, which would normally include taking suitable advice.

In writing reports for employment purposes OH professionals should avoid disclosing unnecessary clinical detail. In general, the information required for employment purposes relates to functional capacity and workplace adjustments rather than specific medical information. There is, however, often a need to put the report into context with non-specific information about the nature of a health problem and complete avoidance of all medical issues can render a report so bland as to be meaningless.

Workers may ask for disclosure of their OH records and full disclosure should be made as speedily as practicable provided there is no perceived risk of harm to a third party. It should be noted that 'harm to a third party' does not include the risk of criticism of or malpractice litigation against OH staff or colleagues. People acting on behalf of a worker (e.g. solicitors, trade unions) may seek the disclosure of information but the consent of the individual should nevertheless be sought. The BMA and the Law Society have produced a standard form of consent, designed for use in England and Wales, for the disclosure of health records.[26]

Consent

Consent is a process whereby an individual agrees to a proposed action after having been provided with full information about it and understanding the consequences—it may be implied or express. Implied consent should only be relied upon in circumstances where it is obvious, routine and generally accepted. In most OH practice express consent is required and this should be documented contemporaneously in the worker's record. Consent is a continuous process which is only valid for the stipulated purpose and which can be withdrawn at any time. Some OH professionals provide treatment, including immunization, and comprehensive guidance on consent has been produced by bodies such as the UK GMC[27] but for most the issues arise in relation to the preparation and release of an OH report.

The overriding principle which OH staff should apply in producing reports on workers is one of 'no surprises'. The reason for a referral and the content of the assessment should be explained at the beginning of a consultation in a way that the worker understands and express consent to proceed should be obtained. The content of the report should be explained during the consultation and it is good practice for the OH practitioner to offer to show the worker a copy before sending it to the recipient. This latter element has been included in GMC guidance on disclosing information for insurance, employment, and similar purposes[28] since 2009. It is becoming common practice to copy all reports to workers as a routine in the interests of openness and transparency.

There can be practical difficulties associated with the advance release of reports and there may be unintended consequences if the worker then withdraws consent for release. Problems can be minimized by having clarity throughout the process, demonstrating integrity in behaviour and firmly resisting attempts to alter opinion. If a worker withdraws consent for the release of a report having had the opportunity to read it then the OH professional must accept that and advise the commissioning body of what has happened. The employer, or other body, must then act based on the information available to them and this may not be in the best interests of the worker. Where consent to release a report is withdrawn, a copy should be retained within the OH record, clearly marked that consent has been withdrawn and that it has not been and will not be released. The Faculty of Occupational Medicine has given consideration to some of the issues relating to this matter and has produced a set of 'frequently asked questions'.[29]

Social media

The use of social media is expanding rapidly at home and at work with the boundaries between the two sometimes blurred. Workers and occupational physicians may use networking sites to communicate with friends, colleagues, and customers as well as to seek information and to answer specific queries. OH practitioners should not be deterred from using this technology appropriately but should be aware of the potential dangers of mixing personal and professional activities.

Workers for whom one has a professional responsibility should not normally be accepted as 'friends' on social sites and privacy settings should be set conservatively. If professional discussion forums are used, care should be taken in relation to the release of information regarding individual cases and details that would allow the identity of a worker to be determined must not be given.

Covert surveillance

Increasing use is being made, particularly in benefit and personal injury cases, of covert recording. OH professionals should not be party to commissioning such evidence, since (by definition) it is obtained without consent. They should also be very wary of commenting on it as a substitute for a properly constituted assessment since they cannot determine the relevant background in an impartial way. If an OH practitioner does comment on surveillance material relating to a worker of whom they have no previous professional knowledge then there can be no disclosure and consent is not required. Consent would, however, be required if the OH professional is asked to comment on material concerning a worker whom they had previously assessed or obtained confidential reports upon, unless the request is simply to confirm the identity of the individual.

Working with others

Many OH professionals work in multidisciplinary teams which may be purely clinical or may include colleagues with a non-clinical background. The qualities and values that should be displayed with colleagues are set out in the Faculty of Occupational Medicine's publication *Good Occupational Medicine Practice*.[30]

Clinical and non-clinical teams

Sharing information within a clinical team for the benefit of a worker's health is invariably good practice but the 'need to know' principle should be applied and it should be clear to those accessing a service that this is the unit's way of working. OH staff should brief workers not just of the requirement for information sharing to support care provision but also for professional supervision and clinical audit. Sharing clinical information within a wider non-clinical team, without specific informed consent, is not acceptable ethically. Work organization is a major determinant of health and sharing appropriate information with non-clinical colleagues can not only generate substantial health benefits but failure to do so could constitute a culpable act of omission. Where information obtained in a clinical setting is shared for use by non-clinical colleagues it must be anonymized and presented as group data. Care should be taken to ensure that sample sizes are large enough and that other identifiers do not compromise confidentiality.

Other health professionals

It is likely to be beneficial to a worker for their primary care physician to be aware of work-related facts which may have a bearing on their health. OH staff should therefore obtain consent to share information in this way when appropriate but consent must not be assumed. Requests for information to a worker's own practitioners should be specific, relate only to the matter in hand, and explain the context of the enquiry. Blanket requests for a complete set of records can rarely be justified in occupational medicine practice. Written consent for the provision of a report must be obtained from the worker in advance of a request being made and should make it clear what information is being sought. In the UK, the Access to Medical Reports Act 1988[31] will normally apply. The same provisions apply to information sought or provided by telephone, email, or any other media.

Others in the workplace

Workers sometimes ask to have a friend or trade union representative accompany them to an OH consultation. Most OH professionals would normally agree but it is prudent to clarify the role of the representative, which is to provide support to their colleague rather than to act as a spokesperson. OH services are often funded by the employer which can jeopardize both the perception and the reality of impartiality. Some employers may not understand that impartiality is a fundamental tenet of ethical practice in OH; practitioners therefore need to highlight the issue and demonstrate by their behaviour that it is practised consistently.

Legal departments in organizations have no greater right of access to OH records than any other representative of the employer and worker consent is required before disclosure. Non-clinical managers of services should not normally require access to clinical records; if there are concerns about the ability to maintain appropriate privacy in a department managers may be asked to sign a confidentiality agreement. Similarly, auditors of an OH service (as opposed to those undertaking clinical audit) should not be given access to clinical records without the subjects' consent; the information required for a service audit should be obtained from other sources even if this is administratively less convenient for the auditor.

Others outside the workplace

Normal ethical principles should be applied to dealings with government officials and information obtained in confidence should normally only be disclosed with suitable consent. The number of agencies with powers to seize documents has increased significantly in recent years and legal advice should be sought if seizure is attempted. Any court order to release records must be complied with. OH professionals may become aware of information relating to adverse health effects arising from an organization's operations. In such circumstances a public interest disclosure may be considered and it would be prudent to take appropriate advice. It would be rare to make such a disclosure without having discussed matters fully with the organization concerned. Disclosure of this type may attract legal protection but may still result in adverse consequences for the 'whistle blower'. OH professionals may be approached by the media to comment on issues and it should be established in what capacity they are being asked to act. In general, information given should be limited to scientifically determined facts and evidence based opinions. On no account should the health of individuals be discussed. It is unusual to be offered any form of editorial control after comments are made and editing can distort messages. Clarity and simplicity in comment is therefore indicated.

Occupational health research

Research is central to the development of evidence-based practice in OH. The need to undertake research may be a training requirement or arise as part of professional practice, for example, investigating a cluster of disease or emerging occupational risk factors. There is increasing regulation and heightened societal expectation that research will respect the rights and privacy of the individual, even if there is potential for public benefit. Most funded research in OH is carried out through academic centres that should have established procedures and access to expertise in ethics but all OH professionals should have an understanding of the main issues that might arise.

A common area of difficulty for OH professionals is deciding whether the activity they wish to undertake constitutes research or not. Problems may arise in differentiating research from clinical audit and service evaluation since there can be considerable overlap. However, for the purposes of determining whether an activity is ethical these distinctions matter little. The main issue for most OH professionals is determining if there is the need for an *independent* ethical review of the work, generally by a research ethics committee. This will arise if there is a specific statutory requirement (e.g. under the UK Human Tissue Act) or if the governance arrangements of the controlling organization require independent ethical review. The majority of universities and the UK NHS require independent ethical review for research but not for audit and service evaluation. It is therefore essential to consider ethical issues from the outset in relation to all programmes. This is a precursor to deciding whether reference to a research ethics committee is warranted and independent review is not a substitute for reflective analysis.

The decision on whether it is ethical to embark on a particular study involves weighing the risk of potential harm to the research participant against the possible benefits to society. The four ethical principles form the basis of such an evaluation and these have been supplemented by various international codes and guidelines. Emanuel and colleagues have defined seven requirements that provide a systematic and coherent framework for determining whether clinical research is ethical[32] and these can form a useful template for potential researchers.

Those recruited to a research study must give free and informed consent. Issues can arise in a workplace setting in relation to whether participation is truly 'voluntary'. Coercion must not be used and attention should be paid to whether workers might feel that participation would affect their employment position. Similarly, misrepresentation of the societal importance of the research or the possible impact on workers' personal health status is unethical.

If it is proposed that routine OH records or personal exposure data might be used to generate anonymized information for research purposes, the OH professional must ensure that employees are informed prospectively. Effective communication is important not just at the point of recruitment into a study but throughout the research. In particular there should be a plan for communication of results as part of the study protocol. Where the research topic is sensitive and of interest to the public, there may be pressure from the media to disclose information when the full implications are not clear. In such cases it is particularly important to handle the timing of communication to workers in relation to the media release. In general, individual results from studies are not disclosed. However, the individual worker should have the right of access to their own results and procedures should be put in place to communicate those appropriately.

References

1 Beauchamp TL, Childress JF. *Principles of biomedical ethics*, 6th edn. New York: Oxford University Press, 2008.

2 General Medical Council. *List of ethical guidance*. [Online] (<http://www.gmc-uk.org/guidance/ethical_guidance.asp>)

3 British Medical Association. *Medical ethics*. [Online] (<http://www.bma.org.uk/ethics/index.jsp>)

4 World Medical Association. *International Code of Medical Ethics*, 2006. [Online] (<http://www.wma.net/en/30publications/10policies/c8/>)

5 Faculty of Occupational Medicine of the Royal College of Physicians. *Guidance on Ethics for Occupational Physicians*, 6th edn. London: Faculty of Occupational Medicine of the Royal College of Physicians, 2006.

6 Nursing & Midwifery Council. *The code: standards of conduct, performance and ethics for nurses and midwives*, 2008. [Online] (<http://www.nmc-uk.org/Publications/Standards/The-code/Introduction/>)

7 International Commission on Occupational Health. *International code of ethics for occupational health professionals*, 2002. [Online] (<http://www.icohweb.org/site_new/multimedia/core_documents/pdf/code_ethics_eng.pdf>)

8 Faculty of Occupational Medicine. *Good occupational medicine practice*, 2010. [Online] (<http://www.facoccmed.ac.uk/library/docs/p_gomp2010.pdf>)

9 General Medical Council. *Good medical practice: probity*, 2006. [Online] (<http://www.gmc-uk.org/guidance/good_medical_practice/probity_information_about_services.asp>)

10 Faculty of Occupational Medicine. *Qualifications and training in occupational medicine.* [Online] (<http://www.facoccmed.ac.uk/about/qualstra.jsp>)

11 Nursing and Midwifery Council. *Specialist community public health nursing.* [Online] (<http://www.nmc-uk.org/nurses-and-midwives/specialist-community-public-health-nursing/>)

12 British Psychological Society. *Becoming an occupational psychologist.* [Online] (<http://www.bps.org.uk/careers-education-training/how-become-psychologist/types-psychologists/becoming-occupational-psychol>)

13 Safe Effective Quality Occupational Health Service (SEQOHS). Occupational health standards for accreditation: <http://www.seqohs.org/>

14 World Health Organization. *Mental health: a state of wellbeing,* 2011. [Online] (<http://www.who.int/features/factfiles/mental_health/en/index.html>)

15 Health and Safety Executive. *Line manager competency tool,* 2009. [Online] (<http://www.hse.gov.uk/stress/mcit.htm>)

16 Kieselbach T, Triomphe TE, Armgarth E, *et al. Health in restructuring,* 2009. [Online] (<http://www.workinglives.org/londonmet/fms/MRSite/Research/wlri/WORKS/HIRES%20New%20engl%20FR%20FIN.pdf>)

17 World Health Organization. *Global status report on non-communicable diseases,* 2011. [Online] (<http://www.who.int/nmh/en/>)

18 World Economic Forum. Workplace Wellness Alliance: <http://www.weforum.org/issues/workplace-wellness-alliance>.

19 British Medical Association. *The occupational physician,* 2011. [Online] (<http://www.bma.org.uk/employmentandcontracts/3_occupational_medicine/occphybooklet.jsp>)

20 Data Protection Act. 1998, s. 1. Data protection principles. http://www.ico.gov.uk/for_organisations/data_protection/the_guide/the_principles.aspx

21 UK National Screening Committee. *Programme appraisal criteria,* 2012. [Online] (<http://www.screening.nhs.uk/criteria>)

22 Faculty of Occupational Medicine. *Guidance on alcohol and drug misuse in the workplace,* 2006. London: Faculty of Occupational Medicine.

23 Human Genetics Commission. *Genetics and employment.* [Online] (<http://www.hgc.gov.uk/Client/Content.asp?ContentId = 123>)

24 MacDonald C, Williams-Jones B. Ethics and genetics: susceptibility testing in the workplace. *J Business Ethics* 2002; **35**: 235–41. (<http://www.biotechethics.ca/wgt/index.html>)

25 General Medical Council. *Good medical practice: duties of a doctor.* [Online] (<http://www.gmc-uk.org/guidance/good_medical_practice/duties_of_a_doctor.asp>)

26 BMA and the Law Society. *Consent form for the release of health records,* 2011. [Online] (<http://www.bma.org.uk/ethics/health_records/bmalawsocform.jsp>)

27 General Medical Council. *Consent guidance: part 2: making decisions about investigations and treatment,* 2008. [Online] (<http://www.gmc-uk.org/guidance/ethical_guidance/consent_guidance_part2_making_decisions_about_investigations_and_treatment.asp>)

28 General Medical Council. *Confidentiality: disclosing information for insurance, employment and similar purposes,* 2009. [Online] (<http://www.gmc-uk.org/Confidentiality_disclosing_info_insurance_2009.pdf_27493823.pdf>)

29 Faculty of Occupational Medicine. *GMC guidance on confidentiality and occupational physicians FAQ,* 2010. [Online] (<http://www.facoccmed.ac.uk/library/docs/m_gmcconf_qa.pdf>)

30 Faculty of Occupational Medicine. *Good occupational medicine practice,* 2010. [Online] (<http://www.facoccmed.ac.uk/library/docs/p_gomp2010.pdf>)

31 Access to Medical Reports Act. 1988, c.28. (<http://www.legislation.gov.uk/ukpga/1988/28/contents>)

32 Emanuel EJ, Wendler D, Grady C. What makes clinical research ethical? *JAMA* 2000; **283**: 2701–11.

Chapter 6

Neurological disorders

Richard J. Hardie and Jon Poole

Introduction

This chapter deals mainly with common acute and chronic neurological problems, particularly as they affect employees and job applicants. The complications of occupational exposure to neurotoxins and putative neurotoxins will also be covered in so far as they relate to the fitness of an exposed employee to continue working.

In addition to a few well-known and common conditions, many uncommon but distinct neurological disorders may present at work or affect work capacity. Fitness for work in these disorders will be determined by the person's functional abilities, any comorbid illness, the efficacy or side effects of the treatment, and psychological and social factors, rather than by the precise diagnosis. This will also need to be put into the context of the job in question, as the basic requirements for a manual labouring job may be completely different from something more intellectually demanding. Indeed, even an apparently precise diagnostic label such as multiple sclerosis (MS) can encompass a complete spectrum of disability, from someone who is entirely asymptomatic to another who is totally incapacitated. Similarly, the job title 'production operative' may be applied to someone who is sedentary or who undertakes heavy manual handling.

Furthermore, reports by general practitioners, neurologists, or neurosurgeons may describe the symptoms, signs, and investigations in detail, but without analysing functional abilities. These colleagues may also fail to appreciate the workplace hazards, the responsibilities of the employer, or what scope exists for adaptations to the job or workplace.

Size of the problem

Neurological disorders are an important cause of disability in modern Western society.[1] Estimates from the Neurological Alliance, an umbrella organization of the main neurological charities in the UK, suggest that about 10 million of the UK population have a neurological condition that has a significant impact on their lives.[2] Most are able to manage their lives on a daily basis, but over 1 million of them, 2 per cent of the population, are disabled and are likely to be excluded from full-time employment. About one-quarter of those aged between 16 and 64 with a chronic disability have a neurological condition.

With the exception of malignant brain tumours and motor neurone disease, relatively long survival rates mean that prevalence and disability rates of neurological diseases tend to be greater than their incidence. Neurological conditions, including headache, account for about 5 per cent of sickness absence.[3]

Occupational causes of neurological impairment

The occupational physician is more often involved with job adaptation and rehabilitation of patients with neurological disabilities than with eliminating the few known occupational neurotoxins from the workplace; but he or she should be aware of possible work-related factors that may exacerbate a pre-existing neurological disorder. Potential occupational exposure to organic solvents or heavy metals, for example, needs to be carefully considered in an employee who has a neurobehavioural problem, a tremor, or a peripheral neuropathy.

Clinical assessment

This should include an assessment of the person's alertness and mental functioning, as well as their posture, balance, coordination and gait. Neurobehavioural disorders following head injury, stroke, encephalitis, or a neurotoxin may range from mild and transient effects that can only be detected by psychometric tests to severe and permanent impairment. Someone may be left with communication disabilities from dysarthria or dysphasia, a visual field defect, or more global cognitive problems of which they lack insight. Dysphasia can preclude employment that requires good verbal communication and dyspraxia may preclude work that requires good dexterity. Disturbance of spatial relationships may prevent the patient from driving, and the efficient integration of all cognitive functions is important for those with intellectually demanding jobs.

Disturbances of posture, balance, coordination, or gait are relatively easy to establish with appropriate clinical testing. Complaints of dizziness, light headedness, unsteadiness, or spatial disequilibrium should be distinguished from vertigo, which is a sensation of movement of the surroundings or of the patient. Parkinson's disease (PD) is a classic example of a movement disorder. Anti-Parkinsonian drug treatment may minimize work problems, but jobs that involve rapid or coordinated hand movements, good mobility, or fluent speech may still be difficult. Similarly, muscle spasticity associated with upper motor neurone disorders may prevent manual work, or even the ability to stand for long periods.

The consequences of neurological dysfunction may be different for manual and non-manual workers. Manual jobs require good muscle power, good coordination, and peripheral sensation, but a degree of impairment in intellectual function might be tolerable. Lifting or moving objects— particularly if repeated frequently—can be a problem for those with disorders of muscles, the neuromuscular junction, or peripheral nerves. If there is a radiculopathy, specific movements of the vertebral column may exacerbate symptoms or disability. By contrast, an employee with paraplegia or a hemiparesis may still be able to undertake a desk job, although commuting to work may be a bigger problem than doing the job itself.

The impact of prognosis and rehabilitation on work

The impact of neurological symptoms on work can be considered broadly in three stages. The first stage covers workers with no previous health or disability problems who develop a condition, whether or not it is work related, that has the potential to affect job performance in the future if their condition deteriorates. The second stage is reached when the condition affects job performance, for which adjustments can be made. At the third, performance and attendance at work are adversely affected, but no further reasonable adjustments can be made.

Some slowly progressive neurological conditions may move predictably through the three stages, but in others the clinical course may be unpredictably episodic, transient, or static. Such prognostic considerations are important to employment considerations. Although some diseases such as epilepsy (Chapter 8) have their own unique, statutory, medico-legal implications, with which the physician must be familiar, most disorders should be dealt with on an individual basis.

For example, the prognosis of MS is difficult to evaluate at the outset. The disease may never cause more than a transient episode of blurred vision or it may progress rapidly and inexorably to tetraplegia. Similarly, cerebrovascular disorders may range from a catastrophic intracerebral bleed to a transient ischaemic episode with full resolution. Most stroke patients recover at least partially, so it is important wherever possible to keep their original job open, albeit if necessary in a modified form. Such modifications may be temporary or permanent and will require periodic re-evaluation. Comorbid obstacles to returning to work such as depression or unhelpful beliefs or perceptions need to be identified and addressed. The occupational physician should be actively involved in matching the job to the disabled worker and in advising on appropriate rehabilitation interventions.

After an acute episode the neurologically impaired employee should not expect, or be expected, to have made a full recovery before work is resumed. The rehabilitation process will be enhanced if the patient can return initially to a modified or part-time job. The process of going to work and performing a job is an important outcome in itself, and ongoing rehabilitation will allow problems to be identified at an early stage. Therapy at the place of work can be of benefit to both employees and employers, but rarely occurs. Recruiting and training new employees can be expensive and it may be more cost-effective to rehabilitate a trained but disabled worker. Small changes in posture, the ergonomics at work, mobility or communication aids, or simple adjustments to workplace layout, can make a big difference to functional capacity.[4]

Similarly, those in whom slowly progressive disability is anticipated deserve careful planning to review their needs at intervals appropriate to the underlying pathology. Continuing at work may be a source of psychological strength to someone recently diagnosed with an incurable neurological disease, but both patient and employer must also be protected from unnecessary risk to health, performance, or productivity. The diagnosis of a neurodegenerative condition may be compatible with full-time working, but usually carries with it the inevitability of progression and, depending on the expected time course, premature retirement.

Specialist vocational rehabilitation services are available and the UK's Rehabilitation Council has drawn up rehabilitation standards.[5] Disability Employment Advisers at local Jobcentres and Access to Work teams have financial and practical resources to help disabled people back to work and to make adjustments to the workplace. The integration of occupational health services into mainstream National Health Service (NHS) provision has also been recommended as a way of supporting workers with health problems.[6]

How neurological illnesses may influence work

The disability that a patient suffers is dependent on the symptoms and signs that the disease produces and not the disease itself. Certain disorders, and particularly brain injuries caused by a variety of pathologies, can lead to loss of function anywhere in the nervous system. The following headings provide a checklist to ensure comprehensive consideration of the key potential clinical aspects of a given neurological disorder. The physician should identify those clinical features that may be present, and actively seek to exclude their presence or assess the extent of any impairment in order to evaluate the occupational implications. Often it is not possible with brain disease to decide how much of the employee's disability is physical and how much is psychological, and it may not always be helpful to attempt to separate them.

Higher cerebral functions

Many neurological diseases affect mental functions, but their influence on work depends very much on the job. A labourer, for example, can continue to work with a moderate or sometimes even a severe intellectual impairment, but an executive cannot. There are no guidelines that can be used universally and each case will need to be judged on its own merits.

Cognitive function and psychometrics

Possibly the most important consideration is the likelihood of a person with cerebral pathology suffering cognitive impairment that may render them unreliable or unsafe at work. In one community-based occupational survey, frequent or very frequent cognitive failures (e.g. problems of memory, attention, or action) and minor injuries were reported by about 10 per cent of workers, and work accidents requiring treatment by almost 6 per cent.[7] The extent to which these could be attributable to organic neurological disease is not known.

Detailed and objective psychometric evaluation may be necessary in the presence of some neurological disorders affecting the brain, depending on the person's responsibilities. For those with unskilled jobs, it may be sufficient for a line manager to be satisfied that an employee can understand and follow basic instructions satisfactorily. On the other hand, a person may require careful assessment to protect themselves from the risk of making errors and to protect their employer from claims of negligence. An important feature of some cerebral pathology, such as dementia, is lack of insight into one's own limitations, so it is imperative not to rely wholly on the patient's self-report.

The patient may already have undergone cognitive assessments, in which case the relevant reports should be obtained. It will be necessary to distinguish between results of screening tests, often administered by occupational therapists, and more definitive standardized neuro-psychological tests such as the Minnesota Multiphasic Personality Inventory used by clinical psychologists. In recent years symptom validity (effort) tests have been developed by neuropsychologists to evaluate the validity of reported psychological or cognitive symptoms such as memory loss. The best test to use will depend on the type of impairment being assessed, but the most popular in the UK are the Test of Memory Malingering and the Word Memory Test.[8]

The physician should consider the available data and when they were obtained in the light of the pathology, natural history, and trends in functional capacity. The relevance of the results should be considered in the light of the demands of the specific job under consideration.

The term 'ecological validity' has been coined to refer to the relevance of performance under formal test conditions to the patient's behaviour in 'the real world', which may of course be better or worse than expected from the tests. For example, a patient may perform well on specific tests of verbal memory in quiet conditions in an outpatient setting, but be incapable of taking telephone messages reliably in a noisy hectic office environment. Poor performance on tests thought to be sensitive to frontal lobe dysfunction may be irrelevant to someone's ability to return to undemanding work which they have been doing for many years, and scores worse than chance may be due to deception. It may often be better if practicable, to allow an employee the opportunity for a work trial under careful but unobtrusive observation and supervision. This may promote insight and lead to better acceptance of a negative decision, and precautionary safeguards can be formalized or dispensed with. Memory loss can seldom be improved pharmacologically, but it can arise or be made worse by drugs such as anticonvulsants or psychotropic medication, in which case reduction in medication may be beneficial.

Simple memory aids are universally used at home as well as in the workplace, from the basic written 'to do' list or note stuck in a prominent position, to sophisticated paper-based organizers, 'smart' mobile phones, and computer software. The demands of many jobs require such powers of cognitive processing that they would be beyond most average people without such aids. Paradoxically, their greatest limitation is in the person who loses their portable aid or just forgets to use it, which is by no means confined to those with organic neurological disease! Nevertheless, behavioural approaches can be beneficial for the cognitive rehabilitation of those with memory impairment.[9]

Behaviour and impulse control

Even when rigorous neuropsychological testing reveals no abnormality, a cerebral pathology can still give rise to disturbances of normal behaviour and impulse control with serious implications for employability. Sometimes these are obvious to lay colleagues and managers, particularly if they knew the employee before a traumatic brain injury or the onset of a neurological condition. Lack of attention to personal hygiene, appearance, and presentation at work may be a clue to the onset of frontal lobe dementia. Occasionally, and especially in MS, euphoria may limit an employee's work potential.

Other changes can be more subtle and unpredictable, with outbursts of offensive language, physical aggression, or sexually inappropriate behaviour towards colleagues or customers giving rise to serious concern and perhaps disciplinary action. Such neuro-behavioural changes can be associated with secondary problems that may be mistaken for the primary cause (e.g. marital breakdown, substance misuse), unless the connection is made by gathering information from a variety of sources with the necessary consent.

Disturbances of arousal and consciousness

Fixed deficits of alertness and attention are usually obvious, but certain conditions can give rise to variable deficits, particularly where sleep is disturbed. Epilepsy is dealt with in Chapter 8. Here the key occupational considerations are the risk of lapses in attention or awareness occurring at work, and the possible adverse effects of medication.

Sleep

We live in an increasingly sleep-fragmented society with up to 20 per cent of the population working outside the regular 08.00–17.00-hour day. Some major accidents have been related to sleep deprivation while the daily toll on the roads is such that lack of sleep is as much a contributor to injury as alcohol is—and the combination is particularly lethal.

Sleep disturbance is not uncommon in neurological conditions affecting cerebral function or associated with chronic pain or immobility, effects that can be magnified by stimulants and anti-Parkinsonian drugs. The use of drugs to treat insomnia is rising despite evidence of harm and little meaningful benefit, and the correlation of psychopathology with poor sleep satisfaction is strong. Accurate diagnosis of the causes of poor sleeping is seldom achieved and simple effective measures are often not tried first.[10]

Obstructive sleep apnoea (4 per cent men, 2 per cent women) is of increasing importance, given its neurocognitive and cardiovascular sequelae. It is associated with day-time fatigue, increased sickness absence, and accidents. Early treatment can also be justified on economic grounds.[11,12]

Shift work causes a disruption of circadian rhythms. Older employees tend to fare less well, but there is great variation between individuals. Night work may cause sleep deprivation but there are no neurological disorders that present an absolute contraindication to night or shift work. However, because sleep deprivation is epileptogenic, epilepsy is a relative contraindication. Prevention of jet lag is increasingly well understood and simple measures to reduce fatigue are available for those who travel as part of their work.[13]

Pain disorders

Certain neurological conditions may be entirely benign and yet associated with intense paroxysms of pain. Trigeminal neuralgia, for example, is characterized by lancinating facial pain that is difficult to treat. Post-herpetic neuralgia and migraine are other common pain disorders. Here the key occupational considerations are the risk of incapacitation occurring at work and the possible adverse effects of medication. Chronic regional pain syndrome (reflex sympathetic dystrophy) is frequently overdiagnosed in the presence of unexplained pain, but should normally be restricted to patients with localized allodynia, changes in skin colour or sweating, and, if prolonged, with muscular wasting.

Speech, language, and communication

Speech disorders, whether dysphasia, dysphonia, or dysarthria, can be helped by speech therapy, but it is rare for major improvement to occur without recovery of the underlying condition. Those who earn their living by talking will be most affected. It is often more effective to reduce the importance of speech in the job and to provide aids such as a word processor with text-to-speech software. A microphone and speech amplifier can be used if the voice is very weak, as can occur in laryngeal dystonia or functional dysphonia. Dysphasia can be associated with other language problems such as dyslexia, dysgraphia, and dyscalculia, and therefore in such cases the communication needs as a whole must be considered with a speech and language therapist.

Emotional state

Changes in mood state may occur with neurological disease. It is not uncommon to develop secondary depression if a condition is incurable, and progressive disability tends to be very frustrating. This can be helped by psychological support or antidepressant tablets, particularly those with stimulant rather than sedative properties, provided that unwanted effects on mental function can be avoided. Patients with PD are prone to depression and those with MS may exhibit euphoria and denial of their problems as part of a psychological defence mechanism; it may also be a sign of incipient cognitive failure with frontal lobe dysfunction.

Symptoms related to cranial nerves

Problems relating to the nerves of the eye and ear are considered in Chapters 9 and 10 respectively. Impaired olfaction from a neurological cause occurs most commonly after head injuries, although local rhinological conditions or heavy smoking and advancing age are more likely causes in the general working population. In occupations using noxious substances, an employee with impaired olfaction might be at greater risk of hazardous exposure. Few jobs specifically require a good sense of smell, but with anosmia there is usually a concomitant loss of taste. Cooks and professional tasters would therefore be handicapped by such impairment.

Lesions of the trigeminal nerve rarely influence work capacity, although the risk of corneal trauma should be considered when sensation is impaired. In contrast, the pain of trigeminal neuralgia, combined with the sedative effects of analgesia, can interfere with concentration at work.

Bell's palsy is a fairly common cause of acute painless unilateral weakness that involves the orbicularis oculi, frontalis and other facial muscles. There should be no sensory loss. It usually improves with time, but is disfiguring and can be embarrassing if the work involves talking to and meeting the public. The only danger is to the eye, when the cornea is at risk from drying and abrasion due to problems with lid closure and the tear mechanism. Fortunately eye closure nearly always recovers, even if the lower facial paralysis does not. Bell's palsy and other facial palsies should rarely be a cause of a long-term inability to work. Synkinesis and facial spasm, common features of partial recovery, can be effectively managed with botulinum toxin injections. Plastic surgery techniques such as weighting of the upper lid may improve eye closure and cosmesis too.

After either trigeminal or facial nerve deficits, corneal protection is important in employees working with machinery or in dusty atmospheres. They should be educated to report new findings such as eye pain, discharge, or change in vision. Wearing goggles or large protective glasses with side guards helps exclude draughts and dust. Lubricating drops can be applied regularly by day and a simple eye ointment used at night. Those occupations necessitating the wearing of face masks or breathing apparatus may require special assessment.

The lower cranial nerves principally control swallowing and articulation. The development of portable ventilators has enabled some people with high cervical cord injuries and paralysis of the respiratory muscles to return to work part-time with the appropriate safeguards.

Motor symptoms related to the trunk and limbs

Patients with problems related to their trunk and limbs often find it difficult to describe their symptoms. Often the word 'weakness' is used to describe incoordination and sensory symptoms and 'numbness' is used to express weakness when there is no sensory change. Careful clinical assessment is necessary.

Weakness can be due to many causes including lesions of the upper or lower motor neurones or neuromuscular junction, muscle disease (myopathy), or psychological mechanisms. These can usually be distinguished from one another clinically. The management of the different causes and their effects on work capability are different.

Upper motor neurone lesions, extrapyramidal disorders, and hypertonia

In acute upper motor neurone lesions, for example, after a stroke, difficulties can often be helped by rehabilitation. Physiotherapy aims to retrain movement patterns, posture and trunk control as the central nervous system (CNS) adapts, and hence function can be improved. Pure muscle strengthening exercises are usually contraindicated. Hypertonia in long-standing upper motor neurone lesions leads to poor posture and clumsiness of movement that often affects fine hand movements or gait. Spasticity is often present, and causes problems with pain, involuntary spasms, and contractures that may require specific treatment or workplace adjustments, such as with botulinum toxin, splinting or a keyboard guard.[4,14]

In PD and other Parkinsonian syndromes, increased tone and rigidity is associated with bradykinesia. It is the slowness of movements that is usually the greatest disability. For example, a patient may walk easily for long distances in the open but with great difficulty in a crowded workshop where frequent changes of direction may be needed. Fine motor skills can be considerably impaired and unfortunately are not easily helped by physiotherapy. Drug treatment is usually more rewarding.

Employers sometimes assume that a lighter or sedentary job will be easier to perform, but this is not always true as weakness may not be the problem. Instead the patient may need a job requiring less skilful movements: for example, assembling small components would be more difficult than a heavier but less precise activity. Safety to drive should also be considered.

Ataxia and incoordination

The effects of ataxia and incoordination can be similar to those of peripheral sensory loss, but the disability is likely to be worse because other sensory input, for example, vision, cannot be used in compensation. Unless the cause of the ataxia can be corrected, no amount of retraining will help. Loss of joint position sense is also very disabling and will make coordinated movements unsafe. In these circumstances, where practicable the workplace should be adapted.

Lower motor neurone lesions

With lower motor neurone diseases the situation is different. Unless there is very severe weakness and joint instability, the main difficulty is loss of power rather than decreased tone. In contrast to upper motor neurone lesions, physiotherapy should aim to strengthen the appropriate muscles. If there is complete paralysis of a muscle, other muscles may be strengthened and trick movements learnt. The long-term prognosis depends on the pathology. In acute Guillain–Barré syndrome full recovery can occur. In progressive diseases where treatment cannot halt the decline, excessive physiotherapy can lead to exhaustion and worsen symptoms but orthoses such as a wrist or foot drop splint may help localized sites of weakness.[4]

Disorders affecting the neuromuscular junctions

Disorders affecting the neuromuscular junctions, such as myasthenia gravis, are much less common than other neurological diseases. They are characterized by fatigability. Exercise makes the weakness worse and so muscle-strengthening exercises are inappropriate. The pattern of weakness is typically proximal and may also affect eye muscles causing ptosis and diplopia. Sedentary workers may have little or no difficulty apart from coping with stairs, low toilet seats and reaching files from high shelves, but manual workers will have most difficulty and will need adjustments.

Somatosensory impairments

The effects of somatosensory loss in the limbs can be more disabling than motor lesions. Humans rarely exert their maximum muscle power but all modalities of sensory input are often used to the full. It is difficult to compensate for even mild cutaneous sensory loss in the fingers caused by a neuropathy or cervical myelopathy, and no amount of therapy or retraining will restore normal function. Employees with sensory loss are likely to encounter difficulty with skilled movements of the hands or unsteadiness of gait, but may be helped by using a different type of pen or a word processor, or a walking stick.

Loss of spinothalamic pain and temperature sensation produces different problems. If light touch and position sense are preserved, the patient's skilled use of the hands and walking are unaffected but the normal protective response of withdrawing from dangerous stimuli may be impaired. Those with loss of pain sensation are at risk of thermal injury if they come into contact with particularly hot or cold materials at work and remain exposed without realizing. Similarly, ill-fitting footwear may not be appreciated, resulting in skin damage. These difficulties occur most frequently in diabetic patients or those with other chronic neuropathies.

In more severely disabled employees with paraplegia, loss of sensation in the buttocks and legs results in increased risk of pressure sores. Proper seating to prevent trauma, both in the wheelchair and at the workstation, is important. Occupational therapists specialize in prescribing posture aids, seating cushions, and appropriate chairs.

Loss of sphincter control

Poor sphincter control is a feature of many neurological diseases. A catheter with a drainage bag or intermittent self-catheterization may be necessary where there is urinary retention or incontinence, but some patients learn how to stimulate their bladder to empty by abdominal pressure or other means and thereby regain control of micturition. Neuropathic bowel dysfunction may result in extremes of faecal incontinence or chronic constipation, sometimes alternating unpredictably between the two. Laxatives help to overcome constipation but may be avoided because they are assumed to make incontinence more likely. One method is to use bulk softeners or laxatives and to aim for a regular bowel action at a conveniently planned time. This may rarely require an enema or digital rectal stimulation, but can usually be achieved with regular suppositories.

Fatigue

Fatigue is a vague and imprecise term, and a normal emotional and physiological consequence of work. Rather than weakness, which is the inability to activate muscle power, physical fatigue denotes the inability to sustain power output and so can theoretically be measured objectively. However, fatigue can also affect mental performance and be influenced by factors such as motivation, mood and arousal. It is also a subjective symptom that can be pleasant, but is usually regarded as unpleasant tiredness, weariness, or even exhaustion. Chronic fatigue syndrome is discussed later in this chapter.

Fatigue affects many people with neurological disorders, simply because mental and physical performance may already be impaired physiologically. For example, people recovering from simple concussion, let alone severe traumatic brain injuries, commonly complain of mental fatigue that is made worse by any form of sustained concentration. Those with corticospinal motor impairment from myelopathy or after stroke suffer from inefficient contraction of agonist and antagonist muscles and spasticity. PD, other involuntary movement disorders and cerebellar ataxia are all associated with greater energy demands, and of course myasthenia is characterized by objective muscle fatigability. However, it is MS that is most commonly associated with complaints of disabling fatigue, even in the absence of severe physical disability, either due to inefficient neurotransmission in the presence of demyelination, or to psychological factors.[15,16]

Simple measures may assist a neurological patient who is struggling to cope at work because of excessive fatigue. They may benefit from extra assistance at home with personal care that may be unduly time-consuming, or with mobility aids and transport. Sometimes gentle persuasion to accept provision of a wheelchair or motorized scooter can help someone previously determined to remain ambulant at all costs. Cardiovascular fitness can sometimes be improved with an appropriate exercise programme, and relative immobility is not an exclusion criterion because paraplegics can work out using a hand bicycle, for example. Flexible work practices should be considered, with reduced hours and increased rest periods. Relaxation techniques, sleep hygiene, and psychological interventions may also be beneficial.

Drug management

Patients with neurological disease are sometimes overmedicated, which can limit their capacity for work. As a general rule, any drug acting on the CNS will interfere with arousal, awareness, and cognitive function to some degree, particularly when given in higher doses. Therefore, it is important to review any medication and liaise with medical colleagues responsible for the clinical management about stopping non-essential treatment. Not infrequently, drugs are initiated by specialists in an acute setting, but not tapered off when the patient is discharged. Antiepileptic medication is a conspicuous example. The occupational health consultation prior to a return to work may be the ideal opportunity to rationalize medication. Analgesia requires particular care, as patients do not always appreciate the potential adverse effects as much as the benefits. The underlying cause of the pain must be treated, but skill is required in selecting the correct analgesia.[17] Working whilst taking an opiate such as morphine or tramadol should be avoided, or only permitted where safeguards are in place. Certain types of neuropathic pain may respond to particular therapies, such as carbamazepine. Hypnotics can be particularly helpful when taken at night for a few weeks to improve sleep, which itself may ameliorate pain. Tranquillizers should be used with caution during the daytime as drowsiness can make driving or other safety critical work dangerous and reduce efficiency at work.

Explicit advice must be given about dose frequency, because some patients tend to take too much, while others take inadequate pain relief. If the pain is continuous or regular then the therapy needs to be taken regularly. An employee who waits to take analgesia until breakthrough pain impedes their work has probably waited too long. On the other hand, medication overuse may be a significant factor perpetuating, for example, chronic headache.

Antispasticity medication with baclofen or tizanidine can relieve painful and disabling muscle spasms. The dose may have been carefully titrated against functionally relevant criteria, but not infrequently is increased simply because spasticity is still detectable on examination without taking into account possible adverse effects. These include increasing muscle weakness, which is actually the mechanism of action, and sedation that may interfere with work capacity.

Drug treatment is relatively straightforward in the early stages of PD, but special neurological expertise is required to manage longer-term complications of anti-Parkinsonian medication, such as fluctuations in motor response and drug-induced dyskinesia.

Although rare in absolute terms, immunosuppressive therapy is being used more frequently for certain neurological disorders. There is increasing evidence of its efficacy in some acquired neuropathies, as well as inflammatory myopathies and autoimmune conditions such as myasthenia and vasculitis. The occupational physician will need to be mindful of relevant potential side effects such as anaemia, leucopenia, skin changes, steroid-induced diabetes, myopathy, and osteoporosis in those who return to work on this treatment.

Driving

In the interests of road safety, those who suffer from a medical condition likely to cause a sudden disabling event at the wheel or who are unable to safely control their vehicle from any other cause, should not drive. Decisions on fitness to drive can be extremely difficult for patients with neurological conditions.[18] This is particularly true for Group 2 licences for which the regulations are stricter. The standards of medical fitness to drive and the role of the Driving and Vehicle Licensing Agency (DVLA) are discussed in Chapter 28, and the particular problems arising in relation to epilepsy are discussed in Chapter 8. With trauma or other pathology affecting the nervous system, the challenge is to determine whether the resulting neurological deficit itself or the future risk of an alteration to consciousness constitutes an unacceptable driving hazard.

The commonest conditions where licence holders should not drive include following any unprovoked seizure or unexplained blackout, and immediately after a craniotomy, severe traumatic brain injury, or acute stroke. Those with either static or progressive or relapsing neurological disorders likely to affect vehicle control because of impairment of coordination and muscle power may continue to drive providing medical assessment at a disabled drivers' assessment centre confirms that driving performance is not impaired. Doctors have a professional duty to advise patients of their statutory obligation to notify the DVLA of any medical condition that may affect their ability to drive safely.

Factors affecting neurological function
Temperature and humidity

Extremes of temperature or humidity may cause illness, but pre-existing neurological disease may also be adversely affected. At high ambient temperatures, the symptoms of MS worsen temporarily as core temperature rises because of slowing of nerve conduction through demyelinated plaques, but recover when the body is cooled. A similar adverse effect occurs with low ambient temperatures, which also slow peripheral nerve conduction and neuromuscular actions generally, posing a particular problem for those with neuropathic or myopathic disorders. Such patients should, wherever possible, avoid working where extremes of ambient temperature are likely to occur.

Little has been written about any clinical consequences of disordered sweating in neurological patients. Excessive facial sweating can occur with cluster headache and after incomplete lesions of the spinal cord, but this is unlikely to present practical problems. Of greater significance may possibly be those with widespread impaired sweating and hence problems of thermoregulation, because of damage to the spinal cord, autonomic pathways, or peripheral nerves. Patients with reflex sympathetic dystrophy may also experience localized areas of excessive sweating.

Light

Poor lighting at work is a particular problem for the visually impaired (Chapter 9). Both poorly lit and dazzlingly bright workplaces may cause headaches. It is thus important that the employee has optimum refractive correction. Photosensitive epilepsy is considered in Chapter 8. Flashing lights can also precipitate migraine. Some patients with dyslexia report sensitivity to bright lights, or the shimmering of black print on a white background, for which the term scotopic sensitivity syndrome has been used and coloured overlays recommended.[19]

Chemical factors

Naturally occurring or synthetic chemical agents in the environment, including the workplace, may sometimes cause changes in neurological structure or function. For example, Parkinsonism can be a feature of poisoning by carbon disulphide, carbon monoxide, and manganese. Chronic mercury exposure is classically associated with tremor, but may also cause cerebellar ataxia and peripheral neuropathy. Many potentially toxic agents can persist for many years in the body, especially those that are lipid soluble. More often non-occupational neurological disorders mimic neurotoxic syndromes such as encephalopathy, movement disorders, and peripheral neuropathy. Patients with a non-occupational neurological deficit may also have their symptoms exacerbated by workplace exposure, or attribute symptoms to their work and seek confirmation or reassurance about their exposures.

Furthermore, there have been several health scares concerning putative neurotoxins, such as aluminium sulphate in drinking water or pesticide crop sprays in air, where numerous factors confound the interpretation of hard facts and fuel considerable controversy. There are some validated biomarkers such as red blood cell acetyl cholinesterase for organophosphates, blood lead, ZPP or ALA-d for inorganic lead, blood atomic absorption spectroscopy for heavy metals, urinary lead for organic lead poisoning, or urinary metabolites for solvent exposure. However, many of the declared symptoms from poisoning need careful evaluation with neurophysiological or psychometric tests. In the meantime adequate protection with personal protective equipment is important whilst, for example, sheep dipping, and crop or solvent spraying. More specialist texts on neurotoxicology are available.[20,21]

Toxic neuropathies

Peripheral neuropathies induced by inorganic lead compounds and the organic solvents n-hexane and methyl-n-butyl-ketone have been well described and predominantly affect motor nerves, but mercury and polychlorinated biphenyls cause a predominantly sensory neuropathy. Regeneration usually follows slowly and uneventfully provided exposure is halted in affected employees. It would be inadvisable for any employee with a pre-existing neuropathy of any aetiology to be exposed knowingly to such an additional hazard, regardless of the standard safety precautions in the workplace.

Heavy metal toxicity and organic solvents

An acute encephalopathy associated with exposure to aluminium was first described in smelter workers. It was known as 'pot room palsy', and characterized by incoordination, poor memory, and impaired abstract reasoning.[20] Permanent neuropsychological impairment has been reported following occupational exposure to high doses of metals such as mercury, arsenic, zinc, and manganese, either by inhalation or after accidental ingestion.

More controversial is whether low-level chronic exposures to metals, either in the workplace or the environment, could be responsible for cognitive dysfunction and dementia. The literature includes various papers assessing neuropsychological function in workers at risk. In some studies, researchers have assessed subclinical endpoints, such as workers having non-specific symptoms or no symptoms. It remains uncertain whether continued occupational exposure may lead to clinical and irreversible problems.[22]

This is also true of organic solvents that are widely used in manufacturing industry, dry-cleaning, degreasing, and paint production and application. The acute effects of organic solvents range from mild fatigue to frank psychosis. The weight of evidence suggests that chronic exposure to hydrocarbon solvents at current limits does not appear to cause adverse neurobehavioural effects. Nevertheless, there is still controversy over the severity of effects that can arise from workplace exposure. Psychosis, dementia, and compensatable disability appear to be more frequent in Scandinavian studies, but less severe effects have been described in other Western countries.[23,24]

Organophosphate pesticides and sheep dips

Well-established acute toxic effects of organophosphate pesticides and sheep dips arise from their capacity to inhibit acetyl cholinesterase in the central and autonomic nervous systems and at the neuromuscular junction.[20] An acute cholinergic crisis, muscle weakness, or a polyneuropathy have been seen, most commonly in agricultural workers in developing countries, after excessive exposure that should not occur if the substances are used with appropriate personal protective equipment. A more controversial possibility is that organophosphates might cause long-term illness even when there has been no obvious acute toxicity. In particular, a syndrome of chronic organophosphate-induced neuropsychiatric disorder has been proposed, including personality changes, impulsive suicidal thoughts, and cognitive impairment.[25]

The Committee on Toxicity concluded in 1999 that subtle and probably clinically insignificant neuropsychological abnormalities probably could occur as a long-term complication of acute organophosphate poisoning, especially if the poisoning was severe.[26] The balance of evidence did not support the occurrence of a peripheral neuropathy from organophosphates following non-severe exposure and neither were they thought to be a major factor in the excess mortality from suicide that had been demonstrated in British farmers. However a recent large longitudinal study of vineyard workers in France has shown impaired cognitive performance in subjects chronically exposed to pesticides.[27]

Identification and prevention of occupational neurotoxicity

A detailed occupational and environmental history is advisable when assessing the potential for chemical exposures to cause or aggravate a neurological condition. This should cover the employee's tasks, use of personal protective equipment and contact with specific chemicals. Specific enquiries should be made and if possible documents, such as risk assessments, safety data sheets and environmental measurements inspected.

Questions about the use of specific natural remedies, recreational drug use, and routine household products as well the source of residential water supply are also important. Obtaining exposure data and estimating the likely dose and duration is part of a risk assessment. A comparison of this dose and duration with available literature from individual, group, or animal data published by regulatory agencies is an important next step. Working with a professional toxicologist or industrial scientist is recommended when managing such a patient.

Preventive procedures may be applied to the chemical process, the workplace, or to the individual worker. Effective engineering controls and devices have included ventilation systems, ergonomic changes, safer tools, and the isolation of areas for dangerous exposures. Education and advice about work hazards and the provision of personal protective equipment may not always reduce accidents and exposures as these garments may not fit properly, or be uncomfortable to wear, and poor compliance may limit protection. Pre-placement medical examinations can identify those with relevant medical risk factors (e.g. diabetics with neuropathy), and reduce their exposure by reassigning work. Health surveillance is also important and should aim to identify early adverse health effects and biological effect markers such as persistently low levels of acetyl cholinesterase.

Assistive technology

With environmental control systems, it is often possible to set up a workstation that will allow the disabled employee to use a word processor or a telephone, and even initiate simple mechanical tasks. An environmental control system is a computer with links to peripheral equipment, such as doors, telephones, and light switches. The patient can control the equipment from a keyboard, hand-held remote infrared controller, or more sophisticated switching devices that, although slower, can be operated by small movements of the limbs, head, lips, or tongue. Regional environmental control coordinators based at major rehabilitation units can advise.[4] The systems are available for home use under the NHS but at work they may allow a disabled person to continue useful work. Such technology might include a lightweight electric wheelchair, a keyboard with large easy-to-use keys, a key guard for a patient with a tremor, keyboard emulation such as a joystick or head pointer, and speech recognition software. A large computer screen, a speech synthesizer, or an electronic reading machine may also helpful.[14] Specialist help from the UK government's Access to Work scheme can be sought when choosing and purchasing such technology.

Specific neurological disorders

Earlier in this chapter the relation between symptoms and signs of neurological disease and work were considered. Although the symptoms and signs give a better assessment of work capability, the neurological diagnosis is also important in assessing prognosis and in guiding decisions about whether a person should be employed, what adjustment(s) should be made, or eligibility for medical retirement.

Headache disorders

Daily in the UK more than 90 000 people are absent from school or work due to headache.[28] Eighty per cent of the population have tension type headache, 2–3 per cent of adults have chronic tension type headache (on more than 15 days per month), 10–15 per cent have migraine, and 4 per cent have chronic daily headache, with 1 in 50 having medication overuse headache. Organic disease is a very uncommon cause unless the headache is of recent origin, has changed its character, or it is associated with symptoms of raised intra-cranial pressure or abnormal physical signs. In the older worker, temporal arteritis should also be considered.

Migraine may occur with or without aura, typically a visual disturbance although other transient focal neurological deficits may occur simultaneously or sequentially, such as dysphasia or sensory disturbance. It then progresses to a unilateral or generalized headache with nausea and/or vomiting. Migraine aura can occur without headache. The manifestations of the migraine can change with time, and migraine is only rarely symptomatic of an underlying localized pathology.

Headache in general and migraine in particular may lead to sickness absence, but workplace underperformance is at least as significant as absence. Conversely, a high proportion of workers attribute headaches to stress, dissatisfaction with work, or worry about losing their jobs. Education about headaches, relaxation, and neck and shoulder exercises have been shown in community studies to be effective in reducing the prevalence of headaches.[29]

In spite of advances in medication and management guidelines, migraine and other forms of headache are underdiagnosed and undertreated. A variety of questionnaire instruments have emerged to manage them better. History taking should pay particular attention to coexisting stress, depression, and anxiety. Thus, depression and stress are often features of morning headaches that prevent people getting to work. A stress-prone personality or an individual's perceived capacity to exercise self-control is a factor in the aetiology of headaches and can be improved with cognitive behavioural therapy.[30] Chronic headaches can also result from medication overuse, including the triptans (5HT-1a agonists), which also needs to be considered.

Precipitating factors such as workplace chemicals (including perfume or deodorant), volatile organic compounds from building materials, extremes of temperature, humidity or light, irregular meals or sleep patterns (particularly sleeping in late) should be elicited in an occupational history. There are many modes of medication delivery including nasal sprays, injectable and sublingual formulations, and suppositories, and regular prophylaxis with beta-blockers or amitriptyline such that effective treatment is available for the majority.

Employees with headaches are unlikely to fall under the disability provisions of the Equality Act 2010 as normal day-to-day activities are possible between attacks. Workplace adaptation might require a change to ambient lighting, humidity, or temperature and a quiet, dark room when a sufferer needs to rest. Migraineurs are likely to be precluded from safety-critical jobs that have a minimum incapacitation rate set by their industries, as is the case for airline pilots, air traffic controllers, and aerial climbers.

Disorders of awareness and sleep

Disturbances of awareness include blackouts, seizures, and fluctuations in wakefulness. A patient who has lost consciousness must be advised not to drive and to inform the DVLA, which will decide on their eligibility to continue to hold a driving licence according to published guidelines that can reasonably be applied in occupational settings where incapacitation risks must be minimized.

Daytime somnolence can be a normal physiological phenomenon, particularly after a heavy lunch. However, obstructive sleep apnoea is increasingly being recognized as a cause of excessive daytime somnolence. This is important to recognize because of its neurocognitive and cardiovascular sequelae and potential to interfere with work or give rise to accidents.[31] Sleep disruption is frequent with hypoxaemia and hypercapnia, causing headaches on waking, poor concentration, and consequent impairment of work. It can also cause drowsiness at the wheel. Establishing a diagnosis of obstructive sleep apnoea can be difficult and depends on clinical suspicion and the results of polysomnography. Patients frequently contend that night-time sleep is normal—the problem, in their view, is in the daytime, unless their partner complains of loud snoring, which is not an invariable feature. Sufferers are particularly intolerant of rotating shiftwork, and should lose weight and avoid alcohol. In severe cases continuous positive airways pressure at night is often very effective in relieving symptoms and reducing risk of simulated accidents.[32]

Screening tools such as the Epworth Sleepiness Scale are available and early treatment can be justified on economic grounds.[12] In an occupational context, a two-stage approach has been recommended in a workforce of commercial drivers, using symptoms plus body mass index for screening everyone for the presence of severe sleep apnoea, followed by overnight oximetry that can be done at home for those at high risk.[33]

The classical narcolepsy syndrome is very rare, comprising cataplexy, hypnogogic hallucinations, and sleep paralysis as well as an irresistible desire to sleep. Cataplexy is the sudden decrease or loss of voluntary muscle tone following emotional events. Effective treatment involves optimizing nocturnal sleep duration, and allowing planned daytime naps as well as appropriate medication such as modafinil, sodium oxybate, and amphetamines.

Return to work following stroke and transient ischaemic attacks

The effects of an acute stroke are determined both by the extent and location of damaged brain tissue.[34] This combination will also determine the rate of recovery and the occupational prognosis.

Cerebrovascular disease results in two different pathologies, ischaemia or haemorrhage, with infarction, gliosis, and atrophy as the end result of both. Typically haemorrhage is intracerebral, but it can be subarachnoid from either aneurysms or vascular malformations. Acute stroke management depends as much on the clinical state as on the underlying pathology.

Transient ischaemic attacks (TIAs) cause focal neurological disturbance for less than 24 hours and have more limited occupational implications, such as no ordinary driving for a month and no vocational driving for 12 months. However, it is not uncommon for incomplete neurological assessment or clinically silent cerebral infarction to occur in this context. For these reasons, the occupational physician should adopt a systematic approach for any employee who has suffered a cerebrovascular event. Such an assessment needs to take into account the following factors.

Risk factors

These include: smoking, hypertension, obesity, diabetes, hyperlipidaemia, cardiac pathology, arrhythmias, and carotid stenosis.

Risk of recurrence/incapacitation

It would be wrong to prevent a person returning to work just because the employer is concerned that a further episode might occur. Each employee needs to have their prognosis assessed and reasonable adjustment made to work practices. The absolute risk of a first stroke following a single TIA, or of a second stroke following a first one, is statistically quite low. Nevertheless, the risk of recurrent TIAs is highest within the first 6 weeks of an initial event, and the lifetime risk of a second stroke is double compared with those who have never had a stroke. Such analysis may have implications for those who work in isolation or alone. There is a small but significant risk of sudden incapacitation from recurrence, hence the DVLA medical standard of at least 1 month off driving depending on clinical features and the nature of the licence (see Chapter 28).

Medication

As with all employees, any potentially adverse effect of prescribed medication should be identified. For safety reasons, postural hypotension and cognitive slowing are particularly important. There may be a need to assess those who are on anticoagulants for risk of injury and subsequent haemorrhage. For example, members of the uniformed services might be restricted to administration and training, rather than frontline duties. Access to facilities for measurement of blood clotting time may also be relevant.

Functional deficits

The time to maximum recovery after a stroke varies widely, but can be a year or more. However, after about 4 months it is usually possible to give a reliable prognosis, as by then the functions that are recovering can clearly be discerned and any function that has not started to recover is unlikely to do so completely. Ideally, a final prognosis should not be given until the employee has received optimum rehabilitation.

Physical deficits such as a residual hemiparesis are usually apparent to everyone, including the employee, their managers, and work colleagues. Assessment should determine any reasonable adjustments to the workplace or job, for which advice may need to be sought from Access to Work or an occupational therapist. Subtle deficits of cognitive function may occur, particularly following non-dominant hemisphere strokes affecting frontal lobe executive functions and non-verbal abilities. Those who have had a dominant hemisphere lesion may not only have residual dysphasia with word-finding difficulties apparent in normal conversation, but also coexistent dysgraphia, dyslexia, and dyscalculia which should be sought where appropriate with the help of a clinical psychologist. Visual field deficits, whether absolute, or for simultaneous stimuli presented in opposite visual fields, may require careful assessment, together with other tests for visual agnosia or other perceptual difficulties. This is particularly important where driving or other safety critical work is undertaken.

Cerebral tumours

Unlike tumours elsewhere in the body, primary cerebral and spinal cord tumours do not metastasize outside the CNS. Their histological grade can still vary from benign to rapidly malignant, but ultimately the anatomical site determines prognosis. Even the most benign tumour can be incurable if it is deeply inaccessible within the brain. Fortunately most benign tumours can be treated successfully by surgery, some of the malignant ones can be halted by radiotherapy, and a few are sensitive to chemotherapy.

After treatment, an assessment of the employee's functional ability and information about the prognosis usually facilitates decisions about work. Return to work will be determined by:

- The natural improvement that will occur with rehabilitation and recovery after treatment such as surgical excision, not dissimilar to recovery from a stroke.
- The natural history of the tumour, which has a worse long-term prognosis if malignant or likely to recur.
- The liability to seizures from the tumour or as a consequence of craniotomy.
- The nature of the job, with driving and other safety critical work needing to be considered.

Parkinson's disease

PD is, after stroke, the second most common cause of acquired physical disability from a neurological condition in later life. Its incidence increases progressively with age, and it affects about

Box 6.1 Causes of Parkinsonism

◆ Any acute cerebral pathology, e.g. encephalitis, traumatic brain injury, anoxia, or ischaemia.

◆ Parkinsonism-plus syndromes associated with non-Lewy body neurodegenerative disease.

◆ Chronic exposure to prescribed medication that blocks dopamine receptors in the brain, e.g. major tranquillizers, and other phenothiazines such as prochlorperazine and metoclopramide given as antiemetics or for vertigo.

◆ Environmental toxins such as manganese.

1 per cent of the population above retirement age. Nevertheless, a significant minority of cases occur at younger ages, occasionally even under 40 years. The cardinal features of Parkinsonism are the classical triad of slowness of movement or bradykinesia, resting tremor, and cogwheel rigidity, together with impairment of postural righting reflexes.

Before reaching a diagnosis of primary Parkinsonism, i.e. idiopathic PD characterized by Lewy body neuropathology, the physician must attempt to rule out other causes of Parkinsonism (Box 6.1).

Environmental neurotoxicity hypotheses

Although the aetiology of idiopathic PD is unknown, one popular hypothesis concerns one or more hitherto unidentified environmental toxins, perhaps affecting only those exposed subjects with a genetic susceptibility. Epidemiological studies have suggested that drinking well water, exposure to industrial chemicals or living near industrial chemical plants, or exposure to pesticides or herbicides increases the risk of PD.[35,36] Of interest, 1-methyl-4-phenyl-1,2,3,6-tetrahydropyridine (MPTP), a selective dopaminergic neurotoxin, was industrially developed as a potential herbicide, but instead has been used to produce an animal model of PD. It may also be a contaminant of heroin, sufficient to cause severe PD. The herbicide rotenone has also been used to produce an animal model of PD.

The occupational physician should consider any potential neurotoxic exposure in the employee's workplace. For example, manganese poisoning was first described in 1837 from France in men grinding manganese dioxide, and continues to be the subject of reports from several parts of the world. Long-term exposure to manganese dust may cause Parkinsonism (manganism) and clinical progression continues even 10 years after cessation of exposure.[37] A current controversy with medico-legal implications has arisen because of this and the finding of a tenfold increase in the prevalence of Parkinsonism in a sample of male welders in Alabama compared with the general male working population[38] as well as a report of a group of heavily exposed welders with manganism.[39]

Occupational considerations

The main fitness for work considerations in someone with PD are:

◆ The worker's functional capacity in relation to the degree of motor impairment and tremor, and the need for workplace adjustments.

◆ Concomitant cognitive and emotional factors.

◆ Ensuring optimal symptomatic control with medication while minimizing adverse side effects.

◆ Periodic review to monitor disease progression.

In the early stages, motor impairments may be completely corrected with dopamine replacement therapy, although problems with micrographia and a slow shuffling gait may gradually become more apparent. In those occupations dealing directly with members of the public, prominent tremor can be embarrassing for all, although patients are sometimes remarkably resourceful in disguising their disabilities using various trick manoeuvres. When speech is impaired through dysphonia, speech therapy and the use of a voice amplifier, for example, on the telephone, may be needed. A keyboard guard and adjustments to the 'stickiness' of the keys may also be helpful.

Cognitive impairment is rarely a feature of PD, unless it has been present for a decade or more, but depression is remarkably common and may have a similar neurochemical basis of catecholamine deficiency to the motor impairment. Antidepressant medication can improve quality of life.

As the underlying disease progresses slowly after the first few years, the requirement for medication may increase. A significant proportion of patients, particularly younger ones, also develop fluctuations in motor performance during the course of a day that often coincide with cycles of drug absorption and metabolism, resulting in its extreme form in the 'on–off phenomenon'. This can result in spectacular oscillations between someone who is immobile and frozen one minute, and moving freely the next. Sometimes this latter phase is associated with drug-induced dyskinesia, with involuntary movements that can be embarrassing and disconcerting to colleagues. Titration of the timing of oral medication may be insufficient to control these fluctuations. Specialist neurological advice should be sought concerning other available strategies, such as the use of longer-acting dopamine receptor agonist drugs; modified-release levodopa formulations; the use of subcutaneous apomorphine, either by intermittent injection or by infusion; and even deep brain stimulation.

Most anti-Parkinsonian drugs, particularly with the larger doses required in the later years of the condition, have the potential to cause psychiatric side effects including impaired attention, confusion, visual hallucinations, and overt delusional states. These can arise idiosyncratically with certain powerful dopamine receptor agonists, and may resolve completely following withdrawal of the drug.

Although disability in PD does steadily progress, normally it does so only slowly over the course of a decade or more. This may be sufficient for the employee to reach retirement age. The occupational physician should be proactive in arranging to review the employee and his changing circumstances at appropriate intervals. Parkinson's UK takes a particular interest in providing advice and support for sufferers who are still in active employment, and its regional network can provide information and training for employers locally.

Essential tremor

Essential tremor is an idiopathic condition, often familial and dominantly inherited, that is ten times more common than PD, but not associated with bradykinesia or rigidity. It almost always affects both upper limbs symmetrically, and less commonly the head, lower limbs, tongue, and voice. Older textbooks refer to it as benign, but it is a lifelong disorder that gradually worsens. It can cause significant interference with handwriting, employment, and activities of daily living, and also with social function because of embarrassment.

Many patients with essential tremor require nothing more than an accurate diagnosis and reassurance that a more sinister disease is not present. The impact of social embarrassment, depression, and anxiety must be considered. The avoidance of stimulants such as caffeine and the judicious consumption of ethanol at social events are helpful to some patients. Approximately half benefit from either primidone or beta-adrenergic blockers such as propranolol. Response to one drug does not predict response to the other, but complete suppression of tremor is rare.[40]

Dystonia

There are various forms of dystonia but, rather like essential tremor, they are probably underdiagnosed, usually idiopathic but with a significant genetic component, and poorly understood. Primary generalized dystonia normally starts in childhood and gives rise to severe motor dysfunction ('dystonia musculorum deformans') that is seldom compatible with work. Secondary causes are extremely rare except as a side effect of drugs such as major tranquillizers.

However, focal forms of adult-onset dystonia are probably more common than PD in those of working age, and are classified according to their anatomical involvement. They usually cause irregular involuntary muscle spasms such as dystonic writer's cramp, torticollis, dysphonia, or blepharospasm. They are usually persistent and remission is uncommon, but they do vary in severity and can be controlled to some extent by voluntary strategies such as trick movements. Formerly, they were classified erroneously as psychogenic conditions, but there is now good evidence that they are associated with basal ganglia dysfunction. Focal dystonias respond poorly to anticholinergic medication such as benzhexol, but the introduction of botulinum toxin treatment has revolutionized their management.

Return to work after traumatic head and brain injuries

The first step when assessing an employee's capacity to undertake their duties after head injury is to estimate the severity of the injury to the brain, which is the best indicator of prognosis (Table 6.1). Most people use the term 'head injury' loosely to refer to any traumatic event, but the term 'traumatic brain injury' is preferred to underline this distinction. Various data can be used to estimate the severity, of which the Glasgow Coma Score (GCS), and the durations of coma and of post-traumatic amnesia (PTA) are most useful prognostically, providing they are not prolonged by anaesthesia, sedative medication, or systemic factors. PTA of 2 weeks or more generally predicts measurable residual cognitive problems, of variable impact as far as employment is concerned; a month of PTA predicts at best a reduced work capacity and PTA of 3 months makes voluntary or supported work a likely best outcome, while at worst residential placement may be needed. Younger adults and those with more years of education have a better outcome.[41]

Table 6.1 Severity grading of traumatic brain injuries

Severity	Initial GCS	Duration of coma (GCS <9)	Duration of PTA	Duration in hospital	Duration of recovery	Return to work
Complete recovery usual						
Very mild	14–15	<5 min	<5 min	0	<1 month	<1 month
Mild	13–15	<15 min	5–60 min	<2 days	1 month	<2 months
Moderate	9–12	15 min–6 h	1–24 h	7 days	1–3 months	1–4 months
Some permanent impairment expected						
Severe	<9	6–48 h	1–7 days	>7 days	3–9 months	6–12 months
Very severe	<9	>48 h	>7 days	>7 days	9–12 months	>12 months
Extremely severe	<9	>48 h	>28 days	>14 days	24 + months	Never

GCS, Glasgow Coma Scale; PTA, post-traumatic amnesia.

However, there are many patients whose injuries are not obviously very severe yet have difficulty returning successfully to their previous work. There are two possible explanations for this: either the severity of the underlying brain injury has been underestimated, or there are associated non-organic factors that are contributing to a vicious cycle of ongoing cognitive difficulties, low mood, negative perceptions, muscular deconditioning, and medico-legal issues. The eventual outcome will be the result of interactions between injury severity, intrinsic recovery, and individual personal and environmental factors.

Even with concussive injuries involving little or no period of loss of consciousness, injuries to the brain can occur with focal contusions and disruption of cerebral connections secondary to diffuse axonal injury. However, the physical signs of organic disease can be minimal, and accurate estimates of PTA may be confounded by a prolonged period of sedation during and after surgical interventions and intensive care. Diagnostic pointers include other features of high kinetic energy impact (e.g. high-speed collisions, craniofacial fractures, spinal or proximal long bone limb fractures, visceral rupture). Magnetic resonance imaging (MRI) can usually demonstrate brain injuries objectively long after the event, provided that the correct sequences are requested and the films reported by an experienced neuroradiologist. Finally, formal neuropsychological assessment may help distinguish between focal cognitive impairments, general intellectual under functioning compared with estimated pre-morbid ability, deficits more in keeping with anxiety and depression, or even deliberate exaggeration of difficulties (see symptom validity testing, discussed earlier).[42]

Approving return to work after concussion and minor brain injury

In certain occupations, for example, safety-critical jobs or professional sportsmen, even a minor head injury requires careful assessment before allowing the person to resume their usual activities. The potentially fatal risks of so-called 'second impact syndrome' have been exaggerated, but clearly carry enormous medico-legal implications. The national governing bodies of certain sports in many countries now insist upon a medical examination as part of a 'return to play' protocol. Indeed in the USA, a normal brain scan may be a mandatory prerequisite, even though poorly evidence-based.[43]

The basic requirement is that the person is fully recovered from whatever effects they may have suffered, but this is sometimes hard to confirm with certainty. After a minor head injury, there are three main areas for the physician to consider: symptoms, physical signs, and cognitive functioning.

Symptoms
Seemingly, it should be easy to be satisfied that someone has returned to their pre-injury state—just ask the patient! However, those doctors who manage elite sports athletes know only too well that patients' accounts can sometimes be misleading. Incentives exist for the professional athlete to conceal the truth if the consequences of not competing are likely to affect their prize money or chances of being picked for the national squad. Similar motives may influence other workers, especially those involved with litigation.

Signs
Unfortunately, the neurological examination is not sensitive enough to identify people who are still symptomatic. Minor abnormal neurological signs are uncommon even after moderately severe traumatic brain injury, and after milder injury findings are more likely to reflect pre-existing conditions. Perhaps one of the most sensitive signs of impaired recovery is subtle impairment of coordination and balance. Although not usually part of the standard examination, stringent tests

of high-level balance such as the sharpened Romberg and Unterberger tests, single-leg stance, and walking along a low beam, as well as standard heel-to-toe gait will be examined routinely by sports physicians and physiotherapists. In practice, vocational tests in a protected training or simulator environment should be undertaken before allowing, for example, pilots to return to work or professional athletes to return to competition.

Cognitive functioning

Neuropsychological tests have long been thought to be the most sensitive and objective measure of recovery after minor head and brain injury. Simple tests of orientation, attention, and recall have been incorporated into standardized concussion assessment tools such as SCAT2 by consensus groups, but they have not been scientifically evaluated. They can be used for contact sports on the sidelines during a match, or by the roadside after an accident and can be extended to evaluate satisfactory recovery.[43] More detailed pencil and paper tests can also be used to chart and confirm recovery, and do not necessarily require a trained clinical neuropsychologist. However, the selection of appropriate tests that can be administered repeatedly to the same subject while avoiding practice effects does require special expertise.

Computerized neuropsychological test batteries have also been developed that claim to minimize practice effects while remaining sensitive to significant slowing of information processing speed and other relevant impairments. By using such instruments in a comprehensive programme of pre-season baseline testing, governing bodies such as the English Rugby Football Union and the Jockey Club have established databases for participants in their respective sports that can be used to compare an individual's performance after a single head injury. They may also identify those with a trend of deteriorating performance that might provide evidence of cumulative harm from repetitive head injuries.[43]

Vocational rehabilitation after moderate–severe brain injury

Early liaison with relevant healthcare professionals and support organizations such as Headway is highly desirable. Psychometric testing will usually establish the extent of any organic impairment which may be integral to a person's rehabilitation back to work.[44] Participation in a brain injury education programme may be beneficial to increase insight into residual difficulties, anticipate areas of potential difficulty at work and identify compensatory strategies. The information can usefully be communicated to colleagues and line managers to facilitate understanding and adjustment. Ideally, this should be an integral part of a formalized managed process of vocational rehabilitation.[45,46] Employees should be advised to do as much as they can for themselves, take regular meals, go to bed at reasonable hours, and adjust their lifestyle. Alcohol should be avoided, both because of reduced tolerance to intoxication and increased adverse neurobehavioural effects.

As with other organic lesions of the brain, functional improvement does occur but takes time and may be incomplete. Shift work is best avoided and medication that might impair concentration or cognition should be stopped unless absolutely necessary. For many employees after prolonged absence, returning to work too abruptly can be counter-productive and a graduated return is preferable, taking on limited responsibilities at first and then adding to them. This is because of a combination of physical deconditioning, particularly if commuting involves long journeys, and mental fatigue induced by cognitive inefficiency and increased multitasking.

Meningitis and encephalitis

Most infections of the CNS begin acutely over the course of hours or a few days, and involve both the meninges and brain to some extent. Many different viral, bacterial, and even fungal pathogens can cause an identical acute neurological syndrome with intense headache, fever, malaise, and drowsiness that may progress to coma and seizures, depending on the extent of cerebral involvement. After the first few days and appropriate timely antimicrobial treatment, the course is mostly one of slowly progressive improvement over several days or weeks. The prognosis and influence on work capacity vary according to the organism and extent of underlying cerebral damage. Herpes simplex encephalitis, the most common cause of severe sporadic encephalitis in the Western world, can cause considerable memory impairment and these patients may never return to intellectually demanding occupations. Other less severe infections usually result in full recovery.

Better treatment for opportunistic infections and the development of highly active antiretroviral therapies has greatly reduced morbidity and mortality in those infected with HIV, and a marked decrease in the incidence of HIV-associated dementia. Nevertheless, because of their high prevalence, a high index of suspicion must be kept for neurological disorders in the HIV or AIDS patient (Chapter 23).

Alzheimer's disease and other pre-senile dementias

Dementia usually develops insidiously, most often after retirement, but poses a diagnostic and management problem when it arises in someone of working age. If the employee has been in the same job for many years, cognitive failure may be less obvious. They can work relatively well in familiar surroundings at routine tasks, but new tasks are difficult. Colleagues may become aware of deterioration in driving safety or work performance.

Dementia from occupational neurotoxic exposure is considered earlier in this chapter. Unfortunately, reversible causes of dementia (e.g. metabolic, normal-pressure hydrocephalus, and certain drugs including alcohol) are uncommon. (HIV-associated dementia is dealt with in the section on meningitis and encephalitis.) Degenerative dementias such as Huntington's disease are progressive by definition, and decisions about continuing employment must be based objectively on competency and reasonable adjustments. Any safety-critical activities should be prohibited, and administrative safeguards instituted at diagnosis if medical retirement is not effected immediately.

Sporadic Creutzfeldt–Jakob disease (sCJD) generally presents after age 50 years with much more rapid progression over weeks or months (although cases aged below 40 years have been described), and 10 per cent of cases are familial with autosomal dominant inheritance. A new variant of the disease (vCJD) due to an abnormal prion protein was first described in 1996 by the UK National CJD Surveillance Unit based in Edinburgh, which maintains a website with up-to-date research and advice.[47]

Neurological disorders of childhood

Cerebral palsy includes a group of childhood syndromes (historically classified as either spastic or dystonic) resulting from genetic and acquired insults to the developing brain, causing abnormalities in tone, posture, and movement. It is important to appreciate that cerebral palsy includes a wide range of infectious, hypoxic–ischaemic, endocrine, and genetic conditions. Other developmental disorders of the posterior fossa and spinal cord, such as Chiari malformations and spina bifida, may cause similar disabilities, not least because of their association with hydrocephalus. Poliomyelitis should be approached in a similar way.

At the start of employment it is advisable to have a full medical and functional capability assessment so that work can be adjusted to allow the employee to use their skills most efficiency.

A systematic approach to a prospective employee, often a young school leaver, allows accurate identification of the key occupational considerations and prognosis, and avoids the danger of stereotyping, as someone with severe physical disability may have no intellectual impairment at all and vice versa.

Employment prospects are usually established during education and training, enabling a young person to develop their potential abilities and attain appropriate vocational qualifications. It is usually valuable to obtain previous statements of educational needs that document the subject's abilities systematically. Minor motor impairments rarely pose a problem except during highly skilled activities. Machinery, office equipment, and vehicles can usually be adapted.

Spinal cord injury and disease

The commonest neurological disease affecting the spinal cord itself is multiple sclerosis (described in the next section). Primary tumours arising within the spinal canal are rare and are usually benign, the commonest being a neurofibroma. However, the commonest cause of acute myelopathy is trauma, which tends to affect younger adults engaging in risk-taking activities and a significant proportion occur at work. Some patients return to work after spinal cord injury with the help of adaptive technology, particularly those who need to work and who are in sedentary jobs.[48] The employee may require reasonable time and space to use a standing frame during the working day, or to self-catheterize intermittently. The occurrence of autonomic dysreflexia with postural hypotension or hypertensive storms also needs to be considered in those with high thoracic injuries.

Multiple sclerosis

MS is the commonest neurological disorder affecting young adults. The diagnosis traditionally requires two or more CNS lesions separated in time and space, not caused by other CNS disease. The manifestations vary enormously because lesions can occur anywhere in the CNS. Common presentations include a single episode, lasting only a few weeks, of visual impairment, ataxia, or focal motor or sensory disturbance.

MRI and cerebrospinal fluid analysis are abnormal in more than 95 per cent of definite cases. MRI has also become essential to rule out conditions that could mimic MS. Updated diagnostic criteria use new MRI lesions to define separation in time and space.[49] These criteria are helpful after a clinically isolated demyelinating syndrome, such as optic neuritis or transverse myelitis, when the risk of later evolution into MS is far greater in those with abnormal brain scans at presentation.

The majority present with relapsing and remitting disease, but MS is progressive from onset (primary progressive MS) in about 10 per cent of cases, particularly with later age of onset. More typically, there are three phases: initially relapses with full recovery, then relapses with persisting deficits, and later secondary progression. There is cumulative loss of oligodendroglia and neurons, with increasing demands on compromised surviving cells. In the progressive phase clinical remissions disappear, but constant low-grade immune activation continues or worsens.

The time course is extremely variable, as some patients may spend years or even decades in each phase, whereas about 10 per cent rapidly become severely disabled. About 25 per cent of patients have a benign form of MS that is not disabling. The prognosis is relatively good when sensory or visual symptoms predominate and there is complete recovery from individual relapses, a pattern commonest in young women. Negative prognostic predictors include cerebellar or pyramidal signs; frequent early attacks, development of secondary progression, or a primary progressive course, and age over 40 years at onset. Later onset MS is more common in men and often primary progressive; even when it begins as relapsing-remitting disease, secondary progression occurs earlier.

After a single episode with full recovery an employee should be able to return to normal work. If recurrent attacks are infrequent with full recovery, the amount of time off work over a period of years should be small. In more chronic cases regular assessment will be required to decide about capability, adjustments, and medical retirement. Most patients with established disease will have attended hospital and their diagnosis and management policy been determined. If this has not occurred, referral to a specialist should be made before the employee's future work situation is decided. Beta-interferon and other disease-modifying treatments may be used, but their long-term value is uncertain.

The initiating event for the first attack is unknown, but genetics and environmental factors both interact. Epidemiological studies have found an association between MS and residential latitude in different parts of the world, but the significance of those factors remains unclear. Trauma and stress have been implicated anecdotally as causing MS or triggering exacerbations, but the occurrence of any specific exacerbation cannot yet be causally linked to any specific stressor. However, if a patient has not made a full recovery it is possible that certain environments may make the symptoms greater or more obvious, although no particular work environment should affect prognosis.

Fatigue is one of the most common complaints among patients with established and disabling MS, typically magnification of post-exertion fatigue with sensitivity to heat and humidity. Some studies have shown modest benefit from treatment with amantadine and from energy conserving courses.[50] High temperatures are not well tolerated and some patients like to work in slightly colder environments than is usually desired by other employees as this reduces their symptoms.[17]

Poor sleep, worry, or depression, as well as cognitive deterioration due to demyelination, also need to be considered by the physician. Euphoria can be an early sign of frontal lobe dysfunction, causing abnormal contentment with physical disability. This has advantages for the sufferer as a patient, but not as an employee, as increased commitment is needed to overcome the disability and to continue to cope.

The factors relating to remaining in work are mainly disease related, such as balance and walking abilities, but the physical requirements of the job and the motivation of the employee to remain at work are also relevant. Financial and practical help with travel is available from the UK government's Access to Work scheme. To remain in work people with MS need good healthcare management such as an orthotic support for foot drop, or an indwelling catheter for urinary incontinence, as well as workplace or job adjustments such as wheelchair access, or adjustments to their role.[51,52] Flexible working hours, time off work for physiotherapy or medical appointments, and increased absence due to MS are also reasonable adjustments that will help patients remain in work. Regular occupational screening for visual field loss or cognitive decline may be necessary for employees in safety critical jobs. Employees should be encouraged to join self-management groups run by the MS Society.

Multidimensional scales for objectively assessing impairment and disability of patients with MS have been developed, such as the Kurtzke Expanded Disability Status, the Multiple Sclerosis Functional Composite, and the Incapacity Status Scales, but they all have their limitations, such as the need for self-reported information and maximal effort by the patient when assessing walking, using the arms, or doing mental arithmetic.[53] Unfortunately this may not be the case when fitness to work or eligibility to a medical pension is being evaluated!

Miscellaneous genetic disorders

A small but significant proportion of neurological disease is caused by single-gene mutations, which can present at working age. Neurocutaneous genetic syndromes share a dominantly inherited predisposition to developing tumours of the nervous system. Such a diagnosis is compatible with working, but the risk of developing complications is unpredictable and may justify some form of regular occupational screening, such as for acoustic neuromas in type 2 neurofibromatosis or for visual acuity or field loss due to haemangioblastomas in von Hippel–Landau disease.

An employee with limb-girdle or facio-scapulo-humeral muscular dystrophy affecting the shoulder or pelvic girdle may need adjustments to their job or workplace if, for example, they have difficulty lifting their arms above their shoulders, climbing stairs, or rising from a squatting position. Someone with dystrophia myotonica will have difficulty releasing their grip in cold weather, so will need to be moved indoors and, because of their propensity to develop cataracts, regularly screened for deteriorating visual acuity.

Motor neurone diseases

The term 'motor neurone disease' describes a family of rare disorders resulting from selective loss of function of lower and/or upper motor neurones controlling the voluntary muscles of the limbs or bulbar region. Four main syndromes are recognized—amyotrophic lateral sclerosis, progressive muscular atrophy, bulbar, and pseudo-bulbar palsy. Some forms progress rapidly, in which case medical retirement is appropriate, whereas others are more benign and compatible with work with the help of adaptive technology. Mental ability is unimpaired so the patient may be able to control their environment and, for example, operate a telephone or computer with assistive technology.

Peripheral neuropathy

Neuropathy is a common condition with a very broad differential diagnosis (Box 6.2). It is typically insidious in onset with glove and stocking sensory loss and produces gradually increasing disability. Progress is usually slow and many cases are asymptomatic or have little disability. The main exception is acute idiopathic inflammatory polyneuropathy or Guillain–Barré syndrome, in which symptoms develop rapidly over days and then resolve, usually completely, within weeks or months. Return to work is usually possible when the patient becomes fully ambulant, although occasionally residual muscle weakness may persist indefinitely so each case will need to be assessed for functional capacity.

About 15 per cent of all patients with diabetes mellitus have significant peripheral neuropathy. Symmetrical sensory or autonomic neuropathy with postural hypotension, incontinence, and impotence, or isolated peripheral nerve lesions, or multifocal neuropathies may occur and mixed syndromes are common. Walking aids such as ankle–foot orthoses may be helpful when there is foot drop.

Hereditary neuropathies, such as Charcot–Marie–Tooth disease, usually affect both motor and sensory nerves and present during school years with foot deformities or difficulty in walking. A family history makes the diagnosis easier, but sporadic cases may arise by recessive inheritance or new mutations.

Peripheral neuropathy is a recognized complication of many toxic chemicals and therefore the onset of a peripheral neuropathy should always alert the doctor to the possibility of toxic chemical exposure at work (see 'Toxic neuropathies').

Regardless of the cause, neuropathies are seldom a reason to cease work and as progression is slow the patient may be able to continue to work for several years. Care of the feet is vitally

Box 6.2 Causes of peripheral polyneuropathy

- Cryptogenic, undetermined.
- Alcohol misuse.
- Metabolic and endocrine disorders: diabetes, uraemia, amyloid, myxoedema.
- Genetic: hereditary neuropathies, inherited neurometabolic diseases.
- Inflammatory and post-infectious neuropathies: Guillain–Barré syndrome, critical illness polyneuropathy.
- Nutritional deficiencies: vitamins B1, B6, B12, E, folate.
- Chronic inflammatory demyelinating polyneuropathy.
- Toxins: acrylamide, carbon disulphide, arsenic, inorganic lead, mercury (hatters' shakes), thallium, triorthocresyl phosphate, organic solvents such as MBK and n-hexane.
- Drugs: mainly cytotoxic agents, isoniazid, amiodarone.
- Paraproteinaemia: monoclonal gammopathies of undetermined significance.
- Connective tissue disorders: polyarteritis nodosa, rheumatoid arthritis, etc.
- Neoplastic and paraneoplastic.
- Infections: HIV, hepatitis B, *Borrelia*, herpes zoster
- Hand–arm vibration syndrome.

Box 6.3 Occupational checklist for employees with peripheral neuropathy

- Motor function: check walking ability and balance is adequate for the job.
- Proprioception: this is an important component of balance, particularly if employee is working at heights.
- Pain and temperature impairment: footwear must be fitted with extra care, and restrictive footwear or protective garments and extremes of temperature avoided.
- Avoid activities that are hard on the feet, such as running and jumping, and standing or walking for prolonged periods without adequate rests.
- Reinforce quit smoking advice to minimize concomitant peripheral vascular disease.

important in any sensory neuropathy, to prevent minor injuries being left untreated, the development of chronic ulceration, and possibly even amputation. Other occupational considerations are listed in Box 6.3.

Neuromuscular junction disease

Neuromuscular junction diseases are rare. The most prevalent is myasthenia gravis, an auto-immune disorder in which antibodies interfere with normal neuromuscular transmission. Repeated or sustained exercise induces focal weakness, usually affecting limb girdle muscles, the extra-ocular muscles, or bulbar-innervated muscles, so an employee may first complain of proximal weakness when asked to do physical work, or of transient diplopia, or difficulty with chewing. Myasthenia is difficult to diagnose in its early stages, when it may be misdiagnosed as psychogenic because objective weakness varies from one day to the next. If suspected, examination should be carried out before and after exercise, and positive serum acetylcholine receptor antibodies are diagnostic, but seronegative cases require more specialist investigation.

Provided the correct diagnosis is made, few cases become gravely ill nowadays because most respond well to treatment with the anticholinesterase drug pyridostigmine and immunosuppressants, including steroids. Most patients then enter remission, but may require treatment indefinitely and adverse drug effects need to be monitored. Certain classes of drug such as D-penicillamine and aminoglycosides aggravate myasthenic weakness so should be avoided, and muscle-strengthening exercises are inappropriate. A small proportion of cases require thymectomy, either because of an associated thymoma, or thymic hyperplasia in early-onset seropositive subjects. Unless the job is particularly physically demanding, the majority of employees with myasthenia should be able to continue working.

Muscle diseases

Muscle disease is less common than CNS disease. Some acquired myopathies are associated with drug treatment (e.g. statins, corticosteroids), or some other endocrine or malignant disease, on which its prognosis will depend. Polymyositis appears to be a syndrome of diverse causes that often occurs in association with systemic autoimmune diseases, viral infections, or connective tissue disorders such as lupus and rheumatoid arthritis. Chronic polymyositis can give rise to mainly proximal weakness with periodic flare-ups that may require increasing doses of steroids and other immunosuppressant therapy.

Persistent muscle weakness and fatigue may affect survivors of acute respiratory distress syndrome and other critical illnesses, who may encounter apparently unexplained difficulties upon returning to work apparently fully recovered. The possibility of myopathy, polyneuropathy, or muscular deconditioning secondary to critical illness should be considered in anyone who has had a prolonged stay on an intensive care unit.

Entrapment neuropathies

The median nerve may be compressed in the carpal tunnel of the wrist causing nocturnal pain and paraesthesiae in the affected hand or forearm. Sensory loss in the hand will be in a median nerve distribution and if severe, associated with wasting and weakness of abductor pollicis brevis in the thenar eminence (carpal tunnel syndrome (CTS)). Phalen's wrist flexion sign may also be positive. Occupational risk factors for CTS are highly repetitive flexion and extension of the wrist allied to a forceful grip >4 kg force, or daily exposure to >3.9m/s^2 of hand-transmitted vibration,[54,55] which is a 'prescribed disease' for Industrial Injury Disablement Benefit purposes. Aspects of management are covered in Chapter 13.

A cervical rib from the seventh cervical vertebra may produce a similar picture by compressing the C8 and T1 nerve roots causing pain down the medial aspect of the forearm and weakness of abductor pollicis brevis.

The ulnar nerve is most commonly compressed in the cubital tunnel of the elbow, but may also be damaged in Guyon's canal between the pisiform and hammate bones in the wrist to cause the hypothenar hammer syndrome (HHS) in which there is damage to the ulnar nerve or ulnar artery as a consequence of trauma to the heel of the hand, as may occur in some manual jobs when this part of the hand is used as a tool. The ulnar nerve divides into superficial and deep branches in the canal causing sensory loss in an ulnar nerve distribution or weakness of the intrinsic muscles of the hand when damaged. A ganglion in the wrist may produce similar symptoms. HHS needs to be distinguished from hand–arm vibration syndrome.[56]

The lateral cutaneous nerve of the thigh may be compressed as it passes under the inguinal ligament causing burning or numbness over the anterior thigh (meralgia paraesthetica), the common peroneal nerve may be compressed against the neck of the fibula causing foot drop and the posterior tibial nerve may be compressed in the tarsal tunnel causing pain and numbness in the sole of the foot.

Chronic fatigue syndrome

A degree of limiting fatigue has been reported by 27 per cent of working adults, but the prevalence of chronic fatigue syndrome is 0.1–2.6 per cent depending on the criteria used. The underlying mechanisms remain poorly understood, but psychosocial factors are thought to be relevant. Chronic fatigue syndrome should be diagnosed when fatigue sufficient to interfere with normal physical and mental functioning has lasted for more than 6 months and no medical (as opposed to psychological) cause for the fatigue has been found. The only treatments that have been shown in clinical trials to work are cognitive behavioural therapy and graded exercise therapy.

Adjustments to work such as a phased return, a reduction in workload, the resolution of interpersonal difficulties and additional support are helpful when rehabilitating someone with chronic fatigue back to work. As such patients are usually relatively young, medical retirement is rarely justified on the grounds of permanent incapacity. Prognosis is highly variable but many patients improve spontaneously or sufficiently with treatment to return to work or normal functioning, although they may still report feelings of fatigue. Medical retirement should not be considered until these adjustments and treatments have been explored and engaged with.[57]

References

1 Langton Hewer R, Tennant A. The epidemiology of disabling neurological disorders. In: Greenwood RJ, Barnes MP, McMillan TM, *et al.* (eds), *Handbook of neurological rehabilitation*, 2nd edn, pp. 5–14. Hove: Psychology Press, 2003.

2 The Neurological Alliance. *Neuro numbers: a brief review of the numbers of people in the UK with a neurological condition.* London: Neurological Alliance, 2003. (<http://www.neural.org.uk>)

3 Local Government Employers. *Local Government sickness absence levels and causes 2008-9.* [Online] (<http://www.lga.gov.uk>)

4 Fyfe NCM, McClemont EJW, Panton LE, *et al.* Assistive technology: mobility aids, environmental control systems, and communication aids. In: Greenwood RJ, Barnes MP, McMillan TM, *et al.* (eds), *Handbook of neurological rehabilitation*, 2nd edn, pp. 231–44. Hove: Psychology Press, 2003.

5 United Kingdom Rehabilitation Council. *Rehabilitation Standards* 2009. [Online] (<http://www.rehabcouncil.org.uk>)

6 Black C. *Working for a healthier tomorrow: review of the health of Britain's working age population.* London: TSO, 2008. (<http:// www.workingforhealth.gov.uk>)

7 Simpson SA, Wadsworth EJ, Moss SC, *et al.* Minor injuries, cognitive failures and accidents at work: incidence and associated features. *Occup Med* 2005; **55**: 99–108.

8 Professional Practice Board. *Assessment of effort in clinical testing of cognitive functioning for adults.* Leicester: British Psychological Society, 2009.

9 Wilson BA, Herbert CM, Shiel A. *Behavioural approaches in neuropsychological rehabilitation: optimising rehabilitation procedures.* Hove: Psychology Press, 2003.

10 Morgan K, Kucharczyk E, Gregory, P. Insomnia: evidence-based approaches to assessment and management. *Clin Med* 2011; **11**: 278–81.

11 Smith IE, Quinnell TG. Obstructive sleep apnoea: relevance to non-sleep clinicians. *Clin Med* 2011; **11**: 286–9.

12 Pelletier-Fleury N, Meslier N, Gagnadoux F, *et al.* Economic arguments for the immediate management of moderate to severe obstructive apnoea syndrome. *Eur Respir J* 2004; **1**: 53–60.

13 Herxheimer A, Waterhouse J. The prevention and treatment of jet lag: It's been ignored, but much can be done. *BMJ* 2004; **326**: 296–7.

14 Poole CJM, Millman A. Adaptive computer technology. *BMJ* 1995; **311**: 1149–51.

15 van Dijk FJH, Swaen GMH. Fatigue at work. *Occup Environ Med* 2003; **60**(Suppl. 1): i1–2.

16 Johansson S, Ytterberg C, Hillert J, *et al.* A longitudinal study of variations in and predictors of fatigue in multiple sclerosis. *J Neurol Neurosurg Psychiatr* 2008; **79**: 455–7.

17 Holdcroft A, Power L. Management of pain. *BMJ* 2003; **326**: 635–9.

18 Drazkowski JF, Sirven JI. Driving and neurologic disorders. *Neurology* 2011; **76**(Suppl. 2): S44–S49.

19 Evans BJ, Cook A, Richards IL, *et al.* Effect of pattern glare and colored overlays on a stimulated-reading task in dyslexia and normal readers. *Optom Vis Sci* 1994; **71**: 619–28.

20 Massaro EJ (ed). *Handbook of neurotoxicology: volume 1.* Totowa: Humana Press, 2010.

21 Dobbs MR. *Clinical neurotoxicology: syndromes, substances, environments.* Philadelphia, PA: Saunders Elsevier, 2010.

22 Genuis SJ. Toxicant exposure and mental health—individual, social, and public health considerations. *J Forensic Sci* 2009; **54**: 474–7.

23 Jin CF, Haut M, Ducatman A. Industrial solvents and psychological effects. *Clinics Occup Med* 2004; **4**: 597–620

24 Dick F, Semple S, Osborne A, *et al.* Organic solvent exposure, genes, and risk of neuropsychological impairment. *Quart J Med* 2002; **95**: 379–87.

25 Roldan-Tapia L, Nieto-Escamez FA, del Aguila EM, *et al.* Neuropsychological sequelae from acute poisoning and long-term exposure to carbamate and organophosphate pesticides. *Neurotoxicol Teratol* 2006; **28**: 694–703.

26 Committee on Toxicity of Chemicals in Food, Consumer Products and the Environment. *Organophosphates.* London: Department of Health, 1999.

27 Baldi I, Gruber A, Rondeau V, *et al.* Neurobehavioural effects of long-term exposure to pesticides: results from the 4-year follow-up of the PHYTONER study. *Occup Environ Med* 2011; **68**: 108–15.

28 British Association for the Study of Headaches. *Guidelines for all doctors in the diagnosis and management of migraine and tension-type headache,* 4th edn. Exeter: British Association for the Study of Headaches, 2010. (<http://www.bash.org.uk>)

29 Mongini F, Evangelista A, Rota E, *et al.* Further evidence of the positive effects of an educational and physical program on headache, neck and shoulder pain in a working community. *J Headache Pain* 2010; **11**: 409–15.

30 Marlowe N. Self-efficacy moderates the impact of stressful events on headache. *Headache* 1998; **38**: 662–7.

31 Chan AS, Phillips CL, Cistulli PA. Obstructive sleep apnoea—an update. *Intern Med J* 2010; **40**: 102–6.

32 Mazza S, Pépin JL, Naëgelé B, *et al.* Driving ability in sleep apnoea patients before and after CPAP treatment: evaluation on a road safety platform. *Eur Respir J* 2006; **28**: 1020–8.

33 Gurubhagavatula I, Maislin G, Nkwuo JE, *et al.* Occupational screening for obstructive sleep apnoea in commercial drivers. *Am J Respir Crit Care Med* 2004; **170**: 371–6.

34 Warlow CP, Dennis M, Van Gijn J, *et al.* Which arterial territory is involved? Developing a clinically-based method of sub-classification. In: Warlow CP, Dennis M, Van Gijn J, *et al.* (eds) *Stroke: practical management,* pp. 106–50. Oxford: Blackwell, 2008.

35 Tanner CM, Ross GW, Jewell SA, *et al.* Occupation and risk of parkinsonism: a multicenter case-control study. *Arch Neurol* 2009; **66**: 1106–13.

36 Park J, Yoo CI, Sim CS, *et al.* Occupations and Parkinson's disease: a multi-center case-control study in South Korea. *Neurotoxicology* 2005; **26**: 99–105.

37 Huang CC, Chu NS, Lu CS, *et al.* Long-term progression in chronic manganism: ten years of follow-up. *Neurology* 1998; **50**: 698–700.

38 Racette BA, Tabbal SD, Jennings D, *et al.* Prevalence of parkinsonism and relationship to exposure in a large sample of Alabama welders. *Neurology* 2005; **64**: 230–5.

39 Bowler RM, Nakagawa S, Drezgic M, *et al.* Sequelae of fume exposure in confined space welding: a neurological and neuropsychological case series. *Neurotoxicology* 2007; **28**: 298–311.

40 Hardie RJ, Rothwell JC. The management of tremor and ataxia. In: Greenwood RJ, Barnes MP, McMillan TM, *et al.* (eds), *Handbook of neurological rehabilitation*, 2nd edn, pp. 171–8. Hove: Psychology Press, 2003.

41 Sherer M, Struchen MA, Yablon SA, *et al.* Comparison of indices of traumatic brain injury severity: Glasgow Coma Scale, length of coma and post-traumatic amnesia *J Neurol Neurosurg Psychiatr* 2008; **79**: 678–85.

42 McCauley SR, Boake C, Pedroza C, *et al.* Correlates of persistent postconcussional disorder: DSM-IV criteria versus ICD-10. *J Clin Exp Neuropsychol* 2011; **30**: 360–79.

43 McCrory P, Meeuwisse W, Johnston K, *et al.* Consensus statement on concussion in sport: the 3rd international conference on concussion in sport held in Zurich, November 2008. *Br J Sports Med* 2009; **43**: i76–i74.

44 British Society of Rehabilitation Medicine and Royal College of Physicians. *Rehabilitation following acquired brain injury: national clinical guidelines*. London: Royal College of Physicians, 2003.

45 Department of Work and Pensions. *Building capacity for work: a UK framework for vocational rehabilitation*. London: Stationery Office, 2004.

46 British Society of Rehabilitation Medicine, Jobcentre Plus, and Royal College of Physicians. *Vocational assessment and rehabilitation after acquired brain injury: inter-agency guidelines*. London: Royal College of Physicians, 2004.

47 The National Creutzfeldt–Jakob Disease Research & Surveillance Unit (NCJDRSU): <http://www.cjd.ed.ac.uk>

48 Tomassen PCD, Post MWM, van Asbeck FWA. Return to work after spinal cord injury. *Spinal Cord* 2000; **38**: 51–5.

49 Polman CH, Reingold SC, Banwell B, *et al.* Diagnostic criteria for multiple sclerosis: 2010 revisions to the McDonald criteria. *Ann Neurol* 2011; **69**: 292–302.

50 Lee D, Newell R, Ziegler L, *et al.* Treatment of fatigue in multiple sclerosis: A systematic review of the literature. *Int J Nursing Practice* 2008; **14**: 81–93.

51 Wade D. *NHS services for people with multiple sclerosis: a national survey*. London: Royal College of Physicians and Multiple Sclerosis Trust, 2011.

52 Roessler RT, Rumrill PD. Multiple sclerosis and employment barriers: a systemic perspective on diagnosis and intervention. *Work* 2003; **21**: 17–23.

53 Amato MP, Portaccio E. Clinical outcome measures in multiple sclerosis. *J Neurol Sci* 2007; **259**: 118–22.

54 Palmer KT, Harris EC, Coggon D. Carpal tunnel syndrome and its relation to occupation: a systematic literature review. *Occup Med* 2007; **57**: 57–66.

55 Van Rijn RM, Huisstede BM, Koes BW, *et al.* Associations between work-related factors and the carpal tunnel syndrome—a systematic review. *Scan J Work Environ Health* 2009; **35**: 19–36.

56 Cooke RA. Hypothenar hammer syndrome: a discrete syndrome to be distinguished from hand-arm vibration syndrome. *Occup Med* 2003; **53**: 320–4.

57 Cairns R, Hotopf M. A systematic review describing the prognosis of chronic fatigue syndrome. *Occup Med* 2005; **55**: 20–31.

Chapter 7

Mental health and psychiatric disorders

Richard Heron and Neil Greenberg

Introduction

In recent years there has been much published about the substantial impact that mental health disorders have upon the productivity and well-being of the working population. Organizations have moral, legal, and economic reasons to support the mental health of their workforce and the issue is one of such importance that in 2009 the National Institute for Health and Clinical Excellence (NICE) issued public health guidance on promoting mental well-being through productive and healthy working conditions. The consequences of organizations failing to pay 'due consideration' to the impact of mental health disorders at work are often expressed financially. For instance, a 2007 report from the Sainsbury Centre for Mental Health noted that impaired work efficiency, as a result of mental disorders, costs the UK £15.1 billion a year with mental health related absenteeism costing an additional £8.4 billion annually.

However, the relationship between work and health, in particular mental health, is often complex. Whilst some of the more serious mental health disorders, such as chronic schizophrenia, are associated with clear impairments of function which are likely to limit the work options for afflicted individuals, the picture is less clear for those who suffer from the much more common and less severe disorders of mental health, including anxiety and many types of clinical depression. In their review, *Is Work Good For Your Health and Well-being?*, Waddell and Burton[1] summarize the theory and evidence base indicating that work is generally beneficial for physical and mental health and well-being. For many, probably the majority, the social environment of work, allied to a predictable daily routine, is positive for health and well-being.

Concurrent with the realization that being employed is good for most people is an increasing awareness of the harmful effects to health associated with long-term 'worklessness'. While recognizing that for a small number of people (5–10 per cent) work may contribute to poor health, overall, the beneficial effects of work outweigh the risks and are greater than the harmful effects of long-term unemployment and prolonged sickness absence. Encouragingly, a recent survey 'Attitudes of working age adults to health and work' showed that most working age adults share in this belief—over eight in ten respondents in a survey by the Department for Work and Pensions felt that paid work was generally good or very good for both physical and mental health.[2] Work for all, or at least the vast majority, regardless of the presence of a mental health disorder should also be possible since almost all organizations, advised by occupational health professionals, are legally required, (under the disability provisions of the Equality Act 2010) to consider how reasonably to adjust the workplace to accommodate people with mental health disorders.

The aim of this chapter is to consider how work and mental health interrelate and how employers can ensure the mental health needs of their workforce are dealt with appropriately to maximize opportunities for productivity and minimize psychological morbidity. The chapter will follow a preventative medicine format by considering primary, secondary, and tertiary prevention of mental health disorders at work. Primary prevention equates to the prevention of mental ill health within a workforce and working environment; it is the responsibility of line managers and organizational policies and procedures. They may be advised by occupational health professionals who have a role to play in assuring the content of such policies and practices, and raising awareness about them. Secondary prevention refers to the early identification of the warning signs likely to indicate that mental health problems will develop. Early identification allows for either the prevention of progression of a disorder through management interventions or to ensure that personnel receive early treatment leading to a rapid return to occupational effectiveness which may involve healthcare professionals in some cases. Tertiary prevention refers to treatment and recovery which aims to prevent longer-term disability in those who have a diagnosed mental health disorder. Whilst is it beneficial for line managers to support tertiary prevention interventions, the responsibility for delivering them is likely to rest with healthcare professionals.

The extent of the problem

Mental ill health is common and many people will experience mental health disorders themselves or within family or work colleagues during their life. At any one time, up to one in six adults have mental health conditions, and a further sixth will experience symptoms associated with poor mental health, including problems with sleeping, fatigue, irritability, and worry. An increasing number also report that work causes stress or makes it worse.

Since the early 1990s, household surveys conducted by the Office for National Statistics (ONS, formerly OPCS) have established the prevalence of and trends in common mental disorders.[3,4] Between 1993 and 2000, the proportion of people with depression and anxiety increased to 16 per cent of those aged 16–64 years; there was no significant change when reviewed in 2007. When segmented by gender, ONS found that the increase from 1993 to 2007 was significant for women (19.1–21.5 per cent), but not for men (see Figure 7.1).

Interestingly, during the same period the proportion of people with the more severe psychiatric disorders remained steady at around 1 per cent.

Looking specifically at the impact of mental health disorders in the working population, as opposed to those of working age who may or may not be working, a report carried out for the Department for Work and Pensions[5] in 2011 showed the most common symptom suffered by respondents (10 per cent in total) was depression/bad nerves/anxiety. This was also one of the most likely symptoms to be reported as being caused by work, which clearly has implications in terms of potential litigation.

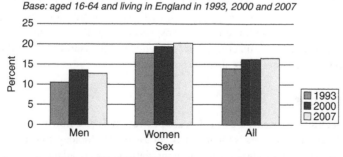

Figure 7.1 Prevalence of common mental disorder, by sex and survey year. Reprinted from Sally McManus et al. (eds), *Adult psychiatric morbidity in England, 2007: Results of a household survey*, Copyright © 2009. Re-used with the permission of The Health and Social Care Information Centre. All rights reserved.

The employment statistics among the mentally ill make grim reading. Patients with severe, enduring mental health problems account for 8 per cent of long-term disabled people of working age. Of these only 18 per cent are in some form of employment (even though 30–40 per cent are thought capable of holding down a job) compared with 52 per cent of non-mentally long-term disabled according to a report by the Royal College of Psychiatrists.[6] Even the more minor, and less severe, mental disorders are associated with poor employment statistics. Adults with neurotic disorders are four to five times more likely to be permanently unemployed compared with the rest of the population: 61 per cent of males and 58 per cent of females with a single neurotic disorder are in work compared with 75 per cent and 65 per cent respectively in the general population. Comorbidity is common in psychiatry and further reduces employment prospects. In patients with two concomitant neurotic disorders the proportions in work fell further to 46 per cent of males and 33 per cent of females. Patients with phobic disorders had the bleakest employment record: only 43 per cent of males and 30 per cent of females were working. This does not mean the mentally ill are 'work-shy', and despite these high rates of unemployment as many as 90 per cent of patients state they would like to return to work if the opportunity presented itself. Among those with neurotic disorders who were unemployed, and actively seeking work, 70 per cent had been unemployed for more than 1 year.[7]

The economic burden of mental illness

Approximately 80 million working days per year are lost in the UK as a result of mental illness with an estimated cost to employers of £1.2 billion. This figure is almost certainly an underestimate given that mental health problems are often undetected or misdiagnosed. On average approximately 3000 people in the UK per week move on to Incapacity Benefit; musculoskeletal disorders account for 28 per cent of these, with psychiatric disorders coming a close second at 20 per cent. In a recent survey, 1 in 5 days of certified sickness absence was due to psychiatric illness, accounting for 92 million lost working days.

Overall direct costs of mental illness vary and have been estimated by some to be about £32.1 billion: this comprises £11.8 billion in lost employment, £4.1 billion in costs to the National Health Service (NHS), and £7.6 billion in Social Security payments.[8] The Royal College of Psychiatrists estimated the annual cost of poor mental health in Great Britain is more than £40 billion a year.[6] Some of the more difficult to measure costs of mental health disorders amongst the workforce come from what is called *presenteeism*. In this chapter we use this term to refer to the loss of productivity as a result of poor performance because of impairment as a direct result of a mental health disorder. However, it is also possible that mental health disorders may lead to loss of productivity in other ways, such as the increased propensity for accidents amongst members of the workforce with impaired concentration or other aspects of cognitive function. Whilst a potentially complex area it is fair to say that the impact of mental health disorders on productivity is not wholly a function of employees being absent from work.

Some definitions

One of the difficulties experienced by healthcare professionals and non-medical personnel in discussing mental health disorders is the inconsistent use of terminology. In order to ensure that this chapter uses terminology clearly, the following definitions are adapted to aid the reader's understanding:

- ◆ *Mental healthcare*: healthcare provision which aims to treat established or incipient mental health disorders (such as, but not limited to, clinical depression, post-traumatic stress disorder

(PTSD), or alcohol dependency). Such care is ordinarily delivered by medical professionals including but not limited to general practitioners (GPs), psychiatrists, mental health nurses, and psychologists.

◆ *Mental health*: a state of emotional and psychological well-being in which individuals are able to function effectively at work and in the wider society, and meet the ordinary demands of everyday life without being hampered by cognitive and emotional difficulties.

◆ *Mental well-being*: a positive state of mind and body in which an individual feels safe and able to cope with day-to-day pressures, has a sense of connection with others including the local community and the wider environment.

As is evident from the given definitions, neither mental health nor mental well-being is reliant solely upon the work of healthcare professionals for their equilibrium. Rather, both are moderated by line managers and the wider organization's approach to psychological health. Healthcare professionals do, however, have a significant role to play in advising organizations about how best to promote mental health and mental well-being, even if they are not responsible for providing it.

Primary prevention of mental health disorder

The accountability for primary prevention falls clearly in the non-medical domain. The focus of such efforts should be on the actions which organizations can take to minimize the potential for personnel to develop mental health disorder; this is sometimes known as having a psychologically resilient workforce. An individual's psychological resilience is a product of individual factors (such as education, upbringing, family circumstances) and organizational factors (such as control of work delivery (methods and timing) and the support of management and co-workers). A substantial evidence base demonstrates that personnel in well-led, mutually supportive companies can endure substantially higher levels of psychological pressure than personnel in less well-led and less cohesive groupings. The main role of primary prevention is thus to provide personnel, and leaders, with the knowledge and skills which will enable them to enjoy the highest levels of resilience.

Primary prevention of mental health disorders can be facilitated through several processes. Firstly, given that there are often conflicting and strong beliefs held by personnel in the same organization about the origins and management of mental health disorders, a role exists for preventative mental health training. In the main, this is best focused on providing relevant information to those with leadership positions and raising their awareness about mental health conditions, their recognition, and optimum management. For instance, whilst some managers might think that people who are showing some signs of mild emotionality or who have been exposed to a potentially traumatic event should be given a period of leave, the best evidence suggests that granting such discretionary leave may often be counter-productive. Doing so may deprive employees of a valuable source of social support which has been repeatedly shown to be beneficial for mental health and may also leave those sent home with the sense that they have let colleagues or the organization down. Evidence, primarily from military populations, has shown the benefits of keeping people working, albeit in a temporarily less stressful role, can greatly assist recovery.

Evidence of the spread and popularity of mental health training can be found on many respectable health-related websites including those of the World Health Organization (WHO), NICE, the UK Psychological Trauma Society Group, the Institute of Psychiatry, the National Centre for PTSD and the Uniformed Services University of the Health Sciences (USUHS). There have been, however, few studies which have examined whether such training is effective. Some studies have found benefits from providing mental health training to a military workforce,[9,10] particularly in the prevention of psychological ill health after exposure to traumatic situations. Civilian evidence of providing similar self-help information to emergency department attendees, without any further follow-up, found those who received self-help information did less well than those in the control arm who did not receive such information.[11]

Another aim of mental health training is to debunk the associated myths. Stigma is a term used to describe the set of beliefs which prevent people who may benefit from accessing support, including but not limited to formal mental healthcare, from doing so. Much evidence shows that stigmatizing beliefs are highly prevalent in Western cultures and that stigma is one of the reasons why people do not seek support. Stigmatic beliefs which may prevent seeking help include a fear of what one's colleagues will think and the potential effect of seeking help on an individual's career prospects. Whilst it is easy to sometimes think of stigma as only being an issue for typically macho workplaces such as the emergency services, the media, or the military, there is good evidence that it is a societal issue, rather than one limited to any specific occupational setting.[12] Organizational policies and programmes which aim to reduce the stigma associated with mental health conditions may increase health and well-being of employees by encouraging them to seek collegial support before the need for professional support or medical treatment.

Another important mechanism through which organizations can support the mental well-being of employees is the provision of high-quality work-focused training. When a police force teaches junior police officers how to deal with public disorder, or an oil company inducts prospective oil workers to deal with the hazards associated with living on a drilling platform, the skills that the employee acquires allows them to exert some control over their work environment. One well-accepted model of occupational stress is known as job-demand control.[13] This model proposes that *stress*, (the adverse reaction a person has to excessive pressure or other types of demand placed upon them),[14] can result from workers being unable to exert control over their work environment. High-quality, work-focused training should not only provide employees with the ability to do what is asked of them, but should also support their well-being. Another potential benefit of training, especially training in groups, is that it can engender camaraderie amongst employees which is a key resilience factor; highly cohesive occupational groupings are more likely to deal effectively with pressures than less mutually supportive ones.

Another important model of stress at work is the Effort Reward Imbalance model[15] which proposes that stress-related problems occur where there is an imbalance between high efforts spent and low rewards received. Working hard without appreciation is therefore a recipe for a stressful work environment and 'active distress' in employees. Furthermore the model suggests that highly committed individuals may be at increased risk.

There are many ways in which organizations can reward employees including using the regular appraisals process as a way of ensuring that they remain effective and motivated. Whilst organizational appraisal processes might not be thought of as a mental health support tool, the evidence suggests that they should be. Whilst other rewards such as financial bonuses or extra leave entitlement may be more often thought of as rewards for good service, the evidence suggests that however positive feedback is provided, the effect it has is to support the mental well-being of employees. This may be especially true after particularly pressured periods such as working towards completion of a contract or in the aftermath of a traumatic event.

Secondary prevention of mental health disorders

Whilst the opportunities for primary prevention within an organization may be optimized by ensuring that effective line management processes are put in place and that managers/leaders are appropriately selected, trained, resourced, and enabled to perform their role, it is inevitable that some personnel will develop mental health disorders. There are many factors which determine whether incipient problems will progress to more established mental health disorders. These are often split into predisposing factors such as personality or having experienced adverse childhood experiences, precipitating factors such as the break-up of a relationship or substantial difficulties within the work environment and perpetuating (or maintaining) factors such as poor social support or comorbid alcohol misuse.

Secondary prevention is concerned with the early detection of at-risk employees in order to allow organizational level interventions, including but not limited to temporary changes in duties and increased provision of informal social support, which may return individuals to a good state of psychological health without the need for professional help. Where simple interventions are not successful then referral on to professional help should be undertaken.

One of the challenges with providing secondary prevention at an organizational level is that most systems of early detection of disorder rely on the detection actually being made. The default is that such identification is made by a healthcare professional during a routine consultation, periodic medical, or as a result of a specific screening programme. However, research suggests that many employees do not routinely seek help about work-related problems. This may be because they themselves do not recognize that their difficulties result from mental health problems, their mental health problems go un-noticed by co-workers and managers, or that they do not seek care because of perceived barriers to care, including but not limited to stigma.[16] Furthermore, there is now mounting evidence which suggests that, in the main, most people prefer to use informal mechanisms of support than seek professional help—especially for problems which they consider as being minor. Reluctance to seek help at an early stage is not necessarily a problem for most people who have good support available to them and who will, in any case, recover. However, even those who will go on to make a full and rapid recovery may be temporarily unable to carry out some or all of their duties. The impact of so called presenteeism has been well described as accounting for more loss of productivity than absenteeism.

How best to detect and manage persisting low-grade symptoms or more severe symptoms which are self-limiting and unlikely to come to the attention of health professionals remains a substantial challenge for managers. One mechanism which has gained popularity over recent years is the introduction of peer support programmes.[17] The rationale for this often includes the goals of meeting the legal and moral duty to care for employees, as well as addressing multiple barriers to care (including stigma, lack of time, poor access to providers, lack of trust, and fear of job repercussions). Peer support programmes may take a number of forms ranging from training non-professionals to deliver basic counselling interventions in the workplace, to more formalized early detection and management support processes which are designed to support personnel who have been exposed to traumatic events.[18] Although high-quality research into the effectiveness of peer support programmes in supporting the mental health and well-being of employees is generally lacking, what evidence there is suggests that such programmes are well accepted and may improve occupational function especially in the aftermath of a traumatic event.[19]

Another mechanism which an organization might consider employing to detect the early signs of impending mental health difficulties is screening. Mental health screening often takes the form of asking employees to complete questionnaires which have the capability of measuring psychological distress if answered honestly or, in some organizations, (e.g. the US military) may involve face-to-face interviews with a healthcare provider.

However, there is currently a lack of evidence that screening for mental disorders is effective. Screening programmes assume that effective treatments for mental health conditions that they might detect, e.g. anxiety disorders such as post-traumatic stress or depressive disorders, will work for a screened population as they have been demonstrated to do in controlled trials in a help-seeking group of patients. For instance, in the UK NICE supports the use of both cognitive-behavioural therapy and eye movement desensitization and reprocessing as being effective treatments for PTSD in clinical settings.[20] It is a conceptual leap, however, to suggest that screened populations would experience similar benefits. Those identified using screening techniques differ from patients seen in routine clinical care in terms of severity, interest in accessing health services, and commitment to treatment.[21] Furthermore, whereas healthcare-seeking patients may be likely to engage with multiple sessions of therapy, the effects of screening positive, including stigma, may have a strong influence on an individual's propensity to act upon the results. Therefore even if personnel can be correctly identified by a screening process as needing professional help, they may still not access this help.

Another important issue is that a sensitive screening tool might generate considerable numbers of personnel incorrectly labelled as suffering from mental health conditions which a subsequent clinical interview finds are in fact self-limiting or simply manifestations of their personality. Large numbers of inappropriately identified patients would place substantial demands upon mental health and primary health services if a screening programme were implemented without evaluation and incorrect labelling of employees as suffering from a mental health condition may lead to harm.

Whilst managers and colleagues are often well placed to detect the early signs of mental disorder, not infrequently an individual's friends and family will also be aware of a change in character or clear-cut symptoms of distress. Families and indeed co-workers may either not be aware of how to let employers know of their concerns. They may also perceive that informing employers about the mental health status of friends or loved ones will prejudice a positive work outcome. Secondary prevention measures can only be successful if either the organization is able to detect problems early on or if they are made aware of problems. Therefore, it follows that facilitating family–employer liaison should be a helpful mechanism which should aide secondary prevention measures.

The secondary prevention stage is also critical from an employment law perspective. Once an employee is known to the employer to have a mental health condition or even the conditions which may predispose to it, the issue of foreseeability of potential harm arises. The employer may be therefore required in law to ensure that they make reasonable adjustments for the employee and do not unreasonably discriminate against the employee. In *Dickins* v. *O2PLC* [2008] EWCA Civ1144, an employee had complained of job stress to her manager. The claimant was referred to a counselling programme but adjustments were not made. The Court of Appeal found in favour of Mrs Dickins. This case is also important as it further emphasized that referral to a counselling service in itself does not constitute a defence.

Reasonable adjustments to working arrangements such as changes in working hours, responsibilities, or even work location and team may be required. This is a two-way responsibility. Reasonable adjustments can only be made if the condition is known to the employer. In the case of *Wilcox* v. *Birmingham CAB Services Ltd*, the Employment Appeal Tribunal upheld an Employment Tribunal's decision to dismiss the claimant's claims of constructive dismissal and disability discrimination on the grounds that the employer was never made aware of agoraphobia and travel anxiety suffered by the claimant (*Wilcox* v. *Birmingham CAB Services Ltd* [2011] UKEAT 0293/10/DM).

Tertiary prevention

Tertiary prevention concerns itself with the provision of rapid and effective treatment for those suffering with mental health disorders in order to either return them to full fitness or to minimize long-term disability. The boundaries between incipient mental health problems and an established mental health disorder can at times be blurred. The difficulty in distinguishing between disorders that should be medically treated and those which are likely to resolve without professional intervention may be less of a concern for the so called serious mental illnesses such as schizophrenia and bipolar affective disorder (also known as manic depression) than is the case for conditions that were previously termed 'neurotic disorders' (such a depression and anxiety). However, during the early presentation of someone who will go on to develop a serious mental illness, it can often be unclear whether someone is becoming ill or just acting a little oddly. In many cases the onset of serious disorders may be associated with behaviour that employers regard as being contrary to that which is compatible with being employed and the individual may leave their job or in some cases their contracts of employment may be terminated. This is part of what is known as social drift which is a term used to describe the progressive loss of status, finances, and lifestyle which often precedes the onset of a frank serious mental health problem. Social drift is often accepted as the reason why many people who suffer from serious mental illnesses are part of the lower social strata of society. People in higher social strata who develop serious mental disorders tend to drift towards the lower strata before or shortly after their illness develops.

Tertiary prevention then is most effective if treatment can be provided for the unwell individual in a timely manner before social drift has occurred or before its progression is advanced. The NHS provides a wide range of treatment for mental health conditions; however, it is fair to say that the majority of its provision is targeted towards those individuals who are suffering from serious disorders rather than the much more prevalent 'common mental health disorders' which whilst not likely to be a cause of serious long-term psychiatric morbidity may well be important in terms of occupational function. NICE have issued a variety of guidelines on the management of mental health conditions including depression, obsessive–compulsive disorder, and PTSD.

Mental healthcare is often delivered from a multidisciplinary team usually lead by a consultant psychiatrist, but other mental healthcare professionals may also lead (e.g. psychologists may lead teams of clinicians dedicated to treating personality disorders). The first stage of mental healthcare delivery is the initial 'holistic' assessment which needs to consider not just the presenting complaint but also the wider psychosocial factors related to the disorder. In some cases physical health complaints may directly cause mental health disorders, (e.g. a severe chest infection may lead to low blood oxygen saturation and an acute confusional state may result), but more commonly a combination of factors is associated with the onset of a psychiatric disorder. Most importantly, where workplace relationships are part of the precipitating cluster of factors, then it is unusual for mental healthcare in itself to lead to a return of occupational fitness. Failure to resolve the intra-workplace relationship will also prevent a return to work, especially in the case of a perceived poor relationship with the affected individual's manager/supervisor.

Mental healthcare, especially for the less serious disorders, is likely to involve some psychotherapeutic work. Psychotherapy is a term that is used to describe a wide range of 'talking' treatments. Whilst 'classic' (or Freudian) psychotherapy may involve exploration of an individual's past life, interpretation of dreams, and fantasy-world can take many months or years to complete. Most modern healthcare providers focus on providing more short term psychological intervention such as cognitive-behavioural therapy (CBT) or eye movement desensitization and reprocessing (EMDR) which have a considerable evidence base for their use. There are also other time-limited therapies which may be helpful in some cases, and which have an evidence base supporting their use, such as interpersonal therapy and behavioural activation. The type of therapy deemed to be helpful for the individual in question depends very much on the outcome of the initial 'holistic' assessment; some therapies are likely to suit some individuals (and conditions) but not others. One important factor which is common to almost all psychotherapeutic interventions is the establishment of the therapeutic alliance. Should the patient not be able to feel they can trust, confide in and work with their therapist after having had a few sessions then it is usually unwise to continue with the talking treatment. Most evidence-based therapies are likely to show effectiveness over six to 12 sessions (each lasting around an hour and often delivered once per week) although some more complex cases may need considerably more sessions. It is often helpful to have the clinician who is providing the overall monitoring of care distinct from the person providing the therapy. This helps ensure that an objective view is taken of how an individual is progressing.

Over recent years and since the 2002 Court of Appeal decision in the case of *Hatton* v. *Sutherland* supported their use, employee assistance programmes (EAPs) have grown in popularity (*Hatton* v. *Sutherland and other appeals* [2002] EWCA Civ76). EAPs provide confidential counselling services to employees (and in some cases to their families). Most EAPs provide only a limited number of sessions and the evidence available suggests that the vast majority of the problems EAPs deal with are not work related. There is also a lack of evidence showing the EAPs improve the mental health or well-being of employee. However, not all EAPs work in the same way and it is possible that some are more effective than others. From an employer's perspective it should also be noted that the authority of the Hatton judgment has waned.

Whilst the use of time-limited professionally delivered therapy for specific conditions has been relatively well researched, and found in many cases to lead to an improvement in mental health status, there are also many non-evidenced based treatments on offer for the unwary to avail themselves of. This is particularly so in the matter of PTSD where there is a distinct lack of any high-quality trials (randomized controlled trials (RCTs) in particular) which have examined the effectiveness of 'alternative' treatments, in contrast with a very considerable body of high quality evidence (including numerous RCTs) that show that trauma-focused CBT and EMDR are both highly effective for the treatment of PTSD. It therefore seems to make little, if any sense, in providing non-evidence based therapies to people suffering from conditions, such as, but not limited to PTSD, when there are other evidence-based alternatives which are known to work. There are numerous other examples of similarly non-evidence-based therapies offered as proposed treatments for various mental health conditions which, whilst they may or may not be harmful if provided, may delay someone receiving an evidence-based intervention which may get the individual better.

How mental health problems might interfere with work

Diagnostic labels in themselves may do little to assist occupational health professionals in making decisions regarding an individual's employment potential. The mentally unwell, like the rest of us, have their individual strengths and weaknesses and a thorough appraisal of abilities, deficits, and functional capacity should be integral to any occupational assessment. Excluding an individual on the basis of diagnosis alone is not only discriminatory but also excludes a lot of potential talent from the workplace. However, where diagnosis can help is in determining a management plan and also in helping clinicians make firm prognostic statements which can help organizations determine the long-term likelihood of returning to work or whether someone might be eligible for a disability pension.

One of the areas of potential confusion is in the language used by the various health professionals involved in an individual's case. For instance, occupational health professionals may not always understand the technical jargon used by mental health professionals particularly when trying to 'decipher' recommendations made in reports which comment on the employment prospects of someone who is unwell. Mental health professionals may rely on an 'illness' model which can be highly useful within acute psychiatric environments and in planning mental health service provision, but may be less helpful in the occupational environment where a disability model, focusing on enduring problems, strengths, and weaknesses, is likely to be more useful. The 'disability' model informs the changes and adjustments that might be necessary in the workplace to enable the individual to successfully return to work. The expectation is that others will take steps to facilitate a return to work rather than passively waiting for an individual to simply 'get better'. Disability highlights the interaction between impairment (be it physical or sensory handicap or the lack of self-confidence found in depression) and the obstacles that might exist in the workplace including attitudes, working practices, policies, and the physical environment that may exclude an individual with that impairment from full participation.

The use of a social model of disability is not only consonant with government policy but can also help establish a joint understanding of the types of problems that an individual who is suffering from mental health disorders might be experiencing and help the individual, their line manager, and medical personnel involved in their care approach the problem from a single direction. This is important because the Equality Act 2010 requires employers to act reasonably and focus on preventing discrimination and social exclusion which many mental health service users perceive to exist. Ideally, ensuring that where it is reasonably practicable to do so, keeping the mentally unwell working will provide both the best opportunity for them to recover social role and status[22] and ensure that organizations meet their moral and legal obligations.

Psychiatric disorders may impair one or more domains of psychological or social functioning and it is important to systematically assess each of these in turn.

Impaired concentration and attention

Any mental illness may significantly impair concentration and attention. This may be due to the distractibility and preoccupying worries associated with anxiety states and hypomania, the often slowed thought processes seen in depressive disorders and states of relative malnourishment associated with eating disorders, or the poverty of thought or thought disorder associated with problems such as schizophrenia. Many psychotropic drugs used in the treatment of these disorders can also be associated with marked behavioural effects such as reduced concentration and attention span. Performance, concentration, and attention deficits are best assessed by an occupational therapist using '*in vivo*' tasks that resemble those required in the workplace. Paying proper attention to deficits in concentration may be especially important for people who work in safety critical tasks.

Impaired motor skills

Abnormal involuntary movements as well as a paucity of movement may hamper work performance. Psychomotor slowing is seen in many depressive disorders and the tremor associated with anxiety may impair skilled motor tasks as well as be associated with increased self-consciousness especially in social situations such as meetings. Movement disorders can be a feature of conditions such as schizophrenia and are not only disfiguring but also disturbing to others. Antipsychotic drugs (including many of the newer atypical agents) may produce marked extra pyramidal symptoms, which themselves may become a cause of significant disability.

Impaired communication and social skills

The ability to communicate effectively and get on with colleagues is one of the most important predictors of success at work. Because of their difficulty in taking part in routine social interactions at work, many people who suffer with severe and enduring mental health problems (where they are fortunate enough to find work) may work in either isolated roles (e.g. a security guard) or in low-paid manual roles where they are not called upon to have to relate to other co-workers. For some who suffer with such conditions, it may be that such employment is nonetheless enjoyable, providing a degree of self-sufficiency. In other cases, placing those who become severely unwell in such roles may merely be a means of discharging obligations under disability legislation while keeping their mentally ill employees isolated from the rest of the workforce. Many patients, especially with long-term disorders, have significant difficulties interacting with others. This may be due to the illness itself, for example, the lack of self-confidence associated with depression, or simply lack of practice.

Risk to self and others

A risk assessment is now an integral and explicit part of any psychiatric examination and a written statement regarding risk should form the outcome of all such examinations. Often the severity of the risks to self and others is couched in rather vague terms (often low, moderate, or high) which may not, in itself, convey sufficient information to allow employers to effectively deal with the risks. It is worth noting that whilst the risks of harm to self and others can be associated with mental health conditions, many episodes of self-harm and/or violence are not a result of formal mental health disorders. Both alcohol use (and misuse) and impulsive personality traits also increase the risks of such behaviours.

In terms of risks of suicide, there can be no doubt that the high rates are associated with certain occupations such as veterinary medicine and farming and that the increase in such risks are, in part at least, attributable to the ready availability of lethal means.

The risk to others associated with mental illness is often overstated and grossly exaggerated by the media. The mentally ill are far more likely to harm themselves than others. Indeed deliberate harm to others is also far more likely to be imparted by the mentally well. Nevertheless, occupational physicians have a duty to reassure employers and expect a clear and unequivocal assessment of risk from the psychiatric team.

The effects of abnormal illness behaviour

Motivation, commitment, and willingness to work are perhaps the best predictors of success (or otherwise) in the workplace, irrespective of any psychiatric diagnosis. Many individuals with significant psychopathology are punctual, reliable, and hardworking employees who perform their duties to the satisfaction of all and without giving any hint that they may be suffering from a significant disorder (illness denying abnormal illness behaviour). Indeed some mental health conditions may actually be associated with especially high levels of conscientiousness, e.g. obsessional personalities. It may be difficult at times for occupational physicians to decide what proportion of poor working practice is attributable to illness and what proportion is a function of poor motivation. In the main, most mental health conditions should not be regarded as providing an excuse for poor behaviour but neither should their effects upon motivation and aptitude be ignored. Whilst mental health conditions may be associated with decreased occupational effectiveness, some minority of cases will be simply malingering.

Why work matters: the psychosocial benefits

For most people, work is integral to their sense of personal identity, self-esteem, and worth. A fulfilling job promotes mental well-being, and in the mentally ill, remaining in employment is an important long-term prognostic indicator.[23] Long-term, involuntary, unemployment, conversely, is associated with despair, mental illness, and in some cases suicide.[24] Employment provides income to the individual and with it an improved standard of living to them as well as improving the economic productivity of society. It reduces the financial burden on the state, increases consumer spending, tax revenue, and economic output. However, work brings with it a number of less tangible advantages to the individual such as social status and recognition, contact, social support and an important forum for establishing supportive social relationships, a daily routine and an excuse to get out of bed in the morning.[25] One's role at work is frequently an important part of an individual's identity.

Obstacles to employment

There is little evidence to demonstrate whether particular types of services or interventions are effective in getting the mentally ill back to work. The employment of disabled people in general depends on the state of the economy, including the rate of growth, overall employment rate, and extent of any labour shortages. The mentally ill, and individuals with significant learning disabilities, experience greater difficulty obtaining paid work than any other disabled group. Although a number of voluntary sector employment schemes exist that work in collaboration with mental health services, the poor employment statistics suggest that there is a clear gulf between these resources and the open labour market. Stigma and discrimination over and above that shown towards other disabled groups is the barrier that pervades society. The welfare system can discourage employment because of the benefit trap and the need to limit any (poorly paid) work for fear of compromising state benefit entitlements. GPs, employers, and even mental health professionals have typically poor expectations of the capabilities of the mentally ill as well as overestimating the risk to employers of employing individuals with mental health problems.[26] They may also have a poor understanding of the workplace.

Fit for work? Assessment for employment

Assessment requires skill and experience and can be an important intervention in its own right. People with mental health problems suffer from a mutual lack of understanding between occupational physicians and mental health professionals. The dichotomy between illness and disability models of illness has already been described. In practice this means that psychiatric reports are often unhelpful to occupational physicians and fail to provide the necessary information needed to determine whether an individual is employable in a given work environment. Past behaviour is often the best predictor of future performance and detailed work histories often give a better indication of an individual's employability than any diagnostic label or measure of psychopathology. Personal objectives, motivation, and confidence are far better predictors. The person most likely to succeed is the individual who *really* wants the job! Motivation predicts success in the workplace; however, getting a job itself can be a powerful motivating factor, particularly for individuals who have been repeatedly unsuccessful. Frequent failure though will demotivate.

A comprehensive occupational assessment has three key ingredients: an appreciation of the individual and their strengths and weaknesses; the nature of the workplace and demands of the job; and the desired outcome for both individual and employer. Individual factors to be considered include: past employment history, skills, and work performance, and individual factors including motivation, confidence, and personal aspirations. Finally, the workplace itself should be considered in terms of the expectations of peers and managers, opportunities for supervision, training and development, and links to other employee development programmes.

It should be realized, however, that there are circumstances in which some caution in job placement should be exercised. For example, fitness assessment must consider the risk to the public, third parties, and personal safety in safety-critical jobs (e.g. airline pilots, train drivers, lorry drivers, fire fighters, perhaps even electricians and engineers employed by railway companies). In the NHS there has been a lot of discussion about pre-employment screening of nurses for psychiatric illness; this has become a factor following unexpected patient deaths. Where a pre-screening process is put in place, recent case law emphasizes the importance of specificity when defining pre-employment questions. In the case of *Cheltenham Borough Council* v. *Laird* [2009] EWHC 1253 (QB), the claimant had a past history of several episodes of depression related to work-stress and was taking antidepressants at the time of assessment. After a further depressive episode in a new job, the question of disclosure failure at pre-employment was raised. The High Court found in favour of the claimant who had answered that she was normally in good health, did not have a physical or mental health impairment, absent family history, and that she did not have an ongoing condition which could affect her employment.

The General Medical Council has similar concerns about mental illness and poor performance in doctors; questions of fitness to practice should be asked in the early phases of treatment for florid psychoses, etc. However, blanket judgements should be resisted, provided that there are no legal considerations that apply.

Back to work: reintegration into the workplace

A successful return to paid work is perhaps one of the most meaningful yet least used measures of health outcome, in addition to being an important positive prognostic indicator, irrespective of psychiatric diagnosis. Too many patients with mental health problems make a good clinical and functional recovery only to find themselves living in social exclusion, and become aimless, underoccupied, and unfulfilled. This existence not only potentially undermines an already fragile self-esteem but is itself a harbinger of further mental health problems. There is considerable opportunity for improving social inclusion that has not been adequately addressed at a statutory or policy level. Moreover, traditional mental health services themselves are focused on symptomatic improvement and pay too little attention to occupational outcome and success in the workplace.

While a variety of schemes are provided by both the statutory and voluntary sector to help reintroduce mental health service users to the workplace, there is little evidence to demonstrate their effectiveness. Anecdotally, it is far easier for service users with an established pre-morbid work record to secure employment compared with those who have never been in work and for whom opportunities remain poor. The effectiveness of any employment scheme provided by the statutory and voluntary sector designed to return service users to the labour market will be limited unless employers are more incentivized to be proactive in recognizing the special needs of those recovering from mental illness and doing more to accommodate these within the workplace.

Recovery and return to work

Individuals who have held down a job but have been on a period of (often lengthy) sick leave and are recovering from mental health problems may face some difficulties when returning to work. An occupational health service can maximize the likelihood of a successful outcome. First, it is important to establish whether the mental health team anticipates a return to pre-morbid functioning and, if not, what residual disabilities there are? Would an early return to normal duties help or hinder recovery? In particular, would a period of part-time employment or restricted duties be helpful in enabling the individual to rebuild confidence and re-acclimatize themselves to the work routine? It is especially important to evaluate the extent to which the demands of the employee's job itself may have been contributory to the development of mental health problems, and a decision made on whether or not it is either safe or appropriate for the individual to return to their former job and working environment.

The Equality Act 2010 requires that 'reasonable adjustments' are made where an individual's health needs to be taken into consideration. The occupational physician can do a great deal to help with rehabilitation by putting the case for modified hours, working from home on a temporary basis or even as a permanent arrangement on some days. Occasionally, it helps employees settle back into work more efficiently if tasks can be selected initially which are relatively simple in nature, to reduce any pressures that might otherwise cause difficulty.

There are occasions, of course, where the employee may blame the organization, the system of working, or their manager for their health problem. This is often the case following an absence related to stress with resulting anxiety and/or depression. There may be a need for the manager to sit down and discuss the circumstances. On occasions, a different job or relocation may be a sensible solution.

Work schemes and sheltered employment

For those with more serious mental health problems or those never before employed, a variety of schemes exist which are intended to ease the transition into the workplace. Sheltered employment and occupational rehabilitation are not new concepts and were historically an integral part of the asylum regime. With the advent of community care and the closure of large mental hospitals, much of this activity sadly failed to move into the community with the patient. This resulted in the provision of employment schemes in community settings being increasingly provided by the voluntary sector and becoming haphazard and patchy, both geographically and in terms of quality and meeting local need. One of the few surveys conducted has shown a 40-fold variation in provision across health authority areas. Unfortunately, but not surprisingly, the highest levels of provision are generally found in the most affluent areas.[27] Across the UK more than 130 different organizations offer some form of sheltered employment, including 77 providing open employment and with approximately 50 set up as 'social firms'.[28,29]

Models

A variety of models exist to facilitate a return to work. Sheltered workshops and factories (e.g. Remploy) provide mostly unskilled manual work for individuals with severe enduring mental illness. They are useful in introducing individuals to the work situation in a safe environment. Very few individuals in these schemes, however, move into the open employment market and the organizations themselves often experience difficulty in maintaining profitability. A more recent variant of sheltered employment is the 'social firm' where a business is developed as a commercial enterprise with mental health service users employed throughout the organization and not simply as manual labour. Social firms are not primarily engaged in rehabilitation and employees are paid the going rate. A further variation to this model is the 'Social Enterprise'; a semi-commercial concern that also has the clear objective of providing training and rehabilitation.

Pre-vocational training enables individuals to have a period of preparatory training and a gradual reintroduction to the workplace with the expectation of them moving into the open employment market. 'Supported employment' aims to place individuals directly into the workplace without lengthy preparation or training. Service users are expected to obtain work directly in the open employment market. The employee is hired competitively and employed on the same basis as other employees, with full company benefits, but with supervision and mentoring from the support organization to maximize the likelihood of a successful outcome.[30] Assessment is on the job and support is continued indefinitely. Perhaps this, more than any other model, most effectively bridges the gap between mental health services and the employment community.

User employment programmes

Many NHS Trusts now employ current or former (health) service users in jobs that demand a history of mental health problems as part of the personal specification for the post. Service users are employed on terms and conditions of service identical to other employees and additional support is made available for those who need it. Many of these posts involve patient advocacy where the insight and personal experiences of former service users can clearly be brought to bear for the benefit of patients. Service users are increasingly employed in major service development roles such as National Service Framework Local Implementation Teams and increasingly serve as members of senior medical staff on Appointments Advisory Committees. Indeed, service user involvement has become a key performance indicator with which all Mental Health Trusts are required to comply. This active participation of service users in high-profile positions of obvious importance within the NHS is of immense symbolic value, challenging stigma, prejudice, and the widely held poor expectations about the employability of mentally ill people in positions of responsibility in the workplace.[31]

Common psychiatric disorders

Psychiatric disorders are ordinarily classified according to one of two classification manuals, the WHO International Classification of Disease (ICD—currently Volume 10 is the one in use) and the US psychiatry-specific Diagnostic and Statistical Manual (DSM—currently the fourth volume is in routine use). However, not all healthcare professionals use either classification manual rigidly and there are plenty of examples of ill-thought out diagnostic labelling to be found. This may be more common in primary care rather than secondary care settings; however, since psychiatric disorders cannot usually be diagnosed using 'hard' tests, even mental health specialists do not always come to the same conclusions about the nature of a psychiatric disorder even when provided with the same information. Another problem with classifying psychiatric disorders is that many diagnostic labels can also be found in lay use within everyday language. For instance, diagnostically depression requires at least a 2-week history of the relevant symptoms; however, the term depression is often used by lay people to describe unhappiness and some confusion may arise between the diagnostic and lay use of the term.

The rest of this section includes a brief overview of some of the more common mental health conditions which occupational physicians might encounter.

Adjustment disorders

Adjustment disorders describe a group of extreme short- and medium-term reactions to stressful events. They occur more commonly in people who suffer with other mental health vulnerabilities and may continue for many months after exposure to the stressor ceases or longer where exposure continues. Individuals typically feel overwhelmed or unable to cope and may experience marked symptoms of anxiety or depression as well and exhibit a range of unhelpful behaviours. Adjustment disorders may also lead to individuals presenting with a variety of somatic complaints including headaches, dizziness, abdominal pain, chest pain, and palpitations. People suffering from an adjustment disorder may misuse alcohol or illicit substances to help them (ineffectively) deal with their symptoms of distress. Whilst most of these reactions are self-limiting, it is important to note that the severity of emotions and behaviours may be extreme and even though the disorder may resolve within a relatively short time period, the damage done to an individual's relationship (including their work relationships) can be severe and enduring. Whilst medication, including antidepressants and anxiolytics, may be helpful to some degree to alleviate the more severe symptoms, often providing some respite from continuing stressful circumstances (including the workplace if that is the source of the distress), it may be appropriate only for a short period. Where the workplace is a major source of the problem, it is often helpful to keep people working in alternative roles. Whilst clinicians should ensure that someone suffering with an adjustment disorder is prevented, as far as is possible, from causing themselves longer-term harm, a gradual return to normal functioning is itself generally therapeutic and the expectation should be one of full recovery. Adjustment disorders may evolve into more chronic illnesses such as major depression and other anxiety states in some cases; however, the absence of any past psychiatric history and the presence of a 'robust' pre-morbid personality generally predict a good outcome.

Depression

Clinical depression is a common mental disorder which can be potentially disabling but is also eminently treatable in the majority of cases. Depression is often categorized as mild, moderate, or severe; people who suffer with mild depression can usually continue with their usual pattern of life without substantial impairment, moderate depression impairs but usually does not completely prevent an individual's usual routine. Those suffering with severe depression will have experienced a very marked change in their pattern of life. Presentationally, the three key features of depression are low mood, an inability to enjoy life, and pervasive feelings of tiredness/fatigue. Associated features include disturbance of sleep, appetite and concentration, negative views of the future, lowered self-esteem, feelings of worthlessness, and thoughts of self-harm. Because suffers of depression find it difficult, or embarrassing, to discuss their emotions, it is not uncommon for patients to present with various physical complaints such as fatigue, pain, or anxiety. Depression may also be triggered by physical disorders where it may pass undetected, yet nevertheless can be a major obstacle to recovery. Direct questioning may identify the classic signs of depression. Symptoms may develop insidiously and it may only be with hindsight that an underperforming employee is recognized as suffering from a depressive disorder. Predictors of long-term outcome include pre-morbid personality, the presence of ongoing stressors, and the presence of comorbid disorders, particularly substance misuse.

There are a number of effective treatments for depression including antidepressant medications and a number of psychotherapies such as CBT, interpersonal therapy, or behavioural activation. Many depressed patients also are helped by non-specific interventions which help them adjust their lifestyle and minimize the impact of any major psychosocial stressors. The prospect of work can be intimidating for many depressed patients who may lack confidence and motivation; moreover many perceive their employment (rightly or wrongly) as contributory to their disorder. However, a successful (most likely graded) return to work package can assist recovery through bolstering self-esteem and improving social contacts.

Post-traumatic disorders including post-traumatic stress disorder

The majority of people who are exposed to traumatic events do well and recover without formal assistance from health professionals. However, a minority will be at risk of developing more persistent disorders including PTSD (and depression, other anxiety disorders, or substance misuse). PTSD is a persistent psychiatric condition which occurs in people who have been directly involved in, or witnessed, a traumatic event. People who suffer from PTSD report re-experiencing symptoms, avoidance symptoms and arousal symptoms (see Box 7.1). It is quite normal to report some post-traumatic stress symptoms after exposure to potentially traumatic events; most symptoms resolve spontaneously. In a minority these symptoms fail to improve or deteriorate and individuals may go on to develop a post-traumatic disorder (PTD).

PTSD should not be diagnosed until the symptoms have been present for at least 1 month; most people who develop PTSD will do so within 6 months of the potentially traumatic event.

Box 7.1 Major symptom clusters of post-traumatic stress disorder

Following exposure to a significant traumatic event which is associated with helplessness, horror or fear, the individual reports:

At least one re-experiencing symptom:

1 Recurrent and intrusive distressing recollections of the event, including images, thoughts, or perceptions (in young children, repetitive play may occur in which themes or aspects of the trauma are expressed).

2 Recurrent distressing dreams of the event (in children, there may be frightening dreams without recognizable content).

3 Acting or feeling as if the traumatic event were recurring includes a sense of reliving the experience, illusions, hallucinations, and 'flashbacks' (in young children, trauma-specific re-enactment may occur).

4 Intense psychological distress at exposure to internal or external cues that symbolize or resemble an aspect of the traumatic event.

5 Physiological reactivity on exposure to internal or external cues that symbolize or resemble an aspect of the traumatic event.

At least three symptoms of persistent avoidance of trauma-related stimuli and/or a new onset of numbing of general responsiveness:

1 Efforts to avoid thoughts, feelings, or conversations associated with the trauma.

2 Efforts to avoid activities, places, or people that arouse recollections of the trauma.

3 Inability to recall an important aspect of the trauma.

4 Markedly diminished interest or participation in significant activities.

5 Feeling of detachment or estrangement from others.

6 Restricted range of affect (e.g. unable to have loving feelings).

7 Sense of a foreshortened future (e.g. does not expect to have a career, marriage, children, or a normal life span).

> **Box 7.1 Major symptom clusters of post-traumatic stress disorder** *(continued)*
>
> ## At least two or more new-onset persistent symptoms of increased arousal:
>
> 1 Difficulty falling or staying asleep.
> 2 Irritability or outbursts of anger.
> 3 Difficulty concentrating.
> 4 Hypervigilance.
> 5 Exaggerated startle response.
>
> And:
>
> Symptoms last for more than 1 month and cause clinically significant distress or impairment in social, occupational, or other important areas of functioning.

PTD, (including PTSD) is of particular interest to employers, not least because the traumatic event may have been the result of exposure to occupational factors and be the subject of future litigation. As such, a proactive employer, especially if operating in high-threat environments, may consider how best to prevent PTSD in employees who have been exposed to a potentially traumatic incident. Historically, the use of single-session critical incident stress debriefing or psychological debriefing was popular but randomized controlled trials have failed to demonstrate any benefit for single-session psychologically focused debriefings[20] which have actually been found to cause harm in some cases. However, more recent, less psychologically focused interventions delivered within an organization by appropriately trained non-mental health professionals (such as the peer support programme TRiM (trauma risk management) developed in the UK Armed Forces) have shown promise and are now routinely used in military services, emergency services, and other organizations which routinely deploy personnel to high-threat environments.[32] Such programmes may help mobilize informal social support for those at increased risk of developing a PTD and help ensure that the minority who need professional interventions are treated. Other interventions which organizations might consider using include post-incident education[33] and formal post-incident mental health, both of which have been found of limited effectiveness or even harmful.[34] At times, the treatment of PTDs can be complicated by litigation and it is noteworthy that lengthy legal proceedings and repeated examinations for legal reports are often unhelpful and can impede recovery. Whilst the symptoms of PTSD typically fluctuate and may deteriorate on anniversaries and following reminders of traumatic events, from an occupational health perspective it is important to encourage a timely return to a supportive workplace, to ensure that suffers get evidence-based treatments and avoid potentially harmful interventions (such as single session debriefings).

Chronic fatigue syndrome

The term chronic fatigue syndrome (CFS) describes a heterogeneous group of disorders of varying severity all characterized by reduced energy levels, varying degrees of fatigue, and a variety of other somatic and psychological symptoms. Fatigue by itself is a common symptom and is a feature of a wide range of physical and psychiatric disorders; most fatigue is not a result of CFS. CFS, in the UK, may affect up to about 0.4 per cent of the population and according to the NICE guidelines about half of those who meet the diagnostic criteria are likely to need specialist services. There are several definitions of CFS, but the NICE guidelines suggest that a diagnosis of CFS should be considered in someone who presents with fatigue which has a specific onset and has lasted for at least 4 months (that is, it is not lifelong), is persistent and/or recurrent, is unexplained by other conditions, and has resulted in a substantial reduction in activity level. This is characterized by post-exertional malaise and/or fatigue (typically delayed, for example, by at least 24 hours, with slow recovery over several days) and is associated with one or more additional symptoms such as sleep problems (including hypersomnia and a disturbed sleep–wake cycle), muscle and/or joint pain that is multisite, and without evidence of inflammation, headaches, painful lymph nodes without pathological enlargement, sore throat, and cognitive complaints such as difficulty thinking, inability to concentrate, impairment of short-term memory, and difficulties with word-finding, planning/organizing thoughts, and information processing. Some people who have CFS also report frequently experiencing 'flu-like' symptoms, dizziness and/or nausea, and palpitations in the absence of identified cardiac pathology. It is important to ensure that patients have been adequately investigated to exclude occult underlying physical pathology, particularly where there is associated weight loss, any other unexplained physical signs or a history of foreign travel.

It is worth noting that the terms used to describe the syndrome vary and sometimes the term post-viral fatigue or myalgic encephalitis (ME) may be used when the onset of fatigue appears to follow a specific trigger such as a viral illness. Many people who suffer with CFS have developed their own ideas about what led to their problem and have often tried numerous 'alternative' treatments which they have found to be useful in the short term.

There are a number of evidence-based interventions which have been shown to be effective in this condition including graded exercise and cognitive behavioural psychotherapy; it is perhaps noteworthy to mention that whilst the use of antidepressants for comorbid depression may well be justified, these medications are not helpful for the treatment of CFS per se. When assessing future employability it is important to ensure that every patient has a clear management plan with the expectation of recovery. Lack of motivation can be a problem for the treating physician as well as the patient and it is important to avoid 'therapeutic nihilism' when recovery does not occur rapidly.

Discussions about ill health retirement should not take place until all reasonable treatment options have been tried; this may take a number of years in more complex cases.

Chronic mixed anxiety and depression

Low mood, sadness, and anxiety are occasional features of normal life. Many individuals experience symptoms severe enough to impair normal daily activities but which are insufficient to meet diagnostic criteria for either a depressive episode or other anxiety disorders. They are described and classified using various terms such as dysthymia (a persistent mood disorder characterized by long-standing feelings of being sad, 'blue', low, 'down in the dumps', and little interest or pleasure in usual activities) or with the diagnostic term mixed anxiety and depression. People who suffer with low-grade mood symptoms (which may include some people who suffer from adjustment disorders or mild depression) tend to be considered as grumpy or persistent complainers and their presence in a workplace may negatively affect the well-being of colleagues. Whilst it is important not to miss a treatable mental health disorder, occupational physicians should be careful not to 'medicalise' mild symptoms. Instead, good management and taking a pragmatic approach to handling such individuals (who may be highly productive whilst they grumble) can be more useful. Medication is of uncertain value in more minor disorders and if used should be started as a trial and continued only if of clear benefit. Supportive counselling may be useful if people with these conditions do not have adequate social networks but people who suffer with less serious mood problems need to retain full responsibility for their own recovery. Brief cognitive approaches challenging unfounded worries and challenging negative assumptions, problem-solving approaches, and relaxation techniques may also be useful in some cases. There are a variety of computerized CBT packages which may also be helpful (e.g. <http://www.livinglifetothefull.com>) Motivation on the part of the individual, and their employers, and the willingness to accept responsibility for this is probably one of the best predictors of a successful outcome.

Bipolar affective disorder (also known as manic depression)

This disorder, along with schizophrenia, is often termed a serious mental illness (SMI). Bipolar affective disorder is characterized by episodes of depression, mania, or an admixture of both. Mixed affective states are common and mood, disordered thought (including flight of ideas—which is where the topic of conversation jumps in a non-predictable way), motor behaviour (overactivity or retardation), arousal (irritability or withdrawal), perceptual abnormalities (including mood congruous delusions or hallucinations—that is to say bizarre beliefs or perceptions in the absence of a stimulus which are in keeping with the presenting mood), or behavioural disturbances (retardation or disinhibition) may fluctuate and vary independently of each other. Patients may manifest predominantly depressive or manic symptoms (often depressive presentations are more common with age) and presentations may change over time. Although full recovery from major mood swings is the norm (often as a result of medical and social management) many patients display lesser degrees of emotional instability requiring treatment between episodes.

Factors to be considered in assessing the employability of bipolar patients include frequency of relapse, functional capacity during periods of well-being (remissions), and adherence to any long-term treatment plan, particularly their compliance with mood-stabilizing medication. Comorbid substance misuse during episodes is generally a poor prognostic sign. Disturbed sleep and sleep deprivation are important triggers for episodes of mania and shift work or work involving long-distance air travel may be unsuitable for individuals with bipolar disorders. Whilst, when well, there may be a wide range of roles available for well-controlled individuals who suffer with this condition, suitability for safety critical roles should be considered very carefully.

Schizophrenia

Schizophrenia is usually a chronic serious mental health condition that causes a range of different psychological symptoms. These include hallucinations (experiencing perceptions in the absence of a stimulus), delusions (unusual beliefs that are not based on reality and often contradict the evidence for them), and muddled thoughts based on the hallucinations or delusions with associated (usually negative) changes in behaviour. Schizophrenia is a psychotic illness in which sufferers may not be able to distinguish their own delusions from reality. The exact cause of schizophrenia is unknown. However, it is most probably a result of a combination of genetic, environmental, and neurochemical factors.

Schizophrenia is one of the most common serious mental health conditions, although less than 1 per cent of the population probably suffer from the condition; men and women are equally affected. In men, schizophrenia usually begins between the ages of 15 and 30. In women, schizophrenia usually occurs later, beginning between the ages of 25 and 30. Contrary to statements made in the lay press, the risk of violence from someone who suffers with schizophrenia is small; violent crime is more likely to be linked to alcohol or other substance misuse than to schizophrenia. A person with schizophrenia is far more likely to be the victim of violent crime than the instigator.

From an occupational viewpoint, people who suffer with chronic schizophrenia (about one-third of cases may recover completely) are likely to find highly demanding work far more challenging than people who do not suffer with the condition; stress may be one of the reasons why someone who suffers from well-controlled schizophrenia relapses. However, with good support, an understanding employer and good liaison between occupational health professionals and specialists, there is no reason why people who suffer with schizophrenia cannot be highly effective employees when they are in remission. Specialists may be able to help employers understand the 'relapse signature' for the condition which is often unique to that individual. For instance, it might be that before relapsing, someone who suffers from schizophrenia become less socially integrated, spends more time mumbling to themselves, and begins to wear strange combinations of clothes at work; an employer who was aware of the implications of the changes in behaviour would be able to assist the relapsing employee to seek help before they become floridly unwell.

Acute psychotic disorders

All psychotic disorders are SMIs, not all are enduring. Whilst a first episode of a psychotic condition may be the initial presentation of what will become a chronic schizophrenia or bipolar affective disorder, some psychoses are transient and can occur as a result of extreme stress or be brought about by illicit drug use. People who are suffering with an acute psychotic disorder for any reason are highly unlikely to be suitable for work; active psychosis may lead to unpredictable behaviour and whilst the exact nature of the psychosis is being determined observation is often the best occupational health strategy.

Personality disorders

Personality disorders are maladaptive patterns of behaviour which manifest in late adolescence or early adult life, endure, cause difficulties for the person themselves and/or those around them, and represent the extreme ends of the normal spectrum of personality. Estimates of the prevalence of personality disorders vary from as low as 10 per cent in the general population or up to 40 per cent (or more) in prison settings. Whilst there are many different types of personality disorder, the term should not be used loosely and diagnosis should only follow a high-quality assessment by an appropriately experienced mental health professional. The impact of personality disorder within the workplace also varies and extreme personality traits may be highly adaptive in some environments (e.g. obsessionality as a trait in a quality assurance professional) but less so in others (obsessional individuals working in organizations undergoing significant changes). From an occupational health perspective, employees who suffer from a personality disorder are likely to be highly susceptible to pressure within the workplace (or from other sources) and their enduring personality traits may cause considerable difficulty amongst those who have to work with them. Treatment of these disorders is possible in some cases, (usually through a psychotherapeutic process), but is often lengthy and within the workplace, they are likely to benefit especially from a patient and sensitive line manager.

Conclusions

All employers should have plans in place to optimize the well-being of their employees and to manage mental health conditions as they arise. Being one of the commonest ailments to affect employees and their performance at work, a proactive and evidence-based approach makes economic sense for the employer seeking to attract, motivate, and retain a talented workforce.

The health adviser to the employer has a significant role to play in each of the strategic pillars that positively influence outcomes for employee and employer.

At the primary prevention level: have the risks to mental health from the context and content of work been reasonably assessed and addressed? At the secondary prevention level: are employees and their managers equipped and have time to recognize the signs of mental ill health at work, and guide their employees in the direction of support? At the tertiary level: are the processes in place to accommodate those returning to the workplace after mental health problems, and are co-workers and managers equipped to receive them, and are timely evidence-based interventions readily available? A proactive employer, who takes care to ensure that all levels of prevention are catered for, is likely to reap the productivity, as well as the moral, dividends from doing so.

References

1 Waddell G, Burton AK. *Is work good for your health and well-being?* London: TSO, 2006.

2 Health, Work and Well-being Strategy Unit. *Health, work and well-being: baseline indicators report*, 2010. (<http://www.dwp.gov.uk/docs/hwwb-baseline-indicators.pdf>)

3 Meltzer H, Gill B, Petticrew M. *OPCS surveys of psychiatric morbidity in Great Britain, bulletin no.1: The prevalence of psychiatric morbidity among adults aged 16-64, living in private households, in Great Britain.* London: OPCS, 1994.

4 McManus S, Meltzer H, Brugha T, *et al. Adult psychiatric morbidity in England, 2007: results of a household survey.* London: National Centre for Social Research, 2009.

5 Young V, Bhaumik C. *Health and wellbeing at work: a survey of employees.* Research report 751. London: Department for Work and Pensions, 2011. (<http://research.dwp.gov.uk/asd/asd5/rports2011-2/rrep751.pdf>)

6 Lelliott P, Tulloch S, Boardman J, *et al. Mental health and work.* London: Royal College of Psychiatrists, 2008. (<http://www.dwp.gov.uk/docs/hwwb-mental-health-and-work.pdf>)

7 Meltzer H, Gill B, Petticrew M, *et al. Economic activity and social functioning of adults with psychiatric disorders. OPCS surveys of psychiatric morbidity in Great Britain.* Report No. 3. London: HMSO, 1995.

8 Patel A, Knapp M. Costs of mental illness in England. *Ment Health Res Rev* 1998; **6**: 4–10.

9 Iversen AC, Fear NT, Ehlers A, *et al.* Risk factors for post-traumatic stress disorder among UK Armed Forces personnel. *Psychol Med* 2008; **29**: 1–12.

10 Mulligan K, Jones N, Woodhead C, *et al.* Mental health of UK military personnel while on deployment in Iraq. *Br J Psychiatry* 2010; **197**: 405–10.

11 Turpin G, Downs M, Mason S. Effectiveness of providing self-help information following acute traumatic injury: randomized controlled trial. *Br J Psychiatry* 2005; **187**: 76–82.

12 Woodhead C, Rona RJ, Iversen A, *et al.* Mental health and health service use among post-national service veterans: results from the 2007 Adult Psychiatric Morbidity Survey of England. *Psychol Med* 2011; **41**(2): 363–72.

13 Mausner-Dorsch H, Eaton WW. Psychosocial work environment and depression epidemiologic assessment of the demand-control model. *Am J Public Health* 2000; **90**(11): 1765–70.

14 Health and Safety Executive. *Working together to reduce stress at work: a guide for employees.* London: HSE, 2008.

15 Van Vegche N, De Jonge J, Bosma H, *et al.* Reviewing the effort-reward imbalance model: drawing up the balance of 45 empirical studies. *Soc Sci Med* 2005; **60**(5): 1117–31.

16 Wang J. Perceived barriers to mental health service use among individuals with mental disorders in the Canadian general population. *Med Care* 2006; **44**: 192–5.

17 Levenson RL Jr, Dwyer LA. Peer support in law enforcement: Past, present, and future. *Int J Emerg Ment Health* 2003; **5**: 147–52.

18 Greenberg N. Managing traumatic stress at work. An organisational approach to the management of potentially traumatic events. *Occup Health Work* 2011; 7(5): 22–6.

19 Greenberg N, Langston V, Iversen AC, *et al*. The acceptability of trauma risk management within the UK armed forces. *Occup Med* 2011; **61**(3): 184–9.

20 National Institute for Clinical Excellence. *Post-traumatic stress disorder (PTSD): the management of PTSD in adults and children in primary and secondary care*. London: NICE, 2005.

21 Raffle AE, Muir Gray JA. *Screening: evidence and practice*. Oxford: University Oxford Press, 2007.

22 Oliver M. *The politics of disablement*. Basingstoke: Macmillan, 1990.

23 Schneider J. Work interventions in mental care: some arguments and recent evidence. *J Ment Health* 1998; **7**: 81–94.

24 Bartley M. Unemployment and ill-health: understanding the relationships. *J Epidemiol Community Health* 1994; **48**: 333–7.

25 Warr P. *Work, unemployment and mental health*. Oxford: Oxford University Press, 1987.

26 Warner R. *Recovery from schizophrenia. Psychiatry and political economy*, 2nd edn. London: Routledge, 1994.

27 Crowther RE, Marshall M. Employment rehabilitation schemes for people with mental health problems in the North West region: service characteristics and utilisation. *J Ment Health* 2001; **10**: 373–82.

28 Grove B, Drurie S. *Social firms—an instrument for economic improvement and inclusion*. Redhill: Social Firms UK, 1999.

29 Crowther RE, Marshall M, Bond GR, *et al*. Helping people with severe mental illness to obtain work: systematic review. *BMJ* 2001; **322**: 204–8.

30 Becker DR, Drake RE, Concord NH. Individual placement and support: a community mental health centre approach to rehabilitation. *Community Ment Health J* 1994; **30**: 193–206.

31 Perkins RE, Buckfield R, Choy D. Access to employment. *J Ment Health* 1997; **6**: 307–18.

32 Greenberg N, Langston V, Everitt B, *et al*. A cluster randomized controlled trial to determine the efficacy of trauma risk management (TRiM) in a military population. *J Trauma Stress* 2010; **23**(4): 430–6.

33 Mulligan K, Fear NT, Jones N, *et al*. Psycho-educational interventions designed to prevent deployment-related psychological ill-health in armed forces personnel: a review. *Psychol Med* 2010; **16**: 1–14.

34 Rona RJ, Hooper R, Jones M, *et al*. Would mental health screening of the UK Armed Forces before the Iraq war have prevented subsequent psychological morbidity? A follow up study. *BMJ* 2006; **333**: 991–4.

Chapter 8

Epilepsy

Ian Brown and Martin C. Prevett

Introduction

Epilepsy is a common condition that affects large numbers of working people. In about one-third, epilepsy is the only condition, and in others there are additional neurological, intellectual, or psychological problems. Uncontrolled epileptic seizures can lead to injury and may impact on education and employment, but antiepileptic drug (AED) treatment is effective in approximately 70 per cent of people with epilepsy.

Definitions

Epileptic seizures

Epileptic seizures are the clinical manifestation of an abnormal excessive discharge of cerebral neurons and may involve transient alteration of consciousness and, motor, sensory, autonomic, or psychic phenomena. Epileptic seizures are caused by a wide variety of cerebral and systemic disorders, and may be *provoked* (acute symptomatic seizures) or *unprovoked*.

 ◆ Provoked or acute symptomatic seizures occur during an acute cerebral or systemic illness and do not constitute a diagnosis of epilepsy.

 ◆ Unprovoked seizures may be the late consequence of an antecedent cerebral disorder such as meningitis, head injury, and stroke (remote symptomatic seizures), or there may be no clear antecedent aetiology.

Epilepsy

Epilepsy is defined by a tendency to recurrent unprovoked epileptic seizures.

Classification of epilepsy

The international classification of epilepsies and epileptic syndromes[1] incorporates anatomical, aetiological, and syndromic features, but includes many rare syndromes and can be difficult to apply to clinical practice. Another more commonly used approach is to classify epilepsy by seizure type (Table 8.1). In the classification of seizures proposed by the International League Against Epilepsy (ILAE) in 1981, seizures were divided into two main categories: partial and generalized.[2] Partial seizures were subdivided into simple partial, complex partial, and secondarily generalized seizures. Distinguishing between simple and complex partial seizures was sometimes difficult and the term 'secondarily generalized' was used inconsistently. In the revised 2010 ILAE classification, seizures are divided into focal and generalized, but focal seizures are not subdivided.[1]

Table 8.1 Classification by seizure type

I	**Generalized seizures**
	Tonic–clonic
	Absence
	Myoclonic
	Atonic
	Tonic
	Clonic
II	**Focal seizures**

Adapted with permission from Berg *et al.*, Revised terminology and concepts for organization of seizures and epilepsies: Report of the ILAE Commission on Classification and Terminology, 2005–2009, Epilepsia, Volume 51, Issue 4, pp. 676–685, April 2010, Wiley Periodicals, Inc., Copyright © 2010 International League Against Epilepsy.

Focal seizures

In focal seizures the abnormal neuronal discharge starts in a localized area of the brain. Clinical manifestations vary widely depending on anatomical localization and spread of neuronal discharge. As there is no agreed subclassification, the clinical features should be described. Focal seizures may occur with or without impairment of consciousness and may evolve into a bilateral convulsive seizure.

Generalized seizures

In generalized seizures the abnormal neuronal discharge is widespread and involves both cerebral hemispheres from the onset. Generalized tonic–clonic (*grand mal*), absence (*petit mal*), and myoclonic seizures are the commonest types of generalized seizure in people without other neurological or learning problems. Tonic, atonic, and clonic seizures tend to occur in people with diffuse cerebral disorders associated with learning disability. In all generalized seizures there is abrupt onset without any warning or aura.

Incidence and prevalence

A British study of treated epilepsy showed an incidence rate of 81 (95 per cent confidence interval (CI) 77–85) per 100 000 per year.[3] Between the age of 16 and 65 years, new cases of treated epilepsy occurred at a rate of approximately 75 per 100 000 per year. The lifetime risk of having a seizure is estimated to be 2–5 per cent.

The prevalence of treated epilepsy in England and Wales in 1995 was estimated to be 5.15 cases per 1000.[3] The National General Practice Study of Epilepsy (NGPSE) found that 52 per cent of patients had focal seizures and 39 per cent had generalized seizures. Tonic–clonic seizures were the most common form of generalized seizure, other types being rare. Overall tonic–clonic seizures (either generalized or of focal onset) occurred in 62 per cent of patients.[4] Seizure frequency varies enormously between individuals with about a third experiencing less than one seizure per year and about 20 per cent more than one per week.

Causes of epilepsy

A cause can be confidently established only in a minority of new cases of epilepsy (20–40 per cent). The most common causes of epileptic seizures in adults are listed in Table 8.2. The proportion of patients in whom a cause is identified depends on the extent of investigation, particularly neuroimaging (computed tomography or magnetic resonance imaging (MRI)). Advances in MRI technology have allowed identification of more subtle structural causes, such as disorders of cortical development. Among patients with drug-resistant epilepsy, detailed MRI can detect a potential cause in up to 75 per cent.[5]

The proportion of patients with symptomatic epilepsy increases with age. In the NGPSE, cerebrovascular disease was the most common aetiological factor in 15 per cent (49 per cent in patients over the age of 60 years), 6 per cent of seizures were attributed to a cerebral tumour, 3 per cent to trauma, 2 per cent to infection, and 7 per cent to other causes.[4]

Toxic causes of epilepsy are rare. Seizures may very occasionally occur as a result of lead encephalopathy, almost always in children. Seizures have occurred in employees overexposed during the manufacture of chlorinated hydrocarbons, and ingestion of or gross overexposure to organochlorine insecticides, (dichlorodiphenyltrichloroethane or DDT), has resulted in status epilepticus.[6] DDT is known to interfere with potassium, sodium, and calcium transport across the neuronal membrane, leading to repetitive discharges in neurons and tremors, seizures, and electrical activity triggered by tactile and auditory stimuli. Epileptiform abnormalities on electro-encephalography (EEG) have been recorded in asymptomatic individuals exposed to methylene chloride, methyl bromide, carbon disulphide, benzene, and styrene, although the significance of these observations is uncertain.

Recurrence of seizures

Estimates of recurrence rates after a first seizure have varied from 27 per cent to 84 per cent, the variation reflecting selection bias in the study population.[7] Aetiology has an important influence on the risk of recurrence. In the NGPSE, seizures associated with neurological deficits presumed to be present from birth had a 100 per cent rate of relapse within the first 12 months, whereas seizures associated with a lesion acquired postnatally carried a risk of relapse of 75 per cent by 12 months.[8] The presence of generalized spike and wave activity on EEG also appears to increase the risk of recurrence.

Table 8.2 Common causes of adult onset epileptic seizures

Cerebrovascular disease
Head injury (and neurosurgery)
Cerebral tumour
Vascular malformation (cavernoma, arteriovenous malformation)
Disorders of cortical development
Perinatal injury and hypoxia
Central nervous system infection (meningitis, encephalitis, cerebral abscess)
Genetic
Degenerative disorders (e.g. Alzheimer's disease)

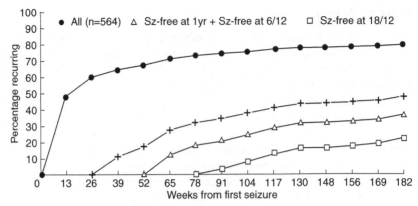

Figure 8.1 Actuarial percentage recurrence rates after a first seizure for those still free of recurrence at 6, 12, and 18 months, and for all patients.[8] Reprinted from *The Lancet*, Vol. 336, Issue 8726, Hart YM *et al.*, National General Practice Study of Epilepsy: recurrence after a first seizure, pp. 1271–74, Copyright ©1990, with permission from Elsevier.

The risk of recurrence decreases as time elapses after the first seizure, a fact that is of importance in resolving concerns about safety at work. In the NGPSE (in which only 15 per cent of patients with a first seizure received treatment), the 3-year risk of recurrence after a seizure-free period of 6 months was 44 per cent, after 12 months seizure-free the risk was 32 per cent, and after 18 months seizure-free the risk fell to 17 per cent (Figure 8.1).

Randomized studies have shown that the risk of recurrence after a first seizure is reduced by AED treatment.[9,10] Patients started on treatment after a first seizure are, however, no more likely to achieve remission than patients in whom treatment is delayed until after two or more seizures, and Bonnett et al. undertook a further analysis of the multicentre study of early epilepsy and single seizures and concluded that at 6 months after the index seizure, (for those taking AEDs), the risk of recurrence in the next 12 months was 14 per cent (95 per cent CI 10–18 per cent). For those patients that did not start AED treatment, the risk estimate was 18 per cent (95 per cent CI 13–23 per cent). These data have resulted in a change to the driving restrictions after a first seizure (see 'Lifting of restrictions').

Chances of remission

Although there is a modest and measurable risk of recurrence after a first seizure, most people developing epilepsy become seizure-free. In the NGPSE, if patients with single or provoked seizures are excluded, 62 per cent achieved a 5-year remission after 9 years of follow-up.[11] In another population-based study, the 5-year remission rates were 65 per cent at 10 years and 76 per cent at 15 years.[12] Most patients who enter remission do so within 2 years of diagnosis and, as time elapses without seizure control, the chances of subsequent remission decreases. Age and seizure type do not appear to influence the chances of remission significantly but a syndromic classification can be useful prognostically. Benign rolandic epilepsy (benign epilepsy with centrotemporal spikes) develops in childhood and spontaneous remission occurs in 98–99 per cent of cases by age 14 years. Juvenile myoclonic epilepsy, however, develops in adolescence and although responsive to treatment, is associated with a lifelong disposition to seizures—over 90 per cent of patients will relapse if treatment is withdrawn.

Twenty to 30 per cent of patients continue to experience seizures despite drug treatment.[13] The introduction of more than ten new therapies since 1990 has had little impact on this figure. There is no evidence that the newer drugs are any more effective than standard treatment and a poor response to initial treatment with any drug appropriate to the type of epilepsy, whether standard or new, tends to predict a poor response to other drugs. A recent prospective study found that among previously untreated patients, 47 per cent became seizure-free with their first AED and 14 per cent became seizure-free during treatment with a second or third drug.[14] In only 3 per cent was the epilepsy controlled by a combination of two drugs.

Withdrawal of antiepileptic drug treatment

For those patients who go into remission and remain seizure-free for 2 years or more, withdrawal of treatment is an option. The risk of relapse in this group is 30 per cent (95 per cent CI 25–30 per cent) in the first 12 months after discontinuing treatment.[15] Given the implications of relapse for work and driving, most patients elect to continue treatment indefinitely.

Prevention of epilepsy in the workplace

Primary and secondary prevention

In the workplace, avoidance of head injuries through risk assessment and implementation of appropriate controls is the most important preventive measure. The use of seat belts and safety helmets is important. Where there is a risk of falling objects, netting can be rigged below the work area, warnings given for those in the vicinity, and wearing of hard hats made compulsory. However, a safety helmet will not protect an individual from serious head injury if anything heavy is dropped from a height. The other main preventive measure is the avoidance of precipitating factors, some of which are described next.

Epilepsy does not follow a trivial head injury; if the head injury is associated with a depressed fracture (especially if the dura is torn), an intracranial haematoma, or focal neurological signs, then there is a significant risk of later epilepsy.

A large community survey of a head-injured population[16] confirmed findings by previous workers that the risk of early seizures (within 7 days of injury) and late seizures (7 days or more days after injury) can be determined by assessing the severity of the brain injury. Severe head injuries (loss of consciousness, amnesia lasting more than 24 hours, subdural haematoma, and brain contusion), are accompanied by a substantially increased risk of epilepsy over the next decade (standardized incidence ratio 17.0, 95 per cent CI 12.3–23.6). Because of this risk, patients who have suffered a serious head injury should be treated in a similar way to those that have already suffered a convulsion, including a 6–12-month ban on driving. The use of antiepileptic medication does not affect the risk of developing post-traumatic epilepsy but it does reduce the frequency of early seizures.[17]

Shift work

Seizures are common just before and after waking, especially in idiopathic generalized epilepsy, so it might be supposed that the introduction of a shift system into the work programme of a person with well-controlled epilepsy would predispose them to an increased frequency of seizures. This has not been documented, possibly because people with epilepsy elect to avoid shift work.[18] Many people with well-controlled epilepsy, however, can work on rotating shifts without problems.

Night work may be an exception. Patterns of sleep are disturbed by night work and to a lesser extent by other types of shift work. Night workers sleep for shorter periods during their working week and sleep longer on rest days to make up the deficit.[19] Sleep deprivation is an important precipitant of seizures for some individuals and is best avoided by those with idiopathic generalized epilepsy.

Stress

Stress is a frequently self-reported precipitant of seizures in patients with epilepsy. Changes in brain arousal lead to changes in excitability and this may affect neuronal discharges, particularly of those neurons that surround an epileptic focus. Many patients report that the frequency of their seizures increase when they are exposed to stress, but stress itself may also be associated with other seizure-provoking factors such as drinking alcohol and sleep disturbance and there may be reporting bias as people search for an explanation for exacerbations of their condition. Stress mediators (corticosteroids, neurosteroids, etc.) probably contribute to this phenomenon.[19,20]

Paradoxically, inactivity and drowsiness may also be related to an increased seizure frequency. The possibility that stress and its associated factors may affect seizure control should be considered when employees with epilepsy are moved to different areas of responsibility.

Photosensitivity and visual display equipment

Photosensitivity epilepsy is a form of reflex epilepsy which is rare in adults and usually associated with idiopathic generalized epilepsy. It may need to be considered where a light source flickers. The overall prevalence is 1 in 10, 000 and more common in women; 90 per cent of patients have suffered their first convulsion due to photosensitivity before the age of 25 years.[21-23] Photosensitivity may be increased following deprivation of sleep. Spontaneous seizures may also occur in photosensitive subjects.

The diagnosis of photosensitive epilepsy is supported by performing an EEG recording with photic stimulation eliciting a photoparoxysmal response. This is usually a generalized discharge of spike wave activity elicited by the flickering stimulus and persisting after the stimulus has ceased. False-positive tests can also arise: some individuals have a paroxysmal EEG response to photic stimulation without evidence of having had a seizure.[21-23] Now obsolete electron gun televisions were a precipitant of photosensitive epilepsy. Proximity to the screen was an important factor, as this enabled the viewer to discriminate the line pattern; most television-sensitive patients reveal their sensitivity at a viewing distance of 1 metre or less. Light emitting diode (LED) and plasma screen televisions do not present the same risk. The use of display screen equipment (DSE) in employment constitutes a much smaller risk than that incurred when viewing television. The probability of a first convulsion being induced by DSE is exceedingly small; seizures are unlikely even in an established photosensitive subject. Sufferers of epilepsy are therefore fit to work with DSE unless there is a clear history of photosensitization necessitating further assessment.

Other precipitants include flickering sunlight (e.g. through the leaves of a tree or when swimming), faulty and flickering artificial lights, and helicopter rotor blades and aeroplane propellers.

The Civil Aviation Authority (CAA) has recognized the special risks that may be associated with flying, especially from the slow flicker visible through helicopter blades. The CAA performed an EEG investigation as part of its routine medical screen on helicopter pilots applying for commercial licences. This is now required in the UK for professional fixed-wing aircraft pilots following the harmonization of aviation medical standards throughout the European Union and another 12 states (the Joint Aviation Authorities (JAA)). Introduced on 1 July 1999, it is a mandatory investigation for all professional pilots on initial examination. No requirement exists for the investigation to be repeated, other than when indicated clinically. For fixed-wing aircraft the risk of epilepsy is negligible. Nonetheless, European harmonization requires it.

Other types of reflex epilepsy

Although reflex epilepsy may occasionally be induced by reading, concentrating, being suddenly startled, or auditory stimuli, this is rare.

Alcohol and drugs

Alcohol misuse increases the risk of epileptic seizures. Seizures may be caused by alcohol withdrawal, a direct toxic effect of alcohol, or associated metabolic disturbance, e.g. hypoglycaemia. Seizures may also occur with chronic alcohol misuse in the absence of withdrawal or other identifiable cause. Alcohol misuse may complicate established epilepsy increasing the risk of seizures and other complications.

A number of drugs lower seizure threshold, especially tricyclic antidepressants but also isoniazid, penicillin, lignocaine, and antipsychotics such as chlorpromazine and haloperidol. Some of the newer antipsychotic drugs, notably olanzapine, are associated with epileptiform abnormalities on EEG.

Fluctuating serum levels of AEDs, which may arise from poor adherence to treatment or interactions with other drugs, increase the risk of seizures. Sudden withdrawal of AEDs, especially phenobarbitone and benzodiazepines, may also result in seizures (see Box 8.1).

Box 8.1 What to do if a seizure occurs

If a seizure is likely to occur at work, supervisors and workplace colleagues should be warned and instructed in appropriate first-aid measures. Convulsive seizures are almost always short-lived and do not require immediate medical treatment:

- The person should be made as comfortable as possible, preferably lying down (eased to the floor if seated).
- The head should be cushioned and any tight clothing or neckwear loosened.
- The patient should remain attended until recovery is complete.
- During the attack, the patient should not be moved, unless they are in a dangerous place—in a road, by a fire or hot radiator, at the top of stairs, or by the edge of water, for instance.
- No attempt should be made to open the mouth or force anything between the teeth.
- After the seizure has subsided the person should be rolled on to their side, making sure that the airways are cleared of any obstruction, such as dentures or vomit, and that there are no injuries that require medical attention.
- When the patient recovers consciousness there is often a short period of confusion and distress. They should be comforted, reassured, and allowed to rest.
- An ambulance or hospital treatment is not required unless there is a serious injury, the seizure has lasted more than 5 minutes,[24] the person has had a series of seizures without recovering consciousness between them, or the seizure has features which differ significantly from the patient's usual pattern.

The Epilepsy Action website (<http://www.epilepsy.org.uk>) provides excellent practical advice for those with epilepsy on many aspects of employment. They also produce a card that provides details about an individual's epilepsy and advice about what to do if the person is found unconscious.

Responsibility of the physician in the workplace

The first task is to establish without doubt that a seizure has occurred. The employee should attend the occupational health department as soon as possible and remain off work in the interim. A detailed history of the event should be obtained and information sought from the patient and any reliable witness to try to establish the nature of the event. Interviewing work colleagues and relatives who witnessed the event can be extremely useful, as the subject usually remembers little beyond the first few seconds. It is unwise to rely solely on the patient's account, written reports from witnesses, or second-hand anecdotal information.

The past medical history may reveal risk factors for the development of epilepsy, such as febrile seizures in childhood, previous significant head injury, or stroke. Relevant points about the family history and consumption of drugs or alcohol should also be obtained. The patient should always be fully examined, as a seizure may occasionally be the first symptom of a serious systemic illness such as meningitis, or of a structural cerebral lesion—detailed medical assessment is always necessary.

Permission to contact both the general practitioner and any hospital consultant should be obtained from the patient. It is often useful to contact these physicians informally and discuss the situation that has arisen. This should be followed by a formal letter giving a concise account of events and the examination findings, and requesting any further relevant information (with consent).

Not all episodes of unconsciousness are epileptic seizures. The most common differential diagnoses are syncope (vasovagal or cardiac) and dissociative seizures (pseudoseizures) with an underlying psychological basis. Other possible diagnoses include transient ischaemic attacks (TIAs) and migraine.

Prolonged cerebral anoxia due to syncope may produce some stiffening, twitching, and even incontinence, although a generalized seizure (secondary anoxic seizure) is unusual. The circumstances of the event, prodromal symptoms, and rapidity of recovery will usually allow distinction between syncope and an epileptic seizure. Dissociative seizures can be very difficult to distinguish from epileptic seizures and specialist advice is usually required.

Focal ischaemia of a TIA does not usually involve a loss of consciousness but often causes neurologically deficits such as aphasia or paresis, and only rarely muscle jerking.

Once it has been established as far as possible that a single, unprovoked, seizure has occurred, the procedure listed in Box 8.2 should be adopted.

Box 8.2 Procedure following a seizure

1 The medical notes must state clearly the course of events and that a seizure has taken place.

2 The management should be contacted and given clear and concise recommendations, in writing, regarding the employee's placement. Such written recommendations should be constructed with the agreement of the employee and should observe codes of medical confidentiality. If epilepsy has been confirmed (not just a single seizure) some employees prefer to inform their immediate supervisor. It is worth discussing the possibility of such disclosure, with the patient.

Box 8.2 Procedure following a seizure *(continued)*

3   The occupational physician and occupational health nurse must become familiar with any AED prescribed and have a sound knowledge of potential side effects.

4   Consideration should be given to sensible employment restrictions. This should include advice to the individual on driving and their responsibility to inform the Driving and Vehicle Licensing Agency (DVLA; see 'The driving licence regulations and their effects').[25]

Consideration of potential new employees

The majority of jobs are suitable for those with epilepsy but job placement may require risk assessment of this. The impairment of epilepsy falls within the Equality Act 2010 even if it is medically controlled. However, precedence is given to the Health and Safety at Work Act 1974 (the HSW Act) when safety issues arise. Sufficient thought must be given to the possibility of making 'reasonable adjustments to the workplace or the job'. With epilepsy, this is nearly always possible except where there is a statutory bar (e.g. the driving of large goods vehicles). Often a safe place of work can be found for an employee, unless the hazard and risk is an integral part of the job (e.g. working as a steeplejack or on an oil rig). Similarly, provided that driving is only a small component of the job (less than 15 per cent), an employee should not be refused employment if they do not hold a valid driving licence. The training manual prepared by the International Bureau of Epilepsy[26] provides excellent practical advice, an assessment questionnaire, and some illustrative cases with vocational scenarios.

Sensible restrictions on the work of people with epilepsy

Proposed restrictions must be discussed with the employee and with management. Clear written instructions should be given to management regarding placement, responsibilities, and review. Confidentiality must not be breached. Restrictions should be no more than necessary on common-sense grounds, as would apply equally to any individual subject to sudden and unexpected lapses in consciousness or concentration, however infrequent.

In the USA it is illegal to deny employment to an otherwise qualified applicant because of disability, provided the disability does not impair health and safety standards at the workplace. The Epilepsy Foundation of America (EFA) has developed a comprehensive interview guide summarized by Masland.[27] The guide helps to define the important considerations,

The success rate in placing people with epilepsy is far greater if they have fewer than six seizures per year. In general, minor seizures are less disruptive than major ones, but periods of automatism, (performance of acts without conscious will), may upset colleagues. Other disadvantageous characteristics are prolonged periods of postictal confusion and atonic and tonic seizures where the possibility of serious injury is increased.

Sensible restrictions include avoidance of the following:

◆ Climbing and working unprotected at heights.

◆ Driving or operating motorized machinery.

◆ Working around unguarded machinery.

◆ Working near fire or water.

◆ Working for long periods in isolation.

Hand-held powered tools may be a hazard if they can be left accidentally in the 'on' position.

There are certain jobs with special hazards where the risk of even one seizure may give rise to catastrophic consequences. These jobs fall into two groups:

1 Jobs in transport, including: vocational drivers, train drivers, drivers of large container-terminal vehicles, crane operators, aircraft pilots, seamen, and commercial divers.

2 Jobs that involve work at unprotected heights (e.g. scaffolders, steeplejacks, and firefighters), work on mainline railways, with high-voltage electricity, hot metal, dangerous unguarded machinery, or near open tanks of water or chemical fluids.

The working environment and equipment to be used by the employee with epilepsy should always be inspected by the occupational physician. The safety officer and the employee's immediate supervisor should also be involved in any decisions.

It is important to remind the employee that contravention of agreed restrictions may endanger not only their own safety, but also the safety of their colleagues. The employee should be reminded that it may be impossible to make an insurance claim for financial compensation for personal injuries should an accident occur as a result of evasion of agreed restrictions.

Lifting of restrictions

A policy should be established for terminating any restriction on work practices. This should be made known to the affected employee and altered only in exceptional circumstances. There is little place for partial lifting of restrictions. If a work restriction is removed after a period of freedom from seizures, the employee should be instructed to report any further attack to the occupational health staff or to a personnel officer or manager. If AED treatment is stopped or changed, consideration should be given to close monitoring at work for a period, or to the temporary reintroduction of restrictions.

It may be that following the introduction of medication, control is poor with an unacceptable rate of seizure recurrence. Every effort should be made to improve control before the individual is rejected or restrictions imposed on employment or promotion. There may be specific and avoidable precipitating factors, e.g. alcohol or poor adherence to medication. It may be appropriate to consider whether the diagnosis is correct and the possibility of dissociative seizures (pseudoseizures) has been eliminated. Also that an appropriate AED has been chosen, there is compliance, and adequate blood levels have been achieved (see 'Effect of antiepileptic drugs on work performance').

A planned date for review of restrictions should be offered, as this will affirm that the employee is a valued member of the workforce. In this respect, it seems reasonable to follow, for employment purposes, those guidelines issued by the Department of Transport for ordinary driving licences (see Chapter 28). An employee who is safe to drive a machine as dangerous as a car should be safe to undertake virtually all industrial or commercial duties. (Jobs with special hazards are listed above.) After an initial seizure, the Department of Transport advises that a subject may not drive a car for 6 months (unless there are clinical factors or investigation results that indicate a high risk of recurrence). If there is considered to be a ≥20 per cent risk of recurrence after a first seizure or there has been more than one seizure, a 1-year ban on driving is applied. It seems reasonable to follow the same practice for restrictions relating to physical safety in the work place.

Effect of antiepileptic drugs on work performance

The aim of AED treatment is control of seizures without significant adverse effects, and in most patients this aim is achievable. For others, particularly those requiring combination therapy, a balance must be struck between seizure frequency and adverse effects.

Acute adverse effects are usually rapidly reversible on drug withdrawal or dose reduction. The chronic adverse effects of AEDs are more difficult to control and can potentially impact on work performance but it is often difficult to separate the effects of AEDs from the effects of the underlying aetiology of the epilepsy and of the seizures themselves.[28]

In patients treated with the combination of AEDs, a reduction of drug intake leads to improvements in cognitive function. It is generally considered that adverse cognitive effects are greater with phenobarbitone than with phenytoin, carbamazepine, and valproate. There is evidence to suggest that some of the new AEDs (e.g. lamotrigine, oxcarbazepine) are better tolerated. The wider range of AEDs now available increases the likelihood of achieving a treatment regimen without adverse effects.

Patients with epilepsy often complain of memory impairment. In some cases this is secondary to impaired attention and concentration that may be affected by AEDs. More often, memory impairment is related to temporal lobe dysfunction related to the underlying cause of the seizures.

The occupational physician should work closely with the neurologist to determine whether the patient's drug regimen is appropriate for their job and to explore therapeutic options that match specific employment requirements.

Special work problems

Disclosure of epilepsy to employers

In an ideal world, individuals with epilepsy would freely disclose how their seizures affected them and the occupational physician could then advise about employment in a sector which maximized the employee's potential and minimized any risk to them or their colleagues. However, people with epilepsy may feel they are at a competitive disadvantage and that their choice of vocation is limited. They may have concerns regarding their mobility and promotion within a company, whether they can join the pension fund, and will face suspicion and scrutiny from their fellow workers.

It is not surprising, therefore, that the presence of epilepsy is often concealed from employers. A survey of people in London with epilepsy showed that over half of those who had had two or more full-time jobs after the onset of epilepsy had never disclosed their epilepsy to their employer, and only one in ten had always revealed it.[29] If seizures were infrequent, or usually nocturnal, such that the applicant considered that they had a good chance of successfully concealing it, then the employer was virtually never informed. Among those who declared their condition, two variables correlated with failure to gain employment: frequent seizures and lack of any special skills.

Educational programmes are important in addressing this situation as well as a clear definition of the jobs that can be undertaken as published by the International Bureau for Epilepsy.[30] This considers the vast majority of jobs to be suitable for people with epilepsy, especially where the person possesses the right qualifications and experience. Blanket prohibitions should be avoided and the organization of work practices should be reviewed to reduce potential risk to an acceptable level.

Accident and absence records of those with epilepsy

There is no evidence that people with epilepsy are more accident-prone or have worse attendance records than other workers although many studies are biased as workers with epilepsy tend to get placed in inherently less risky work. The most significant study of work performance that attempted to eliminate this bias was conducted by the US Department of Labour[31] more than 45 years ago. A statistical comparison was made of ten groups with different disabilities, including people with epilepsy, with matched unimpaired controls in the same jobs. Within the epilepsy group, no differences were found in absenteeism and whilst their incidence of work injuries and accident rates was slightly higher this was not statistically significant. The general conclusion was that people with epilepsy perform as well as matched unimpaired workers in the same jobs in manufacturing industries.

In another study, Udell demonstrated that discriminatory practices against the recruitment of people with epilepsy are unwarranted, if based on the notion that as a group they have high accident rates, poor absence records, and low production efficiency.[32] However, any applicant with epilepsy must be assessed individually with regard to seizure control and other associated handicaps. Employers should have a receptive policy for recruitment and job security. This may encourage employees to admit the problem and allow industry an opportunity to appraise their abilities and place them appropriately.

A study of epilepsy in British Steel[18] generally supported these findings. There was no significant difference between epilepsy and control groups with regard to overall sickness absence, accident records, and five different aspects of job performance. Work performance, however, was significantly reduced in people with epilepsy who also had an associated personality disorder. The British Steel study confirmed that, although some degree of selection has to be applied when employing people with epilepsy, the overall performance of those with epilepsy compares well with that of their colleagues. The major task, however, is not to prove that performance at work is satisfactory, but to challenge and change the often firmly held and deeply entrenched prejudices of employers.

Current employment practices

Although sometimes less than ideal, employment practices are increasingly flexible, especially in light of the Equality Act 2010 with a better appreciation of the capacity of people with epilepsy to discharge most work roles. However, certain restrictions apply in situations determined by health and safety regulations.

In the case of new entrants to the Armed Forces, proven cases of epilepsy are not accepted for service and those who have suffered a single seizure less than 4 years before entry are also rejected. For serving personnel, a single seizure after entry necessitates full examination of the individual, restricted activities, and observation for a period of 18 months. Full reinstatement is awarded only after assessment by a senior consultant. Aircrew who have suffered a single seizure after entry are grounded permanently and servicemen who suffer more than one seizure will be considered for discharge on grounds of disability. The Armed Forces also employ a large number of civilians but the policy for these individuals is more flexible than for servicemen. For civilians, the most significant factor is how well qualified an individual is for a particular job and if that job is safe or can be safely adapted to accommodate their medical history.

Epilepsy is also a contraindication for employment in the police force. The police expect all their officers to be fit for all duties. Officers who develop epilepsy during service are usually retired, but only after careful individual assessment (personal communication to I.B.).

Other employment restrictions listed by the Epilepsy Action website as restricted by law include aircraft pilots, ambulance drivers, fire brigade officers, train drivers, large goods vehicle/public service vehicle drivers, taxi drivers, merchant seafarers, and coast guards (a number of these restrictions relate to driving licence restrictions—see 'The driving licence regulations and their effects').

Many of the large and often previously nationalized industries follow sympathetic and accommodating codes of practice. Epilepsy declared at the pre-employment stage may be a contraindication to employment but is rarely an absolute bar. The discretion of the examining physician may allow for some compromise if the applicant has a special skill or quality to offer and if the job is suitable. Epilepsy developing in service can often be accommodated if the employee is willing to be relocated but this may involve some loss of earnings and status. If this is unacceptable to the employee, retirement on grounds of ill health is usually offered.

The Department for Education has a flexible policy for the employment of school teachers with epilepsy and allows its locally appointed part-time medical officers to use reasonable discretion. Difficult cases are referred to the department's medical advisers and each is judged on its own merits.

The National Health Service (NHS) has made considerable progress over the last decade but still has no national guidelines. This is by virtue of the numerous separate employers that collectively form the entity known as the NHS. Guidelines have been constructed by the Association of National Health Occupational Physicians (ANHOPS), which state in respect of epilepsy that all individuals must be assessed on their merit, although emphasizing that the epilepsy should be well controlled and the care of the patient must never be compromised.

The Civil Service has an open and documented policy on the recruitment and employment of people with epilepsy. The health standard for appointment requires that a candidate's health is such as to not disqualify that person for the position sought and that the person is likely to give regular and efficient service for at least 5 years or for the period of any shorter appointment. The Civil Service occupational health service stresses that epilepsy per se is not a bar to holding any established appointment apart from those posts with special hazards.

Getting employers to understand about epilepsy

Many people with epilepsy are unemployed. Epilepsy Action's survey found that 14 per cent of respondents were unemployed, although actively seeking work. This is significantly higher than the International Labour Organization unemployment rate of 8.8 per cent for disabled people. Even if employed, many workers with epilepsy are still frequently denied promotion because of their disability or because of misconceptions about it. In a survey of employers in the USA, it was found that few would employ people known to them to have had a generalized seizure within the previous year.[33] Employers gave the reason that people with epilepsy: 'create safety problems for themselves and other workers'. Such reasoning has not varied for more than two decades, but this assumption is misconceived. An encouraging feature of this study was evidence of a positive change in attitude and changes in the law in the USA and the continued efforts of public and private agencies may well be responsible. A more recent study examining employers' attitudes in the UK[34] revealed that 21 per cent thought that employing people with epilepsy would be a 'major issue' and 16 per cent considered there were no jobs in their company suitable for a person with epilepsy. It is therefore unsurprising that concealment of the condition remains high.

To improve employers' understanding, informal health education seminars could take place at work. A well-thought-out programme that involves the personnel department, occupational health team, and interested union representatives may prevent problems occurring. Topics such as epilepsy, stress, or alcohol misuse should be discussed openly with the benefit of expert advice on hand. Occupational health can play a major part in health education and changing attitudes. Problems such as epilepsy are often treated as a taboo subject. For such a common complaint, with a prevalence of about 5–10 per 1000 of the population, the ignorance still demonstrated is astonishing. Many employees, both on the shop floor and in management, consider that someone with epilepsy also has some degree of mental handicap combined with a lesser or greater physical infirmity. Certainly such problems may coexist but only exceptionally. It is essential that health professionals dispel myths and bring a sense of proportion to the issue.

The hard work of agencies such as Epilepsy Action, Epilepsy Society, and the Employment Medical Advisory Service (EMAS) has done much to inform employers. Misconceptions about epilepsy are slowly disappearing and attitudes changing.

Medical services and opportunities for sheltered work

Most people with epilepsy are capable of normal employment without need for supervision or major restrictions. A minority will have additional health problems and may only be able to work in a sheltered environment. Poorly controlled seizures, physical disability, learning disability, and poor social adaptive skills will pose additional problems. The following specialized facilities are available in the UK for people with epilepsy.

NHS medical services

All patients with a suspected first seizure should be seen as soon as possible by a specialist in the management of epilepsy.[35] Those patients entering remission will usually be referred back to primary care. The care of the 20–30 per cent whose epilepsy proves difficult to control is usually shared between general practice and hospital clinics. Epilepsy nurse specialists attached to hospital services or based in primary care provide support for people with epilepsy. Some regional neuroscience centres provide tertiary epilepsy services with facilities for specialist investigation and surgical treatment.

Residential care

Residential care is required for a small proportion of people with severe epilepsy and is usually provided by social services. In addition, there are epilepsy charities, residential centres, and special assessment centres that cater for the more complex needs of patients with epilepsy, as outlined in the following sections.

Epilepsy charities

Epilepsy Society

Epilepsy Society (formerly the National Society for Epilepsy), founded in 1892, is the UK's largest epilepsy charity. It provides residential care, medical services (in conjunction with the National Hospital for Neurology and Neurosurgery in London), and information, support, and training. A wide range of written information is available including information for patients on epilepsy and work. Epilepsy Society is also committed to campaigning for improved services for people with epilepsy.

Epilepsy Action (British Epilepsy Association)

Epilepsy Action aims to raise awareness about epilepsy and modify regressive attitudes towards epilepsy. It also provides advice and information about epilepsy.

Residential centres and schools for people with epilepsy

In the UK, there are a number of special schools and centres for epilepsy, the largest of which are the Chalfont Centre for Epilepsy, the David Lewis Centre, and the National Centre for Young People with Epilepsy (NCYPE). These provide residential care for people with epilepsy, who are unable to live independently in the community. Some provide sheltered employment. Financial support is usually provided through the local authority, the health service, or private or charitable funds.

Special assessment centres

There are several special assessment centres in the UK providing short-term and social in-patient assessment for people with severe or complicated epilepsy. The largest is the Chalfont Centre for Epilepsy. Others include the Park Hospital in Oxford for children and the David Lewis Centre in Cheshire.

Relationship between the occupational physician, neurologist, and general practitioner

Recommendations received from the neurologist may conflict with the occupational physician's perceptions about the best interests of the patient in their particular working environment. The family doctor, who is likely to have closer knowledge of the patient and their family, can liaise with these two specialists. It is advantageous if all the doctors involved work together to avoid giving conflicting advice. In companies with an occupational health service, an employee with epilepsy should be encouraged to contact the nurse and discuss problems as they arise. The nursing service at work has a special role in counselling and health education. Confidential notes should be kept and the case discussed with the occupational physician at the earliest opportunity. Employees with epilepsy should be reviewed regularly by the occupational health service and at least annually.

Existing legislation and guidelines for employment

For a more detailed discussion of legal aspects, see Chapter 3 and also Carter.[36] The HSW Act makes no reference to the disabled and applies to all employees regardless of their health. People with epilepsy who do not disclose it to an employer may contravene Section 7 of the HSW Act, if they knowingly accept a job that poses unacceptable risks. The Equality Act 2010 protects disabled applicants and imposes a legal duty on the employer to make reasonable adjustments or modifications to working arrangements to accommodate safely the disabled person. Where it is impossible for employers to make such arrangements, or the costs to do so would be prohibitive, the Equality Act 2010 allows the employer to discriminate where the discrimination can be justified by reasons that are 'material to the circumstances of the particular case and substantial'.

Someone who suffers from epilepsy will be considered disabled even if their condition is controlled by medication. Employers, therefore, must be prepared to make reasonable adjustments to accommodate a person with epilepsy. A common example might be an applicant for a job who is presently unable to hold a group 1 driving licence because of a convulsion. The job applied for requires the applicant to hold a group 1 driving licence but the driving component of the job is only about 10 per cent of the duties. Under these circumstances, it would probably be reasonable for the employer to provide an alternative means of transport for the employee. If the driving component was a substantial part of the job, then it would not be reasonable for the employer to provide an alternative means of transport.

For those in employment developing epilepsy, the employer should also consider reasonable adjustments. An example of an employer justifying impracticability occurred in *Smith* v. *Carpets International UK plc* (case no. 1800507/97). Mr Smith, an employee with a history of epilepsy, was employed as a warehouseman in 1994. He had not suffered a seizure for 9 years and the company's occupational physician considered his condition to be well controlled. No restrictions were therefore imposed. Mr Smith then suffered further convulsions and the doctor considered it was dangerous for him to work in the warehouse because of the heavy machinery and forklift truck work. Following a risk assessment it was concluded that no adjustments could be made to the job. An offer of alternative work was not accepted by Mr Smith as it would have been less well paid. The case went to a tribunal and the employer's case was upheld as the circumstances had been appropriately assessed and reasonable investigations had taken place to examine what adjustments could be made to accommodate Mr Smith. Alternative work was offered and the employer was not expected to reorganize totally the way in which the warehouse work was carried out. An employer, though, may be expected to ensure the employee does not suffer any financial hardship and salary preservation is common practice for an agreed time period, often 1–3 years.

Some employers are under the misconception that an applicant with a history of epilepsy will not be accepted into the pension fund. This is generally untrue but the pension scheme assessors will consider all cases on their merits and very occasionally certain restrictions are placed on individuals joining with specific medical problems. Life cover or ill health retirement provision may be reduced if the risk is considered very significant but this will only be in relation to an accident or disability occurring in direct relation to the specific disability described. In most cases, there is no restriction and occupational pension schemes are far more liberal than independent life assurance schemes.

No special insurance arrangements are necessary for a worker with epilepsy. The employer's liability insurance covers everyone in the workplace, provided the employer has taken the disability into account when allocating the individual's work. Failure to disclose epilepsy will render the employer's insurance invalid, and should an accident occur as a direct result of the condition it is unlikely that a claim for compensation will be met.

The driving licence regulations and their effects

The licensing for driving is one of the few areas in which there is legislation related to epilepsy (see also Chapter 28). This was the first medical condition to be declared an absolute bar to driving, although the rules were relaxed in the 1960s. Regulation is deemed necessary because seizures are a potential cause of road traffic accidents in drivers suffering from epilepsy. Although the overall incidence of road traffic accidents may not be higher in people with epilepsy, the risk of serious accidents and fatal accidents is increased.[37] Ideally, legislation should balance the excess risks of driving against the social and psychological disadvantage to the individual of prohibiting driving. In the UK, it is the licensing authority (DVLA), not the sufferer's personal medical advisers, which makes the decision on licensing. The regulations are based, where possible, on research into the risks of seizure recurrence in different clinical circumstances. Licensing is divided into two groups, with more stringent conditions applied to Group 2 licences because more time is spent driving and the consequences of accidents are often more serious.

- ◆ *Group 1 licences* (motorcars and motorcycles): an applicant for a licence who suffers from epilepsy shall satisfy the following conditions:
  - He/she shall have been free of any epileptic attack during the period of 1 year immediately preceding the date when the licence is granted; or
  - In the case of an applicant who has epileptic attack(s) only while asleep, shall have demonstrated a sleep-only pattern for 3 years or more, without attacks while awake.
  - The person complies with advised treatment and check-ups for epilepsy, and the driving of a vehicle will not be likely to endanger the public.

◆ *Group 2 licences* (large goods vehicles and passenger carrying vehicles, i.e. vehicles over 7.5 tonnes, or nine seats or more for hire or reward): an applicant for a licence shall satisfy the following conditions:

- No epileptic attacks shall have occurred in the preceding 10 years.
- The applicant shall have taken no AED treatment in the preceding 10 years.
- There will be no continuing liability to suffer epileptic seizures.

The purpose of the third condition is to exclude people from driving (whether or not epileptic seizures have actually occurred in the past) who have a potentially epileptogenic cerebral lesion, or who have had a craniotomy or complicated head injury, for example.

Following a first unprovoked seizure the regulations require 6 months off driving for group 1 licence holders unless there are clinical features which indicate a high ($\geq$20 per cent per year) risk of a further seizure. For group 2 licence holders, driving can be resumed after 5 years if recent assessment indicates that the risk of a further seizure is $\leq$2 per cent per year and they have taken no antiepileptic medication throughout the 5-year period prior to the granting of a licence.

If a seizure is considered to be 'provoked' by an exceptional condition which will not recur, driving may be allowed once the provoking factor has been successfully treated or removed and provided that a 'continuing liability' to seizures is not also present. For group 1 licence holders, treatment status is not a legal consideration but it is recommended that driving be suspended from the commencement of drug reduction and for 6 months after drug withdrawal.

Van, crane, and minibus drivers will need to be found alternative employment, as with those whose job also involves driving. The safety of forklift truck drivers will depend on individual circumstances.

Conclusions and recommendations

Many people do not disclose a history of epileptic seizures when applying for a job or during a routine examination at the workplace. This may cause major problems for the individual and the employer and, on occasions, inadvertently contravene the HSW Act or invalidate insurance cover. However, the disability provisions of the Equality Act 2010 now confer some protection on those with epilepsy. The unenlightened attitudes of some employers have led to secrecy or denial by those affected. The possibility of dangerous situations arising at work, or dismissal without recourse to appeal, may be the consequence. A competent occupational health service, trusted by both shop-floor and management, can be invaluable in resolving conflicts and giving advice.

Responsibility for the employment and placement of a person with epilepsy rests with the employer and they should take appropriate medical advice. Each case must be judged on its merits in light of the available information, which must include a sound and complete understanding of the requirements of the job. Employees with epilepsy must be regularly reviewed. The development of good rapport and mutual trust will encourage employees to report any changes in their condition or treatment that have arisen.

A sensible approach by managers, with access to medical advice, should help the individual come to terms with their condition, appreciate the reasons for restrictions, and understand that decisions taken on the basis of such medical advice are in their best interests. The employer should discard old prejudices in favour of current knowledge and understanding about epilepsy. This will only occur when all those concerned with epilepsy undertake the responsibility of educating employers, the general public, and perhaps some members of the medical profession.

References

1 Berg A, Berkovic SF, Brodie MJ, *et al.* Revised terminology and concepts for organisation of seizures and epilepsies: Report of the ILAE Commission on Classification and Terminology, 2005-9. *Epilepsia* 2010; **51**: 676–85

2 Commission on Classification and Terminology of the International League Against Epilepsy. Proposal for revised clinical and electroencephalographic classification of epileptic seizures. *Epilepsia* 1981; **22**: 489–501.

3 Wallace H, Shorvon S, Tallis R. Age-specific incidence and prevalence rates of treated epilepsy in an unselected population of 2 052 922 and age-specific fertility rates of women with epilepsy. *Lancet* 1998; **352**: 1970–3.

4 Sander JWAS, Hart YM, Johnson AL, *et al.* National General Practice Study of Epilepsy: newly diagnosed epileptic seizures in a general population. *Lancet* 1990; **336**: 1267–71.

5 Li LM, Fish DR, Sisodiya SM, *et al.* High resolution magnetic resonance imaging in adults with partial or secondary generalised epilepsy attending a tertiary referral unit. *J Neurol Neurosurg Psychiatry* 1995; **59**: 384–7.

6 Davies JE, Dedhia HV, Morgade C, *et al.* Lindane poisonings. *Arch Dermatol* 1983; **119**: 142–4.

7 Chadwick D. Epilepsy after first seizures: risks and implications. *J Neurol Neurosurg Psychiatry* 1991; **54**: 385–7.

8 Hart YM, Sander JW, Johnson AL, *et al.* National general practice study of epilepsy: recurrence after a first seizure. *Lancet* 1990; **336**: 1271–4.

9 First Seizure Trial Group. Randomized clinical trial on the efficacy of antiepileptic drugs in reducing the risk of relapse after a first unprovoked tonic-clonic seizure. *Neurology* 1993; **43**: 478–83.

10 Marson A, Jacoby A, Johnson A, *et al.* Immediate versus deferred antiepileptic drug treatment for early epilepsy and single seizures: a randomised controlled trial. *Lancet* 2005; **365**: 2007–13.

11 Cockerell OC, Johnson AL, Sander JW, *et al.* Remission of epilepsy: results from the National General Practice Study of Epilepsy. *Lancet* 1995; **346**: 140–4.

12 Annegers JF, Hauser WA, Elveback LR. Remission of seizures and relapse in patients with epilepsy. *Epilepsia* 1979; **20**: 729–37.

13 Bonnett LJ, Tudur-Smith C, Williamson PR, *et al.* Risk of recurrence after a first seizure and implications for driving: further analysis of the Multicentre Study of Early Epilepsy and Single Seizures. *BMJ* 2010; 341: c6477.

14 Sander JWAS. Some aspects of prognosis in the epilepsies: a review. *Epilepsia* 1993; **34**: 1007–16.

15 Kwan P, Brodie MJ. Early identification of refractory epilepsy. *N Engl J Med* 2000; **342**: 314–19.

16 Annegers JF, Hauser WA, Coan SP, *et al.* A population based study of seizures after traumatic brain injuries. *N Engl J Med* 1998; **338**: 20–4.

17 Temkin NR, Dikmen SS, Wilensky AJ, *et al.* A randomised double blind study of phenytoin for the prevention of post-traumatic seizures. *N Engl J Med* 1990; **323**(8): 497–502.

18 Dasgupta AK, Saunders M, Dick DJ. Epilepsy in the British Steel Corporation: an evaluation of sickness, accident and work records. *Br J Ind Med* 1982; **39**: 146–8.

19 Joels M. Stress, the hippocampus, and epilepsy. *Epilepsia* 2009; 50(4): 587–97.

20 Wilkinson RT. Hours of work and the 24 hour cycle of rest and activity. In: Warr PB (ed), *Psychology at work*, pp. 31–54. Harmondsworth: Penguin, 1971.

21 Kasteleijn-Nolst Trenité DGA. Photosensitivity in epilepsy: electrophysiological and clinical correlates. *Acta Neurol Scand* 1989; **125**: 3–149.

22 Wolf P, Goosses R. Relation of photosensitivity to epileptic syndromes. *J Neurol Neurosurg Psychiatry* 1986; **49**: 1386–91.

23 Jeavons PM, Harding GFA. *Photosensitivity epilepsy.* London: Heinemann, 1975.

24 Lowenstein DH, Bleck T, Macdonald RL. It's time to revise the definition of status epilepticus. *Epilepsia* 1999; **40**: 120–2.

25 Bonnett LJ, Shukralla A, Tudur-Smith C, *et al.* Seizure recurrence after antiepileptic drug withdrawal and the implications for driving: further results from the MRC Antiepileptic Drug Withdrawal Study and a systematic review. *J Neurol Neurosurg Psychiatry* 2011; **82**(12): 1328–33.

26 Troxell J, Thorbecke R. *Vocational scenarios: a training manual on epilepsy and employment.* Second Employment Commission of the International Bureau for Epilepsy. Heemstede: International Bureau for Epilepsy, April 1992.

27 Masland, RL. Employability, part V111. Social aspects. In: Rose C (ed), *Research progress in epilepsy*, pp. 527–32. London: Pitman, 1983.

28 Kwan P, Brodie MJ. Neuropsychological effects of epilepsy and antiepileptic drugs. *Lancet* 2001; **357**: 216–22.

29 Scambler G, Hopkins AP. Social class, epileptic activity and disadvantage at work. *J Epidemiol Community Health* 1980: **34**: 129–33.

30 Employment Commission of the International Bureau for Epilepsy. Employing people with epilepsy. Principles for good practice. *Epilepsia* 1989; **30**: 411–12.

31 US Department of Labor. *The performance of physically impaired workers in manufacturing industries.* US Department of Labor Bulletin No. 293. Washington, DC: US Government Printing Office, 1948.

32 Udell MM. The work performance of epileptics in industry. *Arch Environ Health* 1960; **6**: 257–64.

33 Hicks RA, Hicks MJ. The attitudes of major companies towards the employment of epileptics: an assessment of 2 decades of change. *Am Correct Ther J* 1978: **32**: 180–2.

34 Jacoby A, Gorry J, Baker GA. Employers' attitudes to employment of people with epilepsy: still the same old story? *Epilepsia* 2005; **46**(12): 1978–87.

35 NICE (National Institute for Clinical Excellence). *The epilepsies: diagnosis and management of the epilepsies in adults in primary and secondary care* (Clinical Guideline 20). London: NICE, 2004.

36 Carter T. Health and safety at work: implications of current legislation. In Edwards F, Espir M, Oxley J (eds), *Epilepsy and employment*, pp. 9–17. London: Royal Society of Medicine, 1986.

37 Taylor J, Chadwick D, Johnson T. Risk of accidents in drivers with epilepsy. *J Neurol Neurosurg Psychiatry* 1996; **60**: 621–7.

Chapter 9

Vision and eye disorders

John Pitts and Stuart J. Mitchell

Introduction—vision, perception, and work

When considering the interaction of the visual system and the working environment, consideration should be given to the effect of vision on work and the effect of work on the eyes.

The effect of vision on work

Vision can affect work by influencing the ease with which information is gathered and by affecting the feedback available for task completion. It therefore has an influence on safety (for example, in transport) and quality control (for example, in manufacturing).

Diseases of the eye or nervous system result in varying degrees of visual dysfunction, which may be compensated to some extent by neural and psychological adaptations. An example would be colour-impaired workers learning to use contrast instead of hue to differentiate colours.

The effect of work on vision

This may be transient or permanent. Visual fatigue, for example, is a temporary effect, whereas in ocular injury the effect may be permanent. Most workplace injuries are preventable, so it is of the utmost importance that workplace assessment takes account of eye protection.

Perception and ergonomics

Perception is more than vision.[1] It is affected by neural processing, which modifies the meaning of a stimulus on the basis of previous experience. Errors, therefore, result not only from defects in the visual system (impaired colour vision, for example) but also from a variety of visual illusions which fool central information-processing mechanisms. Perceptual error rates are greater under the stresses of fatigue and high workload.

The science of ergonomics relates to the interaction between man and machine; it concerns information (display ergonomics) and inputs (control ergonomics).

Good displays are designed to respect the physiological and psychological limitations of the human visual system. Ideally, they should present information in a legible, coherent manner, without crowding, and with intelligent use of icons and colours to convey meaning.

Control ergonomics, in addition to respecting anthropometry and posture, should use labelling, icons, and colours with respect to human visual performance to convey accurately the function of levers, knobs, and switches.

Visual ergonomic factors, such as the use of optical correction and displays, should be optimized to visual physiology and psychology and to the task at hand. This holds true whether the worker has normal vision or is visually impaired. Workplace visual ergonomics is an important topic, as ergonomic support can allow people who are visually impaired to function safely in the workplace in appropriate roles.

Matching visual capability to the task required

Ramazzini, the father of occupational medicine, stressed in 1700 the importance to the occupational physician of knowledge of the workplace. Any professional advising on visual performance must be familiar with the workplace, tasks performed there, and their demands on the employee.

In addition, an assessment of the individual is required to determine whether their visual abilities match the requirements of the job.

If a mismatch exists, there are two possible courses of action:

♦ The task can be adjusted where possible. The Equality Act 2010 is likely to apply, and requires an employer to make 'reasonable adjustments'.

♦ The visual capabilities of the individual can be enhanced by spectacles or other visual aids.

Unfortunately, many occupations have historically prescribed visual standards that are neither evidence-based nor task-related.[2] There are signs that this is now changing. In aviation, for example, the simulator can be used to investigate task proficiency with different degrees of colour vision deficiency.

Vision and driving

The DVLA requirements are published on the Internet.[3] The numerical parameters are not given here, as these are regularly updated.

Counterintuitively, poor vision is not associated with accident rates. While this may be partly due to the fact that accidents do not generally have a single cause and often result from a combination of events, it remains true that the standards used for driving are not based on any hard evidential link with driving performance. Driving simulators and functional driving tests are recommended in cases where clinical vision measurements are borderline.

Aims of this chapter

This chapter is arranged in five sections. Part one introduces the main symptoms and functional effects of vision disorders. Part two reviews the main ocular diseases and uses a tabular approach to link the main symptoms of visual dysfunction to their effect on work—and the adjustments that have to be made as a result. Part three takes a brief look at visual ergonomics—including lighting, DSE, visual fatigue, and the employment of people with visual impairment. Part four reviews the commonest ocular hazards and toxins found in the workplace and eye protection. Part five is a brief introduction to ocular first aid in the workplace.

Symptoms and signs of visual dysfunction

In non-specialist medical practice there is often great fear of involvement in ophthalmological cases. Usually, this is unfounded, as the basic clinical skills of taking an accurate history and carrying out a guided examination (particularly of visual acuity with and without a pinhole) are sufficient to result in an accurate management plan. The main symptoms and signs of eye disease are:

1 Disturbed visual acuity.

2 Disturbed colour vision.

3 Disturbed visual field.

4 Disturbances in binocularity.

5 Visual discomfort or glare.

6 Somatosensory discomfort or pain.

Disturbed visual acuity

Central visual function is measured clinically as a visual acuity (VA). The subject is positioned 6 m from the test chart. 6/6 vision means the subject can see at 6 m what he ought to be able to see at 6 m. 6/60 vision means the subject can see at 6 m what he ought to be able to see at 60 m.

Near VA is measured by using standard printers' font sizes at the standard working distance of 33 cm. It is important to realize that the actual working distance may be greater than 33 cm, e.g. 50, 75, or 100 cm, in which case near VA should be measured at that distance as well.

These methods assess static VA. Specialized tests of dynamic VA may be better at predicting performance at certain tasks. In occupational health settings, optometers are often used to screen employees. While these may be better at assessing function in certain industrial tasks such as inspection of mechanical parts, the Snellen test of VA is more reproducible.

Disturbed colour vision

Colour vision can be assessed by a variety of techniques. The commonest in use for screening purposes is the Ishihara test plate, which was designed to detect the commonest form of *inherited* colour deficiency, red/green confusion.

More detailed methods can also detect acquired colour vision defects, such as the blue/yellow defects, which occur in optic nerve disease or as a side effect of drugs such as amiodarone or ethambutol.

The various lantern tests developed by the navy and matching tests used first in the textiles industry are being superseded by computer-based tests[4] such as the CAD (Colour Assessment and Diagnosis) test, which can quantify the severity of the defect.[5] This is particularly useful in occupational fields where some degree of colour deficiency may be tolerated without significantly affecting visual performance.

A recent review of the 1958 British birth cohort[6] has shown no increase with colour deficiency in the rate of unintentional injuries in driving or in the workplace.

Disturbed visual fields

Visual fields are nowadays almost exclusively measured by static techniques, where the target does not move but instead blinks on and off with varying intensity to construct an accurate map, which includes relative as well as absolute defects.

Peripheral vision is mediated by the rod photoreceptors; these are part of the magnocellular system, which is concerned with movement and balance. Severe visual field defects are therefore associated with disequilibrium; workers so affected should not be permitted to work at height.

Disturbances in binocularity

Although stereoscopic vision enables three-dimensional vision, this is only one of the brain's mechanisms for depth perception.

Beyond approximately 0.5 km, the use of monocular (psychological) cues assumes greater importance in judging depth. These monocular cues are: relative size, perspective, overlapping, position in field, washout due to atmospheric scattering of light (Rayleigh scattering), and parallax. Monocular workers use these psychological clues to depth perception at all distances.

Stereoscopic vision is expressed in seconds of arc. Stereopsis of 120 seconds of arc gives a stereoscopic range of 120 m, 60 seconds gives 240 m, and 30 seconds gives 480 m. Stereopsis is only important for visual tasks relatively close to the subject and in certain specific workers such as forklift drivers.

It is noteworthy that 4 per cent of the general population have amblyopia, and 12 per cent of the population lack stereoscopic vision. Childhood disturbances in vision may prevent stereopsis from developing and increasing age reduces stereopsis; by age 65 it is absent in 33 per cent, and reduced in a further 33 per cent of the population.

Visual discomfort or glare

There are a variety of forms of ocular visual discomfort:

◆ Asthenopia, or eye strain, is due to any imbalance affecting accommodation or convergence.

◆ Glare is due to scattering of light inside the eye and comes in various forms:

  • Pure discomfort glare does not degrade VA but causes distraction, aversion, and fatigue.

  • Disability glare causes a reduction in VA. Three types of disability glare are recognized. In *veiling glare*, due to windscreen reflections, for example, a diffuse light source is superimposed on a retinal image, thus reducing contrast. In *dazzle glare*, due to the headlights of oncoming vehicles, for example, rays from a bright light source are scattered within the eye, thus reducing contrast at the fovea. In *scotomatic glare*, due to arc welding, for example, a brilliant light source temporarily bleaches the photoreceptors.

Somatosensory discomfort or pain

Sensation in the eyes is served by the ophthalmic branch of the Vth (trigeminal) nerve, and so referred pain (e.g. from tooth disease) or neurological disorders (e.g. trigeminal neuralgia) must be considered in all cases of apparently ophthalmic pain.

Because the eyes have such a rich supply of sensory nerves and such a large area of representation in the somatosensory cortex, discomfort and pain in ocular disease can be extremely severe. Discomfort varies from the potentially mild foreign body sensation of tear deficiency to the excruciating 'toothachey' pain of scleritis. The functional importance of severe ocular pain is that it cannot be ignored and therefore acts as a distraction from any occupational task, no matter how safety-critical.

Common eye disorders and their effects on visual function

The occupational physician must avoid making assumptions about an individual's ability based on a disease label, since a particular diagnosis may have a vast range of functional effects depending on individual factors such as severity, personality, and the level of support in the work environment.

Refractive errors and their correction

In *myopia* (short-sightedness), the eye is relatively long, such that rays of light are brought into focus short of the retina. This is corrected by a concave (minus) lens. Myopia is not simply an optical state; it is associated with degeneration of the vitreous gel and peripheral retina, an increased risk of retinal detachment and a higher risk of early-onset macular degeneration.

In *hyperopia* (long-sightedness), the eye is relatively short, such that rays of light have a virtual focus behind the retina. This is corrected by a convex (positive) lens. Hyperopia is associated with an increased risk of squint and amblyopia in childhood and with angle closure glaucoma in later life.

In *astigmatism*, the cornea has different radii of curvature in different axes and is sometimes described to laymen as being shaped like a spoon or a rugby ball. Astigmatism may be myopic, hyperopic, or be a mixture of both. Astigmatism is notorious for causing symptoms of asthenopia as the ciliary muscle has to go through continuous gymnastics between two competing meridians in order to produce a focused retinal image.

Presbyopia is the reduction in accommodation (focusing power for near) which accompanies age. Because of their different starting points, it occurs earlier in hyperopes, and later in myopes. It is easily corrected with a plus lens in spectacles or contact lenses, but accurate correction critically depends on determination of the individual's working distance. Presbyopic symptoms may initially only occur in borderline illumination.

Where spectacles are used to correct refractive errors, they must be compatible with any necessary personal protective equipment (PPE). Contact lenses have the advantages of a more physiological retinal image and almost universal compatibility with PPE, but they may be impractical in dry, dusty or contaminated work environments, where contact lens care is difficult and there is an increased risk of potentially sight threatening complications such as keratitis.

Refractive surgery

Modern techniques of refractive eye surgery, including laser, are not without risk. Photorefractive keratectomy (PRK) has been in existence since 1988 and uses an excimer laser to mould the shape of the cornea. In low myopia it typically removes some 10 per cent of the corneal thickness which, while it does not significantly alter the structural strength of the globe, dramatically alters the measurement of intra-ocular pressure. A sub-epithelial haze peaks at 2–3 months and then gradually disappears at 12 months, after which there may be no visible signs of surgery on slit-lamp examination. The refraction stabilizes at 3 months. Significant regression is more apparent in higher myopes. Glare sensitivity is increased in the first month, and visual function under dilated pupil conditions may remain compromised for a year or more. Haloes occur when the pupil diameter exceeds the ablation zone, which rarely exceeds 6 mm now, and is more of a problem with previously-treated patients and some high myopes and younger patients, who tend to have larger pupils.

Laser-assisted *in-situ* keratomilieusis (LASIK) was developed in 1990. Traditionally it used a micro-keratome mounted in a suction ring to raise a uniform flap of corneal surface tissue and the excimer laser to mould the underlying stroma to the desired shape. In modern LASIK, two lasers are used. The femtosecond laser is used to raise the flap with air bubbles and the excimer laser to reshape the underlying cornea. Because surgery is carried out under intact epithelial surface, haze, scar formation, and pain are minimal. Modern LASIK also uses wavefront-guided technology which has been shown to produce less optical aberration and better night vision. Over 12 million LASIK procedures have been performed worldwide since 1995. It is also possible to treat astigmatism and hyperopia with LASIK, although there is less experience of the technique in these conditions.

A plethora of surgical techniques are emerging for the treatment of presbyopia, such as scleral expansion, corneal inlays and onlays, refractive lens exchange, multifocal LASIK and femtosecond laser reshaping of the posterior corneal surface.

Another common surgical strategy is to use conventional LASIK to render one eye optimum for distance and the other optimum for near. The resulting visual status is known as monovision and it is *specifically banned* in some occupations such as civil aviation (Table 9.1).

Table 9.1 Refractive errors and their management at work

Condition	Dysfunction	Workplace adjustment	Other medical actions
Myopia	DVis		Optometry
Hyperopia	DVis VGla		Optometry
Astigmatism	DVis VGla		Optometry
Presbyopia	DVis (near only)	Test luminance of workplace	Optometry
PRK	VGla ~1 year		Glare testing
LASIK	VGla ~3 months		Glare testing
Monovision	Banned in some occupations, e.g. pilot		Check occupational requirements

DVis, disturbed visual acuity; VGla, visual discomfort or glare.

External eye diseases

Dry eye

Reduction in the amount or degradation in the quality of tears causes discomfort and predisposes to infection. The condition is due to an autoimmune attack on the lachrymal glands and is also seen with poor nutrition and recent emotional upset.

Some working environments exacerbate the symptoms of dry eye. When a worker complains of dry eye symptoms, it is important to measure the relative humidity in the workplace. Some workplaces cannot be humidified, and the worker will need to be placed elsewhere if simple lubricant eye drops do not solve the problem.

Allergy

Allergies are becoming more common in the population. The 'atopic triad' of asthma, eczema, and hay fever also causes allergic conjunctivitis with subtarsal papillae. The condition may be worse in spring, or be present all year round, and can be controlled with the long-term use of mast cell stabilizing agents. Use of long-term steroids should be avoided, as these produce cataract and glaucoma.

Allergic contact dermatitis can occur on the lids, particularly due to secondary contact with sensitizing agents on the hands. Occasionally, one can identify a discrete substance in the working environment which the employee is sensitive to, such as wheat germ protein in bakers.

Infection

Infective conjunctivitis can be bacterial, viral, or chlamydial. Viral conjunctivitis can result in an epidemic that can decimate a workforce ('shipyard eye')[7] and it is mandatory that affected subjects be sent home promptly until the conjunctivitis has recovered.

Infective keratitis is inflammation of the cornea, commonly in the form of a corneal ulcer. Infection may spread into the eye, causing hypopyon (pus in the anterior chamber), and the condition can rapidly result in blindness. Soft contact lens wear is a risk factor for keratitis.

Table 9.2 External eye disorders and their management at work

Condition	Dysfunction	Workplace adjustment	Other medical actions
Dry eye	Mild SDis DVis rarely	Measure relative humidity. Adjust humidity. Remove from unavoidably dry or dusty workplace	Ophthalmological assessment (tear drops)
Allergy	Moderate SDis and/or itch; VGla less commonly	Remove from workplace source of allergen. No work at height or machinery operation if requires antihistamines.	Ophthalmological and/or allergist assessment Try to identify allergen
Infective conjunctivitis	Moderate SDis	Remove from workplace as may be infectious (droplets or fomites)	Ophthalmological assessment • ? antibiotic drops • ? infectious • ? allergic
Infective keratitis	Severe SDis Severe VGla Severe DVis	Consider whether other employees at risk. Re-employ depending on degree of visual disability	Urgent ophthalmological assessment (may need hospital admission)

DVis, disturbed visual acuity; SDis, somatosensory discomfort; VGla, visual discomfort or glare.

Fungal keratitis is seen in agricultural workers, and is sight-threatening.[8] Any such worker must be referred urgently for an eye opinion when they complain of red eye with blurred vision. The key predisposing factor is trauma with implantation of spores into a corneal abrasion (by vegetation, for example, or an animal's tail). Eye protection for agricultural workers should not be neglected[9] (Table 9.2).

Cataract

This term describes opacification of the lens; this may be a normal ageing phenomenon or a form of lens pathology. Visible lens changes are almost universal from the age of 40 but cataract can also be accelerated by a number of factors including diabetes, trauma, and steroids.

Surgery can be performed at any time when the vision deteriorates to the extent that the individual patient is unable to carry out the desired visual tasks. Modern phaco-emulsification surgery is carried out as a day case through a small incision under local anaesthesia and heals very rapidly with a minimum of astigmatism and a minimum amount of time off work

The glaucomas

This family of diseases is characterized by the triad of raised intra-ocular pressure (IOP), optic nerve damage and visual field loss.

IOP is maintained by the balance of production and drainage of aqueous humour. As the pressure rises, perfusion of the optic nerve head falls. This results in ischaemic and direct pressure damage to the fibres serving the visual field. Clinically, this appears as increased cupping of the optic disc and there is a useful nomogram which relates disc size to cup/disc ratio.[10]

Ocular hypertension

In this condition, IOP is raised above 22 mmHg but there is no optic nerve damage or visual field loss. Approximately 10 per cent of patients progress to primary open angle glaucoma, particularly where other risk factors for glaucoma are present.

Primary open-angle glaucoma

In primary open-angle glaucoma (POAG) the rise in intra-ocular pressure is insidious, intermittent, and asymptomatic. Pressure spikes occur in the early morning, so that the raised pressure may be missed in patients seen in clinic in the afternoon. It is now possible to carry out 24-hour pressure monitoring by wireless ocular telemetry to detect these spikes.[11]

Visual loss starts from the physiological blind spot and is asymptomatic. Detection of POAG therefore depends on screening. POAG was traditionally treated with eye drops and surgery was reserved for later in the disease. This gave rise to poor results and a bad reputation for glaucoma surgery. Nowadays, surgery is offered earlier in the disease and the results are much better. POAG is more common in myopes.

Normal tension glaucoma

In normal tension glaucoma (NTG) the disc and field features are identical but the pressure is low or normal. NTG is thought to be due to impaired perfusion in the optic nerve head or primary neural degeneration. The disease is more difficult to treat and this has given rise to the concept of target IOP, which states that one should aim for a pressure reduction of 30–40 per cent of the pressure at diagnosis.

More recently, some specialists in glaucoma have challenged this paradigm and emphasized that 'lower is better', i.e. that the target pressure should only reflect the upper limit of acceptable glaucoma control.[12] There is some evidence that statins are useful in this condition.[13]

Angle-closure glaucoma

In angle-closure glaucoma (ACG), the outflow of aqueous is blocked by contact between the iris root and the peripheral cornea. This is an extremely painful condition, which produces blurred vision, red eye, headache, and vomiting.

Sometimes ACG occurs in a more insidious, chronic form as recurrent headaches. Angle closure is more common in hyperopia, or when early cataract causes the lens to swell. Treatment uses surgery or the YAG laser to make a small hole in the periphery of the iris (a peripheral iridotomy) to allow the aqueous to bypass the pupil block (Table 9.3).

Squint

In this family of conditions, the visual axes of the eyes are not aligned. This may produce double vision if the squint is of recent onset whereas, if the squint is of gradual onset, particularly in a child, the brain learns to suppress the image from the squinting eye to avoid such diplopia. In these circumstances, binocular vision is impossible and stereopsis is absent.

Childhood squint results in amblyopia (lazy eye) if undetected before the age of 5 years. Many adults who have amblyopia as a result of undiagnosed squint in childhood do not have an obvious squint.

Squint can often be treated with surgery to lengthen or shorten the extra-ocular muscles. Modern techniques include adjustable suture surgery and botulinum toxin injection.

There is considerable evidence in the literature that people with squints are subject to discrimination in the recruitment process and in the workplace.[14] This is particularly inappropriate as there

Table 9.3 Anterior segment disorders and their management at work

Condition	Dysfunction	Workplace adjustment	Other medical actions
Cataract	DVis VGla	Usually none necessary. Increase luminance and contrast in inoperable cases with severe DVis	Ophthalmological assessment Time off after cataract surgery, depending on type of operation and type of job[a]
Ocular hypertension	None	None	Ophthalmological assessment
Primary open angle and normal tension glaucoma (POAG and NTG).	DFld DVis (late disease)	Ophthalmological assessment	Assess risks, based on the residual visual field defect
Angle-closure glaucoma (ACG)	Severe SDis DVis DFld	Ophthalmological assessment	Urgent ophthalmological assessment Assess risks, based on residual visual field defect

[a] In all cases of eye surgery in safety-critical occupations, such as aviation, a report must be obtained from the treating clinician that there are no complications and the patient has recovered. The patient must meet the visual requirements of the appropriate regulatory authority.

DFld, disturbed field of vision; DVis, disturbed visual acuity; SDis, somatosensory discomfort; VGla, visual discomfort or glare.

is now some direct evidence that people with squints do as well as orthophoric (straight-eyed) people in complex tasks such as flying.[15]

Adult squint is more commonly due to muscular or neurological disorders and must be investigated. Double vision is disabling and can cause serious danger if, for example, the employee is involved in transport or in working at a height.

Double vision occurs in the direction of action of the weak muscle and, in the chronic situation, this may be occupationally relevant. Diplopia in upgaze (due to weakness of an elevator muscle), for example, would be disabling to a forklift driver but not to an office worker (Table 9.4).

Table 9.4 Strabismus and its management at work

Condition	Dysfunction	Workplace adjustment	Other medical actions
Amblyopia	DVis Binocularity	None after original diagnosis	Do not place in a role requiring stereopsis
Long-standing squint since childhood	Binocularity	None after original diagnosis	Do not place in a role requiring stereopsis
Recent-onset adult squint	Binocularity (diplopia)	Urgent neurological assessment (for cranial nerve palsy)	Placement depends on treatment for diplopia
Squint in particular directions of gaze, e.g. upwards	Binocularity (diplopia)	Placement in role which avoids field of diplopia and avoid forklift driving in diplopia on upgaze	Placement depends on treatment for diplopia

DVis, disturbed visual acuity.

Retinal disorders

Diabetes

Diabetes mellitus causes a spectrum of eye problems due to capillary closure and ischaemia. These problems are seen in both Type 1 and Type 2 diabetes.

Background retinopathy is characterized by dots and blots due to capillary microangiography. *Pre-proliferative retinopathy* is characterized by variation in venous calibre, deep cluster haemorrhages, and cotton wool spots (also called 'soft exudates', although they are, in fact, retinal infarcts). In *proliferative retinopathy* new vessels grow from the venous side of the circulation, commonly from the disc or from the major vascular arcades. These are fragile and prone to bleed. Bleeding causes vitreous haemorrhage; and subsequent organization can cause tractional retinal detachment.

The development of retinopathy is related to diabetic control and is so strongly associated with nephropathy that significant retinopathy rarely occurs in the absence of proteinuria.

Retinal vein occlusion

Venous occlusion may be caused by systemic hypertension, ocular hypertension, and hyperviscosity. These conditions must be excluded and the patient followed in the eye clinic for ischaemic retinal complications.

Retinal artery occlusion

Some patients with retinal artery occlusion (RAO) have prodromal episodes of amaurosis fugax. RAO may be due to emboli from the heart wall, the cardiac valves or the great vessels. The patient must be adequately investigated in order to prevent stroke, as detailed in the following sections.

Posterior ciliary artery occlusion

This causes anterior ischaemic optic neuropathy, a clinical triad of reduced acuity, afferent pupillary defect, and milky swelling of the optic disc ('pale papilloedema'). Posterior ciliary artery occlusion is most commonly due to giant cell arteritis, so all patients should have their erythrocyte sedimentation rate (ESR) and C-reactive protein measured and have temporal artery biopsy.

Retinal detachment

Rhegmatogenous retinal detachment is caused by thinning and degeneration in the peripheral retina combined with degenerative changes in the vitreous.

The vitreous gel undergoes focal liquefaction and becomes more mobile. In other areas the vitreous forms degenerate fibres which have contractile properties. The vitreous pulls on the retina as it contracts, tearing holes in the degenerate area. The fluid vitreous passes through the holes, separating the retina from its normal anatomical support, the underlying retinal pigment epithelium (RPE). When the retina remains separate from the RPE for more than a few hours, the photoreceptors undergo necrosis. A 'macula-on' detachment is, therefore, regarded as a surgical emergency because there is still potential for preserving central vision.

Treatment of retinal detachment is surgical. Fresh holes can be spot-welded with the argon laser. Very peripheral small detachments can sometimes be treated by injecting gas into the vitreous. Larger detachments require an operation to push the sclera on to the hole in the retina to obtain a seal, in combination with localized freezing to cause an adhesive scar.

Modern techniques of vitreo-retinal surgery allow the vitreous to be removed and replaced with gas, fluid or oil. These techniques have dramatically improved the success rate of retinal detachment repair (Table 9.5).

Table 9.5 Retinal disorders and their management at work

Condition	Dysfunction	Workplace adjustment	Other medical actions
Background diabetic retinopathy	None	None	None
Preproliferative diabetic retinopathy	None	None	None
Proliferative diabetic retinopathy	DVis	Depends on other aspects of diabetes diagnosis	Urgent ophthalmological and medical assessment
Retinal vein occlusion	DVis	Depends on extent of visual recovery. May be left effectively monocular	Urgent ophthalmological and medical assessment[a]
Retinal artery and PCA occlusion	DVis	Depends on extent of visual recovery. May be left effectively monocular	Urgent ophthalmological and medical assessment[b]
Retinal detachment	DFld DVis	Depends on extent of visual recovery. May be left with field defect or reduced VA if affecting the macula	Urgent ophthalmological and medical assessment[c]

DFld, disturbed field of vision; DVis, disturbed visual acuity.

[a] Medical assessment should include: blood pressure by 24-hour blood pressure recording if necessary, management of other cardiovascular risk factors, exercise ECG to the Bruce protocol, thrombophilia screen

[b] Medical assessment as per a but also including FBC and ESR; temporal artery biopsy if ESR raised or if otherwise indicated, carotid Doppler scan and echocardiogram

[c] Retinal detachment should be treated before it progresses to affect the macula

Time off work after surgery

This will depend on the nature of the job and the surgeon's recommendations in the individual case; also on whether work is manual or sedentary, and whether it is hazardous or safety-critical (Table 9.6).

Visual ergonomics—lighting, display screens, visual fatigue, and employment of people with visual impairment

Lighting and visibility

Visibility is affected by lighting, by air clarity (often reduced in foundries and mining, for example), and by glare from reflective surfaces. Lighting is extremely important for safety, since the more rapidly a hazard is seen the more easily it can be avoided.

Poor lighting can result in significant costs to a business both as time off work due to injury or accidents and also by reducing productivity.

Lighting in the workplace

Regulation 8 of the Management of Health and Safety at Work Regulations (MHSW) 1992 as amended by the Health and Safety (Miscellaneous Amendments) Regulations 2002 requires

Table 9.6 Time off work after common ophthalmic surgical procedures (NB Suggested times are guidelines for uncomplicated cases only; these may vary in the individual case depending on the clinical circumstances)

Operation	Time off work			
	Manual	**Sedentary**	**Hazardous, e.g. dusty, working at height**	**Safety-critical**[a]
Cataract (phaco)	2 weeks	1 day	2 weeks	3 months
Cataract (ECCE)	2 months	2 weeks	2 months	3 months
Drainage surgery for glaucoma	2 months	2 weeks	2 months	3 months
Pterygium excision	2 weeks	1 week	1 month	3 months
Corneal transplant	2 months	2 weeks	2 months	3 months
Refractive surgery	2 weeks	1 day	2 weeks	3 months
Squint correction	2 weeks	1 week	1 month	3 months
Conventional retinal detachment repair	2 months	2 weeks	2 months	3 months
Vitrectomy retinal detachment repair	2 months	2 weeks	2 months	3 months
Nasolarimal surgery	2 weeks	2 days	2 weeks	1 month
Orbital surgery	1 month	2 weeks	6 weeks	4 months

[a] In all cases of eye surgery in safety-critical occupations, such as aviation, a report must be obtained from the treating clinician that there are no complications and the patient has recovered. The patient must meet the visual requirements of the appropriate regulatory authority.

employers to have lighting which is suitable and adequate to meet the requirements of the workplace. Measurement of available light should be made using an appropriate light meter. Owing to the different frequencies of light sources that are commonly found in the workplace, a light meter with variable light source settings should be used.

Typical light source settings include daylight, fluorescent, mercury, and tungsten. The luminance should be task-related and adjusted for the age of the employee. Due to age-related miosis, lens opacity, and reduced retinal sensitivity, the older employee may require higher levels of luminance to achieve the same levels of visual efficiency. Under the MHSW Regulations there is a requirement to assess possible risks in the workplace. This includes considering whether the lighting arrangements are satisfactory and whether they pose any significant risk to staff. There is also a requirement to provide emergency lighting where people may be exposed to danger.

In addition to general diffuse lighting local lighting at each workstation should be under the control of the employee. Care must be taken, however, to ensure that this does not become the source of glare for other employees working in the vicinity.

Detailed recommendations are given in the Charted Institution of Building Services Engineers (CIBSE) 'lighting handbook'.[16] The Society of Light and Lighting (SLL) publishes a Code of Practice and various useful lighting application standards and guides which can be downloaded from their website.[17]

Display screen equipment

There is no evidence that working with computer screens can harm employees' sight, although the following temporary phenomena may occur:

♦ Display screen equipment (DSE) images are inherently blurred; as blur is a stimulus to the accommodation reflex, the eyes may undergo a constant focussing search, causing eye strain.

♦ Ciliary spasm produces a measurable increase in the resting point of accommodation after DSE use. After 4 hours this produces approximately 0.11D of myopia which can take 15 minutes to resolve.

♦ Concentrating on a VDU also produces a reduction in blink rate, exacerbating dry eye symptoms.

Frequent work breaks are advised to avoid these temporary effects, particularly with visually demanding or repetitive work. The relevant legislation can be found in the Health and Safety (Display Screen Equipment) Regulations 1992 as amended by the Health and Safety (Miscellaneous Amendments) Regulations 2002. The Health and Safety Executive (HSE) website provides free downloads concerning the law on VDUs on their website.[18]

Headaches attributed to eyestrain may be due to ergonomic problems, which result in poor posture and muscular strain. The Display Screen Regulations emphasize the importance of correct seating at workstations.

Equipment should be properly maintained to avoid flicker, glare, and reflection. There should also be flexibility in positioning of the screen, keyboard, and source material to allow the operator to adjust the workstation to meet their visual requirements.

Presbyopic individuals may have difficulty because their reading spectacle correction does not correct their sight for the distance required for DSE work. The Association of Optometrists[19] suggests that operators be able to read N6 throughout the range 75–33 cm and have any phorias at working distances corrected, unless they are well-compensated or suppression is present. The near point of convergence should be normal and any convergence insufficiency should be treated.

'DSE users' should be tested periodically. These are people who:

1 Normally use DSE for continuous or near-continuous spells of an hour or more at a time.

2 Use DSE in this way more or less daily.

3 Have to transfer information quickly to or from the DSE.

This can be achieved by software tests used on the DSE, and the results can be collated on the computer. The directive makes the employer responsible for the provision of an optical correction necessary for the DSE task at the appropriate working distance.

Visual fatigue

The best way to avoid visual fatigue in employees is to optimize the working environment in terms of lighting and ergonomics. Uncorrected astigmatism and defects in accommodation and convergence are notorious for causing asthenopia and should be treated. Spectacles should be optimized for the working distance of the individual employee.

Employment of people with visual impairment

Under the National Assistance Act 1948, blind certification is defined in occupational terms. A person is legally blind if they cannot do any work for which eyesight is essential. Generally, those with VA less than 3/60 can be certified blind. If the vision is better than 3/60, blind registration is possible if there is a contracted field of vision, particularly inferiorly.

There is no legal definition of partial sight. The guideline is that a person can be certified as partially sighted if they are substantially and permanently handicapped by defective vision caused by congenital defect or illness or injury.

Partial sight registration entitles the same help from the local authority department of Social Services as blind registration, but without the financial benefits and tax concessions.

Older workers find it more difficult to adapt to visual loss, as do patients who have a sudden onset loss of vision. There is a bereavement reaction associated with sight loss and loss of sighted employment, and this is rapidly followed by profound depression. It is therefore vital that the occupational physician assists with job replacement as soon as possible.

Ergonomic support can allow people who are visually impaired to function safely in the workplace in appropriate roles in accordance with the Equality Act 2010. Advice for employers is available online from the RNIB[20] and the government.[21]

Ocular hazards, toxicology, and eye protection

Heat

Direct thermal burns to the ocular surface occur with sparks and molten metal injuries. Infra-red radiation can cause damage to the anterior lens capsule, and is implicated in a form of occupational cataract in glassblowers.

Light

Light is hazardous to the eyes and the skin. Photons impacting in tissues produce direct damage to cells and produce free radicals which cause further damage. Chronic exposure to sunlight causes skin damage such as solar elastosis and keratosis, basal cell carcinomas, and squamous carcinomas. These conditions are more common in outdoor workers.

Sunlight can cause an acute keratitis, particularly when it is reflected from sea or snow (Labrador keratopathy). The harmful wavelengths are ultraviolet (UVB) (295–315 nm). Chronic surface exposure causes conjunctival elastosis and pterygium formation. Sunlight also causes damage within the lens and is cataractogenic; the harmful wavelengths are UVA (315–380 nm). Phototoxic damage to the retina by high energy blue light of 400–500 nm is also thought to be a risk factor for macular degeneration.

Light causes glare, as discussed earlier. Good-quality sunglasses protect the eyes from the toxic effect of light by filtering out harmful wavelengths

The light intensity passing through the filters in sunglasses should have a transmittance of 18 per cent, reducing luminance at the ocular surface to 1000 cd/m^2. Neutral grey filters allow the preservation of the spectral composition of light. The transmittance of harmful wavelengths such as UVA/UVB and blue should not be more than 1 per cent.

UV light is a cause of acute keratitis (welder's flash), retinal damage, and maculopathy in arc welding.[22] This has been reported even with short duration exposure or when wearing eye protection, and has also been reported to be potentiated by photosensitizing drugs such as fluphenazine.[23] Welding UV exposure has been implicated as a risk factor for skin and ocular malignancy.

Lasers

Laser is an acronym for light amplification by stimulated emission of radiation. Laser is a monochromatic (single wavelength), collimated (parallel), and coherent (in-phase) beam of light, which delivers high energy over a small area. Applications of laser include: cutting and shaping materials, measurement, recording, displays, communications, holography, remote sensing, surveying, uranium enrichment, medical uses, and as weapons.

Lasers are classified according to their energy levels and the risk of injury. In general, laser bio-effects can be photochemical, thermal, or acoustic. Photochemical effects are generally transient and are a form of scotomatic disability glare. Thermal effects include retinal burns, which cause permanent scotomas.

The site of laser damage is in the posterior segment, where the light is converted to heat by absorption within the pigments of the RPE and retina to produce a burn.[24] The burn has more functional effect if it is at the fovea; this occurs when the patient was looking directly at the laser source at the moment of discharge. Acute eye injuries occur in medical and industrial settings with inadequate eye protection but there is some evidence of more chronic damage in the form of diminished colour vision in workers using lasers over long periods.

Laser hazards can be significantly reduced by proper safety procedures. Multiple types of filter exist to protect against beam-related injuries, and these are not always easy to distinguish, particularly in a dark work environment. It is imperative that the eye protection worn contains a filter appropriate to the wavelength of the laser being used. It is less straightforward to protect certain occupational groups such as pilots from deliberate, criminal assault with hand-held laser pointers, a dangerous occurrence which is reported to be on the increase by aviation authorities around the world.[25]

Non-beam hazards associated with lasers include thermal injury, fire, smoke plume, and electrical hazards. There should be a qualified laser safety officer whose responsibilities include regular inspection and maintenance and training of staff in risk reduction.

An evidence-based protocol should be established for the diagnosis and management of laser injuries. Retinal laser lesions that cause serious visual problems are readily apparent on ophthalmological examination, and do not cause chronic pain without physical signs. Alleged laser injuries can result in lengthy medico-legal claims and therefore full assessment should be carried out on all such cases.[26]

Radiation

Ionizing radiation causes damage to both the lens of the eye (cataract) and the posterior segment (radiation retinopathy). Radiation retinopathy presents clinically as degenerative and proliferative vascular changes, mainly affecting the macula.[27] It is more pronounced in diabetes and is thought to result from oxygen-derived free radical damage and be influenced by endothelial cell antioxidant status.

Although less common, microwave injury has also been documented as causing lens and retinal damage.

Electrical shock

High-voltage shock has been documented to produce cataract, which is amenable to standard surgical treatment.

Chemicals, particles, fibres, allergens, and irritants

Caustic chemicals (acids and alkalis), solvents (alcohols such as n-butanol, aldehydes, and ethers), anionic or cationic surfactants, methylating agents such as dimethyl sulphate, aniline dyes, and toxic vegetable products such as *Euphorbia* saps can all cause damage to the corneal and conjunctival epithelium, which can result in late scarring and opacification.

Exposure may be in the form of a splash, but the conjunctiva of the eye is a mucous membrane and is affected by the same gases (e.g. ammonia) that cause respiratory embarrassment. The pathogenesis of ocular toxic reactions varies with the agent, but, for example, surfactants cause emulsification of the cell membrane lipid layer. An excellent reference work on ophthalmic toxicology is available.[28]

Fibres and dust in the atmosphere also cause irritation. Part of the response to atmospheric irritants is lacrimation, and this reduces VA by a surface effect, as well as being distracting. This may compromise safety in situations such as mining and work at heights.

Allergic reactions have been reported to a vast number of challenges across a wide array of occupational groups. Allergic reactions may be acute or chronic, and can occur as allergic contact dermatitis in the eyelids with chemicals commonly spread from the hands, or as allergic conjunctivitis due to aerosols, pollens, animal dander, and proteins in food manufacture. Adequate ventilation is more effective than eye protection in these situations.

Glass fibres occasionally lodge under the lids or in the lacrimal puncta, where they can be very difficult to visualize due to their virtual transparency.

One study of chemical industry workers in South Africa showed an increased prevalence of ocular disorders including tear film disorders, dry eye conditions, allergic conjunctivitis, and conjunctival melanosis. Forty-one per cent of the ocular disorders in this study were thought to have resulted from occupational exposure.

In veterinary nurses, a prevalence of allergic disorders of 39 per cent was found in one study of attendees at an international conference in Australia.[29] In animal handlers (vets, vet nurses, breeders, trainers, laboratory animal handlers, researchers) who develop allergic symptoms, 80 per cent will report rhino-conjunctivitis (compared with 40 per cent with skin symptoms and 30 per cent with occupational asthma). One prospective study showed the mean time to first symptoms in newly appointed lab workers exposed to rats as 7 months for eye and nose, 11 months for skin, and 12 months for chest. Ocular bites have been reported as another hazard in this occupational group.

ASHRAE (The American Society of Heating, Refrigeration and Air conditioning Engineers) has recommended environmental controls for animal rooms at 10–15 air changes per hour with 100 per cent outdoor air, relative humidity of 30–60 per cent, and a temperature of 16–29°C (61–84°F). Good workplace hygiene aims to reduce exposure to hair, dander, urine, and saliva, as does the wearing of lab coats, gloves, face shields, and respirators. Emergency procedures should be in place for managing anaphylaxis, including staff training in CPR and availability of adrenaline.

Occupational injuries and eye protection

Recent statistics from the USA show that eye injuries at work account for 13 per cent of all eye injuries, compared with 40 per cent at home, 13 per cent on the street, 13 per cent playing a sport, 12 per cent other, and 9 per cent unknown.

MacEwan[30] studied all eye injuries over a 1-year period in Glasgow, and found that 60.9 per cent were due to work, that the majority of work-related eye injuries were due to buffing and grinding, and that in 83 per cent the required eye protection was not being worn.

One study in Hong Kong[31] showed that in 85 per cent of eye injuries in the construction industry, no eye protection had been worn. The following were associated with lower risk:

◆ Longer duration in the current job.

◆ Job safety training before employment.

◆ Regular repair and maintenance of machinery or equipment.

- ◆ Wearing safety glasses regularly.
- ◆ A requirement for wearing eye protection.

Injuries to the eyes can occur in isolation, but the more severe injuries occur in the setting of more widespread trauma, in which case the ATLS® (Advanced Trauma Life Support) principles of rapid primary survey and detailed secondary survey apply.

ATLS® comprises the rapid initial assessment (primary survey) and simultaneous treatment of life-threatening conditions in the sequence of ABCDE:

- ◆ Airways maintenance with cervical spine immobilization.
- ◆ Breathing and ventilation.
- ◆ Circulatory support with control of haemorrhage.
- ◆ (Disability)—neurological status.
- ◆ (Exposure)—examine completely undressed while preventing hypothermia.

Once the patient is stable, a systematic secondary survey is carried out to identify definitive injuries to the brain, head and eyes, face, neck, thorax, abdomen, pelvis, and extremities, so that appropriate specialist care can be instituted.

In an industrial setting, the common eye injuries seen are corneal abrasion, corneal and subtarsal foreign bodies, superficial burns, and chemical burns. Severe blunt injury, penetrating eye injury, intra-ocular foreign body, and compressed air injuries are rare, and their management is essentially to provide rapid first aid and then protect the eye while the patient is transferred to a specialist unit.

Corneal abrasion

In this condition the corneal epithelium is damaged by a scratch. The abrasion can be highlighted with fluorescein drops and blue light. The treatment is antibiotic ointment and padding of the eye. Healing is rapid and complications are rare, but these do include infection and impaired healing with recurrent spontaneous breakdown of the epithelium (recurrent corneal erosion syndrome).

Corneal foreign bodies

These are commonly seen where workers are under a raised platform, or in grinding incidents. The metal is embedded in the epithelium and superficial stroma of the cornea. It is easily removed, but this is best done at the slit-lamp. Metal ions pass into the cornea and oxidize, forming a semi-solid rust ring. This is best removed with a corneal burr, again at the slit-lamp. Removal of the rust ring is sometimes best deferred until the day after the primary foreign body is removed, and several sessions are sometimes necessary to allow the cornea, which is only 0.5–1.0 mm thick, to heal. After each session the treatment is as for a corneal abrasion.

Subtarsal foreign bodies

There is a longitudinal ridge under the upper eyelid where loose foreign bodies become trapped, abrading the cornea with each blink. These are easily removed with a cotton bud after everting the lid. The vertical corneal abrasions on the upper cornea are managed as for corneal foreign bodies.

Superficial burns

These are common in welders, who know them as arc eye or flash. The injury is caused by UV light, but the symptoms of surface cell death are delayed for several hours, and include lid swelling, blepharospasm, ocular pain, photophobia, and profuse lacrimation. Treatment is with topical analgesia, antibiotic ointment, and padding.

Chemical burns

Chemical injury causes direct cell death and ischaemic necrosis, followed by ingress of leucocytes and release of inflammatory mediators such as prostaglandins, cytokines, superoxide radicals, and lysosomal enzymes.

Acids tend to cause superficial effects—due to surface coagulation, the acid does not penetrate the eye. These tend to cause stromal haze and ischaemia affecting less than one-third of the corneal limbus. They are associated with a good visual prognosis.

Alkalis tend to cause deeper effects—the alkali penetrates the eye and the pH in the anterior chamber rises rapidly, damaging intra-ocular structures such as the iris, the drainage angle, and the lens. These cause stromal opacity and ischaemia affecting more than one-half of the corneal limbus. They are associated with a poor visual prognosis.

Immediate irrigation is the priority, using water, saline, Ringer's lactate, balanced salt solution, or, in reality, whatever is available and safe. Ideally, irrigation is continued using an intravenous infusion set while holding the lids open with a speculum if necessary. Following transfer of the casualty to a specialist centre, medical treatment includes steroids, antibiotics, and ascorbic acid, and late surgery may be necessary to deal with scar tissue. Secondary glaucoma is a real risk.

Blunt injury

1 *Haematoma* (black eye) may hide a severe eye injury until the swelling subsides.

2 *Orbital apex fractures* are associated with high-velocity injuries and result in damage to the optic nerve, which can only withstand ischaemia for 2 hours, or pressure-induced disturbance of axoplasmic flow for 8 hours. If such an injury is suspected, the consensus favours systemic steroids and early neurosurgical decompression.

3 *Orbital blowout fracture* describes a situation where the eye is propelled backwards and the walls of the orbit fracture outwards into the ethmoid and maxillary sinuses, leaving the eye and the orbital rim intact. This injury was first described as a sports injury in an officer of the New York Police Department in 1957. Clinical features are enophthalmos, diplopia, surgical emphysema, and infra-orbital nerve anaesthesia. Radiology shows the *hanging drop sign* in the maxillary antrum, and a computed tomography scan may help quantify the bony defect. Management is controversial, with equally vociferous proponents of early surgery and conservative management, and no real clinical trial evidence. In terms of first aid, antibiotics are useful because asymptomatic sinus infection is common, and the patient should be instructed not to blow their nose as this can spread infection to the soft tissues of the orbit and because surgical emphysema can compress the optic nerve.[32]

4 *Contusion injuries of the globe* cause damage at the point of impact and contre-coup injuries. These include hyphaema, iris damage, angle damage, lens damage, vitreous haemorrhage, retinal oedema (*commotio retinae*), retinal breaks and detachment, and traumatic optic neuropathy. Their management is best left to specialist centres, with first aid during transfer consisting of adequate analgesia and anti-emesis and a Cartella eye shield to protect the eye.

Penetrating injury

This is often painless. Signs include a visible laceration, prolapse of intra-ocular contents (iris appearing as a dark knot of tissue, vitreous as a blob of gel) and a collapsed anterior chamber. Extreme caution should be exercised in examining the eye to avoid prolapsing the ocular contents. (One of the authors has encountered a patient whose iris was removed by a well-meaning first-aider who thought that a knuckle of prolapsed iris was a foreign body.)

The eye should be covered with a shield and anti-emetics or sedation given as necessary while preparing for transfer. Some injured eyes do well with primary repair and secondary reconstruction, but an eye damaged beyond repair should be removed within 2 weeks to prevent the development of sight-threatening autoimmune inflammatory disease in the fellow eye (sympathetic ophthalmitis).

Intra-ocular foreign body

This is a special type of penetrating eye injury, where a small metallic body lodges in the eye, leaving a tiny entry wound that may not be apparent on casual inspection. The diagnosis depends on accurate history-taking, with the patient usually hammering metal on metal without eye protection. The diagnosis must be made early to prevent metal ions diffusing into the eye tissues causing late toxicity and blindness. A missed intra-ocular foreign body is a frequent cause of clinical negligence claims, and a negative orbital x-ray does not exclude the diagnosis.

Compressed air injuries

Surgical emphysema can compress the optic nerve[33] and in situations where the vision is deteriorating, emergency decompression of the orbit can be performed with an intravenous cannula or by dis-inserting the lateral margin of the lower eyelid (emergency cantholysis).

Time off work

Table 9.7 provides indicative information on time off work following occupational injuries to the eye.

Eye protection

This is an element of visual ergonomics that follows on from task analysis, and must be part of a programme of continuous staff training within a culture of safety consciousness.

Generally, products should comply with the European Union Personal Protective Equipment Directive, bear the CE mark and be appropriate to the actual hazards of the work undertaken with regard to dimensions, lens quality, optical power, prescription, field of vision, transmittance of infrared and UV, luminous transmittance, signal recognition, frame requirements, mechanical strength, impact resistance, abrasion resistance, resistance to molten metal, and resistance to dust and gas.

Standards exist for different forms of protection, for example, British Standard (BS) EN 166 for personal eye protection, BS EN 169 for personal eye protection used in welding. To give an idea of the complexity and choice available in eye protective equipment, one supplier offers over 200 different products for eye protection!

The following criteria should be used in selection, and employers should consult the legislation and the Health and Safety Executive guidance available on their website.

1 Type of hazard:
  (a) Mechanical (flying debris, dust, or molten metal).
  (b) Chemical (fumes, gas, or liquid splash).
  (c) Radiation (heat, UV, or glare).
  (d) Laser (over a wide spectrum of wavelengths).
2 Type of protector:
  (a) A safety face shield protects face and eyes but does not keep out dust or gas. It can be comfortably worn for long period.
  (b) Safety goggles provide protection for all hazards and may be worn over spectacles.
  (c) Safety spectacles are comfortable but will not keep out dust, gas or molten metal. Prescriptions are easily incorporated.

Table 9.7 Time off work following occupational eye injuries (NB Suggested times are guidelines for typical cases only; these may vary in the individual case depending on the clinical circumstances)

Injury	Time off work			
	Manual	**Sedentary**	**Hazardous, e.g. dusty, at height**	**Safety-critical**
Welder's flash	1 day	–	–	–
Corneal abrasion	2 days	1 day	1 week	2 weeks
Corneal foreign body	2 days	1 day	2 weeks	1 month
Subtarsal foreign body	1 day	1 day	1 day	1 day
Chemical burns—mild, e.g. perfume	1 day to 1 week	1 day to 1 week	1 day to 1 week	1 day to 1 week
Chemical burns—acid	1–3 months	1–3 months	1–3 months	1–3 months
Chemical burns -alkali	1–6 months	1–6 months	2–6 months	May not be able to return to work
Haematoma	1 day to 1 week	1 day to 1 week	1 day to 1 week	1 week to 1 month
Apical orbital fracture with optic nerve involvement	2–6 months	2–6 months	2–6 months	May not be able to return to work
Blow-out fracture	2 months	2 weeks	2 months	3 months
Blunt trauma	Depends on actual injuries and severity	Depends on actual injuries and severity	Depends on actual injuries and severity	May not be able to return to work
Penetrating trauma	Depends on actual injuries and severity	Depends on actual injuries and severity	Depends on actual injuries and severity	May not be able to return to work
Intra-ocular foreign body	2 months	2 weeks	2 months	3 months
Compressed air injury	Depends on actual injuries and severity	Depends on actual injuries and severity	Depends on actual injuries and severity	May not be able to return to work

3 Type and shade of lens:

    (a) Toughened and laminated glass is less impact resistant but more resistant to abrasion.

    (b) Polymethylmethacrylate and polycarbonate offer high impact resistance but are easily scratched.

Ocular first aid at work

Planning

Risk assessment should include the possibility of chemical splashes to the eyes, the number of employees likely to be affected, and the optimum sites for positioning of emergency eye wash stations.[34] Training should be given to staff in the actions to be taken if they or their colleagues are injured. Training must be updated regularly.

In remote workplaces, a prearranged telemedicine service provides an invaluable source of information for the care of casualties including eye injuries.

Assessment

An adequate light with magnification and fluorescein eye drops are necessary to examine eye casualties. Local anaesthetic drops are invaluable in calming the situation down and enabling adequate examination. Proxymetacaine does not sting, but has to be stored refrigerated.

A vision chart should be at hand. The telephone number of the local eye unit should be available with printed and laminated protocols for injury management at the first-aid station, and an emergency management slate for record keeping.

Irrigation

Immediate irrigation is the priority, using water, saline, Ringer's lactate, and balanced salt solution or, in reality, whatever is available and safe. Ideally irrigation is continued using an intravenous infusion set while holding the lids open with a speculum if necessary.

Eye shields

In suspected eye injury, a transparent Cartella shield can be taped over the eye while arranging transfer. Shields should be secured with suitable tape, and Friar's balsam is useful to keep the skin sticky for long transfers in patients who may be sweating profusely.

Medications

Prior to transfer of the casualty to a specialist centre, emergency medical treatment may include antibiotic drops as directed by the telemedicine service. A preparation such as chloramphenicol Minims should be at hand. Ointment should not be used in eye injury as it may enter the eye in penetrating injuries. Preservative-free drops will not cause problems in this situation.

Acknowledgements

The authors would like to thank Dr Ray Johnston for his valuable contribution to the earlier editions of this chapter.

References

1 Dutton GN. Cognitive vision, its disorders and differential diagnosis in adults and children: knowing where and what things are. *Eye* 2003; **17**: 289–304.

2 Clare G, Pitts JA, Edgington K, *et al*. From beach lifeguard to astronaut: occupational vision standards and the implications of refractive surgery. *Br J Ophthalmol* 2010; **94**(4): 400–5.

3 DVLA. *At a glance guide to the current medical standards of fitness to drive*. Swansea: DVLA, 2012. (<http://www.dft.gov.uk/dvla/medical/ataglance.aspx>)

4 City University London. *A new web-based colour vision test*. [Online] (<http://www.city.ac.uk/health/research/research-areas/optometry/a-new-web-based-colour-vision-test>)

5 Rodriguez-Carmona M, O'Neill-Biba M, Barbur JL. Assessing the severity of colour vision loss with implications for aviation and other occupational environments. *Aviation, Space Environ Med* 2012; **83**: 19–29.

6 Cumberland P, Rahi JS, Peckham CS. Impact of congenital colour vision deficiency on education and unintentional injuries: findings from the 1958 British birth cohort. *BMJ* 2004; **329**: 1074–5.

7 Jawetz E. The story of shipyard eye. *BMJ* 1959; **5126**: 873–6.

8 Thomas PA. Fungal infections of the cornea. *Eye* 2003; **17**: 852–62.

9 Pitts J, Barker NH, Gibbons DC, *et al.* Manchineel keratoconjunctivitis. *Br J Ophthalmol* 1993; **77**: 284–8.

10 Garway-Heath D, Ruben ST, Viswanathan A, *et al.* Vertical cup/disc ratio in relation to optic disc size: its value in the assessment of the glaucoma suspect. *Br J Ophthalmol* 1998; **82**: 1118–24.

11 Mansouri K, Shaarawy T. Continuous intraocular pressure monitoring with a wireless ocular telemetry sensor: initial clinical experience in patients with open angle glaucoma. *Br J Ophthalmol* 2011; **95**: 627–9.

12 Singh K, Shrivastava A. Early aggressive intraocular pressure lowering, target intraocular pressure, and a novel concept for glaucoma care. *Surv Ophthalmol* 2008; **53**(Supp 11): 33–8.

13 Leung DY, Li FC, Kwong YY, *et al.* Simvastatin and disease stabilization in normal tension glaucoma: a cohort study. *Ophthalmology* 2010; **117**(3): 471–6.

14 Durnian JM, Noonan CP, Marsh IB. The psychosocial effects of adult strabismus: a review. *Br J Ophthalmol* 2011; **95**: 450–3.

15 Chorley A, Hunter R, Dance C, *et al.* Heterotropia and time to first solo in student pilots. *Medécine Aéronautique et Spatiale* 2011; **52**: 74–9.

16 Chartered Institute of Building Services Engineers (CIBSE). Lighting handbook and training courses: <http://www.cibse.org/>.

17 Society of Light and Lighting (SLL): <http://www.sll.org.uk/>.

18 Health and Safety Executive—guidance and regulations: <http://www.hse.gov.uk/msd/dse/guidance.htm>.

19 Association of Optometrists. *VDU/DSE guidance. Guidance on vision screening.* [Online] (<http://www.aop.org.uk/practitioner-advice/vision-standards/vdu-dse-guidelines>)

20 Advice on visual impairment for employers: <http://www.rnib.org.uk/professionals/Pages/professionals.aspx>

21 Advice on entitlements of disabled people in the workplace: <http://www.direct.gov.uk/en/DisabledPeople/Employmentsupport/WorkSchemesAndProgrammes/DG_4000347>

22 Magnavita N. Photoretinitis: an underestimated occupational injury? *Occup Med* 2002; **52**(4): 223–5.

23 Power WJ, Travers SP, Mooney DJ. Welding arc maculopathy and fluphenazine. *Br J Ophthalmol* 1991; **75**(7), 433–5.

24 Barkana Y, Belkin M. Laser eye injuries. *Surv Ophthalmol* 2000; **44**(6): 459–78.

25 Houston, S. Aircrew exposure to handheld laser pointers: the potential for retinal damage. *Aviat Space Environ Med* 2011; **82**: 921–2.

26 Mainster MA, Stuck BE, Brown J Jr. Assessment of alleged laser injuries. *Arch Ophthalmol* 2004; **122**(8): 1210–7.

27 Archer DB, Gardiner TA. Ionising radiation and the retina. *Curr Opin Ophthalmol* 1994; **5**(3): 59–65.

28 Chiou GCY. *Ophthalmic toxicology.* New York: Raven Press, 1992.

29 van Soest EM, Fritschi L. Occupational health risks in veterinary nursing. *Aust Vet J* 2004; **82**(6): 346–50.

30 MacEwan CJ. Eye injuries: a prospective survey of 5671 cases. *Br J Ophthalmol* 1989; **73**: 888–94.

31 Yu TS, Liu H, Hui K. A case-control study of eye injuries in the workplace in Hong Kong. *Ophthalmology* 2004; **111**: 70–4.

32 Pitts J. Orbital blow-out fractures. *Eye News* 1996; **3**: 12–4.

33 Caesar R, Gajus M, Davies R. Compressed air injury of the orbit in the absence of external trauma. *Eye* 2003; **17**: 661–2.

34 Beaudoin A. Comparing eyewash systems. *Occup Health Saf* 2003; **72**(10): 50–6.

Chapter 10

Hearing and vestibular disorders

Linda M. Luxon and Finlay Dick

Introduction

Hearing loss is common and, when severe, can seriously compromise an individual's ability to understand speech, perceive danger, and communicate. Profound hearing loss can affect the acquisition and development of spoken language,[1] compromise educational attainment,[2,3] reduce employability[4–6] and impair the individual's ability to work in a safety critical environment.[7–9] Indeed, even mild hearing loss has been shown to be associated with reduced scholastic achievement.[10] Similarly, dizziness is a common cause of loss of time from employment and vestibular disorders can affect balance, increase the risk of falls in dizzy individuals[11] and render the sufferer unfit to drive vehicles,[12] use machinery, work at heights,[8] or remain safe where a stumble at work might have serious consequences, for example, onboard ships.

Hearing loss refers to a unilateral or bilateral hearing impairment. Mild hearing loss may be defined as a hearing loss of at least 25 dB, moderate hearing loss greater than 40 dB, severe hearing loss greater than 70 dB, and profound deafness is an average hearing threshold greater than 90 dB, although colloquially the terms hearing loss and deafness may be used interchangeably. Deafness may be present from birth (pre-lingual deafness) or manifest itself after speech has developed (post-lingual deafness).

Hearing loss can be subdivided into conductive loss, reflecting disease in the outer or middle ear; sensorineural hearing loss due to disease in the inner ear, eighth cranial nerve (vestibulocochlear nerve), or auditory nuclei; and mixed conductive and sensorineural hearing losses which may be congenital or acquired, as seen in advanced otosclerosis or chronic suppurative otitis media. Sensorineural losses are commoner than conductive hearing losses. Hearing impairment may also result from neurological disorders (e.g. neuropathy of the eighth nerve, cortical strokes), precluding normal auditory processing, despite normal peripheral auditory function on pure tone audiometry (PTA).

Conductive hearing loss may be due to a number of conditions including impacted cerumen, acute otitis externa, perforated tympanic membrane, chronic otitis media, trauma (e.g. ossicular injury, haemotympanum), otosclerosis, and genetic syndromes.

Causes of sensorineural hearing loss include age-related reduction in hearing acuity, termed presbyacusis,[13] infections such as rubella, measles, mumps, and meningitis, genetic conditions such as Usher syndrome (a leading cause of deaf-blindness characterized by sensorineural deafness, vestibular dysfunction in type 1 and sometimes in type 3 Usher syndrome and retinitis pigmentosa),[14] labyrinthitis, noise-induced hearing loss, head injury with, or without, skull fractures, acoustic neuroma, and ototoxic drugs (e.g. gentamicin, phenytoin, cisplatin, quinine, and loop diuretics).

Dizziness is a common and imprecise symptom, often used synonymously with vertigo, and may be used by patients to describe a range of symptoms associated with disequilibrium and caused by diverse pathology, of vestibular (vertigo), neurological (unsteadiness/ataxia), psychological (light headedness, dizziness), or cardiovascular (presyncope) origin.[15] The assessment and management of the patient complaining of dizziness has been extensively reviewed.[16] Vertigo is defined as an illusion of motion which is either subjective (the patient feels he is moving) or objective (the patient sees the world moving). Dizziness and/or vertigo may be associated with common mental health problems (anxiety, panic disorder, depression), but the relationship is complex as vertigo may result in associated psychological symptoms or be consequent upon anxiety. Many drugs may cause dizziness as a side effect, including cardiovascular agents, antiepileptics, sedatives, hypnotics, anxiolytics, and antidepressants. In those of working age, dizziness may commonly be due to vestibular disorders such as benign paroxysmal positional vertigo, vestibular neuritis, migrainous vertigo, and, more rarely, labyrinthitis and Ménière's disease.[17]

Epidemiology of hearing loss and tinnitus

Hearing loss affects almost 10 million people in the UK of whom some 3.7 million are of working age. This headline figure is expected to rise as the population ages, to reach 14.5 million people with hearing loss by 2031.[6] Over 800 000 people are severely or profoundly deaf and they are four times more likely to be unemployed than the general populace. Although over 6 million people in the UK would benefit from a hearing aid, only about 2 million people have an aid and, of these, only 1.4 million people use their aid regularly.[6]

The prevalence of hearing impairment in the UK, defined as a loss of at least 25 dB across 0.5, 1, 2 and 4 kHz (the speech frequencies), i.e. a mild hearing loss, was found to be 16 per cent in the late 1980s.[18] Using the same definition of hearing loss, the US National Health and Nutrition Examination Survey (NHANES) 1999–2004 found the prevalence of hearing loss was 16.1 per cent among American adults.[19] The prevalence of hearing loss in NHANES was increased among men, those with lower educational attainment, white men, and older people. Exposure to occupational, firearms, and leisure noise increased the risk of hearing loss as did hypertension, diabetes mellitus, and smoking (>20 pack years). More recently, passive smoking has also been shown to be associated with hearing loss affecting the low/mid frequencies (0.5, 1, and 2 kHz) in those who have never smoked and who are exposed to second-hand tobacco smoke where exposure was confirmed using serum cotinine levels (adjusted odds ratio 1.14, 95 per cent confidence interval (CI) 1.02–1.28).[20]

Tinnitus (ringing in the ears) affects approximately 10 per cent of the adult population,[21] although the prevalence varies depending on the definition of tinnitus employed. One Scottish postal survey of more than 15 000 people aged over 14 years of age found a self-reported prevalence of tinnitus, defined as noise in the ears of more than 5 minutes duration, of 17.1 per cent.[22] The prevalence of tinnitus rose with increasing age in both sexes and was higher among manual workers than professional or non-manual workers. A Japanese study[23] of older adults (aged 45–79 years) found an overall prevalence of tinnitus of 11.9 per cent, greater with increasing age. In that study, tinnitus was considered to be present if the respondent described an episode of tinnitus without preceding noise exposure lasting longer than 5 minutes.[23] An analysis using data from the 1999–2004 National Health and Nutrition Examination Survey study [24] found that the prevalence of frequent tinnitus, which was defined as tinnitus occurring at least once a day, rose with increasing age up to 14.3 per cent of the population aged 60–69 years. In that study, tinnitus was associated with ageing, hearing loss, noise exposure, hypertension, history of smoking, and anxiety.

Methods of assessing hearing disability

Brief enquiry as to hearing problems may alert the assessing clinician to an individual with possible hearing impairment requiring further investigation. One study exploring screening for disabling hearing loss in the elderly found that the simple question 'Do you have a hearing problem now?' had a sensitivity of 71 per cent and a specificity of 71 per cent when compared with the gold standard of a 40 dB hearing loss at 1 and 2 kHz in one ear or at 1 or 2 kHz in both ears on screening audiometry.[25] A recent Brazilian study[26] of people of working age found that three simple questions 'Do you feel you have a hearing loss?', 'In general, would you say your hearing is "excellent", "very good", "good", "fair", "poor"?', and 'Currently, do you think you can hear "the same as before", "less than before only in the right ear", "less than before only in the left ear", "less than before in both ears"?' all showed satisfactory sensitivity and specificity (79.6 per cent and 77.4 per cent for question one, 66.9 per cent and 85.1 per cent for question two, and 81.5 per cent and 76.4 per cent for question three respectively) for research use when compared to the gold standard of PTA.[26]

The whisper test is a simple screening test for hearing impairment. A number of techniques are employed for the whispered voice test and a standardized approach is necessary to avoid problems with reproducibility. However, the test–retest reliability and reproducibility of this test have been questioned[27] and the use of the whisper test is not recommended.

Speech recognition tests potentially offer a more robust assessment of the understanding of speech than whisper tests as they are not amenable to lip reading. The UK charity Action on Hearing Loss, the new name for the Royal National Institute for the Deaf, has developed the English language version of a validated Dutch speech recognition test: the 'Hearing Check'.[28] This speech in noise screening test relies on the identification of a series of three digits, presented with varying degrees of masking using background white noise. The test can be conducted over the Internet[29] or over a phone line (see <http://www.rnid.org.uk/hearingmatters>). The test takes 5 minutes and results are presented as: (a) unimpaired; (b) possibly impaired; or (c) definitely impaired.

Neither the Weber nor Rinne tuning fork tests are sufficiently discriminating to be useful in screening for hearing impairment.[30]

Audioscopy is a screening tool used for identifying hearing impairment[27] and is a combined otoscope and audiometer which generates 25–40-dB tones across a range of speech frequencies (0.5, 1, 2, and 4 kHz). This screening tool has been shown to have high sensitivity and good specificity when judged against the gold standard of audiometry.[27,31,32]

PTA is the standard test of hearing thresholds; to distinguish between conductive and sensorineural losses both air and bone conduction testing are required. Note that PTA is a subjective test and the results of PTA are dependent both on the individual's attention and motivation. Screening audiometry, widely used by occupational health practitioners in hearing surveillance programmes (as required by the Control of Noise at Work Regulations),[33] employs air conduction testing alone and so cannot be used for diagnostic purposes. Detailed information on audiometry and audiometric testing methods are available from the British Society of Audiology (see <http://www.thebsa.org.uk/docs/Guidelines/BSA_RP_PTA_FINAL_24Sept11.pdf>).

Evoked otoacoustic emissions is a simple, non-invasive, test of hearing which provides an objective assessment of the integrity of the cochlea. Otoacoustic emissions may be evoked from the healthy cochlea by the generation of tones or clicks which elicit sound from the cochlea and which can be detected by an intra-aural microphone.

Auditory evoked potentials are an objective assessment of hearing thresholds and assess the integrity of the auditory system from cochlea to cortex. These specialist audiological tests are generally used for the assessment of hearing in those unable to cooperate (e.g. young children or the mentally handicapped or those in whom compensation is an issue). A series of clicks or tones are presented through headphones and the brain's responses are recorded using scalp electrodes. Sedation or a general anaesthetic may be required in those unable to cooperate with testing.

Clinical aspects affecting work capacity including accidents

There is some evidence that hearing loss increases the risk of accidents in childhood[34] and both occupational accidents[35-37] and road traffic accidents in adult life.[38] It would seem likely that the inability to hear warnings, moving vehicles, or alarms might play a role in this increased burden of accidents. However, while a recent systematic review identified 15 studies which had explored hearing loss as a risk factor for accidents, the overall quality of research in this area is limited.[39] One large, well-designed, Canadian study of almost 53 000 workers followed up for 5 years from last audiogram found that those with greater than 15 dB(A) mean hearing loss across 3, 4, and 6 kHz in both ears were at increased risk of accidents[37] and that those with severe hearing loss employed in worksites with noise levels at, or above, 90 dB(A) were at three times the background risk of having more than three accidents.[40] An analysis of over 46 000 Quebec workers for whom audiometry data, occupational noise exposures, and road insurance claims were available, found that workers with hearing loss were at increased risk of road traffic crashes. Those with a mean hearing loss of more than 50dB had a prevalence ratio of road crashes of 1.31 (95 per cent CI 1.2–1.42).[38]

Individuals with impaired hearing may experience difficulty with the spoken word, in face-to-face communication, and by telephone. While hearing thresholds are a guide to hearing ability, how well an individual will function for any given hearing loss is influenced by motivational factors (both of the individual and their colleagues), environmental factors (e.g. proximity of the speaker, visibility of the speaker, adequacy of lighting which facilitates lip reading, background noise levels, availability of an induction loop, room acoustics), and the complexity and predictability of speech. Reports of communication difficulties by colleagues and managers are important evidence as to how well an individual may hear, but additional assessment beyond PTA is helpful and an objective measure of hearing is required if there is any issue with respect to an accident, noise exposure, or compensation. As indicated earlier, the whisper test has significant limitations both in terms of reliability and repeatability and instead the use of a validated speech recognition test is preferable. The Maritime and Coastguard Agency recommends that the Action on Hearing Loss speech recognition test (the 'Hearing Check') is used, in conjunction with the results of audiometry, when determining communication abilities in seafarers.[7] Advice from the Driver Vehicle Licensing Agency[12] is that for profoundly deaf applicants for Group 2 licensing (large goods vehicles/ passenger carrying vehicles), 'Of paramount importance is the proven ability to be able to communicate in the event of an emergency by speech or by using a device e.g. a MINICOM. If unable so to do the licence is likely to be refused or revoked'.

Management: hearing aids and other assistive technology

There is a wide range of assistive devices for those with hearing impairments and additional information is available on the Action on Hearing Loss website (<http://www.actiononhearingloss.org.uk/supporting-you/factsheets-and-leaflets.aspx>).

Hearing aids broadly fall into two categories—analogue and digital aids. Modern hearing aids are generally programmable digital aids and offer higher-quality sound and directional resolution than the older analogue aids. In addition, many digital aids can adapt to different sound environments automatically. Most hearing aids are intended for use in sensorineural hearing loss, but bone conduction aids may assist some people with conductive losses. Hearing aids may be placed behind the ear (BTE), in the ear (ITE), or in the canal (ITC). In general, two hearing aids will provide better hearing, better sound location, and improved understanding in noisy situations than a single hearing aid. Most hearing aids have a telecoil or T-setting for use with induction loops and phones with inductive couplers. Digital aids may offer automatic noise reduction (ANR) to reduce constant background noise such as traffic, feedback suppression to reduce the annoying whistling familiar to those with analogue aids and twin or multi-microphones to allow the listener to focus on sound in front of them. In addition, digital aids offer automatic gain control (AGC) which selectively amplifies soft sounds more than loud ones. This is an important feature for wearers who have a reduced dynamic range of hearing (e.g. those with cochlear hearing loss), as they will struggle to hear quiet sounds but perceive louder sounds as uncomfortably loud. For those who are deaf in one ear, a CROS (contralateral routing of signals) hearing aid may be provided which transmits sound from the deaf ear to the hearing ear.

Bone conduction hearing aids amplify sound, but transmit it by vibration, via the mastoid process rather than as sound through the ear canal. Bone conduction aids are used for those people who lack an outer ear, have a small ear canal or have recurrent ear infections and so cannot tolerate a standard air conduction hearing aid. They can also be suitable for some people with conductive hearing losses. The hearing aid is worn on the body and a vibrating conductor is strapped onto the head or fixed onto the leg of a pair of spectacles. An alternative to the traditional bone conduction hearing aid is the surgically implanted bone anchored hearing aid (BAHA).[41] Here the vibrating element is implanted into the skull behind the ear and the digital or analogue sound processor is attached externally using a titanium fixture.

The development of multichannel cochlear implants,[42] initially for use in post-lingually deaf people and then in pre-lingually deaf young children (older children with long-standing pre-lingual deafness do not acquire speech recognition successfully), offers the prospect of speech perception in profoundly deaf individuals with sensorineural hearing losses.[43] While most studies indicate improved reading ability in children with cochlear implants when compared with profoundly deaf children without such implants, their reading ability is still poorer than their hearing contemporaries.[44] For those with sensorineural or mixed conductive losses who do not benefit from hearing aids, middle ear implants such as the Vibrant Soundbridge™ may be of benefit.[45–47] These middle ear implants employ an external sound processor which transmits an electrical signal to an implant which then stimulates the ossicular chain with vibrations generated by a floating mass transducer attached to an ossicle.

While tinnitus masking devices, noise generators, and hearing aids may be of benefit for some with tinnitus, the evidence base is limited and a recent systematic review by the Cochrane Collaboration[48] failed to find strong evidence for such masking in the management of tinnitus.

Some conductive hearing losses are amenable to surgical intervention, including those arising from tympanic membrane perforation (tympanoplasty) or otosclerosis (stapedotomy or stapedectomy with insertion of a piston).

Advice, and in some cases financial support, is available from the Access to Work scheme to assist hearing impaired people in securing and retaining work (see <http://www.direct.gov.uk/en/DisabledPeople/Employmentsupport/WorkSchemesAndProgrammes/DG_4000347>).

A range of assistive listening devices exist including wireless (radio or infrared) listening equipment, portable or fixed induction loops, and conference folders with a built-in induction loop and microphone. Sadly, there is evidence that some induction loop systems are poorly maintained and do not function as intended. One-third of hearing impaired workers who need a hearing loop/infrared system have not been provided with it.[49] Telecommunications devices include textphones such as Minicom, telephones with an amplifier or an inductive coupler (for use with a hearing aid on the T-setting), and videophones. In addition, hearing impaired people can make or receive phone calls via Text Relay, the national telephone relay service (see <http://www.textrelay.org/>).

Other available workplace supports include access to electronic notetakers (a service where an operator produces a typed summary of a meeting or seminar), lip speakers (someone who silently repeats a speaker's words, using clearly intelligible lip movements/facial expressions and, if requested, fingerspelling, to facilitate lip reading by the deaf or hard of hearing person), speech-to-text reporters (who produce a verbatim record—in contrast, electronic notetakers will provide a précis), and registered British Sign Language (BSL)/English interpreters, either face to face or online using a webcam.

This last group are registered with Signature, which runs the National Registers of Communication Professionals working with Deaf and Deafblind People (NRCPD). This is the main registration body for sign language interpreters, lipspeakers, speech-to-text reporters, LSP-deaf-blind manual interpreters and electronic notetakers in the UK. A register of sign language interpreters in Scotland is maintained by the Scottish Association of Sign Language Interpreters (SASLI). These schemes are voluntary except for those professionals undertaking court and police work, who must be registered.

Some profoundly deaf adults (>18 years old) benefit from the use of a dog trained by Hearing Dogs for Deaf People (see <http://www.hearingdogs.org.uk/>). These assistance dogs are instantly recognizable by their burgundy 'Hearing Dog' waistcoat and traces.

Depending on the workplace a hearing impaired worker may require a vibrating pager linked to the building's fire alarm system and/or fire alarms with flashing lights. Worryingly, in a recent UK survey,[49] only half of those who identified a need for a workplace fire alarm pager or flashing fire alarm had been provided with this.

Epidemiology of balance disorders

The paired vestibular apparatus (each comprising three semicircular canals, and two otolith organs, the utricle and saccule) provide information on head motion and position. Disorders of the vestibular organs lead to vertigo (an illusory impression of movement, usually rotatory), imbalance, and falls. Common causes of vertigo include benign paroxysmal positional vertigo, vestibular neuritis and migrainous vertigo.[50] The NHANES 1999–2004 study found that over one-third of those over 40 years of age had impaired balance on the basis that they were unable to maintain balance, with their eyes shut, while standing on a foam padded surface.[11] Poor balance was commoner with increasing age, lower education, and diabetes mellitus.[11] A postal survey of over 2000 adults in London found that 23.3 per cent reported dizziness in the preceding month.[51] Similarly, a Scottish cross-sectional postal survey[22] found that one in five respondents reported ever having suffered dizziness and this increased in men with increasing age.

Methods of assessing balance problems

A careful history and clinical examination, together with a clear understanding of the causation of imbalance, is central to the assessment of anyone reporting dizziness or vertigo and many sufferers can be managed in primary care without further specialist assessment. Indications for specialist assessment include failure of improvement and diagnostic uncertainty. That said, a diagnosis may not be achieved in a proportion of cases referred for specialist assessment.

The clinical examination of balance includes Romberg's test, Hallpike's test, oculomotor examination including assessment of spontaneous and positional nystagmus, and gait assessment. The Hallpike test[52] is particularly useful in assessing benign positional vertigo and its use is described by the British Society of Audiology (see <http://www.thebsa.org.uk/docs/RecPro/HM.pdf>). It is also helpful to check blood pressure (supine and erect) and pulse to detect postural hypotension or cardiac arrhythmias, and anaemia should be excluded as the cause of light-headedness.

Individuals reporting tinnitus and unilateral hearing loss, with or without balance disturbance, require further investigation (PTA, magnetic resonance imaging (MRI) scan) to exclude an acoustic neuroma. The diagnostic yield is low, however, with approximately 3–7.5 per cent of those investigated being found to have an acoustic neuroma. Most people with an acoustic neuroma will experience slowly progressive unilateral hearing loss, but a minority (5 per cent) suffer acute hearing loss. Similarly, those reporting acute onset vertigo and sensorineural hearing loss in whom a cerebrovascular accident is suspected will require brain imaging.[50]

Management: vestibular disorders

Many people with a vestibular disorder will compensate over time for their difficulties and so their symptoms will improve, usually within 3–6 months. Labyrinthitis sufferers may benefit from medication such as cinnarizine or phenothiazines for 2–3 days in the acute phase, but ongoing therapy should not be continued as these drugs delay vestibular compensation.[16] A systematic review of the use of oral corticosteroids for the treatment of vestibular neuronitis found insufficient evidence of benefit for this treatment.[53]

The importance of both maintaining ordinary physical activity and instituting vestibular rehabilitation (e.g. customized vestibular/balance retraining exercises) needs to be emphasized. A Cochrane systematic review concluded that there was moderate to strong evidence that vestibular rehabilitation is both safe and effective for the treatment of unilateral peripheral vestibular conditions, including labyrinthitis, benign positional paroxysmal vertigo, and unilateral Ménière's disease.[54] Those with benign paroxysmal positional vertigo benefit from specific particle repositioning manoeuvres and may require vestibular rehabilitation if there is additional semicircular canal dysfunction or loss of confidence.[54]

Ménière's disease is associated with endolymphatic hydrops and is characterized by acute vertigo, tinnitus, and hearing loss. The evidence for the efficacy of diuretics,[55] betahistine,[56] and intratympanic steroids[57] in Ménière's disease is limited. Two recent Cochrane systematic reviews failed to find evidence to support surgery for Ménière's disease,[58] but concluded that intratympanic gentamicin may be of benefit, although carrying with it a risk of hearing loss as gentamicin is ototoxic.[59]

The treatment of vestibular migraine is the same as that of migraine. Prophylactic migraine therapy can be beneficial in reducing the frequency, duration, and intensity of acute vestibular migraine[60,61] and vestibular rehabilitation helps the background disequilibrium.

Options for the management of acoustic neuroma include: annual MRI scanning to monitor progression (i.e. interval scanning), as not all neuromas will grow after diagnosis, neurosurgery, or radiotherapy.[62] Most cases will be managed by surgery which can achieve a cure in up to 97 per cent of cases with 1 per cent mortality. However, surgery for acoustic neuroma may be associated with significant morbidity, including hearing loss, damage to the facial nerve, balance problems, and, less commonly, hydrocephalus. In a small case series of 53 patients with acoustic neuroma about 80 per cent were able to return to their original job, without adjustments following surgery, but one in five patients had to change jobs owing to post-surgical symptoms.[63]

Clinical aspects of vestibular disorders affecting work capacity

Balance disorders can affect the sufferer's employment, personal safety, attendance at work, and productivity. Vestibular dysfunction in association with dizziness was found to increase the risk of falls twelvefold in one large, well-designed, US study.[11] Another study, which was set in neurology clinics in London and Siena, Italy, explored disability associated with dizziness among 400 patients.[64] Benign paroxysmal positional vertigo, labyrinthitis, and Ménière's disease accounted for 28 per cent of cases in London and 51 per cent of cases in Siena; work disability was not presented by diagnostic group, but 27 per cent of participants had changed jobs and 21 per cent had given up work as a result of their dizziness.[64] That survey found that, on average, sufferers had taken just over 7 days of sickness absence in the previous 6 months, owing to dizziness and that over half reported reduced efficiency at work. A postal survey of 2064 adults, aged 18–64 years, found that, of those with dizziness who were in work (n = 278), 25 per cent reported difficulty doing their job and of those not working (n = 194), more than one in five stated that this was owing to dizziness (sometimes in combination with anxiety).[51]

Summary

Hearing and balance disorders are common in those of working age and become commoner with increasing age. Hearing impairment can adversely affect an individual's education and employment prospects and there is limited evidence that it may compromise their safety. Similarly, vestibular disorders are common, can affect fitness for work, workplace performance, sickness absence, and fitness for safety critical work. While individuals with deafness or severe hearing impairment may be unable to work in safety critical roles, they are able to undertake many jobs subject to reasonable workplace adjustments being made (as required under the Equality Act 2010). Sadly, many people with hearing or balance impairment either do not seek, or do not receive, appropriate workplace adjustments and as a consequence continue to experience significant disadvantage in the employment market.

References

1 Geers AE, Nicholas JG, Sedey AL. Language skills of children with early cochlear implantation. *Ear Hear* 2003; **24**(1 Suppl): 46S–58S.

2 Woodcock K, Pole JD. Educational attainment, labour force status and injury: a comparison of Canadians with and without deafness and hearing loss. *Int J Rehabil Res* 2008; **31**: 297–304.

3 Rydberg E, Gellerstedt LC, Danermark B. Toward an equal level of educational attainment between deaf and hearing people in Sweden? *J Deaf Stud Deaf Educ* 2009; **14**: 312–23.

4 Rydberg E, Gellerstedt LC, Danermark B. The position of the deaf in the Swedish labor market. *Am Ann Deaf* 2010; **155**: 68–77.

5 American Speech-Language-Hearing Association. *Effects of hearing loss on development.* [Online] (<http://www.asha.org/public/hearing/disorders/effects.htm>)

6 Action on Hearing Loss. *Hearing matters,* 2011. [Online] (<http://www.actiononhearingloss.org.uk/supporting-you/policy-research-and-influencing/~/media/Documents/Research%20and%20policy/Hearing%20matters/Hearing%20matters_pdf.ashx>)

7 Maritime and Coastguard Agency. *Guidance for approved doctors ADG 13—hearing, ear disease, disorders of speech and communication.* [Online] (<http://www.dft.gov.uk/mca/mcga07-home/workingatsea/mcga-healthandsafety/mcga-medicalcertandadvice/mcga-dqs-shs-seafarer_doc_inf/ad_guidance/adg_13.htm>)

8 Health and Safety Executive. *Safety critical workers.* [Online] (<http://www.hse.gov.uk/construction/healthrisks/workers.htm>)

9 Civil Aviation Authority. *ATCO hearing requirements: Information on hearing standards for European Class 3 ATCOs*, 2009. [Online] (<http://www.caa.co.uk/default.aspx?catid=49&pagetype=90&pageid=10870>)

10 Teasdale TW, Sorensen MH. Hearing loss in relation to educational attainment and cognitive abilities: a population study. *Int J Audiol* 2007; **46**: 172–5.

11 Agrawal Y, Carey JP, Della Santina CC, *et al*. Disorders of balance and vestibular function in US adults: data from the National Health and Nutrition Examination Survey, 2001–4. *Arch Intern Med* 2009; **169**: 938–44.

12 Drivers Medical Group. *At a glance guide to the current medical standards of fitness to drive—a guide for medical practitioners*. Swansea: Driver Vehicle Licensing Agency, 2011. (<http://www.dft.gov.uk/dvla/medical/ataglance.aspx>)

13 Gates GA, Mills JH. Presbycusis. *Lancet* 2005; **366**: 1111–20.

14 Cohen M, Bitner-Glindzicz M, Luxon L. The changing face of Usher syndrome: clinical implications. *Int J Audiol* 2007; **46**: 82–93.

15 Reilly BM. Dizziness. In: Walker HK, Hall WD, Hurst JW (eds), *Clinical methods: the history, physical, and laboratory examinations*, 3rd edn, chapter 212. Boston, MA: Butterworths, 1990.

16 Luxon LM. Evaluation and management of the dizzy patient. *J Neurol Neurosurg Psychiatry* 2004; **75**(Suppl 4): 45–52.

17 Eckhardt-Henn A, Best C, Bense S, *et al*. Psychiatric comorbidity in different organic vertigo syndromes. *J Neurol* 2008; **255**: 420–8.

18 Davis AC. The prevalence of hearing impairment and reported hearing disability among adults in Great Britain. *Int J Epidemiol* 1989; **18**: 911–17.

19 Agrawal Y, Platz EA, Niparko JK. Prevalence of hearing loss and differences by demographic characteristics among US adults: data from the National Health and Nutrition Examination Survey, 1999–2004. *Arch Intern Med* 2008; **168**: 1522–30.

20 Fabry DA, Davila EP, Arheart KL, *et al*. Secondhand smoke exposure and the risk of hearing loss. *Tob Control* 2011; **20**: 82–5.

21 McFerran DJ, Phillips JS. Tinnitus. *J Laryngol Otol* 2007; **121**: 201–8.

22 Hannaford PC, Simpson JA, Bisset AF, *et al*. The prevalence of ear, nose and throat problems in the community: results from a national cross-sectional postal survey in Scotland. *Fam Pract* 2005; **22**: 227–33.

23 Fujii K, Nagata C, Nakamura K, *et al*. Prevalence of tinnitus in community-dwelling Japanese adults. *J Epidemiol* 2011; **21**: 299–304

24 Shargorodsky J, Curhan GC, Farwell WR. Prevalence and characteristics of tinnitus among US adults. *Am J Med* 2010; **123**: 711–18.

25 Gates GA, Murphy M, Rees TS, *et al*. Screening for handicapping hearing loss in the elderly. *J Fam Pract* 2003; **52**: 56–62.

26 Ferrite S, Santana VS, Marshall SW. Validity of self-reported hearing loss in adults: performance of three single questions. *Rev Saude Publica* 2011; **45**: 824–30.

27 Yueh B, Shapiro N, MacLean CH, *et al*. Screening and management of adult hearing loss in primary care: scientific review. *JAMA* 2003; **289**: 1976–85.

28 Smits C, Kapteyn TS, Houtgast T. Development and validation of an automatic speech-in-noise screening test by telephone. *Int J Audiol* 2004; **43**: 15–28.

29 Smits C, Merkus P, Houtgast T. How we do it: the Dutch functional hearing screening tests by telephone and Internet. *Clin Otolaryngol* 2006; **31**: 436–55.

30 Bagai A, Thavendiranathan P, Detsky AS. Does this patient have hearing impairment? *JAMA* 2006; **295**: 416–28.

31 Lichtenstein MJ, Bess FH, Logan SA. Validation of screening tools for identifying hearing-impaired elderly in primary care. *JAMA* 1988; **259**: 2875–8.

32 McBride WS, Mulrow CD, Aguilar C, *et al.* Methods for screening for hearing loss in older adults. *Am J Med Sci* 1994; **307**: 40–2.

33 Health and Safety Executive. *Controlling noise at work. Guidance on the Control of Noise at Work Regulations 2005.* L108, London: HSE Books, 2005.

34 Mann JR, Zhou L, McKee M, *et al.* Children with hearing loss and increased risk of injury. *Ann Fam Med* 2007; **5**: 528–33.

35 Moll van Charante AW, Mulder PG. Perceptual acuity and the risk of industrial accidents. *Am J Epidemiol* 1990; **131**: 652–63.

36 Zwerling C, Sprince NL, Wallace RB, *et al.* Risk factors for occupational injuries among older workers: an analysis of the health and retirement study. *Am J Public Health* 1996; **86**: 1306–9.

37 Picard M, Girard SA, Simard M, *et al.* Association of work-related accidents with noise exposure in the workplace and noise-induced hearing loss based on the experience of some 240,000 person-years of observation. *Accid Anal Prev* 2008; **40**: 1644–52.

38 Picard M, Girard SA, Courteau M, *et al.* Could driving safety be compromised by noise exposure at work and noise-induced hearing loss? *Traffic Inj Prev* 2008; **9**: 489–99.

39 Palmer KT, Harris EC, Coggon D. Chronic health problems and risk of accidental injury in the workplace: a systematic literature review. *Occup Environ Med* 2008; **65**: 757–64.

40 Girard SA, Picard M, Davis AC, *et al.* Multiple work-related accidents: tracing the role of hearing status and noise exposure. *Occup Environ Med* 2009; **66**: 319–24.

41 Colquitt JL, Jones J, Harris P, *et al.* Bone-anchored hearing aids (BAHAs) for people who are bilaterally deaf: a systematic review and economic evaluation. *Health Technol Assess* 2011; **15**: 1–200, iii–iv.

42 Clark GM. Personal reflections on the multichannel cochlear implant and a view of the future. *J Rehabil Res Dev* 2008; **45**: 651–93.

43 Bond M, Mealing S, Anderson R, *et al.* The effectiveness and cost-effectiveness of cochlear implants for severe to profound deafness in children and adults: a systematic review and economic model. *Health Technol Assess* 2009; **13**: 1–330.

44 Marschark M, Rhoten C, Fabich M. Effects of cochlear implants on children's reading and academic achievement. *J Deaf Stud Deaf Educ* 2007; **12**: 269–82.

45 Dumon T. Vibrant soundbridge middle ear implant in otosclerosis: technique—indication. *Adv Otorhinolaryngol* 2007; **65**: 320–2.

46 Mosnier I, Sterkers O, Bouccara D, *et al.* Benefit of the Vibrant Soundbridge device in patients implanted for 5 to 8 years. *Ear Hear* 2008; **29**: 281–4.

47 Bernardeschi D, Hoffman C, Benchaa T, *et al.* Functional results of Vibrant Soundbridge middle ear implants in conductive and mixed hearing losses. *Audiol Neurootol* 2011; **16**: 381–7.

48 Hobson J, Chisholm E, El Refaie A. Sound therapy (masking) in the management of tinnitus in adults. *Cochrane Database Syst Rev* 2010; **12**: CD006371.

49 Royal National institute for the Deaf (RNID). *Opportunity blocked: the employment experiences of deaf and hard of hearing people*, 2007. [Online] (<http://www.actiononhearingloss.org.uk/supporting-you/policy-research-and-influencing/research/~/media/Documents/Research%20and%20policy/Opportunity%20Blocked.ashx>)

50 Swartz R, Longwell P. Treatment of vertigo. *Am Fam Physician* 2005; **71**: 1115–22.

51 Yardley L, Owen N, Nazareth I, *et al.* Prevalence and presentation of dizziness in a general practice community sample of working age people. *Br J Gen Pract* 1998; **48**: 1131–5.

52 Dix MR, Hallpike CS. The pathology, symptomatology and diagnosis of certain common disorders of the vestibular system. *Proc R Soc Med* 1952; **45**: 341–54.

53 Fishman JM, Burgess C, Waddell A. Corticosteroids for the treatment of idiopathic acute vestibular dysfunction (vestibular neuritis). *Cochrane Database Syst Rev* 2011; **5**: CD008607.

54 Hillier SL, McDonnell M. Vestibular rehabilitation for unilateral peripheral vestibular dysfunction. *Cochrane Database Syst Rev* 2011; **2**: CD005397.

55 Burgess A, Kundu S. Diuretics for Ménière's disease or syndrome. *Cochrane Database Syst Rev* 2006; **3**: CD003599.

56 James A, Burton MJ. Betahistine for Ménière's disease or syndrome. *Cochrane Database Syst Rev* 2001; **1**: CD001873.

57 Phillips JS, Westerberg B. Intratympanic steroids for Ménière's disease or syndrome. *Cochrane Database Syst Rev* 2011; **7**: CD008514.

58 Pullens B, Giard JL, Verschuur HP, *et al.* Surgery for Ménière's disease. *Cochrane Database Syst Rev* 2010; **1**: CD005395.

59 Pullens B, van Benthem PP. Intratympanic gentamicin for Ménière's disease or syndrome. *Cochrane Database Syst Rev* 2011; **3**: CD008234.

60 Baier B, Winkenwerder E, Dieterich M. 'Vestibular migraine': effects of prophylactic therapy with various drugs. A retrospective study. *J Neurol* 2009; **256**: 436–42.

61 Fotuhi M, Glaun B, Quan SY, *et al.* Vestibular migraine: a critical review of treatment trials. *J Neurol* 2009; **256**: 711–16.

62 ENT UK. *Clinical effectiveness guidelines acoustic neuroma (vestibular schwannoma)*, 2001. [Online] (<http://www.entuk.org/members/publications/ceg_acousticneuroma.pdf>)

63 Nikolopoulos TP, Johnson I, O'Donoghue GM. Quality of life after acoustic neuroma surgery. *Laryngoscope* 1998; **108**: 1382–5.

64 Bronstein AM, Golding JF, Gresty MA, *et al.* The social impact of dizziness in London and Siena. *J Neurol* 2010; **257**: 183–90.

Chapter 11

Spinal disorders

Keith T. Palmer and Charles Greenough

Introduction

Non-specific low-back pain (LBP) is one of the commonest conditions afflicting adults of working age. It represents a leading cause of disability and a major cause of sickness absence. The problem posed in assessing fitness for work in back pain sufferers is one that all occupational physicians frequently face. Neck pain and its associated disability are scarcely less common. Collectively, therefore, axial pains affecting the spine pose a major challenge to the decision-maker.

Commonly, a number of placement and fitness questions arise. In assessing the absent worker with a current episode of pain:

◆ When will symptoms improve or resolve? Is this a short- or a long-term problem?

◆ Are any further investigations required to exclude serious pathology? Who (among the many with pain) should be referred for such an assessment?

◆ At what point should the occupational physician intervene to hasten rehabilitation? And how?

◆ Has work contributed to symptom onset? Might it worsen or prolong symptoms?

◆ Is it appropriate to return the worker to the same job or does the work need to be modified?

◆ When is chronic spinal pain serious enough to declare a person permanently unfit for work? Could more be done to avoid or control the demands of work before that point is reached?

◆ Following spinal surgery, when will the patient be fit for work? Should special restrictions be considered and if so when?

At the pre-employment stage the issues are no less difficult:

◆ Are there any specific inquiries (questions, examination findings, and investigations) predictive of future spinal pain leading to serious disability or sickness absence?

◆ How should these be utilized in assessing fitness for work? In particular, how should a past history of spinal pain be regarded? Are any characteristics sufficiently predictive to warrant restrictions?

And more generally:

◆ What steps can be taken to promote fitness for work and to prevent spinal pain?

◆ What obligations exist under health and safety legislation and the Equality Act 2010?

◆ Do current policies on back pain promote well-being and avoid needless work restrictions?

In attempting to answer these questions it is helpful to appreciate the frequency and natural history of spinal pain, the markers of serious pathology, and the evidence on fitness assessment and preventing disability.

It is also important, for simple mechanical LBP, to be aware of evidence-based advances in management and rehabilitation. Adoption of consensus guidelines has led to better coping and faster recovery. Specific guidelines have also been developed for the management of workers and these address, in part, some of the questions posed above.

In this chapter we review these initiatives and the problem of assessing fitness for work in those with spinal pain. Emphasis is given to simple non-specific axial spinal pain as this is the commonest presentation. Only rarely does the clinician make a more specific diagnosis; but occasionally serious pathology underlies symptoms and different responses are needed. Some account is provided of more specific spinal pathologies including prolapsed intervertebral disc, spinal stenosis, fusion surgery, ankylosing spondylitis, Scheuermann's disease, fractures, and spinal cord injury.

Non-specific low back pain

Prevalence and natural history

In the UK, LBP (defined variously) has a point prevalence of 17–31 per cent, a 2-week to 3-month prevalence of 19–43 per cent and a lifetime prevalence of 60–80 per cent.[1] A similar picture exists internationally.

Sciatic leg pain has a lifetime prevalence of 14–40 per cent, although by the strictest clinical criteria only about 3–5 per cent of adults have true sciatica.[1]

Many episodes of LBP are short-lived and go unobserved by doctors. But the picture of development, persistence, recovery, and relapse is a complicated one when related to a person's life course. Young adults entering first employment already report a past history of back pain,[2] as do school children, and the prevalence of symptoms rises only modestly with age thereafter.[1]

In the Manchester Back Pain Study[3] most of those with back pain had consulted their general practitioner (GP) about symptoms. Some 70 per cent of presentations represented fresh episodes, 20 per cent were acute-on-chronic exacerbations, and 10 per cent a continuation of chronic background discomfort. Three months later, 27 per cent of cases had resolved and 28 per cent had improved, but in the remainder symptoms were either static (30 per cent) or worsened (14 per cent).

Among improved cases a high relapse rate ensues. Thus, in the occupational setting Troup et al. found that 50 per cent of incident cases received further treatment and incurred work loss in the first year of follow-up.[4] The likelihood of further attacks is greatest among those with recent symptoms and falls off as the latest episode recedes in time (Table 11.1).[5] In one prospective study

Table 11.1 Likelihood of further back pain according to time from the last episode

Time since last episode	Likelihood of attack in the next year
<1 week	76%
1–4 weeks	63%
1–12 months	52%
1–5 years	43%
>5 years	28%

Adapted with permission from Biering-Sorensen F. A prospective study of low back pain in a general population, I—occurrence, recurrence and aetiology. Scandinavian Journal of Rehabilitation Medicine, Volume 15, Issue 2, pp. 71–80, Copyright © Foundation of Rehabilitation Information 1983.

of nurses initially free of LBP for at least 1 month at baseline,[6] those who reported a more distant previous episode were at increased risk of having a recurrence during follow-up compared to those who did not. When the most recent episode lasted less than a week and occurred more than a year before, the odds ratio (OR) for recurrence was 2.7. At the other extreme, when symptoms had lasted more than a month and occurred within the preceding year, the OR was 7.3.

It has been estimated that 20 per cent of people with LBP will continue to have symptoms of some degree over much of their life, while 5–7 per cent will report these as chronic illness.[1]

Disability and sickness absence

There is only an approximate concordance between the severity of reported symptoms and disability, and likelihood of losing work time or seeking healthcare. In general, patients who consult a GP have a similar pattern of symptoms to non-consulters;[3] and the best predictor of future work loss is the past history of this behaviour.[5,6]

Economically, the impact of LBP is considerable. Although recent trends have been more encouraging, it has been estimated that each year 150 million days of work incapacity occur from this cause; 3.7 million people (7 per cent of the adult population) consult their GP about back pain; 1.6 million attend a hospital outpatient department; 100 000 are admitted to hospital; and 24 000 have spinal surgery.[1]

Figure 11.1 provides an estimate of the distribution of work loss among workers with back pain. Most sufferers take a little time off work, while a small minority take many days off. Thus, 67 per cent of workers with LBP episodes return to work within a week, 75 per cent within a fortnight, and 84 per cent within a month; but 10 per cent exceed 60 days and at 6 months about 4 per cent are still absent.

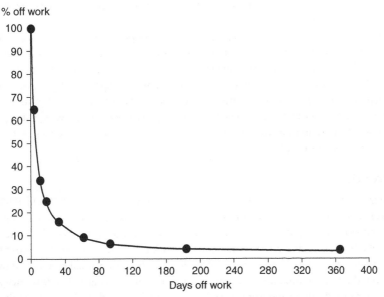

Figure 11.1 Duration of work loss with back pain. Adapted from Clinical Standards Advisory Group. *Epidemiology review: the epidemiology and cost of back pain*, London, HMSO © Crown Copyright 1994.

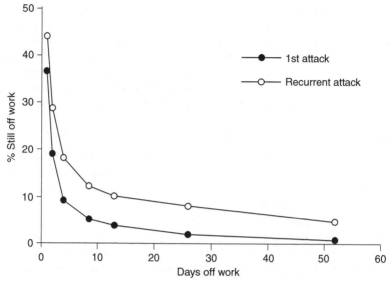

Figure 11.2 Return to work after a first or recurrent back pain attack. Data from Watson P et al. Medically certified work loss, recurrence and costs of wage compensation for back pain: a follow-up study of the working population of Jersey, *British Journal of Rheumatology* 1998; 37(1): 82–6, Copyright © British Society for Rheumatology 1998 and Waddell G. *The back pain revolution*, Churchill Livingstone Edinburgh, Copyright © 1998.

The probability of returning to work is a function of time (Figure 11.2). The longer a person is off the lower their chance of an eventual return, and at 6 months this probability falls to 50 per cent. The curve for those in a recurrent episode of back pain is displaced unfavourably relative to those in their first episode.

It is possible that Figure 11.2 reflects a natural sorting of people according to the severity of illness but another widely held interpretation is that lack of work hardiness becomes self-fulfilling. Reduced mobility, lethargy, and passivity may have effects on muscle strength and tone that raise the physical effort of work; while long-term escape from the responsibilities of work may foster a dependent attitude or erode self-confidence. Whatever the reason, these figures and the two-group absence pattern provide a rationale for encouraging early return to work, with special effort directed towards those in transition from the short-term to the long-term stages. Active intervention at 4–12 weeks is often advocated.

Time trends

The time trends for disability from LBP in the UK are striking. Between 1978 and 1992 inflation-adjusted expenditure on sickness and incapacity benefits rose 208 per cent (vs. 55 per cent for all incapacities) and outpatient attendances for back pain increased fivefold.[1] These changes occurred at a time when the physical demands of work probably lessened. A comparison of two large population surveys a decade apart (1988–1998) found only a small rise in LBP overall with no corresponding rise in functional disability.[7] More recently, during 1997–2007, incapacity benefit awards for LBP declined and were overtaken by mental health disorders as the main reason for award, the change in trend beginning first in London and the South-East and only later spreading to other parts of Britain.[8]

These and other observations suggest that experience of disability may be influenced importantly by culture and prevailing societal beliefs and expectations about health. This idea, which is formalized in the biopsychosocial model of LBP,[9] has been incorporated into management strategies to rehabilitate the affected sufferer (see 'Active rehabilitation').

Risk factors

Many factors can contribute to the onset and severity of LBP, including age, gender, smoking habit, physical fitness, anthropometry, lumbar mobility, strength, psyche and mental well-being, other aspects of medical history, pre-existing spinal abnormalities, and physical demands of work. Evidence on these factors is not always consistent but more comprehensive reviews are published elsewhere.[10,11] Here only a brief overview is given with focus on aspects relevant to fitness for work.

Rates of back pain vary substantially by industry, occupation and job title. In general LBP is reported somewhat more often in people with heavy manual occupations, and workers in these jobs tend to lose significantly more time from work during back pain episodes (Figure 11.3).[12]

Certain physical exposures carry a consistently higher risk of reported back pain. These include lifting, forceful movements, exposure to whole-body vibration, and awkward working postures (Table 11.2).[11] The combination of adverse physical exposures, like lifting and awkward posture, probably carries an even higher risk (Table 11.3).[13] However, back pain is common even in white-collar settings and some authorities consider that physical risk factors only account for a small proportion of the observed overall effect.

Psychosocial factors may be important. In a study conducted within the Boeing Company, psychological distress and dissatisfaction with work were the best predictors of new onset LBP over follow-up.[14] They proved to be more important than any of the physical risk factors studied, although still not highly predictive. In the Manchester Back Pain Study, people free of back pain but more distressed at baseline were more likely to report a new episode over the next 12 months and more likely to see a doctor;[15] those who were dissatisfied with their work were also more likely to report a new episode. Psychological factors, including fear-avoidance beliefs and behaviours, have also been associated with delayed recovery among established cases[16]—these represent risk factors for chronicity and disability. Distress over somatic symptoms, in particular, has been associated with disabling and persistent regional pain, including back complaints.[17]

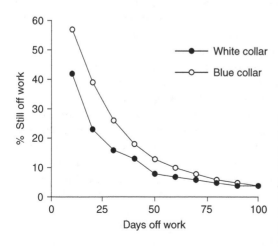

Figure 11.3 Return to work times in blue- and white-collar workers. Reproduced from Waddell G. *The back pain revolution*, Churchill Livingstone, Edinburgh, Copyright © 1998, with permission from Elsevier.

Table 11.2 Evidence for a causal relationship between physical work factors and back pain

Risk factor	Strong evidence (+ + +)	Evidence (+ +)	Insufficient evidence (+/0)	Evidence of no affect (–)
Lifting/forceful movement	√			
Awkward posture		√		
Heavy physical work		√		
Whole-body vibration	√			
Static work posture			√	

Adapted from Bruce P. Bernard (ed) *Musculoskeletal disorders and workplace factors: a critical review of epidemiologic evidence for work-related musculoskeletal disorders of the neck, upper extremity, and low back*. National Institute for Occupational Safety and Health 2007, DHHS (NIOSH) Publication No. 97B141.

Table 11.3 Relative risk of lumbar disc prolapse according to posture and method of lifting

Lifting method	Relative risk	95% confidence interval
Avoids lifting with twisted body	1.0	(reference group)
Lifts while twisting body, knees bent	2.7	(0.9–7.9)
Lifts while twisting body, knees straight	6.1	(1.3–27.9)

Reproduced from Kelsey JL *et al*. Low back pain/prolapsed lumbar intervertebral disc, *Rheumatic Disease Clinics of North America*, Volume 16, Issue 3, pp. 699–716, with permission from Elsevier. Data from Kelsey JL *et al*. An epidemiologic study of lifting and twisting on the job and risk for acute prolapsed lumbar intervertebral disc. *Journal of Orthopaedic Research*, Volume 2, Issue 1, pp. 61–6 © John Wiley & Sons 1984.

Assessing back pain and disability

Pain, by definition, is a subjective personal experience. Therefore, assessing its severity against objective benchmarks is an imprecise process. Several formalized clinical and research approaches have been employed.

Simplest is the use of the visual analogue scale. The pain sufferer is asked to make a mark on a line drawn on a recording sheet and anchored at each end by descriptors such as 'I have no pain at all' and 'my pain is as bad as it could be'. The distance of the mark along the line is measured, and provides a proportionate measure of pain severity, relative to the maximum scale value. This does not circumvent the problem that people's perceptions of pain may differ, but it does offer the opportunity to measure change over time within the same individual.

Other approaches, such as the McGill questionnaire, classify pain by its intensity and a set of adjectives that incorporate the emotional response to pain (throbbing, gnawing, sickening, etc.).

Disability from back pain can be gauged clinically by its interference with activities of daily living—such as sitting, walking, sleeping, and dressing, together with more energetic activities. Well-recognized assessments, such as the Oswestry, and Rowland and Morris questionnaires, are quick, simple, and as robust as more complex approaches to assessing disabling pain.[18]

Another well used, extensively tested, and helpful scale in the occupational health setting is that proposed by Von Korff et al.[19] (Table 11.4). This combines elements of intensity, disability, and persistence in one simple grading scale. Some 4.7 per cent of the Canadian adult population report back symptoms that place them at grade IV and 7.2 per cent at grade III.

One *disadvantage* common to all these approaches is their subjective reliance on the patient's own account. Functional capacity evaluation (FCE) aims to provide independent corroboration of impaired performance. Waddell describes several simple, standardized, quick clinical tests that

Table 11.4 Grading of chronic back pain and disability (after Von Korff et al.[19])

Grade	Degree of disability	Intensity
I	Low	Low
II	Low	High
III	High	Moderately limiting
IV	High	Severely limiting

Reproduced with permission from Von Korff *et al*, Grading the severity of chronic pain, Pain, Volume 50, Issue 2, pp. 133–49, 2002. This table has been reproduced with permission of the International Association for the Study of Pain (IASP). The table may not be reproduced for any other purpose without permission.

can be used (such as the 'shuttle walk' test, the 'five minutes of walking' test and the 'one minute of stand up' tests); but he cautions that FCEs are only semiobjective (reliant still on patient cooperation). Some FCEs, however, have been found in pain management programmes to be good markers of clinical change, which is an attraction. More sophisticated machine-based assessments can produce useful data. But none of these tests is fail-safe in detecting malingering.

Assessing the worker who presents with low-back pain

As work limitation from LBP is frequent across all groups, most occupational physicians will see patients with back-associated sickness absence and will need to assess their prognosis and fitness for work.

Triage assessment and investigation

One aspect of this duty concerns appropriate investigation. Back pain is a symptom and not a diagnosis. However, in an estimated 85 per cent of presentations no underlying pathology can be identified and serious causes are rare. In recent years this has prompted a pragmatic approach to assessment, endorsed in a number of well-respected reports and based on the principles of triage. Cases of LBP should be classified on the basis of a few simple clinical criteria (Box 11.1)[9] into one of three groups:

Box 11.1 Diagnostic triage in patients presenting with low back pain, with or without sciatica

Simple backache (90% recover within 6 weeks):
- Presents at age 20–55 years.
- Lumbosacral area, buttocks, thighs.
- Mechanical in nature: varying with activity and with time.
- Patient well.

Nerve root pain (50% recover within 6 weeks):
- Unilateral leg pain >LBP.
- Dermatomal distribution.
- Sensory symptoms in same distribution.
- Straight leg raising reproduces the pain.
- Motor/sensory/reflex change only in one nerve root.

Box 11.1 Diagnostic triage in patients presenting with low back pain, with or without sciatica *(continued)*

Red flags: possible serious spinal pathology:

- Age at onset <20 or >55 years.
- Violent trauma.
- Constant progressive pain.
- Thoracic pain.
- History of carcinoma, steroid use, drug abuse, or HIV.
- Unwell, weight loss.
- Widespread neurological features.
- Structural deformity.
- Features of cauda equina syndrome (problems of micturition/faecal incontinence; saddle anaesthesia—anus, perineum, genitalia; progressive motor weakness; gait disturbance; sensory level).

From Waddell G. *The back pain revolution*, 2nd edn. Edinburgh: Churchill Livingstone, Copyright © Elsevier 2004.

---

1 Simple backache.

2 Nerve root compression or irritation.

3 Possible serious spinal pathology (less than 1 per cent of all back pain).

The aim is to identify, among the many, the few requiring urgent investigation; and for the rest to follow a conservative approach bolstered, if recovery is stalled, by early active rehabilitation. Urgent specialist referral is required only in exceptional circumstances.

The role of investigation is limited. In the presence of so-called 'red flags' (Box 11.1), plain spinal x-rays, a measurement of the erythrocyte sedimentation rate, or a limited series of magnetic resonance imaging (MRI) in suspected metastatic disease or infection are indicated. In the absence of worrying features investigation is rarely indicated. In particular, the use of computed tomography and MRI is unwarranted and inadvisable in most situations. Usually the prior probability of serious spinal pathology will be low, and in this situation the positive predictive value of the test for serious pathology will be low. However, on many occasions simple age-related changes are reported to the patient as significant pathology, and then a focus on a search for physical pathology in the back may distract from the main emphasis on bio-psychosocial management of symptoms.

Other issues in assessment

More generally, a review commissioned by the UK Faculty of Occupational Medicine[20] has prompted several specific recommendations for occupational physicians assessing workers with back pain (Box 11.2). This advice follows research highlighting:

- The limited value of examination findings, including height, weight, and lumbar flexibility in predicting the prognosis of non-specific LBP.
- The poor correlation of symptoms and work capacity with x-ray and MRI findings.

Box 11.2 Guidance from the Faculty of Occupational Medicine on assessing the worker who presents with back pain

- Screen for 'red flags' and nerve root problems (see Box 11.1).
- Clinical examination otherwise limited in occupational health management and in predicting vocational outcome.
- Clinical, disability, and occupational history important, focusing on impact on work and occupational obstacles to recovery and return to work.
- Screen for 'yellow flags' (Box 11.3) as markers of developing chronic pain and disability; use this assessment to instigate active case management at an early stage.
- X-rays and scans not needed for occupational health management.
- Incident LBP that may be work-related should be investigated and advice given on remedial action and the risk assessment.

From Faculty of Occupational Medicine. Occupational health guidelines for the management of low-back pain at work. Evidence review and recommendations. London: Faculty of Occupational Medicine, 2000.

- The important role of personal and work-associated psychosocial factors in persistence of symptoms, disability, and response to treatment.
- The importance of workers' own beliefs and expectations in their capacity for work.

The evidence-based review identified several relevant prognostic indicators, including age (over 50 years) and a history of the following:

- Prolonged and severe symptoms.
- Radiating leg pain.
- A poor response to previous therapy.

It recommended that an adequate clinical history should cover these aspects, and collect information about the job–to appreciate its physical demands, the scope for job modification, and the attitudes and concerns of the worker and manager.

Psychosocial 'yellow flags' (Box 11.3), should also be sought. Although imperfect indicators, these denote a higher risk of chronicity and disability, and so their presence may suggest the need for early active case management.[21]

Box 11.3 Psychosocial ('yellow flag') risk factors

Factors that consistently predict poor outcomes:

- Belief that back pain is harmful or severely disabling.
- Fear-avoidance behaviour and reduced activities.
- Low mood and withdrawal from social interaction.
- Passive expectation of help (rather than a belief in self-participation).

Managing the worker with a fresh episode of low-back pain

The Faculty's review stresses the importance of following current clinical management guidelines. Several such evidence-based guidelines now exist; from these the Faculty selected the model of the UK Royal College of General Practitioners (RCGP) to align occupational health practice with that of primary care. (A comparison with other guidelines is offered in the following sections.)

Keeping active

A central component of the guidelines is advice to continue ordinary activities of daily living as normally as possible 'despite the pain'. Many trials indicate that this approach can give equivalent or faster symptomatic recovery from symptoms, and leads to shorter periods of work loss, fewer occurrences, and less sickness absence over the following year than advice to rest until completely pain free.

This advice is captured in a user-friendly way in *The Back Book*,[22] an evidence-based booklet developed in conjunction with the RCGP clinical guidelines (Box 11.4). This is a valuable handout to patients.

Box 11.4 Extracts from *The Back Book* which aims to promote self-coping in sufferers through positive evidence-based messages

Back facts:
- ... back pain need **not** cripple you unless you let it!

Causes of back pain:
- ... it is surprisingly difficult to damage your spine.
- ... back pain is usually not due to anything serious.

Rest vs. active exercise:
- ... bed rest is bad for backs.
- ... exercise is good for you-use it or lose it.

Copers suffer less [than avoiders] at the time and they are healthier in the long run. To be a coper and prevent unnecessary suffering:
- Live life as normally as possible ...
- Keep up daily activities ...
- Try to stay fit ...
- Start gradually and do a little more each day ...
- Either stay at work or go back to work as soon as possible ...
- Be patient ...
- Don't worry ...
- Don't listen to other people's horror stories ...
- Don't get gloomy on down days ...

Extracts reproduced from Kim Burton *et al. The Back Book* © Crown Copyright 2002, available from <http://www.tsoshop.co.uk/bookstore.asp?Action = Book&ProductId = 9780117029491>.

Keeping active at work

Continuation of ordinary activities implies encouraging the worker to remain in their job, or to return to it promptly, *even if this still results in some LBP*. Direct evidence that this hastens rehabilitation is limited for the occupational setting (in contrast to primary care and community research), but the same general principles are thought to apply.

Most workers are able to follow this advice and remain at work or return to it within a few days or weeks. In some situations a return to full normal duties may not be possible—as when work requires exceptional levels of physical fitness (e.g. emergency rescue or military combat duties) or unavoidable manual handling of heavy loads. But such circumstances should be unusual. The Manual Handling Regulations require heavy physical tasks to be avoided or minimized, generally, by adaptation of the work and the provision of lifting aids. Guidance that accompanies the Manual Handling Regulations suggests ways in which lighter duties can be constructed.[23,24] The HSE has also developed a risk assessment tool, the Manual Handling Assessment Chart (MAC) (<http://www.hse.gov.uk/msd/>), to support job design and placement.

Any prolonged period off work raises the chance that symptoms will become chronic. It is preferable to find or devise temporary light duties or an adapted pattern of work to encourage uninterrupted employment, and the earliest possible resumption of normal duties should be encouraged.

Whilst doctors and managers commonly employ work restrictions in returning patients with LBP to the occupational environment, evidence for their effectiveness is limited. In 2003, Hiebert et al. reported a retrospective cohort study of patients who experienced absence from work because of LBP.[25] Forty-three per cent were provided with work restrictions. For a fifth of these workers restrictions were never lifted. Restricted duties did not reduce the incidence or duration of sickness absence and no significant reduction was observed in injury recurrence.

The advice given by health professionals is of critical importance. A recommendation to stay off work is often made on the basis of little or no evidence, but can seriously impair the prognosis.

Proper communication between the affected worker, the occupational health team, and line managers, and a shared understanding of the rehabilitation goal are 'fundamental for improvement in clinical and occupational health outcomes'.[20] An organizational culture that secures high stakeholder commitment may also reduce absenteeism and duration of work loss.

Managing the worker who still has problems after 1–3 months

A worker with LBP who is still having difficulty in returning to normal occupational duties at 1–3 months has a 10–40 per cent risk of still being absent at 1 year. By the time 6 months has passed, the risk is higher still. Thus a need exists to identify workers off work with LBP before chronicity sets in. Intervention after 4 weeks is more effective than treatment received much later, and a system should be established to identify absence of this degree.

Active rehabilitation

At the subacute stage an active rehabilitation programme is needed. There is some empirical evidence that intervention can work,[26–28] and guidelines from NICE advocate a proactive approach in which employers and doctors are encouraged to consider referral to a physiotherapist or rehabilitation specialist, psychological interventions such as small group cognitive-behavioural therapy, education in a 'back school', the appointment of a case manager, or intensive multidisciplinary treatment.[29] The evidence from larger and better conducted randomized controlled trials (RCTs) is less strong and benefits seems to be small[30] with uncertainty about cost-effectiveness.

Nonetheless, it has been suggested[20] that certain elements are essential and that effective rehabilitation programmes should:

◆ Include a progressive increase in the amount of exercise to build physical fitness (the precise *type* of exercise being less critical).

◆ Be based on behavioural principles of pain management.

◆ Advise on overcoming fear-avoidance and dependency behaviours (more than the biomedical injury model).

◆ Involve stakeholders in the workplace.

NICE has further suggested that GPs should 'consider offering' an exercise programme, or course of manual therapy or acupuncture; and, in the event of major psychological distress, an 8-week combined physical and psychological treatment programme, including a cognitive-behavioural approach.[31] However, effect sizes, at least for some of these interventions, are likely to be small.[30]

Pre-placement assessment

A past history of symptoms should not be regarded as a reason for denying employment in most circumstances.

Caution should be exercised in placing individuals with a history of severely disabling LBP in physically demanding jobs; but the correct course of action involves a value judgement. Intuitively it may seem obvious that individuals at higher recurrence risk should not be placed in jobs of high physical demand. Unfortunately, this logic has two problems—that of predicting future risk accurately enough, and that of distinguishing recurrence risk in a specific job from recurrence risk in any job (or no job). According to the HSE, the evidence base for matching individual susceptibility to a job-specific risk assessment is insufficient at present to achieve reliable health-base selection. Waddell et al. warn that such judgements carry 'substantial personal, societal, legal, and political implications'.[20]

Investigations and clinical tests

Traditional clinical investigations do little to inform the decision of job placement. The Faculty of Occupational Medicine's evidence review[20] highlighted that future disability from LBP among job applicants is not predicted at all well by the following factors:

◆ Examination findings (e.g. height, weight, lumbar flexibility, straight leg raising).

◆ General cardiorespiratory fitness.

◆ Isometric, isokinetic, or isoinertial measurements of back function.

◆ X-ray and MRI findings.

Symptom-free applicants with single 'yellow flag' histories (Box 11.3) are at a somewhat greater risk of incident LBP, but not to an extent that justifies exclusion.

Collectively these observations suggest a limited role for pre-placement health screening—perhaps just to avoiding the very worst of mismatches between physical demands and back pain history.

Other guidelines

Emphasis has been given in this account on the Faculty's occupational health management guidelines for LBP, but it is instructive to compare these with other sources of advice. Several have been published, including a Canadian version from the Quebec Task Force,[32] an Australian one by the Victorian Workcover Authority,[33] reports from the ACC/National Advisory Committee on Health Disability, New Zealand,[34] and from a working group of occupational physicians in the Netherlands.[35] Other statements have been prepared by the Agency for Healthcare Policy and Research,[36] the Institute for Clinical Systems Integration,[37] and the Preventive Services Task Force[38] in the USA; and the CSAG in the UK.[39]

Generally these agree on the following:

- The need for diagnostic triage, screening for red flags, and neurological complications.
- The identification of potential psychosocial and workplace barriers to recovery.
- Advice to remain at work or to return to work at an early stage, with modified duties as necessary.

More recently, broad consensus has emerged over the importance of screening for 'yellow' (psychosocial) flags as well as flags of other hues (e.g. denoting occupational barriers to a smooth return to work).[40]

Within this broad framework some variations exist, as reviewed by Staal et al.[41] In particular, a few guidelines are more aggressive in their advice on referral, investigation and early intervention. Thus, according to the Quebec Task Force, a referral to a musculoskeletal specialist should occur after 6 weeks of absence; the US guidelines advocate x-ray examination if symptoms fail to improve over 4 weeks; and the US and Dutch guidelines both propose a graded activity programme after 2 weeks of work absence.

None of the guidelines provide a blueprint for implementation. But one clear message that has emerged from public health campaigns in Australia[42] and Scotland[43] is that patient views can be beneficially changed when a single consistent message along the lines of *The Back Book* is given by the media and healthcare professionals. Some employing organizations have also improved awareness and beliefs about the management of LBP among staff and managers, without necessarily reducing LBP-related sickness absenteeism. Various barriers to implementation have been discovered in practice.[44]

Prevention and risk management

Success in preventing spinal disorders depends upon an informed assessment of risk, and a package of risk reduction measures, underpinned by suitable management systems for monitoring and enforcement. A similar approach can help the affected worker to return to work.

A number of preventive measures may have value:

1 Training, to ensure higher risk awareness and better working practices.

2 An induction period, to allow workers in unfamiliar roles to start out at a slower pace.

3 Job rotation and rest breaks, to avoid repetitive monotonous use of the same muscles, tendons and joints.

4 A programme of phased reintroduction to normal work, with temporarily lighter duties or shortened working hours, after sickness absence.

5 Task optimization, e.g. work reorganization to minimize the carrying load, improve the height from which loads are lifted, avoid awkward lifting and twisting, and replace manual handling by employing lifting aids instead.

Some excellent guidelines and case studies from the HSE illustrate this last approach.[22,24]

The case that such job modifications prevent back problems is intuitive and firmly rooted in ergonomic theory. It is also suggested by the research that identifies materials handling as a risk factor for LBP. But the evidence that well-designed workplace and job changes prevent LBP in practice is less clear-cut. Some primary preventive measures have not proved successful.[45] In part this could reflect the difficulty of conducting well-controlled trials in the occupational health setting or of implementing change effectively. Another view is that the scope for preventing disability from LBP is limited, as it has other major non-physical explanations.

However, some well conducted studies have shown a clear benefit. For example, Evanoff et al. examined injury and lost workday rates before and after the introduction of mechanical lifts in acute care hospitals and long-term care facilities.[46] In the postintervention period rates of musculoskeletal injuries, mainly LBP, decreased by 28 per cent, lost workday injuries by 44 per cent, and total lost days due to injury 58 per cent.

In practice, ergonomic theory is likely to hold, at least to the extent that some tasks will aggravate pre-existing and current LBP and hinder the goal of remaining at work. Also in practice, there is a legal mandate to assess risks from manual handling and to minimize unnecessary exposures within reasonable bounds; and simple ergonomic adjustments are likely to be construed as 'reasonable adjustments' within the scope of the Equality Act 2010 for workers with serious back problems.

Neck pain

Prevalence and natural history

By any measure, neck pain, like back pain, is common in the general population. Thus, for example, in a British population survey involving nearly 13 000 adults of working age, 34 per cent recounted neck pain in the past 12 months, 11 per cent reported neck pain that had interfered with their normal activities over this period, and 20 per cent had had symptoms in the past 7 days.[47]

Like back pain, neck pain is often persistent as some 14–19 per cent of subjects report symptoms lasting longer than 6 months in the previous year. Also like back pain, it is commonly recurrent and a source of disability.

Occupational and personal risk factors

Occupational activities are sometimes blamed as a cause of neck pain. One systematic review concluded there was 'some evidence' for a relation with neck flexion, arm force, arm posture, duration of sitting, twisting or bending, hand–arm vibration, and workplace design.[48] A second review, by the US National Institute of Occupational Health, concluded that there was 'strong evidence' for an association with static loading of the neck–shoulder musculature, and 'suggestive evidence' of risks from continuous arm and hand movements and forceful work involving the same muscle groups.[11] A third review found reasonable evidence that repeated shoulder movements and neck flexion were associated with neck pain with tenderness.[49]

Such evidence has tended to accrue from only a few occupations in industry. In community samples the findings have been less consistent. Thus, for example, in a Finnish population study there were no clear-cut differences in neck pain prevalence between blue-collar and white-collar workers[50] and in a UK population survey, no strong associations were found between occupational physical risk factors and neck pain.[47]

Psychosocial factors show a consistent relation to neck pain—in workplaces, in populations, and in patient clinics. Personal feelings of stress and tiredness, and psychosocial stressors like high work pressures and low job control, are both relevant. The situation parallels that of LBP, especially when symptoms are non-specific and unrelated to trauma or serious local pathology.

Assessing and managing the patient with neck pain

Several clinical features predict sickness absence among workers consulting with neck pain. These include short duration, high pain intensity, report of continuous pain, and certain physical signs (pain in the upper limb during rotation of the head and pain in the shoulder during abduction of the arm).[51] Previous sickness absence attributed to neck pain is also predictive of future absence spells from this cause.[52]

Further investigations (e.g. radiology and MRI) are not indicated except in rare circumstances. Changes of osteoarthritis will often be found, but the correlation between symptoms and x-ray appearance is inconsistent, and the predictive performance of such tests for future incapacity is low.

Guidelines on managing neck pain are less developed than those on managing LBP. In principle, and by analogy, the optimal approach should be similar to that for LBP: initial assessment by triage, followed by advice to maintain activity and coping within the limits of pain for simple mechanical neck pain. However, direct evidence on this is sparse.

Complex versions of such advice have been embedded in programmes of multidisciplinary biopsychosocial rehabilitation but there is little evidence at present to justify the effort. Specific exercise programmes, involving strength and endurance training, muscle training, stretching, and relaxation are also of uncertain benefit. Thus, strength and endurance training decreased pain and disability in women with chronic neck problems in one trial, where stretching did not.[53] In another randomized trial, dynamic muscle and relaxation training did not lead to better relief or recovery than continuation of ordinary activity.[54]

Perhaps the best that can be said at present is that most neck pain, like most LBP, does not have a serious underlying cause; that triage is a means of identifying the few cases needing further investigation; that such investigations will rarely aid fitness assessment in the work setting; and that symptomatic relief and advice to remain active is a sensible pragmatic approach, likely in most cases to be followed by an early return to work. Jobs that require workers to crane and twist their necks to an unusual degree (e.g. to inspect overhead electrical equipment in a confined space) and those that require full neck movements to ensure unrestricted field of view in safety critical situations may justify a temporary fitness restriction. However, research evidence is currently lacking to support the view that workplace interventions will reduce the incidence of neck pain.[55]

Spinal surgery

Although back and neck pain episodes are frequent, few patients require surgery. None the less, a small minority undergo such procedures. This chapter will briefly describe the most common spinal surgical procedures.

Surgery for lumbar nerve root compression

The commonest indication for surgery in the lumbar spine is neurological compression, which has two main causes—prolapsed intervertebral disc (PID) and spinal stenosis.

The management of the patient with lumbar neurological compression starts with a clear definition of sciatica. Pain radiating into the leg and foot cannot be considered sciatica unless evidence of neurological dysfunction is also present. Over 70 years ago Kellgren injected hypertonic saline into the supraspinous ligament and described pain referral patterns exactly mimicking dermatomal distribution More recently, studies of patients with mechanical back pain have shown that pain referred below the knee is quite common. To diagnose sciatica, in addition to pain radiating in a dermatomal distribution, some corresponding sensory or motor symptoms and signs must be present.

Asymptomatic disc prolapse can be found in some 20–30 per cent of subjects of working age on MRI scans.[56] The unfortunate patient with a referred pain into the leg and a coincidental asymptomatic disc prolapse on an ill-advised MRI scan is at risk of unnecessary and ineffective surgical treatment.

Prolapsed lumbar intervertebral disc

The commonest cause of nerve root compression in patients of working age is PID. Although the lifetime prevalence of sciatica is high, at 40 per cent, the lifetime prevalence of symptomatic lumbar disc herniation is considerably smaller, at 3–4 per cent and only 1 per cent of patients with acute LBP have nerve root symptoms. The one-year incidence of symptomatic PID lies between 0.1 per cent and 0.5 per cent.[57] Most cases occur at about 40 years of age. Symptoms are equally common in men and women, although men come to surgery 1.5–2 times more often.

So far as aetiology is concerned genetic constitution appears to be of greater importance than mechanical loading.[58] Physical workload, flexion, rotation and whole-body vibration appear to play a role but the effect is not large.

Conservative management

Most cases of PID resolve spontaneously. Initial back pain is usually followed by a dominating leg pain together with neurological symptoms and signs. Leg pain will then tend to improve and approximately 90 per cent of sufferers will experience spontaneous resolution. Between 50 and 70 per cent of conservatively treated cases of disc herniation will resolve completely, often with return to activity within 4 weeks.[59] The natural history of PID is favourable, irrespective of the size or location of the prolapse radiologically. Thus, conservative management is usually appropriate.

Where necessary, epidural steroids or nerve root block can provide pain relief and reduce the need for surgery.[60]

Following a first attack of sciatica, 5 per cent of subjects will experience a recurrence. Following a second attack, the incidence of recurrence rises further to 20–30 per cent, and following the third or subsequent attack recurrences occur in 70 per cent of patients.

Conservative management still requires an active plan. The acute effects of prolapse and the enforced rest lead to significant muscular atrophy. Thus, it is important that normal activity is resumed as soon as pain allows and not left until the pain settles completely. As pain settles, in addition to resumption of normal activities patients should be advised to undertake progressive maintenance exercises to promote muscle endurance and strength (Figure 11.4). In the management of the acute phase effective relief of pain is a vital consideration, as this will allow mobilization and earlier resumption of activities.

As pain settles, in addition to resumption of normal activities patients should be advised to undertake progressive maintenance exercises to promote muscle endurance and strength.

There is little evidence available concerning the return to work following conservative treatment of an acute disc prolapse. However, there is no evidence that resumption of work activities is harmful or capable of precipitating a relapse of symptoms, any more than other normal activities.

Most patients who avoid activity do so because of pain, fear, and negative advice. The key messages, as with simple LBP in the absence of PID, are first that the more rapid the resumption of normal activities the better the overall prognosis and secondly that each incremental increase in activity may cause a temporary increase in discomfort. The patient can be reassured that this is

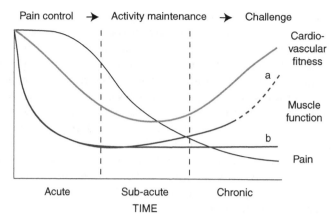

Figure 11.4 Time course of pain, fitness, and muscle function following acute intervertebral disc prolapse. Failure to rehabilitate after the acute stage will result in ongoing decompensation (b) instead of return to normal back function (a).

not dangerous and advised of the difference between hurt and harm. If the patient has not had active management by 6 weeks, then involvement of a physiotherapist for advice, encouragement, and gentle mobilization may be helpful.

Surgical management

The mandatory indication for urgent surgery is worsening neurological deficit. In the absence of profound motor deficit, there is little indication for operative intervention within the first 6 weeks of symptoms. Even in patients with neurological deficit, improvement of sensory loss is unusual following surgery; so the main benefit is in pain relief.

Disc excision surgery is normally an elective procedure. The criteria of Macnab or the 'Rule of Five'[61] have withstood the test of time as indications for such surgery (Table 11.5). Surgery is more successful in relieving leg pain than back pain. Careful examination is required to confirm the presence of neurological deficit and sciatic tension signs according to Macnab's criteria. Early surgery (within 8–12 weeks of symptom onset) under these circumstances results in faster recovery and earlier return to work in the short term, although no difference in outcomes at 1 year.[62]

There has been a trend to admit surgical cases for shorter and shorter periods. Many surgeons now undertake microdiscectomy and fenestration and discectomy without a microscope on a day-case basis, and this works well.

Table 11.5 The 'Rule of Five'

2 Symptoms	1	Leg pain, greater than back pain
	2	Specific neurological symptoms (paraesthesia)
2 Signs	3	Straight leg raising <50% of normal and/or positive crossover test and/or positive bowstring test
	4	Two of four neurological signs (altered reflex, wasting, weakness, sensory loss)
1 Investigation	5	Positive concordant imaging

Modified from McCulloch J, Macnab I. *Sciatica and chymopapain*. Baltimore, MD: Williams and Wilkins, 1983 with permission from Lippincott Williams & Wilkins, Inc.

The postoperative management of patients undergoing surgical treatment for PID is also changing. Fear of recurrence led in the past to postoperative protocols that restricted activity. However, in a study in which patients were allowed to determine their own levels of activity postoperatively, or to return to full activity promptly,[63] the mean return-to-work time from surgery was 1.7 weeks and 25 per cent of patients returned to work the following day; 97 per cent of those working at the time of surgery returned to full duty by 8 weeks. At 2 years no patient had changed employment because of back or leg pain. Recurrent disc prolapse occurred in 6 per cent (three patients) of whom one required surgical intervention. Thus, when freed from restrictions imposed by healthcare professionals, patients returned to activities and work more rapidly and in apparent safety. Magnusson et al.[64] found no rational basis for lifting restrictions after lumbar spine surgery. By contrast, a Cochrane review found strong evidence that intensive exercise programmes commencing 4–6 weeks following surgery were more effective than mild exercise programmes in improving functional status and hastening return to work.[65]

Lumbar spinal stenosis

Spinal stenosis usually results from degenerative change, and is unusual before the age of 50. The commonest symptom is neurogenic claudication (increasing pain or cramping brought on by walking and relieved by sitting). This may be accompanied by symptoms of paraesthesia in the leg or even in the perineum. Eventually the patient is forced to stop walking both by pain and feelings of weakness in the legs. Symptoms appear to arise from restriction of blood flow to the cauda equina and nerve roots. Forward flexion of the lumbar region opens up the intervertebral canals and central canal and explains the typical simian gait adopted by these patients. Symptoms gradually settle on stopping, especially if the patient can sit and flex the lumbar spine. Resolution of symptoms may take 5 minutes or so, and clinically this is a key discriminator from arterial claudication (where the recovery time is substantially less).

Clinical examination at rest may reveal no neurological abnormalities, although subtle weakness and diminution of ankle jerks are present in some 50 per cent of patients.

Conservative management

Non-surgical treatments include the use of non-steroidal anti-inflammatory drugs, prescribed to reduce swelling and inflammation, and for their analgesic effect. However, evidence of effectiveness in neurogenic claudication is not available. Calcitonin and epidural steroid injection have been used, sometimes with positive results. The latter may provide symptom relief for up to 10 months.

Surgical management

Onset of urinary or faecal incontinence is an indication for urgent assessment and operation. Otherwise, surgery for spinal stenosis is dictated by the severity of symptoms.

A comprehensive review from 1992 found that two-thirds of patients undergoing surgery for spinal stenosis had good to excellent results at follow-up.[66] A similar proportion returned to their normal work and a further 12 per cent were able to undertake work of some type. A more recent review concluded that surgery was associated with better outcomes in patients with symptoms lasting more than 6 months.[67] A systematic review published by the US Agency for Healthcare Research and Quality found surgery to be more effective than conservative treatment but noted the evidence base was fair or poor.[68]

There is little agreement on the optimum postoperative regimen, or indeed on the optimum time for return to work duties. However, it would seem reasonable to plan a graduated return to work as an integral part of postoperative rehabilitation.

Surgery for low back pain

A number of procedures exist for the surgical management of LBP, of which the most common is spinal fusion. More recently there has been interest in total disc replacement.

Spinal fusion

Spinal fusion is the gold standard against which other surgical procedures for managing of LBP are judged. However, only a tiny fraction of patients presenting with LBP require surgery. Spinal fusion is a major operation, with success critically dependent on good patient selection. It may be appropriate in patients with chronic symptoms and significant disability, but the patient should already have undergone and failed a formal multidisciplinary intensive functional restoration programme. Psychological distress and compensation claims are recognized predictors of poor outcome.

The efficacy of fusion surgery in appropriately selected patients has been supported by recent systematic reviews and a meta-analysis,[69,70] with benefits sustained over 5 years.

It is clear, therefore, that some chronic back pain patients in whom work restoration is unlikely with conservative treatment may be returned to work by fusion surgery and, moreover, that fusion surgery itself is not a contraindication to employment.

Most surgeons prefer to restrict vigorous activities until bony fusion has been achieved radiologically, a process taking 3–6 months. However, postoperative regimens vary considerably without apparent justification. In a study of spinal surgeons who themselves underwent spinal surgery, 65 per cent had returned to their practice and 42 per cent had resumed operating within 4 weeks following a spinal fusion.[71]

Total disc replacement

The indications for total disc replacement are similar to those for spinal fusion. Disc replacement has several advantages, including the avoidance of bone harvesting from donor sites, preservation of motion (which may reduce degeneration at adjacent levels), and immediate stability (which allows early mobilization). Return to work may thus be accelerated, although policies on postoperative rehabilitation vary and there is no consensus on optimum care. Potential disadvantages include displacement, long-term wear of the prosthesis, and the difficulties and complications of revision.

In a review of nine case series (564 disc replacements) de Kleuver et al.[72] noted that 50 per cent of patients had good results and 81 per cent had excellent results. In one study 31 per cent of patients who were not working prior to surgery were able to return to work, whereas 20 per cent of those working prior to surgery were not working at follow-up.

The cervical spine

Surgery to the cervical spine may be indicated for neurological compression or, more rarely, for cervical pain.

Cervical disc herniation will produce pain and neurological dysfunction in the distribution of the affected nerve root. Like sciatica, neurological compression may be differentiated from referred cervical pain by finding a specific nerve dysfunction. The natural history of cervical disc prolapse is reported as being less benign than for the lumbar region. Up to half of patients treated conservatively continue to experience radicular pain between 2 and 19 years of follow-up.[73] For those patients with insufficient relief from conservative measures, surgery may be considered.

Common procedures (such as anterior discectomy with fusion and decompression with cervical disc replacement) generally give good functional results.

Return to work following cervical surgery, however, is influenced by length of prior sick leave, amount of postoperative pain, age, and claims for compensation.[74]

Postoperative management varies considerably between surgeons and there are no evidence-based reports to guide rehabilitation. However, no adverse effects have been found in patients returning to work within 6 weeks of surgery.[75]

Other spinal conditions

Ankylosing spondylitis

Ankylosing spondylitis (AS) classically presents with an inflammatory onset and involves the sacroiliac and spinal joints. Clinically, the pain is relieved by exercise and not relieved by rest, lumbar spine movement is limited, and chest expansion is decreased. Early morning stiffness taking some time to wear off is frequently observed.

Management relies on analgesics, non-steroidal anti-inflammatory drugs, and disease-modifying antirheumatic drugs such as the tumour necrosis factor (TNF)-alpha inhibitors. Physiotherapy, particularly hydrotherapy, is the mainstay and is clinically effective, although no well-controlled studies have proven its benefit. In the later stages of the disease, where ankylosis is established, pain is a less significant feature.

The National Ankylosing Spondylitis Society comments that 'most people with AS are motivated and reported to have less time off work than average, mostly remaining in full time employment'[76] and evidence exists of this. Nonetheless, AS has an impact on functional work capacity. A study by Boonen et al.[77] found that work disability and incapacity increased steadily with duration of disease. Sick leave was found to vary from 12 to 46 days per year. Work disability increased from 3 per cent at 5 years of disease duration up to 50 per cent at 45 years duration. After 5 years, 96 per cent of patients retained employment, but at 45 years only 45 per cent remained in work.

The difficulties are greater for manual workers. The same researchers found that among those with manual jobs there was a 2.3 fold higher risk of work-related job loss than in those with a non-manual job.[78]

Recently, the more effective pain relief afforded by TNF-alpha inhibitor therapy has improved the vocational prognosis for patients with AS. One RCT reported a significant improvement in work productivity and a reduction in AS-related absenteeism.[79] A caveat is that some TNF-alpha inhibitors are delivered by infusion in hospital outpatient settings, which may require time away from the workplace.

When at work, patients are advised to maintain a good posture, avoid needless forward bending, and to regularly change position. Prolonged car driving may increase pain and stiffness. Patients with rigid or stiff necks may be at greater risk in the event of driving accidents, and the car should be fitted with correctly adjusted head-restraints (and if necessary, additional mirrors to windscreen or dashboard). Disease of mild severity will not preclude vocational driving, although this may not represent the best career choice in the longer-term. Workers with a rigid neck or severe peripheral joint involvement may be unfit to drive vocationally and need to inform the Driving and Vehicle Licensing Agency of their functional limitations.

Patients with AS are at risk of fracture following surprisingly minor trauma. Persistent localized pain in a patient with AS following trauma should be investigated thoroughly. In the ankylosed spine surgical fixation is frequently required to obtain satisfactory union.

About 6 per cent of patients with AS require a hip replacement, which normally restores mobility and relieves pain. The work restrictions that ensue do not differ from those described elsewhere (see Chapter 12), although patients tend to be younger than normal for this surgical procedure.

Rarely, in poorly managed and advanced cases of AS, extreme spinal curvature may occur, limiting normal mobility, posture, and vision. In rare cases surgery is employed to straighten the spine. Other peripheral complications of AS arise sometimes, the most common being uveitis.

Further comments on work limitations can be found in Chapter 13. In most cases, the 'reasonable accommodations' required by the Equality Act 2010 (Chapter 3) should enable AS sufferers to pursue gainful employment, although caution is indicated for occupations where there is an above average risk of trauma (e.g. AS may preclude employment in military combat duties).

Scheuermann's disease

Scheuermann's disease is a kyphotic deformity developing in early adolescence. Estimates of its prevalence vary from 0.4 per cent to 8 per cent. The kyphosis, which is associated with a compensatory lumbar lordosis, is usually noticed clinically, but the diagnosis is radiological with the observation of end plate irregularities, disc space narrowing, and wedging of a minimum of three adjacent vertebrae. Scheuermann's disease can produce a significant kyphosis, normally in the thoracic and thoracolumbar region of the spine.

In general a history of Scheuermann's disease does not suggest the need for job restrictions or adapted work. In a long-term follow-up study, back pain was more common many years later and patients had taken up work with lower physical demands.[80] However, the number of days absent from work with back pain, the interference of pain with activities of daily living, social limitations, level of recreational activities, and use of medication for back pain were not dissimilar from the normal population. The magnitude of the spinal curvature was associated with pain but not with loss of time from work.

Treatment modalities, such as exercise, bracing, and surgery have little impact on work capacity.

Fractures

The thoracolumbar spine

Fractures in the thoracolumbar spine can be divided into three conceptual columns: anterior (anterior body wall and vertebral body), middle (essentially the posterior body wall), and posterior (the posterior elements). Fractures of the anterior column are principally wedge compression fractures and are generally stable. Fractures of both anterior and middle column are often referred to as burst fractures.

Most single column and some two-column injuries are treated conservatively. In general the outcome is very satisfactory even in men still employed in heavy manual labour although job retention seems to be poorer in those claiming compensation.[81]

Burst fractures treated conservatively also have good results. A follow-up by Weinstein et al.[82] found that 90 per cent of patients could return to their pre-injury occupation.

Such fractures may also be treated surgically by internal fixation. Patients with neurological deficit are more likely to undergo surgery, although a meta-analysis[83] concluded there is no evidence that decompression improves neurological outcome. Surgically and conservatively treated cases appear to have a similar long-term outcome, although immediate stabilization reduces immediate pain.[84]

Vertebral fractures occur in cancellous bone and may be expected to heal within 3–4 months. After this period more vigorous activities should be encouraged and work return considered. Surgically treated patients with bone grafting take longer to consolidate but return with restrictions on lifting may be contemplated earlier.

The cervical spine

The recovery from a cervical fracture is mainly influenced by concomitant spinal cord injury. If any significant cord deficit is present then the prognosis is that of the cord injury.

Atlanto-axial injuries are normally treated conservatively with a halo jacket or occasionally by surgical fixation and the results of management are good. The situation is similar for fractures in the subaxial region, although long-term symptoms are more prominent. Fracture dislocations—a source of continuing pain—may be reduced by traction or surgically, to add stability and promote fusion of the injured motion segment.

Following fracture, mobilization may be vigorously commenced once bony union has been obtained, after 8–12 weeks. There is no general consensus on rehabilitation regimens.

Spinal cord injury

Injury to the spinal cord, including major injury to the cauda equina, is rare with an incidence of 20–30 per million per year in the UK. Tetraplegia and paraplegia are now equally common. The age of injured patients is increasing.

Employment rates following spinal cord injury vary from 21 per cent to 67 per cent according to one review.[85] Younger age and greater functional independence predict a positive outcome.

Functional independence is principally determined by the level of neurological injury and residual motor function. The other determinants of individual work capacity include the effects of cord injury on bladder and bowel function, the patient's vulnerability to pressure sores, physical limitations, and various practical barriers to employment (e.g. lack of suitable transportation, lack of work experience and training, physical barriers, disability discrimination).[85] In general, the UK has a poor record of returning patients with spinal cord injuries to work. Just 14 per cent are in employment, versus a European average of 38 per cent and almost 50 per cent in the USA. This substantial underperformance is likely to be a combination of poor expectations among healthcare professionals and inadequate response from employers.

The Equality Act 2010 requires reasonable adjustments by employers to accommodate those with spinal cord injuries—including proper access to the place of work (e.g. ramps, widened doorways, a ground floor work station or access to a lift, special parking rights) and other reasonable assistance (e.g. choosing a job and work schedule to suit the worker's capability, reasonable time off for medical care, adjustments to the work station). Other than access, the most significant practical factor in returning to work is a toilet facility that has enough space and privacy for bladder and bowel management.

Advisors from the Spinal Cord Injuries Centre, the Disability Employment Advisors, together with employers and other training services and educational institutions will be involved and these efforts must be coordinated.

Despite the provisions of the Equality Act 2010, spinal cord injury remains an area where patients in the UK are being significantly failed at present by the work rehabilitation process.

References

1 Clinical Standards Advisory Group. *Epidemiology review: the epidemiology and cost of back pain.* London: HMSO, 1994.

2 Watson KA, Papageorgiou AC, Jones GT, *et al.* Low back pain in schoolchildren: occurrence and characteristics. *Pain* 2002; **97**: 87–92.

3 Croft P, Joseph S, Cosgrove S, *et al. Low back pain in the community and in hospitals.* A report to the Clinical Standards Advisory Group of the Department of Health. Prepared by the Arthritis & Rheumatism Council. Manchester: Epidemiology Unit, 1994.

4 Troup JDG, Martin JW, Lloyd DC. Back pain in industry. A prospective study. *Spine* 1981; **6**: 61–9.

5 Biering-Sorensen F. A prospective study of low back pain in a general population. I—occurrence, recurrence and aetiology. *Scand J Rehabil Med* 1983; **15**: 71–80.

6 Smedley J, Egger P, Cooper C, *et al.* Prospective cohort study of predictors of incident low back pain in nurses. *BMJ* 1997; **314**: 1225–8.

7 Palmer KT, Walsh K, Bendall H, *et al.* Back pain in Britain: comparison of two prevalence surveys at an interval of 10 years. *BMJ* 2000; **320**: 1577–8.

8 Cattrell A, Harris EC, Palmer KT, *et al.* Regional trends in awards of incapacity benefit by cause. *Occup Med* 2011; **61**: 148–51.

9 Waddell G. *The back pain revolution*, 2nd edn. Edinburgh: Churchill Livingstone, 2004.

10 Riihimaki H, Viikari-Juntura E. Back and limb disorders. In: McDonald C (ed), *Epidemiology of work-related diseases*, 2nd edn, pp. 207–38. London: BMJ Books, 2000.

11 Bernard BP (ed). *Musculoskeletal disorders and workplace factors. A critical review of epidemiologic evidence for work-related musculoskeletal disorders of the neck, upper extremity, and low back* (Publication no. 97–141). Cincinnati, OH: US Department of Health and Human Sciences/NIOSH, 1997.

12 Watson P, Main C, Waddell G, *et al.* Medically certified work loss, recurrence and costs of wage compensation for back pain: a follow-up study of the working population of Jersey. *Br J Rheumatol* 1998; **37**: 82–6.

13 Kelsey JL, Golden A, Mundt D. Low back pain/prolapsed lumbar intervertebral disc. *Rheumatic Dis Clin North Am* 1990; **16**: 699–716.

14 Bigos SJ, Battie MC, Spengler DM, *et al.* A prospective study of work perceptions and psychological factors affecting the report of back injury. *Spine* 1991; **16**: 1–6.

15 Croft PR, Papageorgiou AC, Ferry S, *et al.* Psychological distress and low back pain: evidence from a prospective study in the general population. *Spine* 1995; **20**: 2731–7.

16 Burton AK, Tillotson KM, Main CJ, *et al.* Psychological predictors of outcome in acute and subacute low-back trouble. *Spine* 1995; **20**: 722–8.

17 Palmer KT, Calnan M, Wainwright D, *et al.* Disabling musculoskeletal pain and its relation to somatization: A community-based postal survey. *Occup Med* 2005; **55**: 612–17.

18 Roland M, Morris R. A study of the natural history of back pain. Part 1: development of a reliable and sensitive measure of disability in low back pain. *Spine* 1983; 8: 141–4.

19 Von Korff M, Ormel J, Keefe F, *et al.* Grading the severity of chronic pain. *Pain* 1992; **50**: 133–49.

20 Faculty of Occupational Medicine. *Occupational health guidelines for the management of low-back pain at work. Evidence review and recommendations* . London: Faculty of Occupational Medicine, 2000.

21 Kendall S, Burton AK, Main CJ, *et al. Tackling musculoskeletal problems: a guide for clinic and workplace— identifying obstacles using the psychosocial flags framework* . London: The Stationery Office, 2009.

22 Royal College of General Practitioners. *The back book* . London: Stationery Office Books, 2002.

23 Health and Safety Executive. *Manual handling: solutions you can handle.* HSG115. Sudbury: HSE Books, 1994.

24 Health and Safety Executive. *Guidance on Regulations*, 3rd edn. L23. Sudbury: HSE Books, 2004.

25 Hiebert FR, Skovron ML, Nordin M. Work restrictions and outcome of non-specific low back pain. *Spine* 2003; **28**: 722–8.

26 Hillage J, Rick J, Pilgrim H, *et al. Evidence review 1: Review of the Effectiveness and Cost Effectiveness of Interventions, Strategies, Programmes and Policies to reduce the number of employees who move from short-term to long-term sickness absence and to help employees on long-term sickness absence return to work*, 2008. [Online] (<http://www.nice.org.uk/nicemedia/pdf/PH19EvidenceReview1.pdf>)

27 Van Tulber MW, Ostelo R, Vlaeyen JW, *et al.* Behavioural treatment for chronic low back pain: a systematic review within the Cochrane back review group. *Spine* 2000; **25**: 2688–99.

28 Carroll C, Rick J, Pilgrim H, *et al.* Workplace involvement improves return to work rates among employees with back pain on long-term sick leave: a systematic review of the effectiveness and cost-effectiveness of interventions. *Disability and Rehabilitation* 2010; **32**: 607–21.

29 National Institute for Health and Clinical Excellence. *Managing long-term sickness absence and incapacity for work*. NICE public health guidance 19. London: NICE, 2009. (<http://www.nice.org.uk/nicemedia/pdf/PH19Guidance.pdf>)

30 Palmer KT, Harris EC, Linaker C, *et al.* Effectiveness of community- and workplace-based interventions to manage musculoskeletal-related sickness absence and job loss—a systematic review. *Rheumatology* 2011; **51**(2): 230–42.

31 National Institute for Health and Clinical Excellence. *Low back pain: Early management of persistent non-specific low back pain*. NICE clinical guidance 88. London: NICE, 2009. (<http://www.nice.org.uk/nicemedia/live/11887/44343/44343.pdf>)

32 Nachemson A, Spitzer WO, LeBlanc FE, *et al.* Scientific approach to the assessment and management of activity-related spinal disorders. A monograph for clinicians. Report of the Quebec task force on spinal disorders. *Spine* 1987; **12**(7S) (Suppl. 1): S1–59.

33 Victorian Workcover Authority. *Guidelines for the management of employees with compensable low back pain*. Melbourne: Victorian Workcover Authority, 1996.

34 ACC. *New Zealand acute low back pain guide*. Wellington: ACC, 2004 (<http://www.acc.co.nz/PRD_EXT_CSMP/groups/external_ip/documents/internet/wcm002131.pdf>)

35 van der Weidw WE, Verbeek JHAM, van Dijk FJH, *et al.* An audit of occupational health care for employees with low-back pain. *Occup Med* 1997; **47**: 294–300.

36 Agency for Health Care Policy and Research. *Acute low back problems in adults*. Clinical Practice Guideline No. 14. Washington, DC: US Government Printing Office, 1994.

37 Institute for Clinical Systems Integration. *Health care guideline: adult low back pain*. [Online] (<http://www.icsi.org/guide>).

38 Guide to Clinical Preventive Services: *Counselling to prevent low back pain. Report of the U.S. Preventive Services Task Force*, 2nd edn. Washington, DC: US Department of Health and Human Services, 1996. (<http://www.ncbi.nlm.nih.gov/books/NBK15506/>)

39 Clinical Standards Advisory Group. *Back pain*. Report of a CSAG committee on back pain. London: HMSO, 1994.

40 Shaw WS, van der Windt DA, Main CJ, *et al.* for the 'Decade of the Flags' Working Group. Early patient screening and intervention to address individual-level occupational factors ('blue flags') in back disability. *J Occup Rehabil* 2009; **19**: 64–80.

41 Staal JB, Hlobil H, van Tulder MW, *et al.* Occupational health guidelines for the management of low back pain: an international comparison. *Occup Environ Med* 2003; **60**: 618–26.

42 Buchbinder R, Jolley D, Wyatt M.Population based intervention to change back pain beliefs and disability: three part evaluation. *BMJ* 2001; **322**: 1516–20.

43 Waddell G, O'Connor M, Boorman S, *et al.* Working Backs Scotland: a public and professional health education campaign for back pain. *Spine* 2007; **32**: 2139–43.

44 Cunningham CG, Flynn TA, Toole CM, *et al.* Working Backs Project—implementing low back pain guidelines. *Occup Med* 2008; **58**: 580–3.

45 van Poppel MNM, Hooftman WE, Koes BW. An update of a systematic review of controlled clinical trials on the primary prevention of back pain at the workplace. *Occup Med* 2004; **54**: 345–52.

46 Evanoff B, Wolf L, Aton E, *et al.* Reduction in injury rates in nursing personnel through introduction of mechanical lifts in the workplace. *Am J Ind Med* 2003; **44**: 451–7.

47 Palmer KT, Walker-Bone K, Griffin MJ, *et al.* Prevalence and occupational associations of neck pain in the British population. *Scand J Work Environ Health* 2001; **27**: 49–56.

48 Ariens GAM, van Mechelen WV, Bongers PM, *et al.* Physical risk factors for neck pain. *Scand J Work Environ Health* 2000; **26**: 7–19.

49 Palmer KT, Smedley J. The work-relatedness of chronic neck pain with physical findings: A systematic review. *Scand J Work Environ Health* 2007; **33**: 165–91.

50 Takala J, Sievers K, Klaukka T. Rheumatic symptoms in the middle-aged population in southwestern Finland. *Scand J Rheumatol* 1982; **47**: 15–29.

51 Viikari-Juntura E, Takala E, Riihimaki H, *et al.* Predictive validity of symptoms and signs in the neck and shoulders. *J Clin Epidemiol* 2000; **53**: 800–8.

52 Smedley J, Inskip H, Trevelyan F, *et al.* Risk factors for incident neck and shoulder pain in hospital nurses. *Occup Environ Med* 2003; **60**: 864–9.

53 Ylinen J, Takala EP, Nykanen M, *et al.* Active neck muscle training in the treatment of chronic neck pain in women: a randomized controlled trial. *JAMA* 2003; **289**: 2509–16.

54 Viljanen M, Malmivaara A, Uitti J, *et al.* Effectiveness of dynamic muscle training, relaxation training, or ordinary activity for chronic neck pain: randomised controlled trial. *BMJ* 2003; **327**: 475.

55 Aas RW, Tuntland H, Holte KA, *et al.* Workplace interventions for neck pain in workers. *Cochrane Database Syst Rev* 2011; **4**: CD008160.

56 Jensen MC, Brant-Zawadzki MN, Obuchowski N, *et al.* Magnetic resonance imaging of the lumbar spine in people without back pain. *N Engl J Med* 1994; **331**: 69–73.

57 Kelsey J, White A. Epidemiology and impact of low back pain. *Spine* 1980; **5**: 133–42.

58 Battie M, Fideman T, Gibbons L, *et al.* Determinants of lumbar disc degeneration—the study of life time exposure and magnetic resonance imaging findings in identical twins. *Spine* 1995; **20**: 2601–12.

59 Weber H. The natural course of disc herniation. *Acta Orthop Scand Suppl* 1993; **251**: 19–20.

60 Datta S, Everett CR, Trescot AM, *et al.* An updated systematic review of the diagnostic utility of selective nerve root blocks. *Pain Physician* 2007; **10**: 113–28.

61 McCulloch J, Macnab I. *Sciatica and chymopapain.* Baltimore, MD: Williams and Wilkins, 1983.

62 Peul WC, van den Hout WB, Brand R, *et al.* for the Leiden-The Hague Spine Intervention Prognostic Study Group. Prolonged conservative care versus early surgery inpatients with sciatica caused by lumbar disc herniation: two year results of a randomised controlled trial. *BMJ* 2008; **336**: 1355–8.

63 Carragee EJ, Han MY, Yang B, *et al.* Activity restrictions after posterior lumbar discectomy A prospective study of outcomes in 152 cases with no postoperative restrictions. *Spine,* 1999; **24**: 2346–51.

64 Magnusson ML, Pope MH, Wilder DG, *et al.* Is there a rational basis for post-surgical lifting restrictions? 1. Current understanding. *Eur Spine J* 1999; **8**: 170–8.

65 Ostelo RWJG, de Vet HCW, Waddell G, *et al.* Rehabilitation after lumbar disc surgery (Cochrane Review). In: *The Cochrane Library,* Issue 2. Oxford: Update Software, 2002.

66 Turner JA, Ersek M, Herron L, *et al.* Surgery for lumbar spinal stenosis: attempted meta analysis of the literature. *Spine* 1992; **17**: 1.

67 Kovacs FM, Urrútia G, Alarcón JD. Surgery versus conservative treatment for symptomatic lumbar spinal stenosis: a systematic review of randomized controlled trials. *Spine* 2011; **36**(20): E1335–51.

68 Agency for Healthcare Research and Quality. *Diagnosis and treatment of degenerative lumbar spinal stenosis.* [Online] (<http://www.ngc.gov/content.aspx?id = 11306>)

69 Mirza SK, Deyo RA. Systematic review of randomized trials comparing lumbar fusion surgery to non-operative care for treatment of chronic back pain. *Spine* 2007; **32**: 816–23.

70 Ibrahim T, Tleyjeh IM, Gabbar O. Surgical versus non-surgical treatment of chronic low back pain: a meta-analysis of randomised trials. *Int Orthop* 2008; **32**: 107–13. [Correction: *Int Orthop* 2008; **33**(2): 589.]

71 Hall H, McIntosh G, Melles T, *et al.* Outcomes of surgeons who have undergone spine surgery. *J Spinal Dis* 1997; **10**: 518–21.

72 de-Kleuver M, Oner F, Jacobs W Total disc replacement for chronic low back pain: background and a systematic review of the literature. *Eur Spine J* 2003; **12**: 108–16.

73 Gore DR, Sepic SB, Gardner GM, *et al.* Neck pain: a long term follow-up of 205 patients. *Spine* 1987; **12**: 1–5.

74 Bhandari M, Louw D, Reddy K. Predictors of return to work after anterior cervical discectomy. *J Spinal Disord* 1999; **12**: 94–8.

75 Riew KD, Sasso RC, Anderson PA. *Does early return to work following arthroplasty and ACDF result in adverse outcomes?* Annual Meeting of the American Academy of Orthopaedic Surgeons, New Orleans 2010. Paper #539.

76 National Ankylosing Spondylitis Society. *Guidebook for Patients: A positive response to Ankylosing Spondylitis*, 2010. [Online] (<http://www.nass.co.uk/download/4cfcf909bb44a>)

77 Boonen A, De-Vet H, van-der-Heijde D, *et al.* Work status and its determinants amongst patients with ankylosing spondylitis. A systemic literature review. *J Rheumatol* 2001; **28**: 1056–62.

78 Boonen A, Chorus AM, Miedema HS, *et al.* Withdrawal from labour force due to work disability in patients with ankylosing spondylitis. *Ann Rheum Dis* 2001; **60**: 1033–9.

79 van der Heijde D, Han C, DeVlam K, *et al.* Infliximab improves productivity and reduces workday loss in patients with ankylosing spondylitis: Results from a randomized, placebo-controlled trial. *Arthritis Rheum* 2006; **55**: 569–74.

80 Murray PM, Weinstein SL, Spratt KF. The natural history and long-term follow-up of Scheuermann's kyphosis. *J Bone Joint Surg* 1993; **75A**: 236–48.

81 Aglietti P, Di-Muria GV, Taylor TKF, *et al.* Conservative treatment of thoracic and lumbar vertebral fractures. *Ital J Orthop Traumatol* 1984; **9**(Suppl): 83–105.

82 Weinstein JN, Collalto P, Lehmann ER.Thoracolumbar burst fractures treated conservatively, a long-term follow-up. *Spine* 1988; **13**: 33–8.

83 McLain RF. Functional outcomes after surgery for spinal fractures: return to work and activity. *Spine* 2004; **29**: 470–7.

84 Lidal IB, Huynh TK, Biering-Sørensen F. Return to work following spinal cord injury: a review. *Disability and Rehabilitation* 2007; **29**: 1341–75.

85 Krause JS. Employment after spinal cord injury. *Arch Phys Med Rehabil* 1992; **73**: 163–9.

Chapter 12

Orthopaedics and trauma of the limbs

Anne-Marie O'Donnell and Chris Little

Musculoskeletal disease (MSD) remains one of the biggest causes of disability and sickness absence in the working population. As the working population ages, this is likely to continue. The occupational practitioner's role is to reduce the impact of these problems for both employee and employer. This requires not only knowledge of the conditions, but also an understanding of the psychosocial factors underlying sickness absence and an evidence-based approach to rehabilitation. Patients generally do not have to be completely fit to commence, remain in, or return to work, and resuming work may be part of the rehabilitation process (see Chapter 4). Reasonable accommodations under the Equality Act 2010 may help overcome barriers to work to the benefit of workers and their employers (see Chapter 2). Flexible working and well-designed work environments may help retention and facilitate useful and safe work. In this context, fitness for work is a relative concept, dependent on suitable adjustments to the work environment.

The principles of managing musculoskeletal problems at work

Systematic reviews[1,2] have considered absence associated with musculoskeletal conditions. There is a consensus that:

- Absence is related to a combination of medical, psychological, and social factors. To be effective, interventions should consider all factors influencing return to work (see Chapter 4).
- Offering transitional modifications for return is likely to help.
- Interventions should involve the employee and employer in liaison with the occupational case manager, preferably face to face, and relate to the workplace activities as much as reasonably practicable. Contact between the healthcare provider and the workplace may also help.
- Interventions should be implemented in a timely manner. The longer an employee is off work the less likely they are to return.
- If the employee associates the problem with workplace factors, the problems may persist, even with appropriate treatment.
- Ergonomic interventions to reduce an individual's discomfort are generally beneficial and cost-effective, but not in isolation from other interventions.

Ergonomic principles

Advocating specific ergonomic adjustments is problematic in most clinical situations, as generally there is little evidence that one specific ergonomic measure is more effective than another; best practice is more about integrated approaches to control exposure and combinations of ergonomic interventions. In certain employment sectors, the financial benefit of such interventions is

Table 12.1 Ergonomic interventions to limit upper limb pain

Pathology	Painful activity	Possible solution
Shoulder	Shoulder motion/overhead reaching	Reduce reaching/armrest
Epicondylitis	Forceful pronation and grip	Larger handles/lower load Reduce pronation
Carpal tunnel	Flexion of wrist	Ensure neutral wrist position
Finger extensor tendons	Finger extension	Forearm support, a low keyboard

evident.[3] It seems logical to implement adjustments that help the individual avoid a pain-inducing activity (Table 12.1).

Psychosocial factors

Return to work is also influenced by psychosocial factors, i.e. the individual's cognitions, emotions, perceptions, and their interaction with their social environment. Practitioners should assess the individual's level of distress and perception of the workplace and address any factors perpetuating sickness absence. Fear of re-injury is important, particularly if the injury was perceived as work related. Perceived level of control, social isolation, dissatisfaction in the workplace, and multiple comorbidities are factors associated with sickness absence, particularly in non-specific work-relevant musculoskeletal disorders.[4] A 'biopsychosocial' model addressing all contributory elements to absence is recommended (see Figure 12.1).

Return to driving post musculoskeletal surgery

Many employees drive to work and restricting this inhibits their return. The UK Driving and Vehicle Licensing Agency (DVLA) advises that 'drivers should be free from the distracting effect of pain or the sedative or other effects of any pain relief medication. They should be comfortable in the driving position and able to safely control the car, including freely performing an emergency stop'. Licence holders wishing to drive after surgery should 'establish with their own doctor when it is safe to do so'. Many surgeons are conservative in their advice regarding returning to driving postoperatively.[5] Individuals may be safe to drive sooner than guidance would suggest; one study demonstrated good brake response times 2–3 weeks post total knee replacement (TKR)[6] whereas the current advice from the Royal College of Surgeons suggests driving is possible from 8 weeks. Practitioners should advise patients with below-elbow upper limb casts not to drive while immobilized.[7] The most important factors remain that the patient is satisfied that they are safe to drive (in line with DVLA guidance) and have informed their insurance company. If medical conditions (including severe arthritis) are likely to affect safe driving for more than 3 months drivers should notify the DVLA.

Work-related musculoskeletal diseases

The size of the problem

Most musculoskeletal-related sickness absence in Britain arises from complaints that are not attributed to work. Estimating the burden of work-related MSD is difficult because definitions and diagnostic categories vary considerably. However, according to the European Agency for Safety

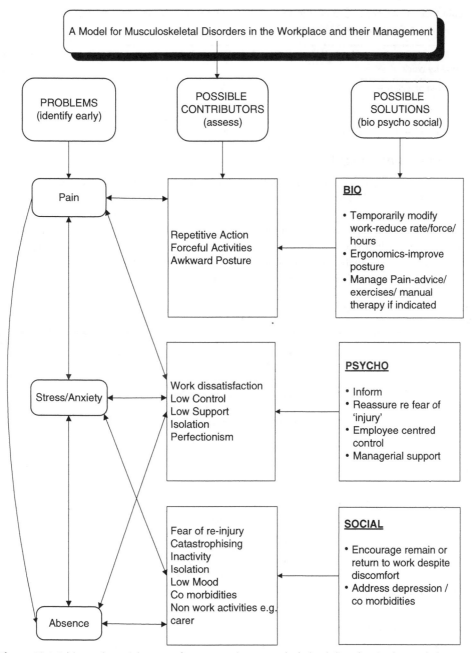

Figure 12.1 A biopsychosocial approach to managing musculoskeletal disorders in the workplace.

and Health at Work[8] MSDs are the most common occupational diseases in Europe. Affected individuals take an average of 13.3 days off work per year due to a self-reported work-related upper limb disorder or injury and 21.8 days with a lower limb disorder. The UK Labour Force Survey[9] estimated the incidence and prevalence of MSDs said to be caused or made worse by work in 2010–2011 (Table 12.2).

Table 12.2 Prevalence and annual incidence of occupational musculoskeletal disorders in the UK Labour Force Survey 2010–2011 (rates per 100 000 in employment)

Conditions caused or made worse by work	Upper Limb/neck	Lower Limb	Back	MSD (total)	All health conditions
Estimated prevalence	660	340	690	1690	3820
Estimated annual incidence	250	100	170	520	1640

Source: Data from Health and Safety Executive (licensed under the Open Government Licence v1.0)

Occupational musculoskeletal disorders

Taking the upper limb as an example, Table 12.3 lists some exposures and occupations that are thought to confer risk. The musculoskeletal section of the Health and Safety Executive website (<http://www.hse.gov.uk>) contains an assessment tool, the ART tool, to identify repetitive tasks that carry significant risks for such conditions and suggests appropriate risk reduction measures. However, although physical exposures can be risk conferring, psychosocial factors are important, and in a recent meta-analysis one of the strongest predictors of upper limb symptoms was a prior history of symptoms, rather than biomechanical work factors.[10]

Table 12.3 Occupational physical risk factors and musculoskeletal symptoms[11,12]

Upper limb condition	Risk factor(s)	Occupations reported to be at risk
Subacromial impingement	1. Lifting (>20kg >10×/day and high hand force >1 h/day) 2. Repetitive shoulder movement 3. Working with hands above shoulder level 4. Hand-transmitted vibration	Fish processing (biceps tendinitis) Slaughterhouse work
Lateral epicondylitis	1. Handling tools (>1 kg/loads >20 kg at least 10×/day) 2. Repetitive forearm movements >2 h/day 3. Low job control/support	Meat cutters Fish processing, foresters, pipe fitter and water/gas suppliers, packers
Medial epicondylitis	1. Lifting (loads >5 kg (2×/min 2 h/day), loads >20 kg at least 10×/day) 2. High hand grip forces >1 h/day 3. Repetitive movements >2 h/day 4. Vibrating tools >2 h/day	
Cubital tunnel syndrome	1. Static load with flexed elbows 2. Ulna nerve pressure	Floor cleaners
Radial tunnel syndrome	1. Static load with extended elbows	
Carpal tunnel syndrome	1. Hand force (>4 kg) 2. Repetitive movements 3. High levels of hand–arm vibration 4. Prolonged work with a flexed or extended wrist	Meat and fish processing, Forestry work with chain saws Electronic assembly work

Source: Data from van Rijn RM et al, Associations between work-related factors and specific disorders of the shoulder-a systematic review of the literature, *Scand J Work Environ Health* 2010; 36: 189–201 and van Rijn RM et al, Associations between work-related factors and specific disorders at the elbow: a systematic literature review, *Rheumatology* 2009; 48: 528–36.

Musculoskeletal disorders of the upper limbs

Disorders of the shoulder

Shoulder pain is common in adults. It may arise from the acromioclavicular (ACJ) or gleno-humeral joint (GHJ), or the rotator cuff, and mixed disorders are common. Limitations in range of abduction indicate subacromial pathology and limitations in external rotation range indicate glenohumeral pathology. In the absence of 'red flag' signs which require urgent investigation and referral (Table 12.4), conservative treatments are recommended, including analgesia, physi-otherapy, and workplace or activity modification (Box 12.1).

Table 12.5 lists some common causes of shoulder pain, their diagnosis, clinical manage-ment, and recommended workplace adjustments. A clinician's diagnostic flowchart and patient information booklet section can be found at the Nuffield Orthopaedic Centre website shoulder and elbow information zone: <www.ouh.nhs.uk/shoulderandelbow/information/patient-information.aspx>.

Physiotherapy

The mainstay of initial treatment is physiotherapy to improve the position of the shoulder blade. Strengthening of the rotator cuff (such as with resistance bands) should commence only *after* scapular posture has been addressed, for fear of worsening symptoms.

Steroid injections

In the absence of a full-thickness cuff tear, the GHJ, subacromial bursa, and ACJ represent sepa-rate cavities. A response to local anaesthetic injections into one of these sites helps to confirm

Table 12.4 Red flag signs in the upper limb

Clinical feature	Possible pathology	Non-sinister causes
Night pain	Tumour; infection; acute rotator cuff tear	Frozen shoulder; arthritis of the ACJ
Significant trauma	Fracture; dislocation; acute cuff tear	
Redness/fever/systemic symptoms	Infection	
Recent convulsion followed by reduced rotation	Unreduced GHJ dislocation (posterior)	
Mass or swelling	Tumour; dislocation or fracture	Ganglion from ACJ

ACJ, acromioclavacular joint; GHJ, glenohumeral joint.

Box 12.1 Work implications—shoulder disorders

The mainstay in the workplace is adaptation of tasks to minimize repetitive forceful shoulder motion, overhead reaching, vibration, and postures that provoke symptoms. Shoulder reha-bilitation may take 12–16 weeks of treatment and exercises. Following surgery, rehabilitation generally involves a period of 4–6 weeks in a sling, followed by restrictions of load-bearing for up to 3–4 months. One-third of patients still have problems 6 months after treatment, particu-larly those with rotator cuff problems.

Table 12.5 Management of shoulder pain

Condition	Typical pain site(s)	Characteristic clinical features	Investigation(s)	Initial treatment	Workplace modifications
ACJ Impingement (also called rotator cuff syndrome or rotator cuff tendinopathy) Usual age: 30–50 years	Deltoid muscle and insertion	Painful abduction arc in mid-to-high zone	Ultrasound MRI	Analgesia Scapular- posture and control physiotherapy Subacromial bursal injection	Reduce: overhead activities Ergonomics to improve shoulder posture, reduce abduction/protraction
Cuff tear Usual age: 50 + years (unless significant trauma)	As above plus resting/ night pains	As above plus possible abduction weakness	Ultrasound MRI	<60 years—consider referral; otherwise as per impingement	Reduce: overhead activities Ergonomics to improve shoulder posture, reduce abduction/protraction
ACJ arthritis Usual age: 50 + years	ACJ	High arc pain; pain on crossing body	X-ray	Analgesia ACJ injection	Reduce: overhead activities Ergonomics to improve shoulder posture, reduce abduction/protraction
GHJ arthritis Usual age: 60 + years	Deep in shoulder	Global restriction of active and passive motion	X-ray	Analgesia; consider GHJ injection	As above and reduce rotation
Recurrent GHJ dislocation	Anterior with provoking motions	Apprehension on provocation testing	MR arthrogram	Proprioceptive retraining and cuff strengthening physiotherapy	Avoid contact/provoking activities, e.g. pulling/ lifting
Frozen shoulder	Deep in shoulder, (sometimes precipitant trauma) Nerve-pattern arm pains, night pain, commoner in diabetics	Global restriction of active and passive motion	X-ray	Ample analgesia (use neurogenic painkillers if radiating pain); GHJ injection; mobilization exercises *after* pain subsides	Avoid pain-provoking activities during painful phase

ACJ, acromio clavacular joint; GHJ, glenohumeral joint.

diagnosis. Injection into the subacromial bursa reduces impingement pain in the short term whilst shoulder posture can be improved by physiotherapy. Steroid injections into the bursa are probably no more effective than alternative treatments (physiotherapy, and non-steroidal anti-inflammatory drugs (NSAIDs)).[13] Steroids can cause atrophy to tendons and joint cartilage, so generally a maximum of three injections is recommended. If no alternative treatments exist (e.g. arthritic joints), surgery may be justified to accelerate symptom relief.

Subacromial decompression

Arthroscopic subacromial decompression surgery improves symptoms in 80 per cent of patients with impingement, particularly if individuals have seen improvement from a steroid injection. Postoperative physiotherapy is essential (as for steroid injections).

Rotator cuff tear

Cuff tears may follow significant trauma, but degenerative cuff tears may be attributed to work when shoulder pain follows minor trauma. Some 25–30 per cent of 65-year-olds have an asymptomatic full-thickness rotator cuff tear which may pre-date a reported injury, although the injury may have caused an extension to a pre-existing degenerative tear. Improvements from physiotherapy can be anticipated over 12–16 weeks (a steroid injection may improve symptoms initially, allowing physiotherapy, so that symptoms abate).

Rotator cuff tears can be repaired (either arthroscopically or by open surgery), although re-tearing is seen in around 25 per cent of cases; newer techniques (e.g. using two rows of securing stitches) may improve healing rates and reduce the duration of rehabilitation. Degenerate cuff tears are less likely to be repairable.

Acromioclavicular joint pain

Pain from an irritable ACJ can improve significantly by improving shoulder posture. Injection into the joint can provide short-lived relief. Surgery to remove the lateral end of the clavicle can be undertaken, generally with a successful return to full activities including work. Ablative surgical procedures (e.g. subacromial decompression or ACJ excision arthroplasty) will require a sling initially for 2–3 days as symptoms allow. Rehabilitation requires restricted load-bearing for 4–6 weeks, with avoidance of overhead activities until symptoms allow.

Replacement of the glenohumeral joint

Severe arthritis of the GHJ may require joint replacement. Following surgery, the discomfort subsides over 6–8 weeks but physiotherapy for scapular posture is essential to avoid impingement. Over 90 per cent of patients experience improvement in pain and range of movement. Loosening of the socket is seen after total shoulder replacement. Thus, workplace loading, including chopping, hammering, digging, strenuous pushing, pulling, and overhead lifting activities should be limited in the long term.

Frozen shoulder

Treatments initially target pain reduction (see Table 12.5). Surgical treatments for frozen shoulder are indicated once the pain has settled if shoulder movement remains very restricted. Treatments to improve motion include: hydro-dilatation, manipulation under anaesthetic, and arthroscopic capsular release. The time course for improvement is unpredictable. The pain generally lessens over 3–6 months. Most symptoms improve over 18–24 months but improvement may extend over 2–5 years. Around a fifth will have residual symptoms, usually not sufficiently intrusive to restrict activities, although some manual tasks at work—especially those involving an extended range of shoulder movement and overhead work—will remain a problem and adjustments may be required.

Glenohumeral joint stabilization

Following stabilization surgery, contact activities must be avoided for 4–6 months. The surgery may be either arthroscopic (which reduces the time in a sling to around 3 weeks) or an open procedure. Movements will generally return towards normal within 2 months, but external rotation will remain restricted initially to around 20–30 degrees, and will improve over 18–24 months. Arthroscopic repairs may have a slightly higher risk of recurrent instability.

Disorders of the elbow

Elbow pain may arise from the joint, the surrounding soft tissue attachments (common forearm flexor or extensor origins, biceps or triceps insertions), or the passing ulnar nerve. Table 12.6 lists some common elbow disorders and clinical and occupational aspects of their management.

Elbow arthritis

Elbow arthritis is usually a consequence of previous trauma or inflammatory arthritis. Patients may complain of pain, stiffness (loss of extension affects reach, loss of flexion affects getting the hand to the face), and intermittent catching or locking (from a loose body or inflamed synovium). There may be hand pain, numbness, and weakness from secondary ulnar nerve entrapment. Restricted forearm rotation limits the ability to place the palm facing upwards producing difficulties with tasks that require cupping of the hands. Compensatory shoulder abduction may cause shoulder impingement when pronation is restricted.

Table 12.6 Management of elbow pain

Condition	Typical pain site(s)	Characteristic clinical features	Investigation	Initial treatment(s)	Workplace modifications
Arthritis	Deep in elbow; more lateral if radio-capitellar	Stiffness with firm end points to motion	X-ray	Activity modification pain relief and physiotherapy	Reduce lifting; workstation changes to accommodate stiffness
Medial epicondylitis	Medial aspect, radiating to hand	Tender CFO; pain on resisted wrist flexion	Ultrasound	as above and brace	Reduced lifting, gripping, and pulling particularly with the arm outstretched
Lateral epicondylitis	Lateral aspect, radiating to hand	Tender CEO; pain on resisted wrist/ middle finger extension		as above and brace	
Cubital tunnel syndrome	Medial elbow; intermittent tingling in little finger	Irritable Tinel sign (tapping) along ulnar nerve in cubital tunnel	Neurophysiology	Restrict elbow flexion; nocturnal elbow extension splint	Avoid prolonged elbow flexion/ direct pressure on flexed elbow

CEO, common extension origin; CFO, common flexor origin.

Treatments

Intra-articular steroids can reduce synovitic pain and locking due to synovitis. Physiotherapy may help overcome early stiffness. Appliances and adjustments to the workstation and work environment can help to overcome problems with reach. Surgery has a limited role (Box 12.2). Arthroscopic removal of loose bodies and a synovectomy relieves intermittent catching or locking. Arthrolysis surgery may improve the range of motion (100 degrees of flexion-extension and forearm rotation enable 90 per cent of tasks of daily living).

Elbow replacement

Elbow replacement has a limited role, as patients should never lift more than 2.5 kg after surgery. This operation is principally indicated for pain control in inflammatory arthropathy.

Box 12.2 Work implications—elbow surgery

Modifications should accommodate the restricted range of motion, and minimize lifting (where this precipitates pain). Following arthrolysis or ulnar nerve decompression gentle activities can be resumed as symptoms allow. Significant lifting is restricted for 6–8 weeks after arthrolysis, and longer (up to 12 weeks) if the triceps tendon has been divided. Procedures vary between patients so liaison with the surgeon about rehabilitation is important.

Epicondylitis

This degenerative tendinopathy affects the common extensor origins (extensor carpi radialis and brevis in lateral epicondylitis) or flexor origins (carpi radialis/pronator teres in medial epicondylitis) of the forearm muscles. Epicondylitis is considered an overload injury and has a prevalence of 3–5 per cent (Box 12.3).

Pain during lifting and gripping initially localizes to the muscle origin at the elbow, later radiating into the forearm. There is local tenderness, maximal 2–3 cm distal to the bony attachment, with pain reproduced on resisted activation of the respective muscle groups. Resisted wrist or finger extension particularly provokes lateral epicondyalgia. Medial epicondylitis is associated with ulnar nerve irritation; lateral epicondylitis is occasionally associated with radial tunnel syndrome.

Symptoms are usually self-limiting and resolve in 80 per cent of cases by 12 months. Activity modifications form the mainstay of long-term management. Braces around the muscle origins, with pads placed over tender points, can reduce symptoms during activities. Physiotherapy should involve deep frictions, stretches of the affected muscles, and eccentric contraction strengthening exercises.

Box 12.3 Work implications—epicondylitis

Forceful activities, high repetition, or awkward posture (particularly gripping) are associated with epicondylitis (see Table 12.3). Reducing load, frequency, gripping requirements, lifting with the palm up, and providing larger-diameter handles to tools in the workplace may help. A vertical mouse may reduce pronation. Low job control and poor social support possibly increase the likelihood of sickness absence and psychosocial factors should be explored.[12]

A single targeted steroid injection may have a short-term effect, confirm the diagnosis, and allow symptom relief until activity modifications are implemented, but physiotherapy or topical NSAIDs are more effective in the long term.[13] Other injection techniques (e.g. dry needling) have limited evidence of efficiency.

Surgery to debride or release the tendon and degenerative tissues can help in resistant cases, good outcomes are reported in 75–80 per cent; forceful gripping and lifting is restricted for 4–6 months. During surgery for medial epicondylitis many surgeons also decompress the ulnar nerve.

Disorders of the wrist and hand

Wrist pain

Pains felt around the wrist may arise from the joint (bones and ligaments) or adjacent nerves and tendons. Carpal tunnel syndrome (CTS) and Wartenberg's syndrome may present with wrist pain.

Pains from the joints are described as 'deep' or as a 'band'; pain from nerves and tendons are described as 'longitudinal'; nerve pain has associated paraesthesia. Tenosynovitis is associated with swelling along the tendons. Ganglion cysts are rarely the source of pain.

Wrist and hand problems affect grip strength which may affect the individual's safety to drive, climb ladders, use cutting tools, or work at heights. In this situation, decisions on fitness to work will depend on the scope for job modification (see Table 12.7) and the safety critical aspect of the work.

Arthritis

Years after an un-united scaphoid fracture or ligament injury, wrist arthritis will ensue because of the altered mechanics of the wrist bones. Widening of the scapho-lunate space can occur in primary arthritic degeneration, hence this sign does not necessarily imply a traumatic origin, as it may pre-date any injury.

Surgical management

If conservative measures are insufficient, surgical options for the wrist may improve pain. Motion-preserving options include denervation (to reduce background aching pains), removal of the radial styloid process (for mechanical impingement pains), excision arthroplasty (to alleviate arthritic pain), and partial wrist fusion (fusing either the radio-carpal or the mid-carpal joint; Box 12.4). Options for joint replacement exist, but are beset by problems of prosthetic loosening.

Thumb-base arthritis

Worsening OA at the thumb base can be reliably addressed by trapeziectomy, debridement, or excision arthroplasty. The long-term outcomes of trapeziectomy are good but pain may take 3 months to settle. In one study the average return to (largely sedentary) work was 5.2 weeks.[14] After joint debridement, work can be considered as symptoms settle. Following excision arthroplasty, healing must occur before manual jobs can be considered (usually at 6 weeks). After fusion surgery, manual tasks can only be undertaken after union (around 8 weeks).

De Quervain's tenosynovitis

This degenerative condition, affecting abductor pollicis longus and extensor pollicis brevis tendons, is found in approximately 1 per cent of the working population. It is more prevalent in females aged 30–50 years, especially during pregnancy or lactation. Forceful grip with wrist pulling and twisting movements aggravate it but the role of occupation in its aetiology is unclear.

Table 12.7 Management of wrist pain

Condition	Typical pain site(s)	Characteristic clinical features	Investigation	Initial treatment(s)	Workplace modifications
Arthritis: thumb-base	Thumb base	Worse on thumb ray compression	X-ray	Splint; analgesics;	Appliances to aid/ avoid grip; (e.g. ball type mouse)
Arthritis: wrist	Deep in wrist	Painful restriction range of motion		intra-articular steroid injection	Reduce flexion/ extension
Tenosynovitis: de Quervain	Radial aspect wrist and forearm	Worse on thumb traction (Finklestein's test)	Ultrasound	Activity modification; splint;	Reduce grip and wrist twisting
					Ball type mouse
Tenosynovitis: flexor	Palmar aspect forearm	Tenderness along affected tendons		analgesics; tendon sheath steroid injection	Reduce wrist flexion
Tenosynovitis: extensor	Dorsal aspect wrist and forearm				Reduce wrist extension
Ulno-carpal abutment	Runs down ulnar side of wrist or forearm	Worse on ulnar deviation of wrist or forearm rotation	Neutral rotation wrist x-ray	Radio-carpal intra-articular steroid injection	Split keyboard; vertical mouse
Scaphoid non-union	Radial-sided	Local tenderness	Scaphoid plain x-rays	Surgical opinion	
Scapho-lunate ligament insufficiency	Dorso-radial	Watson's pivot shift test	MRI arthrogram	Wrist flexor and extensor strengthening and proprioception exercises	

Box 12.4 Work implications—wrist fusion

The most durable solution to wrist arthritis is total wrist fusion, which requires lengthy rehabilitation of 3–4 months. Approximately 70% of individuals can then return to manual duties postoperatively.

Initial management through activity modification and splinting improves mild symptoms. A steroid injection helps around 60 per cent of patients. Physiotherapy aims to stretch the musculo-tendinous unit and reduce irritation. If symptoms persist, surgery to release the tendon from its tunnel has been reported as effective in up to 90 per cent of patients. Complications include tendon instability (a snapping sensation with forearm rotation) and scar tenderness due to irritation of the superficial radial nerve. Return to sedentary work is possible after 1–2 weeks and manual duties by 4–6 weeks after surgery.

Tenosynovitis of the finger flexor and extensor tendons

This usually responds to activity modification and wrist splinting but is associated with systemic poly-arthropathies—hence, systemic steroids may improve symptoms. Steroids, however, can precipitate tendon rupture. Therefore, the patient should avoid heavy (resisted) loading and surgical review should be obtained if there is concern about this or if swelling persists despite treatment.

Ulno-carpal abutment

Some individuals have a relatively long ulna which predisposes to soft tissue and joint surface damage. Soft tissue damage can be debrided arthroscopically, following which manual tasks should be avoided pending wound healing. More significant lesions may require an ulnar-shortening osteotomy, following which delayed union and non-union of the osteotomy may occur, particularly in smokers. Heavy manual tasks will need to be avoided pending union (10 weeks average). Alternatively, excision of the distal ulnar head (a wafer procedure) offers quicker rehabilitation.

Scaphoid non-union

An un-united scaphoid fracture can cause symptoms years later, as arthritis develops. Scaphoid reconstruction with bone grafting and fixation is recommended to reduce the long-term risk of arthritis (Box 12.5). Delayed surgery is less likely to be successful.

Scapho-lunate ligament insufficiency

After a fall onto the wrist, pain, weakness, a 'clunking' or giving way may be due to scapho-lunate ligament insufficiency. Ongoing symptoms, despite physiotherapy, may require ligament reconstruction and/or capsulodesis with a cast or splint for 6–8 weeks, during which time manual tasks must be avoided.

Disorders of the hand

See Box 12.6.

Digital arthritis

Small joint arthritis affecting the digits causes pain and stiffness. Multiple joints are commonly involved, often symmetrically. Initial treatments involve analgesia, physiotherapy, and advice from occupational therapists on the use of appliances. Fusion (or replacing the proximal interphalangeal (PIP) and metacarpophalangeal (MCP) joints) should improve pain and function but will reduce range of motion. Manual work is possible after 8 weeks.

Dupuytren's disease

This affects the fascia in the palm, with nodules and cords forming causing contracture of the digits. The role of occupational trauma in its aetiology is uncertain; systematic reviews suggest

---

Box 12.5 Work implications—scaphoid reconstruction

Postoperatively, splinting will be required for up to 12 weeks, and gripping may need to be avoided for a similar period, depending on the surgical findings. Wrist motion is likely to be reduced in the long term, and discomfort may persist.

Box 12.6 Office adaptations for hand disorders

Keyboard shortcuts can reduce mouse use; reprogrammed 'hot keys' and 'sticky keys' act as multiple keys simultaneously. Input device designs are manifold, including vertical mice (which reduce forearm pronation), ball or bar roller devices, graphics pens and pads, joysticks, and finger-held trackerballs. Voice-activated software helps if hand symptoms affect typing (it can be used in open plan offices but requires careful proof-reading). The Charity Abilitynet advises disabled computer users.

Electric staplers and hole-punchers reduce forceful wrist use. Larger-handled tools generally improve grip comfort for those with arthritic hands.

a possible association with forceful work and hand-transmitted vibration but a case review of nearly 100 000 miners did not show an association between cumulative vibration exposure and prevalence of Dupuytren's contracture.[15] Nodule tenderness usually resolves over 9–12 months but progressive contractures require surgery to divide or excise the cords. Recurrence is common, requiring revision in a 25–30 per cent within 8–10 years. Following surgery, patients must refrain from manual work until wound and graft healing. Less invasive treatments are increasingly used (needle fasciotomy, excision of short segments only, injections of collagenase with manipulation), comparative long-term outcomes are presently unclear.

Trigger digit

In this condition a degenerative swelling catches in the mouth of the flexor tendon sheath in the palm, painfully catching with the finger flexed (the thumb may lock in extension). It is commoner in diabetics. Flexor sheath steroid injections (with or without nocturnal extension splintage) help 80 per cent of cases, but surgical division of the flexor sheath's mouth is sometimes required. Postoperatively, manual tasks should be avoided for 2–3 weeks, as stiffness and discomfort may occur.

Hypothenar hammer syndrome

This thrombosis of the ulnar artery at the wrist is thought to be due to using the heel of the hand as a blunt instrument. It gives rise to pain, cold intolerance, and sometimes ulceration (in particular affecting the ring finger). Vascular reconstruction may be required.

Disorders of the nerves

Nerve compression is often idiopathic but may arise due to structural anomalies, tenosynovitis, fluid re-distribution (e.g. obesity, pregnancy), or systemic conditions (e.g. diabetes, rheumatoid arthritis, hypothyroidism, alcoholism).

Nerve compression can arise at multiple sites. Assessment of nerve irritation should explore the different potential sites of compression. The neck must be screened in patients with upper limb neurological symptoms; shoulder posture protraction may indicate thoracic outlet plexus irritation.

It is important to remember the potential for nerve compression at multiple sites, termed the 'double crush' phenomenon. This can cause symptoms that are out of proportion to the electrophysiology changes. Treatments usually address distal compression sites first as any surgery is usually less hazardous.

There is considerable overlap between median nerve and ulnar nerve compression symptoms. Asking patients to specify if the little finger or thumb is involved may help differentiate. The presence or absence of resting and nocturnal symptoms distinguishes between fixed structural and dynamic (functional) compression.

Diagnostic tests

Conduction studies help diagnosis, but with dynamic compressions, if no permanent nerve changes exist, the results may be normal. With brachial plexus lesions, normal electromyograms of muscle groups that are not clinically implicated help localize the lesion to the plexus as opposed to a peripheral nerve.

Treatment

In the absence of objective neurological loss (clear weakness, muscle wasting, sensory loss, altered sensory threshold) initial treatment involves modifying activities (e.g. care with posture, pacing) (Table 12.8). Splinting also has a role. By placing the wrist in a neutral position, the volume of the

Table 12.8 Management of upper limb nerve entrapments

Syndrome (nerve and site involved)	Typical pain site(s)	Characteristic clinical features	Investigation	Initial treatment(s)	Workplace modifications
Carpal tunnel (median nerve at wrist)	Hand and radial-sided digits (spares little finger)	Phalen's test positive	NCS if doubt	Activity modification Wrist-neutral splintage Carpal tunnel injection	Reduce force/ vibration/ repetitive flexion; pacing advice
Pronator (median nerve around elbow)	As for CTS, but more forearm pain and no night symptoms	Reproduced by resisted muscle activation (depends on site)	EMG (but may be normal)	Activity modification	As above
Anterior interosseous (AIN branch of median nerve in forearm)	Forearm; may be motor loss only	cannot oppose tips of thumb and index	EMG	Observation	
Cubital tunnel (ulnar nerve at elbow)	Medial elbow; ulnar forearm and hand	Elbow flexion test	NCS	Provocation avoidance	Reduce elbow flexion and direct elbow pressure
Ulnar tunnel (ulnar nerve at wrist—Guyon's canal)	Ulnar-side digits	No specific	NCS; imaging to look for cause (space-occupying lesion; hamate hook non-union)	Rest/splintage if no underlying structural cause Surgery (to address cause)	

Table 12.8 (continued) Management of upper limb nerve entrapments

Syndrome (nerve and site involved)	Typical pain site(s)	Characteristic clinical features	Investigation	Initial treatment(s)	Workplace modifications
Wartenberg's (superficial radial nerve compression in forearm)	Dorso-radial hand	Tinel's test provocation with forced pronation	Diagnostic anaesthetic injection	Wrist-neutral splintage (avoiding direct nerve pressure)	Avoid provoking activities
Posterior interosseous (PIN) (radial nerve at elbow, including radial tunnel)	PIN palsy: motor loss only Radial tunnel-proximal forearm	PIN palsy: wrist drop Radial tunnel-resisted wrist/middle finger extension	PIN palsy: imaging to exclude space-occupying lesion	PIN palsy: surgical if mass lesion Radial tunnel-activity modification; wrist-neutral splintage	Pacing advice
Saturday night palsy (radial nerve in arm)	Motor and sensory (dorsum hand) loss	Wrist drop	NCS	Observation; wrist splint; maintain passive motion	
Thoracic outlet syndrome (neurogenic or vascular)	Arm symptoms	Roo's test	Imaging (for cervical rib; arterial assessment if vascular symptoms; chest x-ray to exclude Pancoast tumour)	Shoulder posture and proprioception; surgical if vascular lesions	Ergonomics and pacing advice
Parsonage–Turner (neuritis of the brachial plexus)	Initial marked shoulder pains	None specific	EMG	Shoulder posture	

EMG, electromyography; NCS, nerve conduction studies.

carpal tunnel is maximized. Any objective neurological loss should prompt referral as delay may impair recovery, even following technically successful surgery.

Carpal tunnel syndrome

Predominantly nocturnal symptoms may be relieved by a wrist-neutral splint. A steroid injection (with or without local anaesthetic) into the carpal tunnel (avoiding intraneural or intratendinous injection) temporarily alleviates symptoms in up to 80 per cent of cases, with sustained improvement in 20 per cent. Injections are useful if there is a clear reversible cause (e.g. pregnancy), early in the course of the syndrome, or if there is diagnostic doubt (a transient response indicates that surgical treatment may be helpful).

Surgery is usually effective. It may be open or endoscopic; endoscopic release allows slightly earlier return to work but has a higher rate of permanent nerve damage than open release (Box 12.7).

Box 12.7 Work implications—carpal tunnel surgery

In one study, the surgeon's recommendation was the strongest predictor of return to work time and workers could return to work in less than 3 weeks, particularly to sedentary roles, once wound healing was assured.[16] Scar tenderness generally resolves over 2–3 months, grip strength returns over 3–6 months (pinch grips earlier than power grips). Physical activities including many manual tasks, while initially uncomfortable, can aid scar desensitization. Recurrence after surgery is rare. One study found that pre-surgical work-role functioning, having confidence in managing symptoms, and a supportive organization offering the ability to modify activities in the workplace correlated with better postsurgical work function; depression or pursuing compensation were poor prognostic factors.[17]

Pronator syndrome

Pronator syndrome refers to compression of the median nerve around the elbow by either pronator teres, flexor digitorum superficialis (FDS) or biceps. Nocturnal symptoms are rare (unlike CTS). Provocation clinical testing of the three muscles individually against resistance helps identify the compression site: elbow flexion with forearm supinated (biceps); forearm pronation with elbow extended (pronator); middle finger PIP joint flexion (FDS). Conservative treatments should be tried—modifying activities, using a splint, and NSAIDs—as surgical treatment is extensive (requiring release of the nerve at all the above sites) and the reported outcomes are variable. Fifty per cent of cases managed conservatively resolve within 4 months. Up to 90 per cent of those undergoing median nerve decompression surgery report good to excellent results.[18]

Cubital tunnel syndrome

Ulnar nerve compression most commonly occurs at the elbow, where it passes through the cubital tunnel into the forearm through flexor carpi ulnaris. If the nerve is unstable it subluxes anteriorly over the medial epicondyle with flexion (generally with a palpable snap at around 100 degrees of elbow flexion) and is more likely to require transposition surgery to move it anteriorly. In the absence of nerve instability or permanent neurology, initial conservative management includes: reducing elbow flexion during activities (e.g. using a headset for telephone use), nocturnal elbow extension splints, and avoiding pressure from a desk or arm rest on the back of the elbow. Surgery decompresses the nerve; transposition is controversial, and reserved for cases where there is demonstrable nerve instability, an unhealthy nerve bed or in revision surgery.

Musculoskeletal disorders of the lower limbs

General workplace adaptations for lower limb problems

Lower limb problems may significantly limit work attendance. Maintaining work is important however as employees who cease working whilst waiting for operative procedures are less likely to return. In one study of patients awaiting hip or knee surgery, 30 per cent were off work because of their joint problems. The additional workplace flexibility afforded by larger employers may improve the patient's ability to keep working.[19]

Support for employees may include: altered hours to avoid rush hour travel, provision of a parking space, temporary office relocation, and alteration of duties to reduce the distances walked or the time spent standing. Access to fire escapes, toilets, and dining facilities must be considered. Individuals with a chronic disability may approach the Access to Work fund to pay for taxis into work and specialist workplace adaptations. Arrangements for home working may help an individual awaiting surgery or convalescing. An individual with foot problems may struggle to wear safety footwear but a trainer-type safety shoe is sometimes suitable. Work using ladders or at heights may not be safe if there is concern about coordination, strength, or weakness of the lower limb.

Simple equipment (e.g. a trolley or chair) may significantly improve an individual's comfort or safety. If there is hip stiffness a higher stool may be more comfortable than a low chair. A footstool can help if foot or ankle swelling is a problem. All equipment (including crutches) requires sufficient space to manoeuvre safely. Under the Equality Act 2010 employers have a duty to make reasonable access adaptations for the less mobile employee and for those with chronic health conditions.

Conditions of the hip

Hip osteoarthritis

Predisposing factors include: genetic predisposition, age, female sex, obesity, rheumatoid arthritis, and biomechanical factors such as joint injury, occupational and recreational usage, reduced muscle strength, joint laxity and joint misalignment (e.g. congenital dysplasia or dislocation, slipped upper femoral epiphysis of hip).[20] There is an increased risk for hip osteoarthritis (OA) in farmers and those undertaking prolonged heavy lifting (at least 10–20 kg) over many years and an even greater risk from obesity and trauma. High loads, unnatural body position, and jumping may contribute (Box 12.8). There is insufficient evidence that climbing stairs or ladders causes hip OA.[21] Divers and compressed air workers have an increased risk secondary to aseptic osteonecrosis.

Pain is typically felt around the groin, the greater trochanter, and thigh, or referred to the back or knee and is characteristically worse after exercise. Stiffness worsens after resting. Painful internal rotation with reduction in the range of movement may be an early sign.

Hip replacement

Total hip replacement (THR) or resurfacing significantly reduces pain and increases mobility. The majority of employees return to work postoperatively, particularly if they were in work before

---

Box 12.8 Work implications—hip osteoarthritis

Conservative management consists of pain relief, avoiding exacerbating activities, reducing biomechanical stressors (e.g. weight), use of walking aids, and cushioning footwear. Work-related activity that produces or maintains pain should be avoided. Deterioration to hip replacement often occurs over 1–5 years[20] with increasing functional limitation and absence from work.

Patients with advanced hip OA, who are limited by pain on weight bearing and walking, may struggle to undertake work in which these elements are prominent. By contrast, job retention while awaiting joint replacement is better in sedentary employment, with the opportunity to mostly sit rather than to stand.[19] Reasonable accommodations should always be considered, in line with the provisions of the Equality Act 2010.

Box 12.9 Work implications—hip replacement

After cemented THR, light and clerical duties are possible at 6–8 weeks, heavier manual work at 3 months. In one study, 98% had returned to their original posts by 6 months (50% by 6 weeks). Standard postoperative movement restrictions include: avoiding hip flexion beyond 90 degrees, hip adduction beyond neutral and excessive hip rotation for 6–8 weeks to reduce dislocation risk.[23] Employees may need regular stretch breaks. A raised chair may help initially (chairs with wheels may be too unstable). Kneeling is usually possible. Flying is not recommended for 3 months postoperatively because of risk of deep vein thrombosis. Patients may try to drive from 6 weeks (see DVLA guidance); most drive by 12 weeks. Many patients use ladders successfully but there is a risk of dislocation if the patient falls or lands heavily. The risk depends on the size of the prosthesis. A posterior approach and a small femoral head size (less than 32 mm) have higher dislocation rates. Most dislocations occur within 3 months of surgery.

Over the longer term, higher impact activities that may cause joint loosening (e.g. jogging, contact sports, military combat) are not recommended. By contrast, swimming and cycling are encouraged and many forms of light manual and non-manual work are entirely possible.

surgery. Revision rate following primary hip replacement are 0.6 per cent at 1 year and 1.2 per cent at 3 years[22] (lower with cemented prostheses and higher after resurfacing). Revision surgery requires more prolonged convalescence (Box 12.9).

Conditions of the knee

Bursitis

Bursitis is inflammation of the bursal sac accompanied by a fluctuant swelling arising over hours or days. Pain is felt on flexion of the knee as the bursa is compressed. Aspiration may be necessary to differentiate septic from aseptic bursitis. Bursitis may be related to acute trauma from a fall, inflammatory conditions such as gout or rheumatoid arthritis or repeated minor trauma related to occupation. An increased rate of recurrent bursitis has been shown in occupations involving prolonged practice of the following:

- Kneeling—e.g. suprapatellar bursitis, 'housemaid's knee', in cleaners, roofers and plumbers.
- Leaning against the knee—e.g. fishermen resting against a boat side using their knees.
- Crawling—e.g. 'miners' knee'.[24]

In the carpet and floor laying industry rates of up to 20 per cent have been noted, particularly if 'knee kickers' (tools to smooth the carpet into the wall) are used.

The pain of bursitis usually settles within a few weeks with rest, ice, NSAIDs, and analgesia. In work, adaptation of the role or the use of cushioning knee pads may help, although the design of these must be appropriate. Aspiration and steroid injections are possible. Recurrence is common. Incision and drainage or excision of the bursa is not advised acutely, but may improve chronic symptomatic bursitis.

Knee osteoarthritis

Radiographic changes of knee OA occur in about 25 per cent of adults aged 50 years and older. There is an association between severity of pain and stiffness and the presence of radiographic

Box 12.10 Work implications—knee osteoarthritis

Employees may struggle with squatting, kneeling, climbing stairs, and walking on uneven ground. This may limit work participation in manual occupations more than sedentary ones, although moderate exercise is thought to have a role in clinical management and therefore not contraindicated within the limits of pain.

Some evidence exists that symptomatic knee OA is less common in workplaces with the flexibility to allow job switching.[27] Severe cases awaiting surgery may well be covered by the provisions of the Equality Act 2010, requiring consideration of reasonable workplace accommodations—e.g. transfer of some responsibilities to colleagues, lifting aids, relocation to a sitting job, etc.

osteoarthritis.[20] In the UK, 40 per cent of knee replacement operations are performed on patients of working age. Although most employees return to work after knee replacement, a significant proportion may have already left work because of their joint disorder (Box 12.10).[19]

Risk of knee OA is related to genetic constitution, female sex, obesity, increasing age, and injury to the joint (particularly meniscal tear, anterior cruciate ligament rupture, or intra-articular fracture). There is also an increased risk in mining, forestry, farming, carpet and floor layers, and construction, with evidence for a relationship between kneeling, squatting, and heavy lifting.[25] High loads, unnatural body position, climbing, and jumping may also contribute. Elite rugby players and those undertaking high-impact sports have a higher risk, but recreational non-contact exercise (e.g. running) seems not to be associated with an increased prevalence.

Symptoms of OA include knee and anterior tibia pain on movement (e.g. going up or down stairs), difficulty kneeling, stiffness after rest which eases with movement ('gelling'), and night pain (late severe OA). Symptoms may worsen in damp weather and periods of low atmospheric pressure. Physical signs include crepitus, effusions, cysts, quadriceps wasting, stiffness, and valgus or varus deformity.

Initial management includes pain control, avoiding exacerbating activities, and maintaining function through activity (providing it is not painful), knee strengthening (particularly quadriceps) exercises, cycling, or swimming, and weight loss. Paracetamol should be used initially in sufficient doses.[20] Assistive aids and management of sleep disturbance and mood are important. Knee taping may ease symptoms. There is insufficient evidence that heel wedges, knee braces, acupuncture, and hyaluronic acid are helpful.

Over several years about a third of cases improve with active management, a third stay the same, and a third of patients develop progressive symptomatic disease. Age, varus knee alignment, presence of OA in multiple joints, radiographic features, and obesity in particular predict progression.[26]

Surgery for knee osteoarthritis

Arthroscopy is indicated if there is a clear history of mechanical locking (suggesting a loose body). Newer techniques (e.g. microfracture, autologous chondrocyte implantation and osteochondral grafting (OATS)) may preserve articular cartilage in younger patients but longer-term studies are required. A realigning high tibial osteotomy may be used for compartment arthritis in younger active patients, delaying the need for joint replacement for up to 10 years. Pain relief is comparable to that of joint replacement. These procedures require lengthy rehabilitation. Return to weight bearing may take 6–12 weeks. Running is restricted for a year.

Knee replacement

Referral for joint replacement should occur before prolonged established functional limitation and severe pain, refractory to non-surgical treatment occurs. Over 90 per cent of knee joint replacements are total knee arthroplasties (TKAs; Box 12.11). Studies indicate a 95 per cent or better survival rate for TKAs at 10 years and over 90 per cent at 15 years. Partial or unicompartmental knee arthroplasty (UKA) selectively replaces the damaged compartment, but is less commonly performed and has higher revision rates than TKA.

Meniscal tears

The menisci function as shock absorbers and allow gliding action of the joint. They are at risk if the knee is twisted suddenly in a flexed position (e.g. playing rugby, football, skiing). This often results in concurrent injury to the anterior cruciate ligament (ACL) and delay in ACL repair increases the rate of subsequent medial meniscus tears. Degenerative tears on minimal impact (e.g. getting up from a chair) occur in older individuals. Industries recognized as having higher rates of meniscal disorders include mining and carpet-laying.[24]

Acute knee pain follows the injury but this may settle initially. Subsequent symptoms include pain, particularly on straightening the leg, stiffness and swelling, the sensation of giving way, and loss of range of motion. Patients may report a sudden painful 'catch' from the joint. A free fragment or a bucket handle tear can cause locking. Initial management includes rest, ice, compression, and elevation. Small lateral tears occasionally heal spontaneously but the majority require surgery.

Box 12.11 Work implications—total knee arthroplasty

Most individuals return to sedentary roles by 6–8 weeks. Manually arduous roles may require 12 weeks off work. One study showed median return to all work was 8.9 weeks and that highly motivated patients can return to carefully managed physically demanding jobs. The ability to modify demanding physical aspects influences return to work times.[28] When sick leave exceeds 6 months the prognosis for return to work is poorer.

Postoperative stiffness is common. Stair climbing is affected if the knee does not flex beyond 90 degrees (and may need manipulation under anaesthetic). Many patients report more difficulty with stairs, heavy domestic duties, and squatting than controls.

Many forms of light manual and non-manual work are compatible with having a TKA and 80–100% of patients manage to return to their original work. Restrictions may include avoidance of kneeling, squatting, twisting, jumping, climbing, prolonged standing, and walking. Very heavy work may not be appropriate after TKA. Similarly, high-impact activities that threaten joint loosening (e.g. jogging, contact sports, military combat) are not recommended, although direct evidence on how type of work affects prosthesis survival and functional outcome over the long term is lacking. Consideration of reasonable workplace accommodations may well be mandated by the Equality Act 2010. (Note that, in the event of medical or surgical treatment, the Act includes the proviso that a person's pre-treatment health status should be used as the yardstick in deciding whether they meet the legal definition of being disabled for day-to-day activities.)

Knee arthroscopy

Arthroscopy is a low-risk procedure with a complication rate of 1 per cent (infection, thrombosis, compartment syndrome, and haemarthrosis being the more severe problems). The patient returns home weight bearing but on crutches. For arthroscopy alone, without surgical repair, most people return to work within 1–2 weeks but remain off strenuous activities for 3–6 weeks.

Menisectomy

Surgery is indicated for persistent mechanical symptoms. Because loss of meniscal surface increases the progression rate of osteoarthritis, surgery removes only the torn elements. If the knee is permanently locked, meniscal surgery should be undertaken promptly. Outcomes are very good and 85–90 per cent of patients return to full function (Box 12.12).[29] Degenerative tears are generally managed conservatively with an exercise programme or, if symptoms do not settle, by partial menisectomy.

Meniscal repair

Young people with recent injuries and peripheral tears of the meniscus are most suitable for repair. Postoperatively they are more cautiously managed than after menisectomy, with partial weight bearing for up to 6 weeks (Box 12.13). The outcomes are good in 70–90 per cent of cases; however, 15–25 per cent of repairs require subsequent menisectomy within 6–24 months. In a young person with no significant arthritis a meniscal transplant might be considered but the value in preventing long-term OA is uncertain.

The anterior cruciate ligament

The anterior cruciate ligament (ACL) controls forward movement and rotation of the knee joint, which are essential for side stepping, pivoting, and landing from a jump. It is commonly injured

---

Box 12.12 Work implications—menisectomy

For a straightforward arthroscopy and menisectomy the leg should be elevated for a few days. Sedentary workers can return after 2–3 days (but most return at 10–14 days) and 4–6 weeks for manual work or complex reconstructive surgery. Postoperative restrictions include avoiding kneeling squatting, crawling, or prolonged standing for at least the first 3 weeks. Kneeling may be uncomfortable for a few months. Patients should avoid long journeys for the first 2 weeks to reduce the risk of deep vein thrombosis.

Box 12.13 Work implications—meniscal repair

After meniscal repair, rehabilitation takes about 3 months depending on the technique used. Patients initially require a brace, crutches, and physiotherapy. Leg elevation may be more comfortable and help reduce swelling. Some patients may have permanent restrictions on kneeling, jumping, and squatting.

> ## Box 12.14 Work implications—anterior cruciate ligament repair
>
> Postoperatively, 90% of patients regain near normal knee function. Sedentary workers may return to work 3–5 days following surgery.[30] Playing sport non-competitively is possible at 4–6 months if adequate rehabilitation of the thigh musculature has occurred.

in sports or traffic accidents and farming. Degenerative tears occur from more minor injuries. Fifty per cent of ACL injuries involve other injuries, particularly to menisci and chondral surfaces.

Acute management includes rest, ice, and elevation. The acute swelling settles over 4–6 weeks and walking is possible. Injury is graded 1–3 where 3 (the majority) represents a complete tear and poor joint stability. Patients usually notice weakness or instability. Episodes of instability result in injury to the cartilages and joint surfaces which eventually lead to osteoarthritis.

In degenerative knees in less-active individuals, conservative management is possible using bracing, joint stabilizing exercises, and pain relief. However the patient may continue to experience symptoms of instability and need to restrict their subsequent activities.

Reconstruction Following complete rupture of the ACL, in an unstable knee, surgical reconstruction is recommended in younger patients. Preoperative joint stability exercises are considered useful. Reconstructive surgery usually involves arthroscopic grafting using autologous grafts such as a bone-patella-tendon or hamstring tendon graft. A satisfactory outcome with return to stability occurs in 90 per cent. Graft failure occurs in approximately 2 per cent. Other complications are rare but include deep vein thrombosis and sepsis.

Rehabilitation and return to work Immediately after ACL reconstruction, weight-bearing is encouraged. The majority of patients undergo day-case surgery with immediate intensive physiotherapy for at least 6 weeks. The majority can walk safely without crutches by 2 weeks postoperatively (Box 12.14). Return to physical activity (e.g. gentle jogging) may not occur until at least 12 weeks postoperatively.

Long-term outcomes

By 10 years postoperatively, the prevalence of radiographic OA can be expected to be about 0–13 per cent in patients with isolated ACL injury, and double with additional meniscal injury. The commonest risk factor for knee OA is meniscal injury.[31]

Conditions of the foot

Ankle osteoarthritis

Most ankle OA is post-traumatic from fractures (particularly malleolar and tibial plafond). Patients are younger than those with hip or knee OA. Symptoms include pain, swelling, stiffness, loss of range of movement, and valgus or varus deformity (end stage). Disability related to ankle OA can profoundly affect quality of life (Box 12.15).

Weight loss, analgesia, immobilization with lace-up boots, or ankle foot orthoses, and physiotherapy to strengthen the ankle all offer benefit. Intra-articular steroid injections are a reasonable short-term measure. Bony spurs that cause impingement can be arthroscopically debrided. Distraction arthroplasty using an external fixator to allow movement has promising short-term results as an alternative to fusion in young patients.

Box 12.15 Work implications—ankle fusion

After fusion patients will be non-weight bearing for 2–6 weeks and unable to drive. Long term, patients may prefer to use a rocker-bottomed shoe. Up to 80% experience difficulty with uneven terrain whilst 60% report difficulty with prolonged standing or walking, reduced speed, and length of stride. Ladder work is only possible if the results of surgery are good.[32]

Ankle arthrodesis (fusion) remains the preferred end-stage treatment option. It controls pain in 90 per cent of cases but in the long term increases arthritis in adjacent joints in up to 60 per cent of cases. The failure rate is approximately 15 per cent (and higher if the patient smokes or has diabetes). Although outcomes are generally good there may be associated pain with limited functional improvement.

Although earlier ankle replacements gave poor results, third-generation prostheses are showing comparable outcomes to fusion. Joint replacement is less suitable for younger active patients (the majority) because of the increased need for revision.

Achilles tendinitis (non-insertional)

This condition is related to degenerative change and excessive tendon loading (e.g. running/jumping activities on hard surfaces and in poor footwear). It is commoner in athletes and men aged in their 30s–40s. It is associated with obesity, biomechanical foot problems, fluoroquinolone use, and increasing age. Seronegative arthritides may present with Achilles tendonitis.

Symptoms and signs of Achilles tendonitis and appropriate eccentric exercises are described on the relevant NHS Evidence Clinical Knowledge summaries Internet page (<http://www.cks.nhs.uk/home>). Tendon rupture must be excluded.

Initial treatment should be conservative, including rest, weight loss, correction of excess pronation, and improved footwear. Eccentric exercises two to three times daily for 3 months reduce pain by 60 per cent. NSAIDS and ice may help initially. Steroid injections can precipitate Achilles tendon rupture and are not recommended. Current treatment modalities include cutaneous nitrate patches, dry needling, large volume injections in the pre-Achilles space, lithotripsy, plaster immobilization, night splints, and plasma rich injections, but evidence on their clinical efficacy is limited.[33]

Surgical management for the most recalcitrant cases usually involves debridement, with or without tendon transfer. Minimally invasive techniques, radiofrequency and laser ablation have similar results to conventional surgery. Most patients wear a splint after surgery with modified weight bearing for 4–6 weeks. Although needs vary, the manual worker will generally require 3–4 months off work and the sedentary worker, 6–9 weeks (Box 12.16). The short-term outcome following surgery is satisfactory in about 60–85 per cent of cases.

Box 12.16 Work implications—Achilles tendinitis

Approximately 75 per cent of cases settle with conservative management (footwear and exercises) over 6–12 months. The prognosis is worse if exacerbating factors are not addressed early on. In the acute phase, 'high-impact' activities (e.g. jumping, running) should be limited.

Plantar fasciitis

Up to 10 per cent of the population experience posterior heel pain, with 80 per cent of cases associated with plantar fasciitis. The aetiology is multifactorial but intrinsic risk factors include age, obesity, and pronated foot posture. Extrinsic factors may include prolonged occupational weight bearing and inappropriate footwear.

Pain starts gradually around the medial or plantar aspect of the calcaneus. It is intense on first walking after a period of inactivity, easing initially then increasing again with activity and exacerbated by prolonged standing. Reproduction of the pain by extending the first metatarsophalangeal (MTP) joint is suggestive of the diagnosis. Ultrasonography and magnetic resonance imaging (MRI) may show a thickened plantar fascia (>4.0 mm) and fluid collection, x-rays may show a subcalcaneal spur.

Conservative interventions concentrate on reduction of biomechanical stressors e.g. weight loss, rest, specific stretching exercises (see ARC website <http://www.arthritisresearchuk.org>: 'Information and Exercise Sheet' HO2), and arch-supporting footwear. Over-the-counter shoe inserts, to prevent excess pronation and custom-made night splints, may be beneficial.[34] A steroid injection may reduce pain but there is a risk of plantar fascia rupture and heel pad atrophy with repeated injections. Extracorporeal shock wave therapy has limited evidence. Current research centres on using platelet-rich plasma injections or glyceryl trinitrate patches.

Surgical plantar fascia release helps a small subset of patients with persistent, severe symptoms refractory to nonsurgical intervention. Surgical options include endoscopic release but success rates are variable. See Box 12.17 for occupational implications.

Box 12.17 Occupational implications—plantar fasciitis

Over 90% of patients recover with non-operative treatment over 6–12 months. Individuals require appropriate orthotics and supportive footwear and physiotherapy to establish an exercise regimen. Some require a move to more sedentary duties for several months as symptoms dictate.

Tibialis posterior tendon dysfunction

This tendon supports the mid-foot arch and can become torn or inflamed by impact activities (e.g. court sports). Eventually this causes arch collapse. It is commoner in the obese, women over 40, and those with systemic inflammatory conditions. On walking and standing the patient experiences pain along the medial border of the foot (or lateral pain if the foot collapses into valgus). There may be: tenderness over the tendon, 'too many toes' seen from behind whilst standing, and difficulty rising onto tiptoe on one leg. Treatment includes rest, ice, and arch support orthotics.

Mild cases may resolve; more advanced disease should be referred early as aggressive management with splinting or early surgical intervention (e.g. debridement) prevents catastrophic tendon failure causing architectural changes in the foot. Surgical reconstructions require 2–3 months in plaster and a further 2–3 months off work for all but the most sedentary jobs. About 30 per cent of reconstructions fail at 7 years, requiring hindfoot fusion.

Bunions/hallux valgus

A bunion is a prominent medial bone and inflamed bursal sac over the first metatarsal head, usually associated with hallux valgus deformity of the first MTP joint; pain is from rubbing and pressure from the shoe. Bunions are commoner in women possibly due to ill-fitting footwear. Early severe pain arises from ligaments despite minimal deformity. Differentiation from hallux rigidus is essential. Increasing deviation of the great toe causes subluxation of the first MTP joint, a 'hammer toe' deformity of the second MTP joint and callosities. Patients complain principally of pain in the second toe. Increased use of the lateral foot area causes generalized metatarsalgia.

Initial conservative management includes use of comfortable footwear, a wide toe box, padding, toe splinting, and reducing the number of hours spent standing. Surgery is indicated if conservative measures fail or if deformity causes a mechanical forefoot problem. Surgery is successful in approximately 90 per cent but 10 per cent may have complications which can be severe, e.g. infection, joint stiffness, ongoing pain. Long-term satisfaction rates drop to 60–70 per cent.

Osteotomy is the mainstay of surgery, requiring 2–6 weeks of heel weight-bearing only in a postoperative shoe or occasionally a plaster/rigid splint using crutches (Box 12.18). Older sedate patients may undergo a bunionectomy with or without Keller's osteotomy (excision of the bony prominence). Recovery usually takes 2–3 weeks.

Box 12.18 Work implications—bunion osteotomy

Postoperatively the individual should elevate the foot periodically and may need crutches. Driving is restricted until the patient can brake safely wearing normal shoes, usually by 6 weeks post osteotomy.[35] Very sedentary work is possible by week 3 or 4 and most people are back to work by 6–8 weeks. Prolonged standing becomes possible by week 8 or 9. Patients having bilateral surgery usually need 1–2 weeks more at each stage.

Hallux rigidus

Hallux rigidus, often confused with bunions, is first MTP joint arthritis. Usually seen at 30–60 years of age, there may be a family history or a history of injury. Occupation is not thought to be causative but it often presents in farmers, sportsmen, and ballerinas. Symptoms include increasing joint pain and stiffness making walking difficult. Shoes which press on the joint or open-backed shoes requiring toe flexion cause discomfort. Examination shows joint swelling and reduced range of movement. X-rays show degenerative joint change and osteophytes.

Conservative management includes wearing flat shoes with a wide toe box. Rigidly-soled footwear with a rocker bottom or a stiff orthotic brace ('shank') under the hallux also improves symptoms. These are available in the high street. Steroid injections, with or without manipulation, may offer temporary relief.

Cheilectomy for mild cases involves excision of obstructive osteophytes, thus allowing extension but preserving the joint. Recuperation involves 2–4 weeks in a rigid-soled shoe but patients can return to sedentary work after 3–4 weeks. Fifteen per cent of cases later require further surgery such as fusion or arthroplasty.

Metatarsophalangeal fusion

Fusion is appropriate in moderate to severe hallux rigidus. It is usually controls pain but may limit footwear. Convalescence includes immediate weight bearing in postoperative shoes (Box 12.19).

Box 12.19 Work implications—metatarsophalangeal fusion

Most cases return to sedentary work after 4–8 weeks but manual workers take longer (8–12 weeks). Some patients require a rocker bottom shoe long term and experience difficulty in squatting.

Morton's neuroma

Morton's neuroma, a common cause of metatarsalgia, is a perineural fibrosis of the plantar digital nerve as it passes between the metatarsal heads. Commoner in women, it may be related to footwear. Characteristic symptoms include pain, burning or numbness in the affected metatarsal space or a 'pebble' feeling under the metatarsus. The third metatarsal space is most commonly involved less often, the second or occasionally the forth space.

Conservative management includes using wide toe box shoes, flat soles and an insole with the metatarsal dome. There is little evidence for the use of supinatory insoles.[36] Ultrasound-guided injections are highly successful and have made surgery virtually obsolete.

Surgical treatment involves removal of the nerve. Success rates of 50–80 per cent have been reported in non-randomized trials. Minor complications are common with recurrence rates of 4–8 per cent and occasional severe refractory neuralgia. After surgery, patients return to full weight bearing over 2–6 weeks.

Trauma

As with all return to work, biopsychosocial aspects may impact significantly on return after trauma, particularly if the original injury was caused at work. A strong belief in recovery, the presence of an isolated injury, education to university level, and self-employment may result in a faster return, whereas the receipt of compensation, pre-injury psychosocial issues, older age, pain attitudes, obesity, and blue-collar work may delay return.[37]

Fractures

With fractures, the associated soft tissue injuries are often more important in determining the long-term outcome (Box 12.20). The clinician must consider whether the fracture needs

---

Box 12.20 Work implications—fractures

Bony union usually takes 6–8 weeks in the upper limb (and twice this in the lower limb). Loading is generally restricted until then. The bone then remodels over many months. Fractured bones can be stabilized with plaster casts, wires, external frames, internal plates, and screws or intra-medullary nails, and these allow earlier motion and loading. For return to work, the ability to accommodate any splint, loading restriction, and the required exercise programme needs consideration, bearing in mind safety in the workplace and the potential for reduction in employee performance. The need to elevate the injured limb (to reduce swelling, particularly if wound healing is not mature) and to restrict limb loading pending union of fractures, may delay return to work.

reduction (perfect reductions are necessary when joint surfaces are involved, to reduce arthritis risk), whether the limb can be mobilized or needs protection, and the rate of rehabilitation.

Removing metalwork

Metalwork can be removed once fracture healing is assured, generally at least 9–12 months after injury. Implant removal may reduce local pressure problems (ulnar and ankle plates), and allay concerns about infection and facilitate future reconstructions (e.g. if joint replacements are needed). Because there is a re-fracture risk, and often a higher complication rate with implant removal, (than insertion), most implants will not be removed; however, employees may require 2 weeks off with initial restriction of high impact activities on return.

Avascular necrosis

Fractures involving or adjacent to joints may disrupt the blood supply to articular bone giving rise to problems with union or avascular necrosis (AVN). Fractures of the scaphoid, talus, or anatomical neck of the humerus or femur carry a risk of this complication. AVN frequently leads to symptomatic osteoarthritis. There are other potential risk-factors for AVN such as human immunodeficiency virus infection, sickle cell disease, alcoholism, chemotherapy, steroid use, and decompression episodes.

Pathological fractures

Pathological fractures occur following lower levels of energy transfer through areas of abnormal bone (e.g. tumour, osteoporosis), or repeated micro-trauma (i.e. a 'stress fracture'). The underlying condition influences the management. Stress fractures follow acute changes to loading patterns—either heavier loading with low repetitions/higher repetition of loading, or changing the way in which a bone is loaded. Increasing, persistent, task-related, and, later, resting pain after a recent change in activities raises the possibility of a stress fracture. Areas most often affected include the femoral neck, the tibial shaft, metatarsals, and the pars inter-articularis of the lumbar vertebrae. The diagnosis is confirmed by isotope bone scan or MRI. Incomplete fractures may respond to rest. Persistent incomplete fractures or complete fractures require immobilization (potentially for months) or surgery, potentially with bone grafting. At work, risk assessment should address the provoking tasks and how to avoid recurrent stress fractures.

Dislocations

After joint dislocation the duration of splinting depends on the subsequent stability of the joint—limited or none if the joint is stable, but longer if the joint remains unstable.

+ *Interphalangeal joint dislocations* without associated fractures can frequently be mobilized immediately with buddy-taping to the adjacent longer digit for 4–6 weeks.
+ *Patello-femoral dislocations* require immobilization for up to 6 weeks for a first dislocation (with or without surgical repairs or reconstructions) before mobilization.
+ *Elbow dislocations* tend to stiffen, so early mobilization is important (surgery to repair bone/ligamentous damage may be required).
+ *Anterior shoulder dislocations* in younger individuals often cause significant soft tissue damage to the labrum and ligaments. The shoulder must be immobilized in a sling for a few weeks to reduce the risk of subsequent instability which is common in patients under 30 years.

However, after any subsequent dislocations, early mobilization is permitted because the damage to the soft tissues has already occurred from the first injury. Older individuals have less risk of recurrent instability, so earlier mobilization is allowed.

Ligament injuries

After joint dislocation, significant ligamentous damage causes medium to long-term problems unless recognized and treated promptly (e.g. tears of the knee ACL, the thumb MCP joint ulnar collateral ligament, or the wrist scapho-lunate ligament).

Tendon injuries

Tendons heal if their ends are apposed, but the associated scarring can cause long-term stiffness. This is prevented by using controlled active mobilization regimens following repair to minimize adhesion formation. If less than 50 per cent of the tendon has been divided, partial tendon injuries are treated by bevelling off any tendon flap that may catch. The surgeon may restrict heavy manual tasks during the initial 4–10-week period, depending on the operative findings (Box 12.21). If more than 50 per cent of a tendon has been divided, full repair is needed.

Nerve damage

This may involve:

♦ *Neurapraxia*: damage to the myelin sheathes surrounding the axons. This usually recovers well over 6–8 weeks.

♦ *Axonotmesis*: damage to the axons, with the nerve remaining in continuity. This requires axonal regrowth to the end organ, so recovery is slow depending on the distance from the site of injury and the skin/muscle innervated by the nerve; regrowth occurs at an empirical rate of around 1 mm of nerve growth per day.

♦ *Neurotmesis*: macroscopic disruption of the nerve itself. This requires surgical repair to appose the damaged nerve ends for any recovery to occur. It carries a worse outcome.

Following nerve injuries, important outcome determinants include: the patient's age, smoking status, systemic conditions such as diabetes (which impair general nerve function), the integrity of the nerve, the likelihood of axonal regeneration reaching the appropriate end organ, and the injury mechanism (traction and crushing injuries damage a greater length of nerve and the neural blood supply worsening the outcome). Sensory recovery to the level of protective sensation should occur with time (Box 12.22). Motor recovery depends on the distance to be covered by the regenerating axons—hence, proximal lesions may not recover before the motor end-plates decay irreversibly.

Box 12.21 Work implications—tendon repair

Following repair to flexor tendons in the hand a patient requires a splint to restrict function for 8 weeks. During this time, no gripping is permitted. Similar rehabilitation is seen after uncomplicated extensor tendon repairs. Repair re-rupture rates are around 5%; re-repair is possible, but should be done promptly and compliance with rehabilitation is essential.

Box 12.22 Work implications—nerve damage

Insensate areas must be protected from inadvertent damage (cuts, abrasions pressure, or thermal injury). This has safety implications in certain work environments (e.g. workshops, manufacturing, and catering industries). After 3–4 years it is unlikely that normal sensation will be restored. This may affect an individual's long-term ability to undertake fine manipulative tasks. After digital nerve repair in an index finger, individuals tend to grip without including the digit because of this impaired sensation, even if motion is unaffected. Joints affected by paralysed muscle groups need splinting and passive mobilization until motor recovery occurs to avoid fixed contractures (particularly important with ulnar and radial nerve lesions).

Cold intolerance

Following injury, particularly nerve or vascular injury or repair, persistent disproportionate discomfort is commonly experienced in the injured part in cold environments. Although symptoms will not necessarily prevent working, they may prevent work in cold environments.

Ankle sprain

This common ligament injury is particularly related to sports activities, slips, trips, or previous strains. Lateral sprains (usually the anterior talo-fibular ligament), caused by foot inversion, account for over 90 per cent of instances.

Ankle sprains are graded depending on severity, from 1 (mild tenderness and swelling), to 3 (complete ligament tear with joint instability). The Ottowa Ankle and Foot Rules are a sensitive index for excluding ankle fractures without the need for radiography.

Ankle sprains should be managed initially with 'PRICE': protection, rest, ice, compression, and elevation for 48 hours with judicious anti-inflammatory medication. A semi-rigid support, e.g. a lace-up boot, and appropriate exercise is preferable to complete immobilization. Physiotherapy (but not ultrasound) may have positive short-term effects. Exercise therapy including wobble boards, may reduce recurrence rates and hence chronic ankle instability (which occurs in 10–20 per cent of acute sprains depending on the injury severity). If significant ligament laxity is present, surgical intervention may be considered.

Most ankle injuries settle by 2 weeks. If symptoms continue the diagnosis needs review to exclude occult injuries (Box 12.23). Orthopaedic referral should occur if symptoms persist beyond 6 weeks.

Box 12.23 Work implications—ankle sprain

Many patients do not require significant time off work with an ankle sprain. Those still absent after 2 weeks warrant further investigation. Patients may benefit from a footstool initially and a change to more sedentary work. Ankle instability may threaten safety at heights and on ladders. Post-sprain exercise therapy may reduce instability rates.

Many patients develop synovitis which causes persistent symptoms. This responds to a steroid injection or arthroscopy. Eighty per cent of osteochondral lesions of the talus improve following arthroscopy and debridement. Lateral ligament repairs have a good outcome in 90 per cent of patients. Patients wear splints for approximately 6 weeks then lightweight splints and physiotherapy for a further 6 weeks. Sedentary workers should be able to return to work by 6–8 weeks and manual workers by 10–12 weeks. Return to running requires 4 months.

Achilles tendon rupture

Acute Achilles tendon rupture classically occurs in men aged 30–50 years undertaking sports activities that load the tendon (e.g. squash). Chronic ruptures are usually seen after age 65, particularly if there is a history of chronic tendinitis and steroid tendon injections. The NHS Clinical Knowledge Summary website summarizes the diagnostic criteria (<http://www.cks.nhs.uk/home>).

Conservative and operative management produce similar outcomes. Early active weight bearing produces better results than immobilization. Surgery is offered to younger more active patients as it has a slightly lower rate of re-rupture but a higher complication rate (wound infection and sural nerve injury). For work implications see Box 12.24.

Fractured calcaneus

Calcaneal fractures are high-impact injuries, often from a fall from height or motor vehicle accident. They are commoner in construction workers. Because of the injury mechanism they are often associated with other fractures (particularly vertebral).

Adverse prognostic factors include significant disruption of the subtalar joint, multiple fragments of bone, and significant widening of the calcaneus. Intra-articular fractures carry a higher morbidity and approximately 10–20 per cent of those injured are still not working a year later (Box 12.25). Patients seeking compensation have a poorer outcome.[38]

Box 12.24 Work implications—Achilles rupture

Patients need casts or braces for 6–8 weeks as well as crutches and protected weight bearing. Manual workers may require 3–6 months off. Long-term outcome depends on the timing of diagnosis and treatment. Most patients regain good function (at least 90% of power) if ruptures are treated in the first few days. Delayed (>4 weeks) treatment of the rupture results in an 80% restoration of power, which may affect function. Almost all younger patients in whom rupture is initially missed will require surgical reconstruction.

Box 12.25 Work implications—calcaneal fracture repair

Return to work is limited by the patient's initial inability to weight bear, usually for 8–26 weeks. Some patients experience severe chronic pain refractory to treatment even after a 'successful' fusion. Long-term complications include OA of the joint and residual pain. Employees may not be able to wear certain footwear or walk on uneven ground.

Closed fractures that do not disrupt the joint may be treated conservatively. The patient is non-weight bearing for 2 weeks in a cast and then partially weight bearing for the next 8 weeks. These fractures usually have a good outcome.

Operative management is required when the subtalar joint is disrupted. Anatomical reduction of the joint postoperatively predicts higher functional scores and reduced subsequent arthritis. Twenty per cent of operatively managed cases go on to secondary arthrodesis and many more have arthritic symptoms. Complication rates are increased by diabetes, smoking, and peripheral vascular disease.

Amputation

Some 2000 new patients of working age are seen in UK limb fitting centres annually, the majority with a lower limb amputation. Amputations typically arise from vascular causes (50 per cent) or because of trauma (25 per cent), neoplasm, or infection. The majority of traumatic amputations occur in men younger than 40 years, often from road traffic accidents or combat situations. Early prosthetic fitting, rehabilitation, and psychological support facilitate successful functional recovery.

Problems in postoperative rehabilitation arise in relation to weight bearing, contractures, choke syndrome (venous pooling at the stump), wound care, and stump dermatitis. Phantom limb pain occurs commonly initially, but generally improves with time. Transtibial (below-knee) amputees begin returning to work after 9 months, but following other major amputations, return to work can take 2 years.[39]

Return to work depends on amputation level, number of amputations, age, comorbidity, mobility level, and ongoing stump or prosthesis problems. Educational level, salary, and employer and social support are also important. Sixty per cent of amputees return to work, often to a more sedentary role, and the majority of these are under 45 years old. Return to work should be phased.

Broadly, lower limb amputation affects mobility and standing whilst upper limb amputation affects manual dexterity and handling tasks. Both affect driving and carrying. The more proximal the amputation, the more functional the impact it has. An individual's pain control, mood, and confidence are substantially modified by their psychological status.

Lower limb amputation

Lower limb amputees take roughly 6 months to be fully weight bearing and return to work takes approximately 14 months.[40] They have a reduced capacity for walking, stamping, turning, and standing. Most prostheses do not allow ankle dorsiflexion, which affects stair climbing. The remaining healthy limb also undertakes significantly more work than in non-amputees and tires easily. Supportive adaptations include easy access to the workplace, and job modification to reduce the need for walking, running, lifting, carrying, and negotiating uneven surfaces. Work at heights or on ladders will be precluded. The functional outcome of a transtibial amputation is generally better than that of a transfemoral or through knee because most amputees can use their prosthesis for a significant time per day. Transfemoral amputees have a less efficient gait and often need crutches or a wheelchair for a proportion of their day. Amputees require restroom facilities to remove their prostheses occasionally. However, there are a wide range of sedentary jobs they can still perform and the provisions of the Equality Act 2010 mandate consideration of reasonable alternative work.

Upper limb amputation

Upper limb amputations are likely to arise from trauma or malignancy. Working-age males predominate, the commonest amputation site being the digits. Upper limb amputation of anything more than a finger significantly hinders undertaking manual work. Loss of the thumb or finger affects fine grip and typing, loss of the hand (particularly the dominant hand) affects grasp and writing. Retaining part of the forearm permits some load carrying which is lost as the amputation level rises. Cosmetic silicone prostheses are helpful if aesthetics are important. Voice-activated software has made returning to administrative work possible.

Return to work

Table 12.9 gives some indicative return to work times following common orthopaedic operations. Timings are approximate and assume recommended adaptations are in place. Return to work times vary in practice, depending on complications, age, and coexistent pathology as well as travel needs, office accessibility, rest, and dining facility access. Safety critical activities, e.g. work at heights or using ladders, require individual assessment.

Table 12.9 Return to work times after orthopaedic surgery

Site	Operation	Return to sedentary role from:	Return to manual role from:
Shoulder	Subacromial decompression	1–3 weeks	3–4 weeks
	Rotator cuff repair	3–6 weeks (once out of sling)	3 months
	Shoulder stabilization	1–3 weeks (as above)	2–3 months
	Shoulder replacement	3–6 weeks (as above)	3 months
Elbow	Ulnar nerve decompression	2–3 weeks	4–6 weeks
	Tennis elbow release	3 weeks	6–8 weeks
	Arthroscopy	1–2 weeks	2–4 weeks
	Elbow replacement	3–6 weeks (sling)	Inappropriate
Hand/wrist	Carpal tunnel decompression	1–3 weeks[14]	3–6 weeks
	Dupuytren's segmental aponeurectomy and/or needle fasciotomy	Up to 1 week (if healing)	Once healed (1–2 weeks)
	Dupuytren's fasciectomy	3–4 weeks	4–6 weeks
	Trigger finger release	1–3 weeks	2–6 weeks
	Wrist arthroscopy (no repair)	1–2 weeks	2–3 weeks
	Arthritis excision surgery	2–4 weeks	6–8 weeks
	Arthritis fusion surgery	1–2 weeks	6–12 weeks (average 16 weeks)
	De Quervain's release	1–2 weeks	4–6 weeks
Hip	Total hip replacement	6 weeks No flying for 3 months	12 weeks
Knee	Total knee replacement	6–8 weeks	12 weeks
	Knee arthroscopy	2–3 days (average 10–14 days)	3–6 weeks
	Knee arthroscopy and menisectomy no repair	2–3 days Average: 10–14 days	Up to 6 weeks

Table 12.9 (continued) Return to work times after orthopaedic surgery

Site	Operation	Return to sedentary role from:	Return to manual role from:
	Meniscal repair	6 weeks (in brace)	3–4 months
	Knee ACL repair	On crutches from 3–5 days	From 3–4 months
Foot	Achilles tendon repair	4–6 weeks in brace (22–28 days median)	3 months
	Bunionectomy	3–4 weeks (5–6 weeks if bilateral)	6–9 weeks
	Ankle fusion	Non-weight bearing before 2–6 weeks	

Acknowledgements

We are grateful to Professor A. Price and Mr R. Sharp of Nuffield Orthopaedic Centre Oxford for their advice on aspects of knee and foot care.

References

1 van Oostrom SH, Driessen MT, de Vet HC, *et al.* Workplace interventions for preventing work disability. *Cochrane Database Syst Rev* 2009; **2**: CD006955.

2 Franche RL, Cullen K, Clarke J, *et al.* Workplace-based return-to-work interventions: a systematic review of the quantitative literature. *J Occup Rehabil* 2005; **15**: 607–31.

3 Tompa E, de Oliveira C, Dolinschi R, *et al.* Systematic review of disability management interventions with economic evaluations. *J Occup Rehabil* 2008; **18**: 16–26.

4 Breen A, Langworthy J, Bagust J. *Improved early pain management for musculoskeletal disorders.* London: HSE Books, 2005.

5 Clayton M, Verow P. Advice given to patients about return to work and driving following surgery. *Occup Med* 2007; **57**: 488–91.

6 Liebensteiner MC, Kern M, Haid C, *et al.* Brake response time before and after total knee arthroplasty: a prospective cohort study. *BMC Musculoskelet Disord* 2010; **11**: 267.

7 Edwards MR, Oliver MC, Hatrick NC. Driving with a forearm plaster cast: patients' perspective. *Emerg Med J* 2009; **26**: 405–6.

8 Schneider E, Irastorza X, European Agency for Safety and Health at Work. *European risk observatory report.* Luxembourg: Publications Office of the European Union, 2009.

9 Health and Safety Executive. *Self-reported work-related illness (SWI) and workplace injuries: results from the Labour Force Survey (LFS).* London: Office for National Statistics, 2011.

10 Burton AK, Kendall NAS, Pearce BG, *et al.* Management of work-relevant upper limb disorders: a review. *Occup Med* 2009; **59**: 44–52.

11 van Rijn RM, Huisstede BM, Koes BW, *et al.* Associations between work-related factors and specific disorders of the shoulder-a systematic review of the literature. *Scand J Work Environ Health* 2010; **36**: 189–201.

12 van Rijn RM, Huisstede BM, Koes BW, *et al.* Associations between work-related factors and specific disorders at the elbow: a systematic literature review. *Rheumatology* 2009; **48**: 528–36.

13 Coombes BK, Bisset L, Vicenzo B. Efficacy and safety of corticosteroid injections and other injections for management of tendinopathy: a systematic review of randomised controlled trials. *Lancet* 2010; **376** (9754): 1751–67.

14 Hofmeister EP, Leak RS, Culp RW, *et al.* Arthroscopic hemitrapeziectomy for first carpometacarpal arthritis: results at 7-year follow-up. *Hand (N Y)* 2009; **4**: 24–8.

15 Burke FD, Proud G, Lawson IJ, *et al.* An assessment of the effects of exposure to vibration, smoking, alcohol and diabetes on the prevalence of Dupuytren's disease in 97,537 miners. *J Hand Surg* 2007; **32**: 400–6.

16 Ratzon N, Schejter-Margalit T, Froom P. Time to return to work and surgeons' recommendations after carpal tunnel release. *Occup Med* 2006; **56**; 46–50.

17 Amick BC, Habeck RV, Ossmann J, *et al.* Predictors of successful work role functioning after carpal tunnel release surgery. *J Occup Environ Med* 2004; **46**: 490–500.

18 Lee MJ, LaStayo PC. Compressions that mimic carpal tunnel syndrome. *J Orthop Sports Phys Ther* 2004; **34**: 601–9.

19 Palmer K, Milne P, Poole J, *et al.* Employment characteristics and job loss in patients awaiting surgery on the hip or knee. *Occup Environ Med* 2005; **62**: 54–7.

20 National Collaborating Centre for Chronic Conditions. *Osteoarthritis: national clinical guideline for care and management in adults.* London: National Institute for Health and Clinical Excellence, 2008. (<http://www.nice.org.uk>)

21 Jensen LK. Hip osteoarthritis: influence of work with heavy lifting, climbing stairs or ladders, or combining kneeling/squatting with heavy lifting. *Occup Environ Med* 2008; **65**: 6–19.

22 Dr Foster Health: <http://www.drfosterhealth.co.uk>

23 Peak LE, Parvizi J, Ciminiello M, *et al.* The role of patient restrictions in reducing the prevalence of early dislocation following total hip arthroplasty: a randomized, prospective study. *J Bone Joint Surg Am* 2008; **87**: 247–53.

24 Reid CR, Bush PM, Cummings NH, *et al.* A review of occupational knee disorders. *J Occup Rehabil* 2010; **20**: 489–501.

25 Vignon E, Valat JP, Rossignol M, *et al.* Osteoarthritis of the knee and hip and activity: a systematic international review and synthesis (OASIS). *Joint Bone Spine* 2006; **73**: 442–55.

26 Chapple CM, Nicholson H, Baxter GD, *et al.* Patient characteristics that predict progression of knee osteoarthritis: a systematic review of prognostic studies. *Arthritis Care Res* 2011; **63**: 1115–25.

27 Chen J-C, Linnan L, Callahan LF, *et al.* Workplace policies and prevalence of knee osteoarthritis: the Johnston county osteoarthritis project. *Occup Environ Med* 2007; **64**: 798–805.

28 Styron JF, Barsoum WK, Smyth KA, *et al.* Preoperative predictors of returning to work following primary total knee arthroplasty. *J Bone Joint Surg Am* 2011; **93**: 2–10.

29 Goodyear-Smith F, Arroll B. Rehabilitation after arthroscopic meniscectomy: a critical review of the clinical trials. *Int Orthop* 2001; **24**: 350–3.

30 Frosch KH, Habermann F, Fuchs M, *et al.* Is prolonged ambulatory physical therapy after anterior cruciate ligament-plasty indicated? *Unfallchirurg* 2001; **104**: 513–18.

31 Oiestad BE, Engebresten L, Storheim K, *et al.* Knee osteoarthritis after anterior cruciate ligament injury: a systematic review. *Am J Sports Med* 2009; **37**: 1434–43.

32 Martin RL, Stewart GW, Conti SF. Posttraumatic ankle arthritis: an update on conservative and surgical management. *J Orthop Sports Phys Ther* 2007; **37**: 253–9.

33 Magnussen RA, Dunn WR, Thomson AB. Nonoperative treatment of midportion Achilles tendinopathy: a systematic review. *Clin J Sport Med* 2009; **19**: 54–64.

34 Hawke F, Burns J, Radford JA, *et al.* Custom-made foot orthoses for the treatment of foot pain. *Cochrane Database Syst Rev* 2008; **3**: CD006801.

35 Holt G, Kay M, McGrory R, *et al.* Emergency brake response time after first metatarsal osteotomy. *J Bone Joint Surg Am* 2008; **90**: 1660–4.

36 Thomson CE, Gibson JNA, Martin D. Interventions for the treatment of Morton's neuroma. *Cochrane Database Syst Rev* 2004; **3**: CD003118.

37 Clay FJ, Newstead SV, Watson WL, *et al*. Determinants of return to work following non life threatening acute orthopaedic trauma. *J Rehabil Med* 2010; **42**: 162–9.

38 Galey S, Sferra JJ. Arthrodesis after workplace injuries. *Foot Ankle Clin* 2002; **7**: 385–401.

39 Burger H, Marincek C. Return to work after lower limb amputation. *Disabil Rehabil* 2007; **29**: 1323–9.

40 Pasquina PF, Bryant PR, Huang ME, *et al*. Advances in amputee care. *Arch Phys Med Rehabil* 2006; **87**(3 Suppl 1): S34–43.

Chapter 13

Rheumatological disorders

Steve Ryder and Karen Walker-Bone

Introduction

Musculoskeletal pain affects up to 50 per cent of the population at any one time. Consequently, low back pain, neck pain, and upper limb disorders are important causes of sickness absence. Spinal disorders, including back pain, are covered in detail in Chapter 11, and will not be discussed further here. Instead this chapter will focus on the other common rheumatological disorders, including upper limb disorders (specific and non-specific), osteoarthritis (OA), inflammatory arthritis, connective tissue disorders, and widespread pain syndromes.

Many rheumatological conditions are chronic and potentially disabling but there have been recent developments in medical therapies, especially in the inflammatory rheumatic conditions, which offer the prospect of controlling disease activity, reducing disability, improving quality of life, and enabling work.

Work-related upper limb disorders

These conditions are confusing and contentious. The term 'repetitive strain injury' (RSI) has justifiably fallen into misuse as the term 'injury', not always true, implies fault. Surveillance case definitions for upper limb disorders were proposed by a UK consensus group using a Delphi process aimed at standardizing classification criteria for research (Table 13.1).[1] In their review, Boocock et al.[2] showed that there remains a lack of international consensus around these conditions. The definitions in this chapter are taken from the Harrington criteria and modified as recommended by Boocock et al. One advantage is that the Harrington criteria formed the basis of a standardized system of examination, 'The Southampton examination protocol', which has been developed, tested, and shown to perform reliably,[3] with face validity for the specified diagnoses.[4] To avoid confusion, the term WRULD is used here to cover both specifically defined upper limb conditions (e.g. tenosynovitis, carpal tunnel syndrome, epicondylitis) and non-specific diffuse forearm pain.

The aetiology of WRULD is complex. Uncontrolled studies from Australia[5] purported to show histological abnormalities in affected muscles of patients with pain from chronic overuse. Other researchers have sought to explain the condition in terms of pain amplification.[6] Factors associated with upper limb pain include: task repetition,[7,8] magnitude of applied forces,[9] velocity of movement, joint movement at the extremes of their range, psychosocial factors,[10] perfectionism,[11] stress,[10] and female sex.[12] There remain no definitive diagnostic criteria based on symptoms, clinical findings, or tests. There may be overlap with conditions presumed to be predominantly neurological, such as focal dystonia or 'writer's cramp', a condition that may qualify for Industrial Injury Disablement Benefit (IIDB), in the UK (Prescribed Disease (PD) A4). PDA8, more clearly defined as tenosynovitis, is a separate entity. It remains to be established whether non-specific arm pain may sometimes constitute the prodromal phase of forearm tenosynovitis.

Table 13.1 Summary of consensus case definitions for upper limb disorders

Disorder	Diagnostic criteria
Rotator cuff tendinitis	History of pain in the deltoid region *and* pain on resisted active movement (abduction—supraspinatus; external rotation—infraspinatus; internal rotation—subscapularis)
Bicipital tendinitis	History of anterior shoulder pain *and* pain on resisted active flexion or supination of the forearm
Shoulder capsulitis (frozen shoulder)	History of pain in the deltoid area *and* equal restriction of active and passive glenohumeral movement with capsular pattern (external rotation>abduction>internal rotation)
Lateral epicondylitis	Epicondylar pain *and* epicondylar tenderness *and* pain on resisted extension of the wrist
Medial epicondylitis	Epicondylar pain *and* epicondylar tenderness *and* pain on resisted flexion of the wrist
De Quervain's disease of the wrist	Pain over the radial styloid *and* tender swelling of the first extensor compartment *and either* pain reproduced by resisted thumb extension *or* positive Finkelstein test
Tenosynovitis of the wrist	Pain on movement localized to the tendon sheaths of the wrist *and* reproduction of pain by resisted active movement
Carpal tunnel syndrome	Pain *or* paraesthesia *or* sensory loss in the median nerve distribution *and one of* Tinel's test positive, Phalen's test positive, nocturnal exacerbation of symptoms, motor loss with wasting of abductor pollicis brevis, abnormal nerve conduction time
Non-specific diffuse	Pain in the forearm in the absence of a specific diagnosis or pathology

There may be predisposing factors for WRULD (e.g. a change in technique or working practices), or sometimes the total amount of repetition may exceed a threshold. Typically, symptoms are relieved initially by a short period of rest, perhaps overnight, but as symptoms become more chronic not even the weekend or the 2–3 weeks of annual holiday are sufficient. Patients describe their symptoms as aching, soreness, or tingling, usually localized to a particular part of the musculoskeletal apparatus—often that required for the physical action in question. Sometimes symptoms become more widespread (shoulder–hand syndrome). The wrist, forearm, and elbow areas are typically involved at the onset. There may be disturbance of sleep patterns and generalized fatigue is common.

These patients have few consistent clinical signs although measurement of grip strength may be helpful.[13] Investigators have reported an alteration in pain threshold measured by algometer, although this has not been independently confirmed.[14] There may be involuntary contraction of muscles and sometimes vasomotor changes, particularly among workers from refrigerating plants.

Figure 13.1 presents an algorithm for assessment of arm pain in working-aged adults. Risk filter and risk assessment worksheets have been developed.[15] The Health and Safety Executive (HSE) website has useful tools to assist with the process (MAC and ART tools). When several individuals have similar complaints, various factors need to be assessed (e.g. work rate, method of pay,

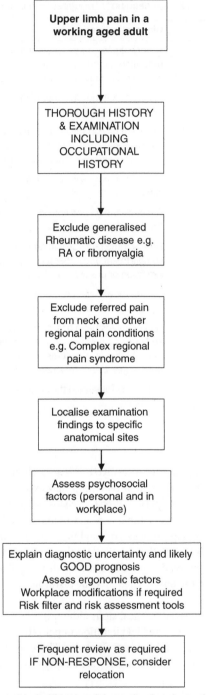

Figure 13.1 Assessment of a patient with a possible work-related upper limb disorder. Reproduced with permission from Graves RJ *et al.*, Development of risk filter and risk assessment worksheets for HSE guidance—'Upper Limb Disorders in the Workplace' 2002, *Applied Ergonomics*, Volume 35, Issue 5, pp. 475–84, Crown Copyright © 2004, published by Elsevier Ltd.

excessive noise, heat or cold, other factors that might increase levels of anxiety, and muscular tension). Individuals should be reviewed until symptoms resolve and, if necessary, be relocated. In practice, management of WRULD has been complicated by medico-legal case law. Specifically, Judge Prosser[16] found against the existence of this condition, a judgment which may have discouraged people from seeking unreasonable damages in courts but also brought into sharp focus conflicting research findings which suggested rates of prevalence for this 'condition' can vary between 5 per cent and 60 per cent. Insightful was the view of Judge Mellow, who recently awarded a record settlement to a typist who developed this condition while working for the Inland Revenue. His apt statement, 'while I do not rule out the existence of some wider diffuse condition, I do not find it proved to exist', acts both as a concise summary and indictment of current medical understanding (and dispute) on the condition.

Whatever the legal viewpoint, the HSE has published guidelines[17] for prevention that employers are well advised to follow. This concentrates on ensuring that all repetitive actions are performed in the position of maximum ergonomic advantage. Appropriate rest breaks should be provided and job rotation may be a means of ensuring this. Workers should be encouraged to report symptoms and be referred early for occupational health assessment to establish the diagnosis, receive advice on prevention, and be referred for specialist treatment where necessary. Intervention in the early stages, when symptoms are reversible, gives the best chance of avoiding chronicity.

Disorders of the neck and upper limb

Cervical spondylosis

Cervical spondylosis is the name given to radiographic changes of OA on cervical spine x-ray. Neck pain with restriction of movement, sometimes associated with headaches and/or dizziness, possibly referred to the upper limb or inter-scapular region, is a common clinical syndrome known by many different names (e.g. cervical myalgia, tension neck syndrome, occupational cervico-brachial disorder, and sometimes, confusingly, 'cervical spondylosis'). Radiographic changes are common in the cervical spine, with prevalence rates as high as 60 per cent at the age of 49 and 95 per cent by age 90 years. However, there is poor correlation between radiographic changes and symptoms and it is unclear to what extent common regional neck pain syndromes are caused by degeneration in the cervical spine. Although there is far less research on neck pain, there are strong parallels with 'mechanical back pain'. It may be that radiographic evaluation is as unhelpful for acute neck pain as it is in the assessment of mechanical back pain.

Conservative treatments focusing on rest, warmth, adequate analgesia, and topical or oral non-steroidal anti-inflammatory drugs, muscle relaxants, and physical treatments such as massage and physiotherapy usually prove effective. Surgical assessment is required only rarely, in cases of persistent neurological symptoms in the arms. Epidemiological studies suggest that at any one time 10 per cent of men and 18 per cent of women aged 20–65 years will report neck pain.[18] Symptoms are less common in sedentary office workers and more common where work requires strenuous use of the arms. Workers on assembly lines seem to be particularly at risk. Only a small minority of subjects will demonstrate 'porter's neck', so-called because bags of meal weighing 90 kg loaded on to the porter's head were clearly linked to radiological changes in the spine, including disc compression. Where a link is demonstrated between symptoms and the workplace, appropriate ergonomic and postural advice is essential in preventing recurrence, but non-occupational factors also need to be excluded.

The frequency and severity of symptoms and degree of functional limitation vary considerably. Severity of changes on cervical spine radiographs is not a reliable guide to prognosis or fitness for work.

Occupational mechanical and psychosocial factors[19,20] may precipitate symptoms or perpetuate chronicity. Work requiring the head and neck to be held in a constrained posture or requiring strenuous physical effort of shoulder girdle muscles (e.g. heavy lifting, carrying or labouring tasks, use of vibratory tools) has been implicated. A systematic review found 'moderate evidence' for a causal relationship between neck pain and exposure to neck flexion allied with repetition and with repetitive movements at the shoulder.[21] Working with the arms elevated above shoulder height or frequently extending the neck to look upwards should be avoided.

For sedentary, desk-orientated work, attention should be paid to seating, spinal posture, and the ergonomic layout of the desk, particularly if display screen equipment is used. All commonly used articles should be within easy arm's reach and the availability of desk lecterns will help to avoid prolonged periods of neck flexion, encouraging an upright neck posture.

In most cases, acute neck pain resolves, but when permanent restriction of neck movement occurs, driving motor vehicles or forklift trucks, or similar activities, may no longer be possible. Degeneration at the cervical spine may be associated with degeneration at the shoulder joint, either of the bony components of that joint or of the fibrous capsule. If the shoulder is unaffected, it can compensate for the restricted range of movement at the neck. When the neck and shoulder are involved together, the disability is greater.

Disorders of the shoulder

The shoulder is a shallow joint with a wide range of movement. To facilitate movement, the joint capsule is loose and the muscles attached to the proximal humerus (the 'rotator cuff') make a major contribution to the joint's stability. Most of the range of movement is achieved by the glenohumeral joint, but symptoms arising from both the acromioclavicular and the scapulothoracic joints may cause shoulder pain. The natural rhythm of elevation and abduction involves synchronized motor function at both the glenohumeral and scapulothoracic joints and the sternoclavicular joint is also stretched. The movements are facilitated by the bursae around the joints that ensure the smooth motion of contracting muscles and their ligaments over the bony prominences.

In patients older than 40 years, osteoarthritic change may occur, causing pain and restricted movements. This is commonest in those engaged in heavy manual work but can occur in divers or compressed air workers after aseptic bone necrosis. The dominant upper limb is more often affected. Local symptoms at the shoulder can be attributable to OA of the acromioclavicular joint, inflammation or tears of the rotator cuff (tendinitis), tendinitis of the long head of biceps tendon, or shoulder capsulitis (frozen shoulder). In occupational terms, shoulder tendinitis and capsulitis are the most important.

Shoulder tendinitis arises from symptomatic inflammation or degeneration of the tendons of the rotator cuff or biceps (Table 13.1).[1] Clinically, features may include: upper arm pain, a painful arc more apparent on active than passive movement, pain that is worse at night, crepitus, subacromial tenderness, referred pain in a C5 distribution, and pain and restriction of abduction of the shoulder beyond 80°. Tendon calcification may be seen on x-ray and magnetic resonance imaging scanning may demonstrate inflammation. Tendon tears may be chronic or acute, partial or full thickness. The preceding traumatic event should be sought in the history, which may or may not be work-related.

If tendinitis arises from acute injury, symptoms may be sudden. For most, however, the onset is more gradual and is presumed to result from eccentric overload, possibly aggravated by instability placing the tendon at a greater mechanical disadvantage. The extent to which ergonomic factors at work contribute to this condition, which can also arise spontaneously, requires careful consideration. Symptoms, when present, can be aggravated by repetitive occupational movements (especially above shoulder height) and healing may be correspondingly delayed if adequate rest is not possible.

Treatment by injection of corticosteroids with lignocaine can be effective in tendinitis and bursitis. The condition can be prolonged, lasting up to 10 months in one survey.[22]

Shoulder capsulitis (frozen shoulder) is characterized by pain in the deltoid region with global restriction of glenohumeral movement in a capsular pattern (Table 13.1).[1] The condition is usually unilateral but there is a 17 per cent chance of subsequently developing it in the other shoulder over 5 years. Underlying diseases such as diabetes mellitus, thyroid disease, infection, stroke, surgery, or cardiac disease may be associated. The prevalence in non-diabetics is 2–3 per cent, but higher, perhaps up to 20 per cent, among diabetics. Adhesive capsulitis is associated with overhead working, lifting weights, poor workplace support and psychological morbidity.[23]

Recovery may be delayed if work requiring shoulder joint movement is continued, although local injection of corticosteroids and analgesics may reduce symptoms. Full movements may not be regained for 12–24 months, which can pose a significant barrier to employment in occupations requiring a good deal of work above shoulder height (e.g. painters, decorators) or heavy lifting (e.g. builders). 'Reasonable' accommodations (e.g. job sharing, allocation to alternative duties, lifting aids) may mitigate the problem, however, while natural recovery evolves.

Prevention

Shoulder pain is common, affecting 21 per cent of the general population in the Netherlands,[24] with similar rates reported in other countries. Shoulder conditions are especially frequent among workers in the following industries: clothing, slaughtering and food processing, fish processing, repetitive assembly line work, and supermarket cashiers.[25] Symptoms are associated with biomechanical factors (repetitive tool use, vibrating tools, and abduction of the arms >90 degrees[26]) and psychosocial factors (monotonous work and poor job control[27]). Prevention and case management in the workplace should be aimed at minimizing these factors: ideally, work should be variable, without continuous repetition, usually achieved by frequent breaks and job rotation, exposure to hand-arm vibration should be limited, and prolonged elevation of the arm above shoulder height avoided. Employees should be given opportunities to change working patterns and develop their jobs.

Epicondylitis of the elbow

Lateral epicondylitis (*tennis elbow*) and medial epicondylitis (*golfer's elbow*) are the commonest soft tissue lesions at the elbow. They should be distinguished from other causes of elbow pain such as OA, olecranon bursitis, or biceps tendinitis. Careful clinical examination is essential. Lateral epicondylitis is associated with lateral elbow pain, tenderness, and pain on resisted wrist flexion[1] (Table 13.1).

At any one time, 1–3 per cent of the population may be affected by epicondylitis,[28] more commonly lateral than medial. A sporting cause is uncommon. Local trauma may play a part, as in an acute wrenching injury, though this is more likely to aggravate established epicondylitis in the older patient. Ageing appears to be associated with anatomical alteration at the enthesis, including changes in collagen content and increasing lipids, which may predispose to injury. Repeated pronation and supination of the forearm, an integral part of some jobs, can aggravate the condition. Whether symptoms can arise *ab initio* from this action is less well established, but reasonable to suppose. Epicondylitis has been associated with the use of heavy tools, and forceful repetitive work, particularly with the wrist in the non-neutral position.[29] In addition to physical workplace factors, psychosocial risk factors can increase the occurrence of elbow complaints.[30]

Epicondylitis is generally considered self-limiting and some patients improve with or without treatment within 1 year, but some still have symptoms after 12 months, particularly if they have maintained the precipitating activity.[31] Recurrence seems more common in manual workers and is attributable to repeated grasping or lifting. Treatment may consist of physiotherapy, acupuncture,[32] use of orthoses, or intra-lesional steroid injection.[33] Whilst steroid injections appear to be more effective at 6 weeks, physiotherapy seems to be more beneficial after 6 months. Surgery can be successful in cases resistant to conservative treatments, but results in litigants can be disappointing.[34] Postural and ergonomic adjustments, task modification, or job rotation may need to be considered to prevent recurrence and help recovery. Less is known about medial epicondylitis but it is thought to have a higher recovery rate (80 per cent at 3 years),[35] and is associated with repetitive bending/straightening of the elbow.[36]

Carpal tunnel syndrome

Carpal tunnel syndrome (CTS) is the commonest peripheral nerve entrapment syndrome. It has an incidence of 99 per 100,000/year in the general USA population[37] and results from compression of the median nerve as it passes through the tunnel formed between the carpal bones and the flexor retinaculum, it typically causes numbness and tingling of the fingers (usually lateral three-and-a-half digits), sometimes experienced more diffusely in the hand. Pain is variable and can extend proximally. Symptoms are often worse at night and in the morning.

Examination includes Tinel's test (tapping over the carpal tunnel, which when positive causes tingling in the thumb and radial three-and-a-half fingers) and Phalen's test (both hands are held tightly palmar-flexed opposite to a prayer position, creating at least a 90-degree angle between the forearm and hand; a positive test is when numbness and tingling are produced when the hands are held in this position for 1 minute). The reported diagnostic sensitivity of these tests is 32–93 per cent[38,39] and the specificity 45–100 per cent.[40,41] Nerve conduction studies are reported to have a sensitivity of 60–84 per cent and a specificity of more than 95 per cent in patients awaiting surgery. Risk factors include obesity, smoking, alcohol use, rheumatoid arthritis (RA) and OA, diabetes, hypothyroidism, local obstruction at the wrist, haemodialysis, pregnancy, and lactation. The condition may be bilateral, particularly if linked to a metabolic cause.

CTS is seen less frequently in patients who do not use their hands substantially and occurs more often in the dominant hand. The balance of probability is now shifting to acceptance that CTS can be a work-associated condition. The National Institute of Occupational Safety and Health (NIOSH), in its systematic review, concluded that there is evidence of a positive association between exposure to highly repetitive work and forceful work.[42] This evidence is stronger if the exposure involves a combination of risk factors (e.g. force together with repetition or force with adverse posture). Musicians and meat cutters who may need to keep the wrist in a flexed position for long periods are susceptible. A stamping or punching action involving the wrist also predisposes, presumably by regular direct compression. A recent quantitative study has confirmed that forceful exertion and repetitiveness are associated with the development of CTS.[43] CTS is a prescribed industrial disease (A12) when associated with work using hand-held vibrating tools, and also in workers whose jobs entail repeated palmar flexion and dorsiflexion of the wrist for at least 20 hours per week (when 'repeated' means more often than every 30 seconds).

Health surveillance may encompass workers with significant exposure to the risk factors described, and some US employers screen for delayed nerve conduction in workers first entering repetitive jobs. The predictive value of this approach is unclear, however, and it is not recommended for routine use.

When the diagnosis has been established, the reduction or avoidance of possible work-associated factors (e.g. abnormal forearm/wrist posture, prolonged wrist flexion, forceful and repetitive wrist movement, direct pressure over the carpal tunnel, and the use of vibratory hand-held tools) may result in reduction or resolution of symptoms. Injection of steroids may relieve symptoms temporarily. The use of a wrist splint is often recommended, but there is limited evidence of benefit while range of motion exercises appear to be associated with less pain and fewer lost days from work.[44] Where delayed nerve conduction is confirmed, surgical decompression of the carpal tunnel may be required. Postoperatively, resolution of symptoms can be expected, enabling a return to unrestricted work activity, but given some uncertainty about the long-term outcome in jobs with continuing exposure, it may be wise to adopt a monitoring brief, with the offer of a follow-up appointment if symptoms recur.

Tenosynovitis of the wrist

This term *tenosynovitis* describes inflammation of the extensor or flexor tendon sheaths at the wrist.[1] Pain, swelling, and pain on resisted movement are pathognomonic (Table 13.1). Inflammation affects the tendon sheath rather than the tendon itself, which is painful on palpation. Crepitus is a fleeting sign and can be associated with triggering or tethering, if the condition becomes chronic.

Treatment involves avoidance of the cause or aggravating movements which are identified at a workplace ergonomic assessment, at least until symptoms settle; topical or oral anti-inflammatory agents, and intra-synovial injection of corticosteroids. Splinting is often recommended but prolonged immobilization should be avoided to prevent muscle wastage and local osteoporosis. If surgery is required to relieve tethering, histopathological confirmation of the condition can be obtained. When the acute phase has resolved (over, say, 4–6 weeks away from the aggravating factor), return to work must be carefully planned over a few weeks if recurrence is to be avoided. Attention must be paid to avoidance of excessive wrist movements, particularly at the extremes of range of motion. Mechanization of the task, time restriction, job rotation, and job transfer need to be considered. In adults with tenosynovitis, there is limited evidence that modified computer keyboards are effective in reducing symptoms.[45] This condition is recognized for compensation (IIDB), in the UK as industrial disease PDA8 when inflammation is caused by manual labour.

De Quervain's tenosynovitis is defined as painful swelling of the first extensor compartment containing the tendons of abductor pollicis longus and extensor pollicis brevis (Table 13.1).[1] The condition should be distinguished from OA of the wrist or first carpometacarpal joint, wrist ligament strains, and a non-united scaphoid fracture. As repetitive movement of the tendon in its sheath is a prime cause the ergonomic case for this being an occupational-related injury is extremely strong. It is more common in women than men. Medical treatment as previously described is appropriate but surgical release may be required.

Trigger finger or *trigger thumb* (stenosing digital tenosynovitis) implies tenosynovitis of one of the flexor tendons to the finger or thumb. Characteristically this occurs with repetitive gripping activities that increase pull and friction on the flexor tendons. Although it can be associated with other conditions (including RA, diabetes mellitus, sarcoidosis, and hyperthyroidism), a clear ergonomic history normally correlates with the anatomical abnormalities. In common with other forms of tenosynovitis, rest is beneficial and too early a return to work (perhaps within 4–6 weeks of withdrawal from the aggravating exposure) delays resolution of the condition. A postural and ergonomic assessment should be undertaken and, where required, alterations made to upper limb movements, work practices, or workplace design. Modifications to hand-held tools may also prove beneficial and, where groups of workers are similarly affected, automation of a process of job rotation may be indicated.

Non-specific diffuse forearm pain

This is a diagnosis of exclusion (Table 13.1). The merit of this diagnostic term as an alternative to RSI or WRULD is that it contains no assumption as to aetiology.[1] Patients complain of forearm pain accompanied by loss of function, subjective swelling, weakness, cramp, muscle tenderness, allodynia, and slowing of fine movements. It should be distinguished from generalized pain syndromes such as fibromyalgia and from referred pain.

Treatment typically involves physiotherapy and, where possible, avoidance of precipitating factors. The guidance laid down earlier with regard to workplace assessment should be followed and measures to minimize exposure to precipitating factors, such as breaks to allow recovery, job rotation, etc. should be considered. In software and computer roles, where a practical dilemma often arises over work restriction for low-grade grumbling symptoms, workstation assessment and the provision of alternative input devices, including voice activated software, may also be helpful.

There is some evidence that a cognitive-behavioural therapeutic approach may be beneficial in non-specific diffuse forearm pain.[46,47] There is limited, but high-quality evidence, that multidisciplinary rehabilitation for non-specific musculoskeletal arm pain is beneficial for those workers who have been absent from work for at least 4 weeks.[45]

Other management pointers in upper limb disorder

A recent review conducted by Burton et al.[47] highlighted the following key points in case management:

- Upper limb disorders can be triggered by everyday activities and over-attribution to work can be detrimental to recovery; over-medicalization and negative diagnostic labels are unhelpful.
- Many cases settle with self-management though some need treatment; intervention should take a stepped care approach, based on biopsychosocial principles.
- Early return to work is important, though some work may be difficult or impossible to perform for a short while; work should be comfortable and accommodating.

Osteoarthritis

OA is the commonest form of arthritis, affecting the knee joints of an estimated 0.5 million people in the UK.[48] When the prevalence of OA is measured using radiological changes, one estimate has suggested that 80 per cent of the population have OA after age 55 years.

The main affected joints are the knees, hips, hands, spine, and, less often, the feet. OA is a metabolically active, dynamic process involving all joint tissues (cartilage, bone, synovium, capsule, ligaments/muscles), responding to injury which causes focal failure of articular cartilage. Damage of the articular cartilage triggers remodelling of adjacent bone and hypertrophic reaction at joint margins, recognized radiographically as osteophytes. This remodelling and repair is efficient but slow and while it takes place, secondary synovial inflammation and crystal deposition can occur. Clinically, the patient experiences pain and stiffness in affected joint(s) with acute episodes of heat, redness, and swelling during secondary inflammatory phases. Longer term, the joint develops permanent structural change leading to functional limitation and disability.

Risk factors for osteoarthritis

OA affects women more than men and is associated with ageing, although it is not uncommon in people of working age. Genetic factors are important, as is obesity. Weight-bearing predisposes to hip and knee OA. Joint injury, recreational or occupational usage, joint laxity, reduced muscle strength, and joint malalignment are all established risk factors. There are also several medical conditions which predispose to secondary OA including: congenital/developmental diseases, inflammatory joint diseases (e.g. RA), endocrinopathies (e.g. acromegaly), metabolic disorders (e.g. ochronosis), neuropathic disorders (e.g. diabetes), and disorders of bone (e.g. Paget's disease).

Occupational risk factors for osteoarthritis

Occupations which entail repetitive use of particular joints over long periods of time have been associated with the development of site-specific OA.[49] Thus, dockers and shipyard labourers have an excess of hand and knee OA; miners have an excess of knee and lumbar spine disease; cotton and mill workers develop an excess of hand OA at particular finger joints; workers using pneumatic drills have an excess of elbow and wrist OA; floor and carpet layers are more affected by knee OA; and farmers have more hip OA. The important exposures for lower limb OA are: kneeling posture, jumping, climbing flights of stairs, and heavy lifting.[50]

Assessment of osteoarthritis

The course of OA varies considerably depending upon cause and the distribution of joints affected. Since OA is essentially a process of repair and regeneration, it can ultimately limit the damage and symptoms in most cases, but rates of progression and symptom severity vary by site (e.g. hand OA generally has a good prognosis except in the first carpometacarpal joints). Once knee OA has started, structural changes rarely reverse, but pain and disability can improve markedly. It has been estimated that over time, one-third of knee OA patients will improve, one-third will stay the same, and one-third will worsen. The prognosis of hip OA has been less well studied but there is evidence that it generally progresses more than knee OA and that over 5 years, a significant proportion of patients require hip surgery.

Most patients with OA consult because of pain but the correlation between pain, disability, and structural changes can be poor, especially early in the disease course. The correlation improves with increasing severity of the structural changes. Within individuals there is an influence of personality, mood, occupation, psychosocial environment, and expectations, both on pain and response to treatment. The National Institute for Health and Clinical Excellence (NICE) guidance for managing OA recommends that the initial assessment should encompass a holistic approach:[51]

- *The patient's thoughts*: what are their concerns and expectations? What do they know about OA?
- *The patient's support network*: is the patient isolated or do they have a carer? If there is a carer, how are they coping and what are their concerns and expectations?
- *The patient's mood*: screen for depression and stresses
- *The patient's attitude to exercise.*
- *The impact of OA on*: occupation, activities of daily living, family responsibilities, hobbies, lifestyle, sleep.
- *Pain assessment*: what self-help strategies are they using? Are they taking medicines? At, what doses, how often, any side effects?

- *Other musculoskeletal pain*: could this be a chronic pain syndrome? Are there other treatable sources of pain (e.g. bursitis, trigger digit, ganglion)?
- *Comorbidities*: are there other medical problems? What impact might comorbidities have on treatment options?

Management of osteoarthritis

Given the variable rate of disease progression, it is always appropriate to take a positive approach at presentation. The patient should be disabused of the misconception that OA universally worsens over time. Initial approaches focus on education, exercise, and self-management (Figure 13.2).[51] Exercise has two main aims: local muscle strengthening and general aerobic fitness. Patients should be advised about the importance of weight loss, which has been shown to reverse large joint progression. Education, given in one-to-one and group contacts, written or even computer-assisted, is an important treatment modality. The emphasis should be on a positive approach, exercise, simple measures such as shock absorbing footwear, heat and ice packs, and the importance of weight reduction. Although popular, there is no convincing evidence that glucosamine or

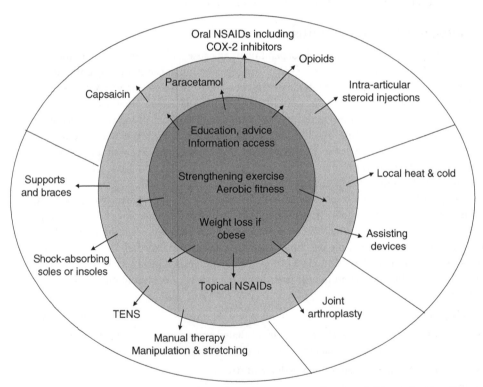

Figure 13.2 An algorithm for the multidisciplinary management of osteoarthritis. National Institute for Health and Clinical Excellence (2008) *CG 59 Osteoarthritis: the care and management of osteoarthritis in adults*. London: NICE. Available from <http://www.nice.org.uk/guidance/CG59>. Reproduced with permission. Information accurate at time of publication, for up-to-date information please visit <http://www.nice.org.uk>.

chondroitin products are beneficial in OA and the NICE guidance for OA recommends that they should not be prescribed.[51]

Treatment approaches should commence at the centre of Figure 13.2 with education and exercise approaches and move outwards as required and appropriate when symptom control is poor.

Management of osteoarthritis in the workplace

Not only do occupational factors contribute to the causation of OA, but people with OA may experience difficulties performing work,[50] decreased productivity, sickness absence, work disability, and early retirement. The Department for Work and Pensions has estimated that around 36 million working days are lost annually because of OA at a cost of £3.2 billion in lost productivity.[52] As the age of retirement increases and the population prevalence of obesity increases, the costs of OA to employers seem set to grow. Measures to reduce the impact of OA on employees are urgent to develop but there is little evidence on exactly what is required.[50] OA features frequently in long-term disability statistics but research rarely considers workplace outcomes, longitudinal data are not available, and few studies inform strategies to prevent sickness absence and early retirement.[50] This is a field where major research is needed.

Pragmatically, work that facilitates movement and encourages flexibility of the affected joints, thus avoiding stiffness, is likely to be of benefit—provided the tasks are not too physically onerous. An ergonomic workplace assessment may help in assessing postural strains and giving appropriate guidance. Where hand joints are affected, the provision of writing aids, the use of a dictaphone, voice-activated control systems for computer work, or grasping aids may be helpful. Where knee joint symptoms are prominent, mobility will be restricted and standing should be reduced, together with work activities requiring climbing, walking over rough ground, kneeling, or crouching.

Inflammatory arthritis

There are many different inflammatory arthritides. These share in common an autoimmune basis in which the immune system triggers systemic inflammation of joints. In the absence of a clear understanding on pathophysiology, most of these conditions are distinguished by their clinical features and/or serological abnormalities. However, as understanding develops, new classification criteria are evolving.

Rheumatoid arthritis

RA is the commonest inflammatory arthritis, with a prevalence of 1–2 per cent. It is a symmetrical polyarthritis, particularly involving the hands, wrists, and feet but can involve any joint. Some of its most disabling features are produced by systemic pro-inflammatory cytokines which cause fatigue, malaise, and low energy levels. When joints are actively inflamed, they are hot, red, and exquisitely tender. Morning stiffness is a prominent feature, lasting from half an hour up to most of the day.

Risk factors for rheumatoid arthritis

RA affects women more than men and has a peak age at onset of 25–50 years, although it can present at any age. Possible independent risk factors for RA include obesity,[53] smoking, and genetic constitution, the last of these contributing to disease susceptibility and/or severity. The higher rate in women has led to the suspicion that female hormonal factors are important in pathogenesis.

In keeping with this, many women experience relative disease remission during pregnancy, but with greater risk of postpartum onset or flare-up; nulliparity and breastfeeding seem to be risk factors; and oral contraceptives may be protective.

Occupational risk factors for rheumatoid arthritis

Several occupational exposures have potentially been implicated in the aetiology of RA, including vibration, exposure to mineral dusts, including silica, during mining,[53-55] farming, and exposure to pesticides.[56,57]

Diagnosis of rheumatoid arthritis

Recently, the diagnostic criteria for RA have been reviewed in light of the emergence of new effective treatments, which need to be started as early as possible after diagnosis to control disease activity and prevent joint damage.[58] A scoring algorithm is applied among patients who have at least one joint with definite clinical synovitis (swelling) that cannot be better explained by another disease (Table 13.2). A score of greater than 6 is required to classify the arthritis as RA.

Table 13.2 Summary of the 2010 American College of Rheumatology/European League Against Rheumatism (ACR-EULAR) classification criteria for rheumatoid arthritis

	Score
A. Joint involvement	
1 large joint	0
2–10 large joints	1
1–3 small joints (with or without large joints)	2
4–10 small joints (with or without large joints)	3
>10 joints (at least 1 small joint)	5
B. Serology (at least 1 test is required)	
Negative RF *and* negative anti-CCP antibodies	0
Low-positive RF *or* low-positive anti-CCP antibodies	2
High-positive RF *or* high-positive anti-CCP antibodies	3
C. Acute-phase reactants (at least 1 test is needed)	
Normal CRP *and* normal ESR	0
Abnormal CRP *or* abnormal ESR	1
D. Duration of symptoms	
<6 weeks	0
≥6 weeks	1

Small joint is fingers or thumbs joint or wrists

Large joint is elbow, shoulder, hip, knee, ankle

CCP, cyclic citrullinated peptide; CRP, C-reactive protein; ESR, erythrocyte sedimentation rate; RF, rheumatoid factor.

Management of rheumatoid arthritis

Various treatments are available to manage RA, including medication, physiotherapy, occupational therapy, and surgery. Guidance from NICE in 2009 emphasized the importance of rapid referral for early assessment in patients suspected of having inflammatory arthritis.[58] Once diagnosed, patients should be commenced on a combination of disease-modifying anti-rheumatic drugs (DMARDs), including methotrexate and at least one other DMARD, plus short-term glucocorticoids. The aim is to obtain control of disease activity, as measured by the Disease Activity Score (DAS28). It is well-established that adequate control of disease activity leads to markedly improved outcomes in terms of joint destruction, function, and disability. Regular monitoring is required until stable control is achieved, and therapy may be escalated as necessary to achieve this aim. After at least two DMARDs have been tried (at therapeutic doses and including methotrexate), and in the presence of ongoing active disease (DAS28 score >5.1 on two occasions at least 1 month apart) and the absence of contraindications, patients become eligible for biological treatment. First-line NICE-approved biologics are the tumour necrosis factor (TNF)-α inhibitors, which are administered by subcutaneous injection weekly (etanercept) or fortnightly (adalimumab or certolizumab pegol) or can be given by intravenous infusion (infliximab). These therapies are usually co-administered with methotrexate and act by lowering levels of circulating pro-inflammatory cytokines which are important to host defences. Treated patients are therefore effectively immunosuppressed. The risk to benefit ratio heavily favours use of these therapies, but the occupational health team should be aware that these patients are at increased risk of infection (or re-infection in the case of tuberculosis) and should receive annual influenza vaccination plus pneumococcal vaccination. They may require antibiotic treatment at a lower threshold than other patients.

Beyond pharmacotherapy, the management of RA is multifaceted and is considerably enhanced by the involvement of a multidisciplinary team including occupational therapists and physiotherapists, podiatric services, and, as appropriate, counsellors, social workers, and pharmacists. NICE emphasizes the role of the specialist nurse in rheumatology in patient advocacy and coordinating case management.[59]

Management of rheumatoid arthritis in the workplace

Work disability is a serious and common outcome for people with RA.[60] In 1999/2000, it accounted for 9.4 million lost working days, equating to £833 million in lost productivity.[48] Age, disease-related factors, and job characteristics have consistently been risk factors for work disability from RA. However, changes over the past two decades, such as improved pharmaceutical treatment,[61] a possibly milder disease course, increased workforce participation of older workers, and decreased physical demands of jobs may have somewhat reduced work disability. Certainly, more recent studies have suggested changing patterns in the prevalence of work disability.[62] Although this remains high, at about 35 per cent after 10 years of disease, it is lower than the 50 per cent reported in earlier studies. In one study work disability was predicted by older age (odds ratio (OR) 1.2, 95 per cent confidence interval (CI) 1.1–1.4) and lower income (OR 1.7, 95 per cent CI 1.0–2.7), worse amongst those with greater functional limitation and RA activity, but not significantly associated with occupational hand use or overall job physical demand.[63]

Traditionally, outcomes in RA have been assessed by monitoring radiographic erosions and by functional measures such as the Health Assessment Questionnaire (HAQ). However, more recently, occupational outcomes have been evaluated using the RA Work Instability Score (WIS), a tool with some validity.[64] Using this instrument, intensive occupational therapy intervention has been shown to improve work-related outcomes among employed RA patients at risk of work disability.[65]

Currently, there is reason for optimism about work-associated outcomes among patients newly diagnosed with RA receiving prompt diagnosis and treatment. The occupational health team should proactively support the employee, working closely with their rheumatologist and other team members, especially occupational therapists. A detailed assessment of permissible work activities, the ergonomic environment and work station are advisable and may need to be repeated. Significant mechanical strain from force, repetition or adverse postures should be avoided. Indoor work requiring skill, rather than strength, is to be preferred. Ergonomic adjustments or the provision of handling aids may be required. In extreme cases, relocation or retraining for less physically arduous tasks may help an individual to remain at work. Expert advice can be obtained from officers of the local Placing, Assessment and Counselling Team or National Health Service occupational therapy department on writing aids, electrically operated devices, or specialized hand-held tools.

Patients rate support from their managers and colleagues as important facilitators of continued working, as well as self-acceptance, self-efficacy, and professional advice on coping at work.[66] When considering the recruitment of an individual with established RA, a detailed history of symptoms and physical limitations, and a careful functional assessment are essential. Although few employers may be willing to recruit an individual with aggressive disease, significant function limitations and an uncertain future, they must consider each case in the light of the requirements of the Equality Act 2010. Similarly, the Act is likely to require proactive attempts at reasonable accommodation if disease develops during employment.

Ankylosing spondylitis

The archetypal inflammatory spondyloarthropathy, ankylosing spondylitis, causes inflammatory low back pain frequently presenting in young men. Ninety-five per cent of those affected will carry the human leucocyte antigen (HLA) B27 genotype. The occupational management of this condition is described in Chapter 12.

Seronegative arthritides

The seronegative arthritides are a group of clinical conditions which share in common seronegativity for rheumatoid factor and certain clinical, epidemiological, and genetic features—e.g. asymmetrical joint involvement, sacro-iliac joint involvement, risk of anterior uveitis, variable association with HLA B27, skin involvement (prominent in psoriatic arthritis), mucosal involvement (urethritis, conjunctivitis), enthesitis, and a variable association with bacteria or bacterial products.

Reactive arthritis

In most cases, reactive arthritis is an acute event, triggered by infection with a causative organism. Although patients may present feeling extremely unwell and with several hot, red inflamed joints, providing the diagnosis is made promptly and appropriate treatment initiated for the causative organism, most cases settle within 6 weeks and the vast majority within 6 months. The prognosis is good and long-term disease-modifying therapy is not required. During the acute phase, the patient may require hospital admission or intensive outpatient management coupled with rest but in the long term, full functional restoration and return to work fitness can be expected.

Psoriatic arthritis

Psoriatic arthritis is a complex clinical entity. Psoriasis is a relatively common skin condition affecting 2 per cent of the population (see Chapter 22) and amongst sufferers of skin psoriasis, it has been estimated that between 1 per cent and 42 per cent develop inflammatory arthritis. (The wide variation in these figures is explained by different methodological approaches to estimation in settings that also differ.)

Psoriatic arthritis is equally common in men and women. It can occur at any age but peaks at age 45–54 years. HLA B27 is seen much less frequently among patients with psoriatic arthritis than ankylosing spondylitis, but more commonly than among the general population. HLA B27 tends to differentiate between those who suffer axial as compared with peripheral involvement. Ethnicity, geography, and workplace factors have an uncertain role but there is some evidence for a viral trigger, and patients with HIV and hepatitis C have an increased prevalence of psoriatic arthritis.

The management strategy for psoriatic arthropathy is modelled on that for RA, ankylosing spondylitis, and skin psoriasis. Assessment of disease activity must include assessment of the skin as well as joint involvement and patient-centred outcomes such as joint pain, disability and function (See 'Management of rheumatoid arthritis'). Only recently have workplace outcomes been evaluated in a few studies of limited methodology.[67] Tillett and colleagues found 'intermediate quality' evidence that rates of unemployment ranged between 20 per cent and 50 per cent and rates of work disability between 16 per cent and 39 per cent in psoriatic arthritis. Unemployment and work disability were associated with longer disease duration, worse physical function, high joint count, low educational level, female sex, erosive disease, and manual work.[68] There was sparse, low-quality evidence that workplace outcomes were worse in psoriatic arthritis than in psoriasis alone.

Among a young cohort (age 18–45 years) with psoriatic arthritis, Wallenius and colleagues found that 32.7 per cent of women and 17.4 per cent of men were receiving a permanent work disability pension.[69] Predictors of work disability were: low educational attainment, long duration of disease, age, radiographic erosions, disability, and female sex. In a cohort of patients with psoriatic arthritis randomized to intravenous infusions of the anti-TNFα infliximab or placebo, those receiving infliximab achieved greater productivity, with a trend towards increased employment and reduced sickness absence.[70] In the UK, prior to treatment with biological therapies, 39 per cent of patients with psoriatic arthritis were work-disabled (vs. 49 per cent of RA patients and 41 per cent of ankylosing spondylitis patients). Prospectively, work disability over 6 months of follow-up was more likely among those with manual jobs and high disability scores.[71]

Since work disability appears to be almost as common as in RA, a similar approach should be taken to the management of this disease group.

Connective tissue diseases

There are a number of heterogeneous multisystem 'connective tissue' diseases that share in common systemic inflammation coupled with immune dysregulation. In most cases, the aetiology is poorly understood and therefore they are classified on the basis of clusters of clinical and/or serological features. All of these conditions are relatively uncommon. Systemic lupus erythematosus (SLE), the commonest, has an estimated prevalence of 1/1000 population.

Systemic lupus erythematosus

SLE affects women nine times more often than men, the highest prevalence being in the West Indies and California. It is notable for its diversity of clinical features which may present in a wide spectrum at onset or over the course of the disease. The commonest features are fatigue, malaise, oral ulceration, skin involvement (particularly the characteristic malar butterfly rash), arthralgia or arthritis, pleurisy, and pericarditis. More serious manifestations may occur in the central or peripheral nervous system or in the kidney. Haematological and immunological disorders are frequently observed, anti-double stranded DNA antibodies being the most specific positive immunological abnormality; positive antinuclear antibodies are less specific but more commonly detectable.

Risk factors for systemic lupus erythematosus

Gender, ethnicity, and genetic factors are the most important risk factors, and twin studies demonstrate a very high rate of concordance among monozygotic as compared with dizygotic twins. Infectious agents have long been implicated in aetiology, especially the Epstein–Barr virus. However, to date, no firm documentation of a viral cause has been shown.

Systemic lupus erythematosus in the workplace

Until recently, there were few data on work outcomes in patients with SLE. In 2009, Baker and Pope undertook a systematic review of the literature and found 26 studies involving over 9500 patients.[72] They estimated a rate of work disability of 20–40 per cent with some 46 per cent of patients in employment. Workplace disability was associated with psychosocial factors and disease factors including age, race, socioeconomic group, educational attainment, activity and, duration of the disease, levels of pain, fatigue, anxiety and neurocognitive function.[72] In a longitudinal study of 394 SLE patients, Yelin et al. found that 51 per cent were in employment at baseline of whom 23 per cent experienced work loss over 4 years of follow-up.[73] Risk factors for job loss included older age, poorer cognitive and physical function, and depression. Over the same 4 years, 20 per cent of the cohort started new work. This was more likely amongst those with fewer lung manifestations, better physical function, and shorter time since last employment. In younger patients (<55 years), low rates of employment were due to lower rates of starting work rather than higher rates of work loss, but after 55 years both work loss and lower work entry were important.

Management of systemic lupus erythematosus

Mild disease often requires simple analgesia, input from the multidisciplinary team, and reassurance with observation. Moderate to severe disease may require hydroxychloroquine, immunosuppression, and glucocorticoids, sometimes over the long term. Renal and central nervous system involvement needs urgent and aggressive management, often involving intravenous cyclophosphamide, a therapy which can cause significant side effects. If antiphospholipid antibody syndrome is present, treatment with aspirin or anticoagulation with warfarin may be required. However, over recent years, targeted immune therapies have been developed. The anti-B cell therapy, (used for lymphoma) and rituximab, seems promising in patients with active SLE affecting important organs.

Management of systemic lupus erythematosus in the workplace

There is little evidence to guide the practitioner beyond general principles. Where the disease is mild, work modifications are unlikely to be required; but in more severe cases, the extreme fatigue may require a change to less onerous, more sedentary and perhaps paced, work. Work disability is common in SLE. Where possible, attention should be paid to potentially reversible factors which seem to increase work disability, particularly depression. Here, good communication with the rheumatology team and support from nursing staff with knowledge and understanding of the disease is likely to be helpful. Among patients requiring immunosuppressive therapy, employment exposing the individual to infective risk (e.g. hospital work, primary school teaching) may be unsuitable.

Chronic widespread pain and fibromyalgia syndrome

Some 13 per cent of the population will report musculoskeletal pain which is chronic (lasting >3 months) and widespread anatomically. Chronic widespread pain (CWP) is one of the core features of fibromyalgia syndrome (FMS), a syndrome which causes high levels of morbidity and high attendant costs to healthcare services. It is characterized by widespread pain, tenderness, fatigue, sleep disturbances, and may overlap with irritable bowel syndrome, tension headaches, and features of the chronic fatigue syndrome.

Since the early 1990s, in order to characterize its epidemiology, risk factors, and the effects of treatment, this widespread pain phenomenon has been called fibromyalgia syndrome and subject to defined diagnostic criteria.[74] Using these criteria, the prevalence of fibromyalgia has been estimated at between 0.5 per cent and 2.0 per cent.

Risk factors for fibromyalgia syndrome

FMS is more common among women and has a peak age at onset of 30–50 years. It is more common among those of lower educational attainment and its impact is greater in this group. Familial clustering of cases has been observed but it is unclear whether this represents shared environmental or genetic factors. In cross-sectional studies, psychological and psychosocial stressors have been found to be more common among patients with FMS, but it is difficult to distinguish cause from effect with this study design. In a prospective study, patients with high baseline scores for depression without evidence of CWP were twice as likely to develop widespread pain at follow-up 7 years later than those without depression.[75] Some but not all studies suggest that patients with FMS are more likely than controls to have a history of childhood physical and sexual abuse. Physical trauma may be a predisposing factor but this has not been evaluated in controlled prospective studies.

Management of fibromyalgia syndrome

A key factor in managing FMS is to recognize and then explain it to the patient. Frequently, patients have considerable fear that they may have a major organic illness and need time and careful counselling to be reassured. Practitioners need to take a positive supportive approach as medical interventions make a limited impact in this condition and self-efficacy is vital. Supervised aerobic exercise training,[76] simple analgesics, antidepressants, and pregabalin and gabapentin can, however, improve control of symptoms and physical function. Management should also focus on ameliorating comorbid complaints such as irritable bowel syndrome. Multidisciplinary rehabilitation is held to be effective although a Cochrane review found only limited data of poor quality to confirm this.[77]

Management of fibromyalgia syndrome in the workplace

The pain and discomfort of FMS are widespread, and patients have significantly poorer health-related quality of life and lower productivity.[78] In one study, FMS patients felt that work needed to be paced so that they could perform their job well and obtain satisfaction whilst maintaining some energy for their home lives.[79] Support from managers and colleagues was rated as very important. A meta-analysis of four large randomized controlled trials of pregabalin versus placebo in

FMS found that effective pain management with pregabalin was associated with reduced sickness absence from 2 days to 0.6 days/week.[80]

Practically, assessment of a patient with FMS should include physical and psychosocial factors, and in particular identify treatable comorbidities such as depression. Workplace assessment should include exploring the workplace demands and facilitating appropriate pacing and flexibility of work schedule. Questioning the veracity and existence of the syndrome is a counterproductive approach. A positive, empathic approach, with emphasis on what the patient *can* do, is likely to be more rewarding.

Conclusion

Musculoskeletal conditions, like back and neck pain, are very common and not infrequently cause significant problems in the workplace. For the most part, symptoms will be benign and self-limiting and need only short-term support and simple workplace measures in the expectation that most work is possible.

This chapter, however, has focused on the more serious spectrum of rheumatic diseases in which biological effects of disease can be greater and more problematic. For such chronic conditions, the approach needs to be more long term and take account of change. Management benefits considerably from good communication between the occupational health (OH) and rheumatology teams, the patient, the manager and the general practitioner. With recent advances in the treatment of inflammatory rheumatic disease, improved workplace outcomes can be anticipated going forwards. Balanced against this, the OH team should remain aware that more aggressive immunosuppressive therapy may carry infective risks in certain working environments.

References

1 Harrington JM, Carter TJ, Birrell L, *et al*. Surveillance case definitions for work related upper limb syndromes. *Occup Environ Med* 1998; **55**: 264–71.

2 Boocock MG, Collier JMK, McNair PJ, *et al*. A framework for the classification and diagnosis of work related upper extremity conditions: systematic review. *Semin Arthritis Rheum* 2009; **38**: 296–311.

3 Walker-Bone K, Byng P, Linaker C, *et al*. Reliability of the Southampton examination schedule for the diagnosis of upper limb disorders in the general population. *Ann Rheum Dis* 2002; **61**: 103–6.

4 Palmer KT, Walker-Bone K, Linaker C, *et al*. The Southampton examination schedule for the diagnosis of musculo-skeletal disorders of the neck and upper limb. *Ann Rheum Dis* 2000; **59**: 5–11.

5 Dennett X, Fry HJH. Overuse syndrome: a muscle biopsy study. *Lancet* 1988; **339**: 905–8.

6 Kellgren JH. Observations on referred pain arising from muscle. *Clin Sci* 1938; **3**: 174–90.

7 Latko WA, Armstrong TJ, Franzblau A, *et al*. Cross-sectional study of the relationship between repetitive work and the prevalence of upper limb musculoskeletal disorders. *Am J Ind Med* 1999; **36**: 248–59.

8 Crumpton-Young LL, Killough MK, *et al*. Quantitative analysis of cumulative trauma risk factors and risk factor interactions. *J Occup Environ Med* 2000; **42**: 1013–20.

9 Arvidsson I, Akesson I, Gert-Ake H. Wrist movements among females in a repetitive, non-forceful work. *Appl Ergonomics* 2003; **34**: 309–16.

10 White PD, Henderson M, Pearson RM, *et al*. Illness behaviour and psychosocial factors in diffuse upper limb pain disorder: a case-control study. *J Rheumatol* 2003; **30**: 139–45.

11 Van Eijsden-Besseling MDF, Peeters FPML, Reijnen JAW, *et al*. Perfectionism and coping strategies for the development of non-specific work-related upper limb disorders. *Occup Med* 2004; **54**: 122–7.

12 Islam SS, Velilla AM, Doyle EJ, *et al*. Gender differences in work-related injury/illness: analysis of workers compensation claims. *Am J Ind Med* 2001; **39**: 84–91.

13 Sande LP, Coury HJCG, Oishi J, *et al.* Effect of musculoskeletal disorders on prehension strength. *Appl Ergonomics* 2001; **32**: 609–16.

14 Mitchell S, Reading I, Walker-Bone K, *et al.* Pain tolerance in upper limb disorders: findings from a community survey. *Occup Environ Med* 2003; **60**: 217–21.

15 Graves RJ, Way K, Riley D, *et al.* Development of risk filter and risk assessment worksheets for HSE guidance—upper limb disorders in the workplace 2002. *Appl Ergonomics* 2004; **35**: 475–84.

16 *Mughal v. Reuters Limited* [1993] IRLR 571.

17 Health and Safety Executive (HSE). *Upper limb disorders in the workplace.* HSG60 (rev). Sudbury: HSE Books, 2002.

18 van der Donk J, Schouten JSAG, Passchier J, *et al.* The association of neck pain with radiological abnormalities of the cervical spine and personality traits in the general population. *J Rheumatol* 1991; **18**: 1884–9.

19 Walker-Bone K, Cooper C. Hard work never hurt anyone: or did it? A review of occupational associations with soft tissue musculo-skeletal disorders of the neck and upper limb. *Ann Rheum Dis* 2005; **64**: 1391–6.

20 Croft PR, Lewis M, Papageorgiou AC, *et al.* Risk factors for neck pain: a longitudinal study in a general population. *Pain* 2001; **93**: 317–25.

21 Palmer KT, Smedley J. Work relatedness of chronic neck pain with physical findings—a systematic review. *Scand J Work Environ Health* 2007; **33**: 165–91.

22 Bonde JP, Mikkelsen S, Andersen JH, *et al.* Prognosis of shoulder tendonitis in repetitive work: a follow-up study in a cohort of Danish industrial and service workers. *Occup Environ Med* 2003; **60**: E8.

23 Walker-Bone K, Reading I, Palmer K, *et al.* The epidemiology of adhesive capsulitis among working-aged adults in the general population. *Rheumatology* 2004; **43**(suppl 1): S143.

24 Bongers PM. The cost of shoulder pain at work. *BMJ* 2001; **322**: 64–5.

25 Leclerc A, Chastang J-F, Niedhammer I, *et al.* Incidence of shoulder pain in repetitive work. *Occup Environ Med* 2004; **61**: 39–44.

26 Svendsen SW, Bonde JP, Mathiassen SE, *et al.* Work related shoulder disorders: quantitative exposure-response relations with reference to arm posture. *Occup Environ Med* 2004; **61**: 844–53.

27 Harkness EF, MacFarlane GJ, Nahit ES, *et al.* Mechanical and psychosocial factors predict new onset shoulder pain: a prospective cohort study of newly employed workers. *Occup Environ Med* 2003; **60**: 850–7.

28 Kivi P. The aetiology and conservative treatment of humeral epicondylitis. *Scand J Rehab Med* 1982; **15**: 37–41.

29 Haahr JP, Andersen JH. Physical and psychosocial risk factors for lateral epicondylitis: a population based case-referent study. *Occup Environ Med* 2003; **60**: 322–9.

30 Van Rijn RM, Huisstede BMA, Koes BW, *et al.* Associations between work related factors and specific disorders of the elbow: a systematic literature review. *Rheumatology* 2009; **48**: 528–36.

31 Binder AI, Hazelman B. Lateral humeral epicondylitis—a study of the natural history and the effect on conservative therapy. *Br J Rheumatol* 1983; **20**: 73–6.

32 Trudel D, Duley J, Zastrow I, *et al.* Rehabilitation for patients with lateral epicondylitis: a systematic review. *J Hand Ther* 2004; **17**(2): 243–66.

33 Smidt N, van der Winde DAW, Assendelft WJJ, *et al.* Corticosteroid injections, physiotherapy, or wait-and-see policy for lateral epicondylitis: a randomised controlled trial. *Lancet* 2002; **359**: 657–62.

34 Kay NRM. Litigation epicondylitis. *J Hand Surgery* 2003; **28**: 460–4.

35 Descatha A, Leclerc A, Chastang JH, *et al.* Medial epicondylitis in occupational settings: prevalence, incidence and associated risk factors. *J Occup Environ Med* 2003; **45**(9): 993–101.

36 Walker-Bone K, Palmer KT, Reading I, *et al.* Occupation and epicondylitis: a population-based study. *Rheumatology* 2012; **51**: 230–42.

37 Von Shroeder HP, Botte MJ. Carpal tunnel syndrome. *Hand Clinics* 1996; **12**: 643–55.

38 Novak CB, Mackinnon SE, Brownlee R, *et al.* Provocative sensory testing in carpal tunnel syndrome. *J Hand Surg Br* 1992; **17B**: 204–8.

39 Grunberg AB. Carpal tunnel decompression in spite of normal electromyography. *J Hand Surg Br* 1983; **8**: 348–9.

40 Seror P. Phalen's test in the diagnosis of carpal tunnel syndrome. *J Hand Surg Br* 1988; **13B**: 383–5.

41 Williams TM, Mackinnon SE, Novak CB, *et al.* Verification of the pressure provocation test in carpal tunnel syndrome. *Ann Plast Surg* 1992; **29**: 8–11.

42 Bernard BP (ed). *Musculoskeletal disorders and workplace factors: a critical review of epidemiological evidence for work-related musculoskeletal disorders of the neck, upper extremity and low back.* Cincinnati, OH: NIOSH, US Department of Health and Human Services, 1997.

43 Burt S, Crombie K, Jin Y, *et al.* Workplace and individual risk factors for carpal tunnel syndrome. *Occup Environ Med* 2011; **68**: 928–33.

44 Feuerstein M, Burrell LM, Miller I, *et al.* Clinical management of carpal tunnel syndrome: a 12-year review of outcomes. *Am J Ind Med* 1999; **35**: 232–45.

45 Dick FD, Graveling RA, Munro W, *et al.* Workplace management of upper limb disorder: a systematic review. *Occup Med* 2011; **61**: 19–25.

46 Spence SH. Cognitive-behaviour therapy in the management of upper extremity cumulative trauma disorder. *J Occup Rehab* 1998; **8**: 27–45.

47 Burton AK, Kendall NAS, Pearce BG, *et al.* Management of work-relevant upper limb disorders: a review. *Occup Med* 2009; **59**: 44–52.

48 Arthritis Research Campaign. *Arthritis: the big picture.* Chesterfield: Arthritis Research Campaign, 2002. (<http://www.arc.org.uk>)

49 Hochberg M. Osteoarthritis. In: Silman AJ, Hochberg M (eds), *Epidemiology of the rheumatic diseases,* pp. 205–29. Oxford: Oxford University Press, 2001.

50 Bieleman HJ, Bierma-Zeinstra SMA, Oosterveld FGJ, *et al.* The effect of osteoarthritis of the hip or knee on work participation. *J Rheumatol* 2011; **38**: 1835–43.

51 National Institute for Health and Clinical Excellence. *Osteoarthritis: the care and management of osteoarthritis in adults.* NICE Clinical Guideline CG059. London: NICE, 2008.

52 Arthritis and Musculoskeletal Alliance. *Standards of care for people with osteoarthritis.* London: Arthritis and Musculoskeletal Alliance, 2004.

53 Silman AJ. Rheumatoid arthritis. In: Silman AJ, Hochberg M (eds), *Epidemiology of the rheumatic diseases,* pp. 31–71. Oxford: Oxford University Press, 2001.

54 Olsson AR, Skogh T, Axelson O, *et al.* Occupations and exposures in the work environment as determinants for rheumatoid arthritis. *Occup Environ Med* 2004; **61**: 233–8.

55 Oliver JE, Silman AJ. Risk factors for the development of rheumatoid arthritis. *Scand J Rheumatol* 2006; **35**: 169–74.

56 Gold LS, Ward MH, Dosemeci M, *et al.* Systemic autoimmune disease mortality and occupational exposures. *Arthritis Rheum* 2007; **56**: 3189–201.

57 Parks CG, Walitt BT, Pettinger M, *et al.* Insecticide use and risk of rheumatoid arthritis and systemic lupus erythematosus in the Women's Health Initiative Observational Study. *Arthritis Care Res* 2011; **63**: 184–94.

58 Aletaha D, Neogi T, Silman AJ, *et al.* 2010 Rheumatoid Arthritis Classification Criteria. an American College of Rheumatology/European League Against Rheumatism collaborative initiative. *Arthritis Rheum* 2010; **62**: 2569–81.

59 National Institute of Health and Clinical Excellence. *Rheumatoid arthritis. The management of rheumatoid arthritis in adults.* NICE Clinical Guideline 079. London: NICE, 2009.

60 De Croon EM, Sluiter JK, Nijssen TF, *et al.* Predictive factors of work disability in rheumatoid arthritis: a systematic literature review. *Ann Rheum Dis* 2004; **63**: 1362–7.

61 Yelin E, Trupin L, Katz P, *et al.* Association between etanercept use and employment outcomes among patients with rheumatoid arthritis. *Arthritis Rheum* 2003; **48**: 3046–54.

62 Wolfe F, Allaire S, Michaud K. The prevalence and incidence of work disability in rheumatoid arthritis, and the effect of anti-tumor necrosis factor on work disability. *J Rheumatol* 2007; **34**: 2211–17.

63 Allaire S, Wolfe F, Niu J, *et al.* Current risk factors for work disability associated with rheumatoid arthritis: recent data from a US National cohort. *Arthritis Rheum* 2009; **61**: 321–8.

64 Tang K, Beaton DE, Gignac MA, *et al.* The Work instability Scale for rheumatoid arthritis predicts arthritis-related work transitions within 12 months. *Arthritis Care Res* 2010; **62**: 1578–87.

65 Macedo AM, Oakley SP, Panayi GS, *et al.* Functional and work outcomes improve in patients with rheumatoid arthritis who receive targeted, comprehensive occupational therapy. *Arthritis Rheum* 2009; **61**: 1522–30.

66 Detaille SI, Haafkens JA, van Dijk FJ. What employees with rheumatoid arthritis, diabetes mellitus and hearing loss need to cope at work. *Scand J Work Environ Health* 2003; **29**: 134–42.

67 National Institute for Health and Clinical Excellence. *Etanercept, infliximab and adalimumab for the treatment of psoriatic arthritis.* NICE technology Appraisal Guidance, T199. London: NICE, 2010.

68 Tillett W, de-Vries C, McHugh NJ. Work disability in psoriatic arthritis—a systematic review. *Rheumatology* 2012; **51**(2): 275–83.

69 Wallenius M, Skomsvoll JF, Koldingsnes W, *et al.* Work disability and health-related quality of life in males and females with psoriatic arthritis. *Ann Rheum Dis* 2009; **68**: 685–9.

70 Kavanaugh A, Antoni C, Mease P, *et al.* Effect of infliximab therapy on employment, time lost from work, and productivity in patients with psoriatic arthritis. *J Rheumatol* 2006; **33**: 2254–9.

71 Verstappen SM, Watson KD, Lunt M, *et al.* Working status in patients with rheumatoid arthritis, ankylosing spondylitis and psoriatic arthritis: results from the British Society for Rheumatology Biologics register. *Rheumatology* 2010; **49**: 1570–7.

72 Baker K, Pope J. Employment and work disability in systemic lupus erythematosus: a systematic review. *Rheumatology* 2009; **48**: 281–4.

73 Yelin E, Tonner C, Trupin L, *et al.* Work loss and work entry among persons with systemic lupus erythematosus: comparisons with a national matched sample. *Arthritis Rheum* 2009; **61**: 247–58.

74 Wolfe F, Smythe HA, Yunus MB, *et al.* The American College of Rheumatology 1990 criteria for the classification of fibromyalgia: report of the Multicenter Criteria Committee. *Arthritis Rheum* 1990; **33**: 160–72.

75 Magni G, Moreschi C, Rigatti-Luchini S, *et al.* Prospective study on the relationship between depressive symptoms and chronic musculoskeletal pain. *Pain* 1994; **56**: 289–97.

76 Busch AJ, Barber KAR, Overned TJ, *et al.* Exercise for treating fibromyalgia syndrome. *Cochrane Database Syst Rev* 2007; **4**: CD003786.

77 Karjalainen KA, Malmivaara A, van Tulder MW, *et al.* Multidisciplinary rehabilitation for fibromyalgia and musculoskeletal pain in working age adults. *Cochrane Database Syst Rev* 2000; **2**: CD001984.

78 McDonald M, DiBonaventura M, Ullman S. Musculoskeletal pain in the workforce: the effects of back, arthritis and fibromyalgia pain on quality of life and work productivity. *J Occup Environ Med* 2011; **53**: 765–70.

79 Bossema ER, Kool MB, Cornet D, *et al.* Characteristics of suitable work from the perspective of patients with fibromyalgia. *Rheumatology* 2011; **51**: 311–18.

80 Straube S, Moore RA, Paine J, *et al.* Interference with work in fibromyalgia: effect of treatment with pregabalin and relation to pain response. *BMC Musculoskelet Disord* 2011; **12**: 125.

Chapter 14

Gastrointestinal and liver disorders

Ira Madan and Simon Hellier

Introduction

Few disorders of the gastrointestinal systems, bar infections, are caused or exacerbated by the work environment. More commonly, gastrointestinal disorders and associated symptoms limit the capacity of individuals to undertake the duties required for their job. The symptoms and treatment of some disorders such as inflammatory bowel disease may lead to the employee requiring periods of long-term sickness absence, to recover from surgery for instance.

Advances in investigation, medical treatment, and surgery should improve symptom control and prognosis in many individuals, enabling them to remain in employment.

Conditions likely to cause employment problems or risks to individuals and the public include:

+ Inflammatory bowel disease
+ Ileostomy and ileo-anal pouch
+ Irritable bowel disease
+ Gastroenteritis and gastrointestinal infections
+ Viral hepatitis
+ Chronic liver disease
+ Obesity.

The Equality Act 2010[1] is likely to apply to disorders affecting the ability to control defecation. Therefore conditions that lead to regular minor faecal incontinence or to even infrequent loss of bowel control are likely to be defined as a disability under the Act. This will include many cases of ulcerative colitis and Crohn's disease. The occupational health practitioner has a key role in supporting employees with this disability who understandably may wish the details of their symptoms to remain medically confidential. Liaison with the employer about the nature of any support or adjustments required will be a key aspect of assessment of fitness to work.

Inflammatory bowel disease

Inflammatory bowel diseases (IBDs) affect four in 1000 people in industrialized countries. The two main types of IBD are Crohn's disease and ulcerative colitis. Crohn's disease is a chronic inflammatory process which may affect any part of the gastrointestinal tract from the mouth to the anus. The inflammation is transmural and may be complicated by fistulas, abscess formation, and intestinal strictures. In contrast, ulcerative colitis only affects the colon; inflammation is superficial, starts at the anus and may extend to the caecum (pancolitis), or affect only the rectum (proctitis).

Ulcerative colitis

Ulcerative colitis classically presents with bloody diarrhoea, colicky abdominal pain, and urgency. The course is one of relapses and remissions with up to 50 per cent of patients relapsing a year. After the first year 90 per cent of patients are able to work fully. There is a slight increase in mortality in the 2 years following diagnosis but this then reverts to that of the normal population. There is a cumulative risk of colorectal cancer of 7.6 per cent at 30 years and 10.8 per cent at 40 years from diagnosis.

Treatment

Aminosalicylates are used in mild presentation and for maintenance, where they reduce relapse rates by up to 80 per cent and reduce the risk of colorectal cancer. Rectal preparations are the first-line treatment for proctitis. Reducing courses of oral prednisolone are used in more severe flares. In steroid-dependent patients, azathioprine or mercaptopurine is used as a steroid-sparing agent. These patients need monitoring because of potential bone marrow suppression. Ciclosporin or infliximab can be used for rescue therapy on an in-patient basis and reduce the need for surgery. Despite medical treatment 20–30 per cent of patients with pancolitis will eventually undergo colectomy.

Ileostomy and ileo-anal pouch

An ileostomy may be fashioned temporarily or permanently. Stomal complications from a permanent ileostomy for ulcerative colitis occur in 75 per cent of patients over 20 years. Stomas have a greater impact on the quality of life of females than males. Ileo-anal pouch procedures are increasingly being performed in patients with ulcerative colitis, with improved social acceptability, work capacity, and quality of life. Frequency of defecation, up to six times per day, may be a problem. There is a significant incidence of sexual dysfunction in males following the procedure. Seventy per cent of patients with a pouch will suffer a complication necessitating hospital admission, up to 30 per cent develop pouchitis, and excision of the pouch is necessary in about 10 per cent.

Crohn's disease

The presentation of Crohn's disease is far more variable than that of ulcerative colitis and depends on the site of the inflammation as well as presence of fistulizing or stricturing disease. Small bowel disease may present with abdominal pain, weight loss, anaemia, and obstructive symptoms. Colonic disease may present in a similar fashion to ulcerative colitis. Perianal disease typically presents with abscesses or discharging fistulas. Crohn's disease is characterized by relapses between spontaneous or treatment-induced remissions; however, about 15 per cent of patients have non-remitting disease and 10 per cent prolonged remission. The prognosis appears to be affected by: the age at diagnosis, disease location, and disease behaviour (Box 14.1); the latter may be genetically determined.

Treatment

Smoking cessation is vital in patients with Crohn's disease. The initial medical treatment of Crohn's disease is usually prednisolone, followed by immunomodulating drugs such as azathioprine, mercaptopurine, or methotrexate. In patients with severe active disease despite the use of standard therapy the anti-TNF therapies infliximab and adalimumab can be used usually in conjunction with azathioprine. Infliximab is given as an infusion with three induction treatments at 0, 2, and 6 weeks followed by maintenance infusions at 6–8-week intervals requiring hospital

Box 14.1 Factors associated with a worse prognosis in Crohn's disease

- Extremes of age
- Extensive small bowel disease
- Fistulating disease
- Stricturing
- Multiple operations
- Smoking.

attendance. Adalimumab is given as a self-administered subcutaneous injection at 1–2 week intervals. Both treatments are usually continued for 12 months with the need for ongoing treatment dependent on evidence of disease activity.

Surgery for Crohn's disease is frequently necessary. Seventy per cent of patients will have an operation within 15 years of diagnosis and 36 per cent will have required two or more operations. The symptoms recur in 30 per cent within 5 years and in 50 per cent by 10 years.

Extra-intestinal manifestations of inflammatory bowel disease

IBD is associated with a range of extra-intestinal manifestations—up to 36 per cent of people with IBD have at least one extra-intestinal manifestation and they occur more commonly in patients with colonic disease.

- *Arthropathy* affects 5–15 per cent of patients, either in the form of sacroiliitis or peripheral arthropathy. There are two types of peripheral arthropathy. Type I affects large joints, often the weight-bearing joints, and occurs at times of IBD activity. This arthropathy affects fewer than five joints and usually resolves within a few weeks as the disease activity decreases, leaving no permanent joint damage. Conversely, type II is a polyarticular, small joint, symmetrical arthropathy, whose activity is independent of IBD activity and usually persists for months or years.

- *Uveitis* and *episcleritis* are probably the most common extra-intestinal manifestations of IBD and are commonly associated with joint symptoms. The reported prevalence is 4–12 per cent with uveitis more common in ulcerative colitis and episcleritis in Crohn's disease. Episcleritis causes a burning and itching sensation in the eye. Anterior uveitis is a serious complication due to acute inflammation of the anterior chamber of the eye. It causes severe ocular pain, blurred vision, and headaches.

- *Skin disorders* are commonly associated with IBD, but have few occupational consequences.

- *Systemic symptoms* are common in people with chronic active IBD and include lethargy, weight loss, and low-grade fever.

Functional limitations

The main problems for individuals with IBD are recurrent or persistent abdominal pain and frequency and urgency of defecation. Extra-intestinal manifestations may increase disability and impact upon work capacity, particularly during relapses. Usually the associated joint disease is mild but pain and stiffness may prevent individuals from undertaking physically strenuous work, including manual handling. Eye disease may cause significant short-term disability until treated. Affected individuals may be unfit to work as a result of pain and visual disturbance.

Mild relapses can be treated as an outpatient with little time away from work. Moderate or severe exacerbations will usually not be compatible with attending work and may require up to several months for recovery with medical treatment. Surgery may result in prolonged absence from work depending on the type of procedure. In many cases the longer-term prognosis after surgery will be favourable; therefore, employers may be prepared to be supportive in accommodating a prolonged period of recuperation.

Adjustments at work

The problem of the frequent, sudden, urgent need for defecation is one of the primary concerns of employees with IBD. Having access to toilet facilities with sufficient privacy and ventilation is paramount. Access to a disabled toilet may be an option. Allowances should be made for frequent toilet breaks and a toilet break after meals. The impact of symptoms will be greater in jobs where rapid and regular toilet access is not possible. This could include those working outside, peripatetic workers, those responsible for the supervision or safety of others, and those undertaking paced work such as production line work where flexible breaks are not possible.

Travel is a key issue for many people with IBD. Frequency and urgency may make travelling by public transport difficult. Employees with IBD may prefer to travel to and from work by car. Employers may wish to consider the provision of a parking space close to work. People with IBD usually do not meet the criteria for disabled permit holders.

Employment issues for workers with intestinal stomas

Physically strenuous work can cause difficulties for some patients with stomas. Development of a parastomal hernia can make manual handling difficult and uncomfortable. Other problems include increased risk of leakage and possible injury to the stoma itself. Work that involves high-risk manual handling, repetitive stooping and bending, and carrying heavy or awkward loads close to the body, may be problematic. However, not all patients will find this to be the case and there are cases of successful employment in safety critical work such as the emergency services. Food handling is not contraindicated in patients with stomas, as there is no evidence of increased cross-infection risk. Providing there is not a problem with leakage and good hygiene is followed, people with stomas should not be excluded from this work.

Work in hot environments could potentially place employees with stomas at greater than average risk because of the increased potential for dehydration and electrolyte imbalance. This should be prevented by ensuring that adequate hydration is maintained. Patients visiting the tropics should be instructed on the use of oral rehydration solutions. Although there is evidence that working life is disturbed for patients after surgery for stoma, there are no absolute contraindications for any work.[2] The nature and siting of the stoma will have an influence on any restrictions so each case should be assessed individually.

Irritable bowel syndrome

Definition, prevalence, and natural history

Irritable bowel syndrome (IBS) is a combination of chronic or recurrent gastrointestinal symptoms not explained by structural or biochemical abnormalities, which is attributed to the intestines and associated with symptoms of pain, disturbed defecation, and/or symptoms of

> ## Box 14.2 Rome III criteria for the diagnosis of irritable bowel syndrome
>
> Recurrent abdominal pain or discomfort on at least 3 days/month in the last 3 months associated with two or more of the following:
>
> 1 Improvement with defecation.
>
> 2 Onset associated with change in frequency of stool.
>
> 3 Onset associated with change in form of stool.
>
> From Drossman DA. The Functional Gastrointestinal Disorders and the Rome III Process. GASTROENTEROLOGY 2006;130:1377–1390.

bloating and distention. The prevalence in industrialized countries is 9–12 per cent. Women are more commonly affected than men and the incidence of the illness is higher in those aged below age 45 than those aged 45 and over. Patients tend to report episodes of IBS, with duration of up to 5 days. Individuals may develop a remission after a series of symptomatic episodes, but there is paucity of literature on the natural history of the illness.[3] The Rome criteria have been developed to standardize diagnosis and aid the selection of patients for clinical trials (see Box 14.2).

Management

The management of IBS is aimed at the individual's symptom profile. Lifestyle advice and dietary modification are important interventions for most symptoms. Antispasmodics are first-line pharmaceutical intervention for variable bowel habit and abdominal pain. If these are ineffective low-dose amitriptyline taken at night is often effective, although this can occasionally cause drowsiness the following day. For diarrhoea-predominant IBS, cholestyramine will be effective in some individuals, otherwise Imodium® (loperamide) is used as necessary. For constipation laxatives are used although both lactulose and Fybogel® (psyllium) can exacerbate bloating. There is a role for cognitive behavioural therapy in those who fail to respond to other measures.

Functional limitations

Many of the symptoms of IBS such as bloating, faecal urgency, incontinence, diarrhoea, flatulence, and borborygmi can impair performance at work and restrict activities of daily living. During functional assessment, the occupational health professional should look for evidence of pain behaviour which would support the diagnosis. Clinicians should acknowledge that the symptoms are real and that other individuals experience similar symptoms.

Adjustments at work

The majority of patients manage to remain in work despite their condition, although exacerbations may lead to up to twice the average absence from work. In severe cases the need for frequent defecation may substantially restrict travel or work and arrangements to facilitate ready access to a toilet at work may need to be put in place. Symptoms may be made worse by perceived occupational stress, job dissatisfaction, or poor working relationships. The possibility of underlying work issues should be explored and, if present, addressed.

Gastrointestinal infections

Distinguishing infectious and non-infectious diarrhoea

Diarrhoea is a very common condition in the community. It usually implies a change in bowel habit with loose or liquid stools which are passed more frequently than normal.

Gastrointestinal infection affects as many as one in five members of the population each year. Symptoms are caused by the organisms themselves or by the toxins that they produce. In the absence of any known bowel disease, a sudden change in bowel habit whereby three or more loose stools are passed in 24 hours is an indication that diarrhoea may be infectious. Other symptoms of infectious diarrhoea include nausea, malaise, and pyrexia, although these symptoms may also accompany other causes of diarrhoea, such as IBD. A thorough medical history should be taken to exclude other common causes of non-infective diarrhoea such as medicines, irritable bowel disease and excess consumption of spicy food or alcohol. The majority of gastrointestinal infections seen in the UK are self-limiting.

The immunocompromised, elderly, and young children are more susceptible and may develop more serious or prolonged infection. There is a strong case for instituting early empirical metronidazole or fluoroquinolone therapy in high-risk patients with moderate to severe diarrhoea of infective type as most will prove to have salmonella, campylobacter, or shigella infections.

Functional assessment and exclusion from work

The symptoms of a gastrointestinal infection such as diarrhoea, vomiting, and pyrexia may result in an individual not being able to work on a temporary basis. But the main risk is that the infected person may infect other employees, the public, or a product such as food. The risk of organisms spreading is highest when the infected person is experiencing diarrhoea and vomiting, because of the high bacterial or viral load. In addition, loose or liquid stools are more likely to contaminate hands and surfaces.

Therefore, individuals with gastrointestinal infections should refrain from work until free from diarrhoea and vomiting for 48 hours. This is particularly important for:

♦ Food handlers
♦ Staff of healthcare facilities in direct contact with susceptible patients (for example, immuno-suppressed patients, children, or the elderly) or their food.

More stringent guidance applies to infection with *Salmonella typhi*, verotoxigenic *Escherichia coli* (VTEC) O157, and hepatitis A. This is discussed in further detail later in relation to food handlers.

If the cause is confirmed as non-infective after the individual was excluded then they can return to work, provided they feel well enough to do so. It is reasonable to presume that a single bout (e.g. one loose stool) or incidence of vomiting is not infectious if 24 hours have elapsed without any further symptoms and this is not accompanied by fever. In this case, as long as there is no other evidence to suggest an infectious cause, the person would only pose a very low risk of being infected and could resume work before the 48-hour limit. On return to work individuals must take extra care over personal hygiene practices, especially hand washing.

The most common infections are summarized in Table 14.1.

Table 14.1 Microbial pathogens responsible for food-borne diarrhoeal disease

	Source	Incubation period	Symptoms	Recovery
Pathogens that colonize the gut				
Salmonella spp.	Eggs, poultry	12–72 hours	Diarrhoea, blood, pain, vomiting, fever	2–14 days
Campylobacter jejuni	Milk, poultry	1–11 days	Diarrhoea, blood, pain, vomiting, fever	7–21 days
Enterohaemorrhagic *Escherichia coli*	Beef	1–14 days	Diarrhoea, blood, pain, vomiting, fever	7–21 days
Vibrio parahaemolyticus	Crabs, shellfish	12–18 hours	Diarrhoea, pain, vomiting, fever	2–30 days
Yersinia enterocolitica	Milk, pork	2 hours–2 days	Diarrhoea, pain, fever	1–3 days
Clostridium perfringens	Spores in food especially milk	8–22 hours	Diarrhoea, pain,	1–3 days
Listeria monocytogenes	Milk, sweet corn	8–36 hours	Diarrhoea, fever	
Preformed toxins				
Staphylococcus aureus	Contaminated food, usually by humans	2–6 hours	Nausea, vomiting, pain, diarrhoea	Rapid, few hours
Bacillus cereus	Reheated food rice, sauces, and pasta	1–5 hours	Nausea, vomiting, pain, diarrhoea	Rapid
Clostridium botulinum	Spores geminate in anaerobic conditions, canned or bottled foods	18–36 hours	Transient diarrhoea, paralysis	Months

Food handlers

Transmission of infection by food handlers

The Food Standards Agency and Health Protection Agency (HPA) estimate that in England and Wales in 2010 food-borne diseases cost the economy just under £1.4 billion, with 5699 cases recorded.[4] According to the HPA, only 1 in 130 cases of food-borne disease are reported. Estimates suggest that infected food handlers cause between 4 per cent and 33 per cent of food-borne disease outbreaks in the UK. The most important infections attributed to transmission from infected food handlers are norovirus, *Salmonella enteritidis* and *Salmonella typhimurium*, which together account for the largest numbers of outbreaks and individual infections. The most common routes of transmission are faecal–oral and via aerosol formation from vomit.

It is important to remember that food handlers not only include those individuals employed directly in the production and preparation of foodstuffs, but workers undertaking maintenance work or repairing equipment in food-handling areas. Managers and visitors to food-handling areas may also be included in the definition.

Guidance and regulations

Regulatory and best practice guidance on fitness to work for food handlers is available online from the Food Standards Agency[5] and detailed, up-to-date guidance on individual infectious agents is available on the HPA website.[6] All cases of food poisoning are notifiable to Local Authority Proper Officers under the Health Protection (Notification) Regulations 2010.[7]

Prevention of microbiological contamination of food

Health screening before food handlers start work is not required by law, but it has been common in the food industry for many years. Such screening usually takes the form of a questionnaire. The Equality Act 2010 precludes health screening before job offer, but the job may be offered on the condition of satisfactory health clearance. If an organization does decide to undertake health screening on food handlers, it is important that they recognize that there is little evidence that health screening by questionnaire will detect a medical problem which is likely to preclude a food handler from work. Some organizations undertake health screening of food handlers when they return from abroad, but like screening before starting work, there is little evidence that such screening will detect a relevant medical disorder. The mainstay of identifying infected food handlers is to ensure that food handlers who develop symptoms of a gastrointestinal infection report their symptoms to their line manager. Local policies should state the procedure that should be followed by food handlers if they develop infection or have been in contact with relevant conditions.

Food handlers must have good personal hygiene and this can be assessed at interview by a manager. Managers should also ensure that food handlers have good access to toilet and washing facilities. Food handlers should be trained in the safe handling of food and have a good understanding of the principles of food hygiene. It is imperative that food handlers are trained to wash and dry their hands before handling food, or surfaces likely to come into contact with food, especially after going to the toilet.

Exclusion from work

Food handlers who develop symptoms of gastrointestinal infection should report immediately to management and leave the food handling area. Excluding infected food handlers from the entire premises should be considered, as this will remove the potential risk of contamination of food via other staff that may use the same facilities (toilets, canteens) as the infected person. It is best to assume that the cause of diarrhoea or vomiting is an infection and the food handler should be excluded until evidence to the contrary is received. As with other workers, food handlers with infectious gastroenteritis should refrain from work until free from diarrhoea and vomiting for 48 hours. However, more stringent guidance applies to infection with *Salmonella typhi*, VTEC O157, and hepatitis A as detailed in 'Infections with special occupational implications'.

A food handler who is in contact with a household member who is suffering from diarrhoea or vomiting does not always require exclusion but they should inform their manager and take extra precautions, such as more stringent personal hygiene practices. If they start to feel unwell they should report this immediately to their manager or supervisor. Cases that may require exclusion are where the household contact has enteric fever, or *E. coli* O157. Detailed information can be obtained from the HPA website.[8] Guidelines on food handlers who have been in contact with a person with hepatitis A are detailed below.

Infections with special occupational implications

Vero cytotoxin-producing *E. coli*

Escherichia coli (*E. coli*) are common bacteria which live in the intestines of warm-blooded animals. There are certain strains of *E. coli* which are normally found in the intestine of healthy people and animals without causing any ill effects; however, some strains are known to cause illness in people. Among these is a group of bacteria which are known as vero cytotoxin-producing *E. coli* or VTEC.

These can cause illness, ranging from mild through severe bloody diarrhoea, mostly without fever, to the serious conditions haemolytic uraemic syndrome and thrombotic thrombocytopenic purpura. The most important property of these strains is the production of one or more potent toxins important in the development of illness. VTEC are relatively rare as the cause of infectious gastroenteritis in England and Wales; however, the disease can be fatal, particularly in infants, young children, and the elderly.

The most important VTEC strain to cause illness in the UK is *E. coli* O157 (VTEC O157). This can be found in the intestine of healthy cattle, sheep, goats, and a wide range of other species. Humans may be infected by VTEC O157 or other VTEC strains when they consume food or water that has become contaminated by faeces from infected animals. Infection may also result from direct or indirect contact with animals that carry VTEC or from exposure to an environment contaminated with animals' faeces, such as farms and similar premises with animals which are open to the public. The infectious dose of VTEC O157 is very low at less than 100 bacterial cells. Infection is readily spread between family contacts, particularly those who may be caring for infected children, and in settings such as children's day nurseries.

People infected with VTEC usually have typical gastroenteritis symptoms, i.e. diarrhoea with or without vomiting, abdominal cramps, and fever. Sometimes there is some blood mixed in with the diarrhoea. Symptoms may last a few days and then disappear within a week or so.

Occupational implications Management of cases is purely supportive. Antibiotics are *not* recommended and might exacerbate the sequelae of infection. Suspected cases must have a stool sample collected and sent to the local hospital laboratory where it will be tested for the presence of presumptive VTEC O157. The case must be reported to the local health protection unit. Screening (contacts of the patient) and exclusion (from school/work) may be necessary upon advice from the health protection unit.

Although the principal reservoir for VTEC O157 in the UK is cattle, therefore making the disease a zoonosis, secondary infections are also acquired, by person-to-person spread by direct contact (faecal–oral). This is particularly important in households, nurseries, primary schools, and residential care institutions. Therefore, efforts are undertaken by public health professionals to control the source of infection. The disease is also under surveillance to increase our understanding of the epidemiology of VTEC in England.

Salmonella infections

The prolonged bacteraemic illness of typhoid is caused by the exclusively human pathogen, *Salmonella typhi*. Annually about 200 cases of typhoid fever are seen in the UK mostly in people after visiting relatives or friends in the developing countries. Watery diarrhoea occurs 12–72 hours after infection, accompanied by abdominal pain, vomiting, and fever. The illness lasts a few days and is usually self-limiting.

Occupational implications Adults excrete the organism for 4–8 weeks but all except food handlers and water workers can resume work after 48 hours symptom free. Food handlers and water workers should not return to work until they have had two consecutive faecal samples free of infection, and have obtained clearance to return to work from the local authority. Food handlers who practice good hygiene are very rarely responsible for initiating outbreaks.

Hepatitis A

The hepatitis A virus is transmitted by the faecal–oral route. In developed countries person-to-person spread is the most common method of transmission, while in countries with poor sanitation faeces-contaminated food and water are frequent sources of infection. Hepatitis A virus is excreted in the bile and shed in the stools of infected persons. Peak excretion occurs during the 2 weeks before onset of jaundice; the concentration of virus in the stools drops after jaundice appears.

The average incubation period of hepatitis A is around 28 days (range 15–50 days). Patients feel unwell during the prodrome but often improve with the onset of jaundice. Lethargy may continue for 6 weeks or for as long as 3 months. The course of hepatitis A infection is extremely variable but in adults 70–95 per cent of infections result in clinical illness. Diagnosis is based on the detection in the serum of immunoglobulin (Ig) IgM antibody to hepatitis A. The presence of IgG antihepatitis A antibody indicates either previous exposure or immunization.

Hepatitis A is usually a mild self-limiting illness but can occasionally result in severe or fatal disease. Fulminant hepatitis occurs rarely (<1 per cent overall), but rates are higher with increasing age and in those with underlying chronic liver disease, including those with chronic hepatitis B or C infection. Hepatitis A does not appear to be worse in HIV-infected patients when compared to HIV-negative persons. Infection is followed by lifelong immunity.

Confirmed case A confirmed case is one that meets the clinical case definition (an acute illness with a discrete onset of symptoms *and* jaundice or elevated serum aminotransferase levels) *and* is laboratory confirmed (IgM antibodies to hepatitis A virus (anti-HAV) positive).

Probable case A probable case meets the clinical case definition (see 'Confirmed case') and occurs in a person who has an epidemiological link with a person with laboratory confirmed hepatitis A.

Occupational implications If a worker is suspected of being infected with hepatitis A, the local Health Protection Unit should be contacted. The index case should be excluded from work until jaundice has disappeared, or for 1 week after the onset of jaundice, whichever is the longer. Those with anicteric hepatitis should remain off work for 1 week after serum transaminases have reached a peak.

Food-borne outbreaks can occur due to the contamination of food at the point of service or due to contamination during growing, harvesting, processing, or distribution. A review of published food-borne outbreaks in the USA found that infected food handlers who handled uncooked food, or food after it had been cooked, during the infectious period were the most common source of published food-borne outbreaks. A single hepatitis A-infected food handler has the potential to transmit hepatitis A to large numbers of people, although reported outbreaks are rare. Such outbreaks often involve secondary cases among other food handlers who ate food contaminated by the index case.

If a food handler has been in contact with an individual who is acutely infected with hepatitis A, a risk assessment should be undertaken as described in Figure 14.1. This algorithm applies if the

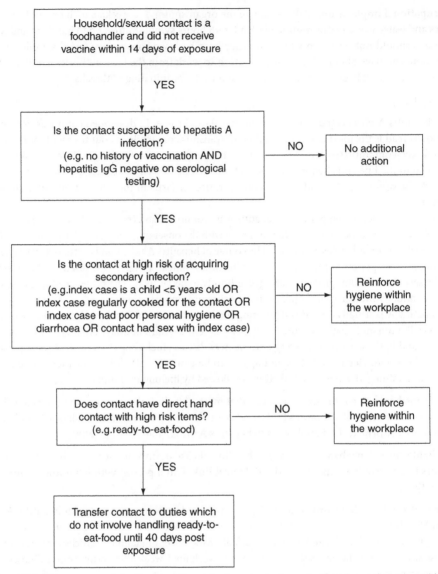

Figure 14.1 Risk assessment for food handlers who have had a household and sexual contact with an individual acutely infected with hepatitis A. Reproduced with permission from *Guidance for the prevention and control of hepatitis A infection*, pp. 13, Copyright © Health Protection Agency 2009 available from <http://www.hpa.org.uk/webc/HPAwebFile/HPAweb_C/1259152095231>.

food handler has not previously received two doses of hepatitis A vaccine (or one dose within the past 6 months), does not have a history of laboratory-confirmed hepatitis A, and is seen within 14 days of exposure to infection.

Prevention of hepatitis A infection Hepatitis A vaccination is recommended for the following at-risk occupational groups:[9,10]

- Laboratory workers: individuals who may be exposed to hepatitis A in the course of their work, in microbiology laboratories, and clinical infectious disease units.

- Staff of some large residential institutions: outbreaks of hepatitis A have been associated with large residential institutions for those with learning difficulties. Similar considerations apply in other institutions where standards of personal hygiene among clients or patients may be poor.

- Sewage workers at risk of repeated exposure to raw, untreated sewage following a risk assessment. There is currently insufficient evidence to justify routinely immunizing all sanitation workers.

- People who work with primates that are susceptible to hepatitis A infection.

Post-exposure immunization Hepatitis A vaccine should also be used to prevent secondary cases and in outbreaks provided that it is given within 7 days from the onset of illness in the index case. Human normal immunoglobulin should be offered in addition or in preference to vaccine for contacts who are more than 7 days from onset of illness in the primary case, and for those at high risk of an adverse outcome. Contacts of the index case include household members and people working in the same area.

Viral hepatitis

Hepatitis B

Epidemiology

The World Health Organization (WHO) estimates that in the UK the prevalence of chronic hepatitis B infection is 0.3 per cent. Hepatitis B is more common in other parts of the world such as South-East Asia, Africa, the Middle and Far East, and southern and eastern Europe. WHO estimates that there are 350 million chronically infected people worldwide. Intravenous drug use is the most frequently reported route of transmission in the UK and is identified as the risk factor in 50 per cent of reported cases. Heterosexual sex is the risk factor in 18.5 per cent, sex with an intravenous drug user in 3 per cent, and men who have sex with men in 8 per cent.

Other recognized modes of transmission include:

- Vertical transmission (mother to baby).

- Receipt of infectious blood (via transfusion) or infectious blood products (e.g. clotting factors).

- Needlestick or other sharps injuries and mucocutaneous exposures (in particular those sustained by hospital personnel).

- Tattooing, body piercing, and acupuncture.

For about a third of cases of acute hepatitis B infection no route of transmission is reported, but many of these may relate to intravenous drug use.

Clinical and laboratory features

Acute hepatitis B Acute hepatitis B has an incubation period of 40–160 days. Many people have no symptoms while others experience a flu-like illness including a sore throat, tiredness, joint pains, and a loss of appetite. Other symptoms may include nausea and vomiting. Acute infection can be severe, causing abdominal discomfort and jaundice. Mortality during the acute phase of infection is less than 1 per cent. Individuals are most infective immediately prior to the onset of jaundice.

When exposed, the immune system is normally capable of clearing the virus and developing natural immunity. However, this depends on the age at which the exposure happens: fewer than 5 per cent of adults will fail to eradicate the virus, but the rate is substantially higher if the infection happens perinatally or within the first 6 months of birth.

Chronic hepatitis Individuals remaining hepatitis B surface antigen (HBsAg) positive for more than 6 months are regarded as having developed chronic infection. HBsAg disappears in about 1–2 per cent of chronic carriers per year. In about 20–40 per cent of chronic hepatitis patients, the virus is active and may progress to end-stage liver disease unless treated. Others may remain healthy and not require treatment but are still infectious.

Treatment

Antiviral agents may be used successfully to treat acute hepatitis B.[11] The treatment for fulminant hepatitis B is transplantation. All patients with chronic hepatitis B should be assessed for treatment with antivirals with the decision being based on serology, viral load, and risk of progressive liver disease following liver biopsy

HBeAg-positive patients There are essentially two goals of treatment for patients who are HBVeAg positive. These are eAg seroconversion and viral DNA suppression to undetectable levels. Pegylated interferon-alfa given for 48 weeks has a seroconversion rate of 30 per cent and a virological response of 25 per cent. However, it is associated with a significant side effect profile, particularly fatigue and depression, and is not used as long-term therapy. Nucleoside/nucleotide analogues lamivudine, entecavir, and tenofovir give a seroconversion rate of 20 per cent at a year although this increases with ongoing use. They give a virological response of 40 per cent, 60 per cent, and 74 per cent respectively. Lamivudine is associated with a 20 per cent/year development of resistance mutations whereas there is very little resistance reported with entecavir and tenofovir.

HBeAg-negative DNA-positive patients The goal of treatment for this group is suppression of viral DNA and is long term. At a year 72 per cent of patients treated with lamivudine, and 90 per cent with entecavir or tenofovir will have had a virological response.

Functional assessment

Approximately 50 per cent of acute infections are mild and may be anicteric. Patients with more severe symptoms will be unable to work during the acute illness. Once recovery has taken place there should be no restrictions on employment (with the exception of some healthcare work, see LIST). Chronic carriers are usually in good health and are able to work normally. There is no evidence of risk of transmission of hepatitis B by casual contact in the workplace.

The individual markers of hepatitis B relevant to occupational health assessment are as follows:

- *Hepatitis B surface antigen (HBsAg)*: HBsAg is a marker of ongoing hepatitis B infection.
- *Hepatitis B surface antibody (HBsAb)*: development of HBsAb is generally associated with immunity. It can develop following infection and disappearance of the virus (natural immunity) or after inoculation with the vaccine. In a small group of people HBsAg and HBsAb may be detectable simultaneously (due to a viral mutation). Therefore, presence of HBsAb should not automatically be interpreted as the individual not being infectious.
- *Hepatitis B core antibody (HBcAb)*: HBcAb will be present in all individuals who have been previously exposed to HBV. Individuals with HBcAb do not need vaccination because they either have chronic infection or natural immunity regardless of the HBsAb level.

♦ *Hepatitis B e antigen (HBeAg)*: HBeAg is a marker of virus replication usually, therefore, an individual with HBeAg has high viral load and is highly infective. Patients without HBeAg but HBsAg positive can still be infectious (usually due to viral mutation).

♦ *Hepatitis B e antibody (HBeAb)*: HBeAb means the proliferation of HBV has been suppressed. It does not mean immunity, nor does it mean that the individual is not infectious. It is of little value in the occupational health setting.

♦ *Hepatitis B virus (HBV) DNA*: HBV DNA is the genetic material of the virus and is assessed by PCR (polymerase chain reaction)—the higher the HBV DNA results the higher the infectivity.

♦ *Natural immunity*: in the majority of people who have been exposed to HBV the natural body defences will eradicate the virus and the individual will acquire natural immunity in which case HBsAg will be negative but HBcAb will remain positive. This group of people will not need HBV vaccination or booster regardless of the HBsAb titre.

♦ *Inactive disease*: an individual with chronic infection (HBsAg positive for >6 months) but low viral load (<2000 IU/mL) and negative HBeAg. They remain healthy but can still transmit the infection.

Prevention of hepatitis B infection

In accordance with the Health and Safety at Work etc. Act 1974[12] and subsequent Management of Health and Safety and Welfare (1999)[13] and Control of Substances Hazardous to Health (COSHH) 2002,[14] it is the employer's responsibility to identify the risks to an individual of exposure to HBV in the workplace and introduce measures to eliminate or reduce the risk. Employees should be provided with information regarding risk of infection and how to prevent it. It is the responsibility of the employer to ensure that the use of universal precautions are facilitated when employees are handling body fluids and it is the responsibility of employees to adhere to the policies instigated by their employer

Hepatitis B immunization Immunization is part of personal protective equipment in the context of risk management. It should be offered to all individuals who are at risk of exposure to HBV.

Hepatitis B immunization is recommended for the following groups who are considered at increased risk:[10]

♦ Healthcare workers including students and trainees who may have direct contact with patients' blood, blood-stained body fluids, or tissues. This includes any staff who are at risk of injury from blood-contaminated sharp instruments, or of being deliberately injured or bitten by patients.

♦ Laboratory staff: any laboratory staff who handle material that may contain the virus.

♦ Staff of residential and other accommodation for those with learning difficulties. Similar considerations may apply to staff in day-care settings and special schools for those with severe learning disability. Decisions on immunization should be made on the basis of a local risk assessment. In settings where the client's behaviour is likely to lead to significant exposures on a regular basis (e.g. biting), it would be prudent to offer immunization to staff even in the absence of documented hepatitis B transmission.

♦ Morticians and embalmers.

♦ Prison service staff who are in regular contact with prisoners.

♦ Emergency services such as the police. In these workers an assessment of the frequency of likely exposure should be carried out. For those with frequent exposure, pre-exposure immunization is recommended. For other groups, post-exposure immunization at the time of an incident may be more appropriate.

The general vaccination course consists of three doses of vaccine given at 0, 1, and 6 months, this achieves a response rate exceeding 95 per cent. A subsequent blood test for hepatitis B surface antibody (HBsAb) 1–4 months after the final dose will determine the development of a protective antibody response. An accelerated schedule may be given to non-immune workers who need to commence a post which may put them at high risk of being exposed to hepatitis B. This consists of three doses of vaccine given a month apart (0, 1, and 2 months) followed by a booster dose to be given after 1 year. HBsAb levels should be checked 1–4 months following the third dose (see Figure 14.2). Risk factors for non-response to hepatitis B immunization include male gender, age over 40, smoking and obesity.

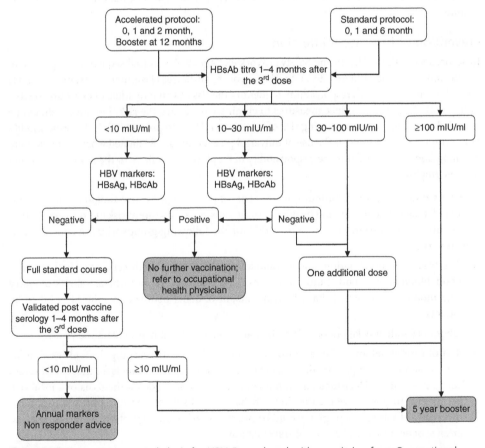

Figure 14.2 Post-exposure prophylaxis for HBV. Reproduced with permission from Occupational Health Department, Guy's and St Thomas' NHS Foundation Trust. Data from Department of Health guidance *HSC 2000/020; hepatitis B infected health care workers*, Department of Health © Crown Copyright 2002 and *Hepatitis B infected health care workers: guidance on implementation of Health Service Circular 2000/020*.

It is preferable to achieve HBsAb level above 100 mIU/mL. HBsAb titre of 10 to 100 are generally accepted as enough to protect against the infection. However, one additional dose of vaccine should be given at the time after which no further post vaccination serology is required. A single booster after 5 years is required once an HBsAb level of greater than 10 is achieved or after an accidental body fluid exposure. Because of strong immunological memory vaccine protection continues after anti-HBs has become undetectable. Therefore, further testing for hepatitis B surface antibody is not necessary. Under the COSHH regulations 2002, the employer must retain records of any workers exposed to blood-borne pathogens for 40 years.[14] Hepatitis B immunization and immunity records should be kept confidentially in occupational health.

Following accidental exposure to HBV in non-immune individuals, passive immunity using hepatitis B hyperimmune serum globulin (HBIg) should be offered. The sooner HBIg is administered the more likely it is to be effective. Ideally, it should be given within 48 hours of exposure, but it can be administered up to 7 days post exposure. Usually two doses of HBIg 1 month apart are recommended. HBV immunization should be started simultaneously, with the first dose given in a site different from the HBIg. An accelerated four-dose immunization schedule (0, 1, 2, and 12 months) is preferred in this setting.

First aid Individuals who undertake first aid in the workplace should be advised that the risk of transmission of blood-borne viruses during normal first aid procedures can be minimized by standard cross-infection control procedures for all casualties. Training should be provided in how to prevent and deal with contamination and protective clothing such as disposable gloves should be provided to reduce the risk of exposure to blood-borne viruses.

Healthcare workers To protect patients against the risk of acquiring hepatitis B from an infected healthcare worker and vice versa, all healthcare workers in the UK whose job involves contact with blood, body fluids, or tissues are offered a course of hepatitis B vaccination on starting work (Figure 14.3) as directed by HSC 2000/020[15,16] and Department of Health guidance on health clearance of new healthcare workers.[17]

A pre-vaccination test is only indicated if there is a reasonable likelihood that the individual may have natural immunity or infection. It is therefore recommended that the following are tested for HBcAb prior to immunization:

♦ Individuals who have lived, or worked as a healthcare worker in China, Africa, Asia, and the Middle East as these places have a high prevalence of hepatitis B.

♦ Workers who recall a history of hepatitis infection.

Non-responders to the vaccine need to take extra care to follow infection control procedures and should report any body fluid exposures immediately as per their local policy as they may require post-exposure hepatitis B immunoglobulin treatment.

Healthcare workers who undertake exposure-prone procedures and dialysis work Very few cases of transmission of HBV from infected health worker to patients have been reported. These have almost exclusively occurred through exposure-prone procedures (EPPs). By definition, EPPs are those where there is a risk that injury to the healthcare worker may result in the exposure of the patient's open tissues to the blood of the worker. Examples of such procedures include those where the healthcare worker's gloved hands may be in contact with sharp instruments, needle tips, or sharp tissues (spicules of bone or teeth) inside a patient's body cavity, wound, or confined anatomical space where the hands or fingertips may not be completely visible at all times. It is also recommended to apply EPP standards of clearance to dialysis

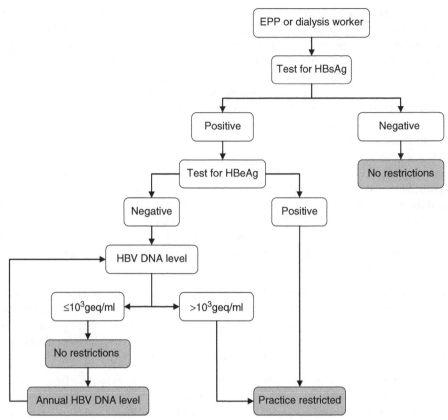

Figure 14.3 Flowchart—investigation of hepatitis B virus status in dialysis workers and workers undertaking exposure-prone procedures. Reproduced with permission from Occupational Health Department, Guy's and St Thomas' NHS Foundation Trust. Data from *Good practice guidelines for renal dialysis/transplantation units; prevention and control of blood borne virus infection*, Department of Health 2002 © Crown copyright.

workers.[18] Dialysis workers are clinical staff recruited to work in renal transplantation unit or dialysis.

Healthcare workers who perform EPP or dialysis work in the UK must have their hepatitis B status checked before starting work. Hepatitis B-infected applicants are only allowed to do EPP or dialysis work if it is confirmed that they have low infectivity (see Figure 14.3 and Table 14.2), i.e. negative HBeAg and HBV DNA level under 10^3 genome equivalents per millilitre (geq/mL). Once an applicant is found to be HBsAg positive a blood sample should be taken for HBeAg. HBV-infected individuals who are HBeAg positive are restricted from EPP or dialysis work.

If a healthcare worker's HBeAg is negative and the viral load is less than 10^3geq/mL, they may perform EPPs, but must repeat this viral load testing on an annual basis. If at any time their status changes, they must have their duties restricted. Once a healthcare worker's viral load has exceeded 10^3 geq/mL, they may not perform EPPs. They cannot resume EPP work until they have had a stable viral load of less than 10^3 geq/mL for more than 1 year off treatment.

Table 14.2 HBV markers and their interpretation

HBsAg	HBsAb	HBcAb	HBeAg	HBeAb	HBV DNA	Immune	Infectious	EPP
−	−	−	N/A	N/A	N/A	No	No	Yes
−	+	−	N/A	N/A	N/A	Yes (by vaccination)	No	Yes
−	+/−	+	N/A	N/A	N/A	Yes (by natural immunity)	No	Yes
+	+/−	+	+	+/−	N/A	N/A	Yes	No
+	+/−	+	−	+/−	$<10^3$	N/A	Very low	Yes
+	+/−	+	−	+/−	$>10^3$	N/A	Yes	No

Healthcare workers with a viral load between 10^3 and 10^5 geq/mL and negative HBeAg may benefit from oral antiviral therapy to persistently suppress their viral load below the cut off level subsequent to which they may become eligible to do EPP or dialysis work. Current guidance indicates that these health care workers need to be assessed individually by an occupational health consultant to discuss possible clearance for EPP or dialysis work.[17]

Non-immune EPP and dialysis workers EPP and dialysis workers, who are not immune against hepatitis B and are HBsAg negative, will be required to have blood tests for HBsAg every 12 months. Any hepatitis B-infected healthcare worker associated with transmission of infection to a patient should cease performing EPP.

Any employee who is discovered to have contracted hepatitis B infection at any stage during their employment (including non EPP workers) should have a full occupational assessment and may require referral to their general practitioner or to a specialist. Hepatitis B is a notifiable disease.

Hepatitis C

Epidemiology and prognosis

The hepatitis C virus (HCV) is the most common chronic blood-borne pathogen. It is an emerging health concern across the world, with 170 million people chronically infected. The prevalence of HCV in England is estimated to be around 0.4 per cent. The most common mode of transmission is intravenous drug use. In the UK blood donations have been screened for hepatitis C since September 1991. However, some people who received blood or blood products before this date could be infected if they received blood from a donor who was carrying HCV. It is also possible to acquire HCV infections by transfusion in a country that does not screen its blood for the virus.

Unlike many other blood-borne viruses, sexual transmission is thought to be relatively rare. Nevertheless, it may occur and people with new or casual sexual partners are advised to use condoms to protect them against all sexually transmitted infections.

Infection is not acquired through normal social contact, but it can occur in situations where blood can be transferred from one person to another, for example, by sharing razors or toothbrushes. It is also possible to acquire hepatitis C infection during body piercing (like tattooing or acupuncture) if sterile needles are not used. The risk of a mother infecting her newborn baby with hepatitis C is estimated to be less than 5 per cent. This risk is highest in mothers who are also infected with HIV and in those who have particularly high levels of virus circulating in their blood.

It is unusual for HCV to present with an acute icteric hepatitis and many people who are infected have no symptoms and are therefore unaware that they are carrying the virus. Chronic infection is defined as infection lasting longer than 6 months. Up to 80 per cent of infected people go on to develop chronic infection. It is estimated that 5–20 per cent of chronically infected people will progress to cirrhosis of the liver over a period of about 20 years. A small number (1–4 per cent of those with cirrhosis) will progress to hepatocellular carcinoma each year.

Treatment

Over the last decade the treatment for chronic HCV infection has consisted of a combination of pegylated-interferon and ribavirin. The aim of treatment is the permanent clearance of the virus. The success of treatment is determined by host factors such as gender, age, weight, underlying liver fibrosis, and concomitant alcohol use, but the most important factor is viral genotype. The standard course for genotype 1 is 48 weeks of combination therapy giving a 50 per cent sustained viral response (SVR) and 24 weeks for genotypes 2 and 3 giving an 80 per cent SVR. More recently the course of treatment has been tailored to individual patients with shorter courses being given to those with a rapid initial drop in viral RNA and longer courses in those who are more resistant to treatment. Treatment is associated with a significant side effect profile, some of the main issues being flu-like symptoms associated with each injection, anaemia and depression. However with the advent of pegylated interferon allowing a once weekly rather than 3-weekly injection, most patients are able to continue their day-to-day activities.

In the last year a new group of protease inhibitors has been licensed for the treatment of HCV which significantly improve outcomes in patients with genotype 1. Cost implications mean they are unlikely to be used universally and only subject to future guidance from the National Institute for Health and Clinical Excellence (NICE).

Functional assessment

Apart from the special problems of healthcare workers there are no specific contraindications for work and no risks of cross-infection in the workplace.

Healthcare workers

Risk to the patients In response to this, the Advisory Group on Hepatitis made recommendations to protect patients. The guidance from the Department of Health states that healthcare workers who embark on, or transfer to, a career which entails EPP (see 'Healthcare workers who undertake exposure-prone procedures and dialysis work') should be checked to ensure that they are free from infection with HCV.[17,19,20] Those healthcare workers who are positive for HCV RNA must not undertake EPP due to the risk of hepatitis C transmission to patients.

Risk to the healthcare worker The risk of an individual surgeon acquiring the HCV has been estimated at 0.001–0.032 per cent per annum. Even in an area with a high prevalence of HCV among its population, the risk of acquiring HCV through occupational exposure is low. There is neither vaccination nor prophylactic treatment available. Rates of viral clearance with treatment of acute HCV infection are considerably higher than treatment of chronic HCV infection.[5] Therefore, it is imperative that healthcare workers follow universal precaution and promptly report all exposures to blood or body fluid exposures according to their local policy.

Risk to patients—healthcare workers undertaking EPPs Although unusual, there have been recorded incidents in which HCV-infected healthcare workers have transmitted the infection to patients. In the UK all healthcare workers new to EPP (as defined previously) are required to be

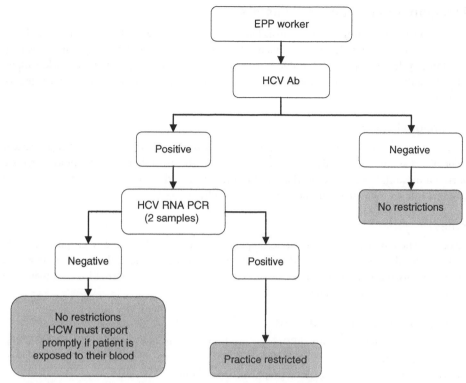

Figure 14.4 Flowchart—investigation of HCV status in a worker performing exposure-prone procedures. Reproduced with permission from Occupational Health Department, Guy's and St Thomas' NHS Foundation Trust. Data from *HSC 2002/010; hepatitis C infected health care workers*, Department of Health © Crown Copyright 2002 and *Hepatitis C infected health care workers: implementing getting ahead of the curve: action on blood-borne viruses*, Department of Health© Crown Copyright 2002.

tested to ensure that they are free from infection with hepatitis C.[17,19,20] If the HCV Ab is positive, the healthcare worker should be tested for HCV RNA PCR. If the HCV RNA PCR is negative on two separate occasions, the healthcare worker may be permitted to perform EPPs. If the HCV RNA PCR is positive, the healthcare worker should not be allowed to perform EPPs (see Figure 14.4). Healthcare workers who already perform EPPs and who believe they may have been exposed to hepatitis C infection should be advised to seek advice from their occupational health department for confidential advice on whether they should be tested.

Cirrhosis of the liver

Prevalence and prognosis

Cirrhosis results from chronic liver injury. The most common causes in the UK are alcohol, chronic viral hepatitis, and non-alcoholic fatty liver disease. The prevalence and prognosis depend on the underlying disease process. Once an individual develops any of the major complications of cirrhosis listed later, the prognosis is generally poor.

Management and functional assessment

There is no specific treatment for cirrhosis itself. Management is aimed at treating the underlying aetiology where possible, and surveillance for, and then treatment of complications as they arise. Initially, fatigue may be the predominant symptom causing impairment at work. Fatigue and intractable pruritis are particularly prominent symptoms in individuals with primary biliary cirrhosis.

Oesophageal varices

The development of portal hypertension is a common sequela of cirrhosis. If oesophageal varices are identified at annual surveillance endoscopy, individuals are started on propranolol to reduce the risk of bleeding. This can exacerbate confusion in those with a tendency to encephalopathy and affect balance particularly in those with an alcoholic aetiology.

Ascites

The development of ascites is a sign of decompensation. It is usually treated with spironolactone which may result in electrolyte disturbance and tender gynaecomastia. Individuals intolerant of, or refractory to, diuretics undergo day case paracentesis and may be referred for a trans-jugular intrahepatic porto-systemic shunt.

Spontaneous bacterial peritonitis

Spontaneous bacterial peritonitis (SBP) is a complication of ascites which can lead to encephalopathy and precipitate hepato-renal syndrome. Consequently it has a poor prognosis. Individuals who recover from SBP require lifelong prophylactic antibiotics.

Hepatic encephalopathy

Hepatic encephalopathy can present as subtle personality changes through varying degrees of confusion to coma. It usually presents as an acute episode often precipitated by infection, constipation, or a gastrointestinal bleed and is reversible if the underlying cause is treated. Some individuals suffer a chronic encephalopathy. Regular lactulose has been the standard treatment, however minimally absorbed antibiotics such as rifaximin are likely to play an increasing role.

Hepatocellular carcinoma

Hepatocellular carcinoma (HCC) usually occurs as a consequence of cirrhosis. However, the relative risk is dependent on aetiology with HBV and HCV giving the biggest risk. Cirrhotic patients therefore undergo surveillance ultrasound scans and alpha-feto protein on a 6-monthly basis. HCC can be treated with radiofrequency ablation, chemo-embolization, resection, or liver transplantation.

Adjustments at work

A specialist should optimize the care of patients with cirrhosis and decompensated liver disease before work is resumed. In patients with oesophageal varices there is no restriction on occupation once the varices have been treated. Patients with ascites may experience difficulty with lifting, bending, or stooping. Although alcohol addiction and dependency are excluded from the definition of impairment under the Equality Act 2010, the complications arising from alcoholism especially ascites, hepatic impairment and depression will require individual assessment, to determine whether the patient is disabled within the meaning of the Act.

Patients with chronic or intermittent encephalopathy should not be employed in intellectually demanding work or jobs requiring a high degree of vigilance, including safety-critical work or operating machinery. Impairment of cognitive functioning is not usually compatible with driving and in most instances a Group 1 and 2 licence will be refused or revoked by the Driver and Vehicle Licensing Authority (DVLA).[21] Patients who have been dependent on alcohol are barred from holding a vocational licence until they can demonstrate evidence of uninterrupted absence of dependency and misuse for 3 years. Individual suitability for driving duties should be discussed with the medical branch of the DVLA.[21]

Liver transplantation

Liver transplantation is the ultimate treatment for cirrhotic patients with end-stage chronic liver failure. The most common indications for transplantation are decompensated cirrhosis secondary to alcohol, hepatitis C, and primary biliary cirrhosis. Approximately 650 liver transplants are carried out each year in the UK. Overall 1-year graft survival rate for first transplants is now 88 per cent.[22] Individuals undergoing liver transplantation remain on lifelong immunosuppressant therapy and require regular follow-up by a hepatologist. General side effects include increased risk of infection and malignancy.

Implications for employment

Physical fatigue is the main symptom limiting work activity in transplant recipients. In general, implantation of a new liver results in significant improvements in cognitive function. In a study of 188 adults who underwent primary liver transplantation at the Mayo Clinic between 1995 and 1998, 44 per cent of respondents indicated they were working full- or part-time 3–5 years after transplant, 21 per cent were retired, 22 per cent were unemployed, 9 per cent were temporarily laid off, students, or homemakers, and 4 per cent did not report employment status. Employment prior to transplant was the strongest predictor of employment post transplant: 82 per cent of those employed pre-transplant were employed post-transplant compared to 20 per cent of those not employed prior to transplant. A small but significant percentage of survivors who were unemployed prior to transplant were successful in gaining employment after transplant. Success in obtaining employment was highly correlated with basic general health and strong mental health status.[23]

Guidelines for employees handling hepatotoxins

In general, patients with chronic liver disease with ongoing inflammation or liver damage should not work with hepatotoxins. All patients working with hepatotoxins should avoid alcohol misuse and enzyme inducing agents such as anticonvulsants, in particular phenobarbitone and phenytoin.

Obesity

Prevalence and definitions

In adults, body mass index (BMI) is frequently used as a measure of overweight and obesity, with overweight being defined as a BMI 25–29.9 kg/m^2 and obesity as a BMI equal to or greater than 30 kg/m^2. In England the prevalence of obesity in adults has trebled during the past 25 years. In 1980, 8 per cent of adult women and 6 per cent of adult men were classified as obese; by 2008 this had increased to approximately 24 per cent of men and women. Furthermore, 0.9 per cent of men and 2.6 per cent of women are classified as morbidly obese, with BMIs over 40 kg/m^2.

In adults, central adiposity is measured by waist circumference, with raised waist circumference defined as equal to or greater than 102 cm in men and equal to or greater than 88 cm in women. Central adiposity is associated with insulin resistance, decreased high-density lipoprotein cholesterol, raised low-density lipoprotein cholesterol and triglycerides, hypertension, and decreased glucose tolerance known together as the metabolic syndrome. Seventy-five per cent of individuals with obesity will develop non-alcoholic fatty liver disease, which can cause progressive liver disease leading to cirrhosis and its complications.

Obesity becomes more common with age and is more prevalent among lower socioeconomic and lower-income groups, with a particularly strong social class gradient among women. Adults at greater risk of becoming obese include those who were previously overweight and who have lost weight, smokers who have stopped smoking and those who change from an active to an inactive lifestyle.

Treatment

This section is based on guidance published by NICE in 2010 on detecting and managing obesity.[24]

The initial management of obesity is dietary modification, increased physical activity, and, if necessary, behavioural interventions. The only drug treatment currently available is Orlistat® which inhibits lipase in the gastrointestinal tract and prevents absorption of 30 per cent of dietary fat. It can cause sustained weight loss of 5–10 per cent over 2 years.

Indications for treatment are:

- BMI >28.0 kg/m^2 with associated risk factors (e.g. type 2 diabetes, high cholesterol).
- BMI >30.0 kg/m^2.

The outcomes of bariatric surgery have improved steadily; the procedures work in one of two ways either by restricting the individual's ability to eat, e.g. gastric banding, or by interfering with the nutrient absorption, e.g. bypass surgery. Drawbacks to surgical therapy are lifelong rearrangement of the gastrointestinal tract, operative mortality (<0.5 per cent), and morbidity (approximately 10 per cent). Nonetheless, surgically induced weight loss is currently the most effective treatment for the severely obese patient (see Box 14.3).

Box 14.3 Summary of NICE criteria for bariatric surgery in people with obesity

- A BMI ≥40 kg/m^2, or between 35 kg/m^2 and 40 kg/m^2 with other significant disease (e.g. type 2 diabetes, high blood pressure) that could be improved by weight loss.
- All appropriate non-surgical measures tried and failed to achieve or maintain adequate, clinically beneficial weight loss for at least 6 months.
- Receiving or will receive intensive management in a specialist obesity service.

From National Institute for Health and Clinical Excellence (2006). *CG 43 Obesity: guidance on the prevention, identification, assessment and management of overweight and obesity.* London: NICE. Available from <http://www.nice.org.uk/guidance/CG43>. Reproduced with permission. Information accurate at time of publication, for up-to-date information please visit <http://www.nice.org.uk>.

Prevention and treatment of obesity in the workplace

Occupational health units are likely to become increasingly involved in the prevention and treatment of obesity in the workplace. Two systematic reviews examined the use of workplace health promotion programmes and found evidence to support this as an effective intervention for overweight and obese adults.[24] As little as a 10 kg weight loss can have a significant benefit on blood pressure, serum lipids, glucose control in diabetics, and mortality. Factors that appeared to be beneficial included dieting, supervision of exercise, and personal counselling. NICE recommends that an organization's policies and incentive schemes should help to create a culture that supports healthy eating and physical exercise (Box 14.4).[24]

Functional limitations

Obese workers are more likely to take more short-term and long-term absence attributable to sickness than their non-obese counterparts.[25] Much of the increased absence from work in obese individuals is attributable to comorbid conditions and obesity-related chronic medical problems. Presenteeism may also be increased in obese workers.

When assessing overweight and obese workers it is important to assess their physical limitations in the context of the job that they are expected to do. Obese workers who are physically fit may be more mobile than slim workers who are unfit. Assessment should take into account comorbid conditions, especially metabolic syndrome and sleep apnoea. There are few jobs that obese workers are not able to do. However, the following need careful consideration:

- A person's mobility and size may affect entry to confined spaces and access into vehicles, use of personal protective equipment or other equipment such as ladders.
- Obese workers may be at increased risk of heat stress when working in high temperatures.
- Some safety critical work requires high levels of mobility.

Box 14.4 Summary of NICE recommendations for prevention of obesity in the workplace

Workplaces should provide opportunities for staff to eat a healthy diet and be physically active through:

- Active and continuous promotion of healthy choices in restaurants, hospitality, vending machines, and shops for staff and clients in line with existing Food Standards Agency guidance.
- Working practices and policies such as active travel policies for staff and visitors.
- A supportive physical environment such as improvements to stairwells and providing showers and secure cycle parking.
- Recreational opportunities such as supporting out-of-hours social activities lunchtime walks, and use of local leisure facilities.

From National Institute for Health and Clinical Excellence (2006). *CG 43 Obesity: guidance on the prevention, identification, assessment and management of overweight and obesity*. London: NICE. Available from <http://www.nice.org.uk/guidance/CG43>. Reproduced with permission. Information accurate at time of publication, for up-to-date information please visit <http://www.nice.org.uk>.

Adjustments at work

In assessing whether obesity would be considered a disability as defined by the Equality Act 2010, the focus should be on whether the obesity has a substantial adverse effect on the person's ability to carry out normal day-to-day activities. The question of what caused the obesity is irrelevant. In most cases, it is likely that the effects will be long term, that is, they have lasted for, or are likely to last for at least 12 months. The employer should, in these cases, consider if reasonable adjustments to the job are required. Even if the obese worker is not considered disabled as defined by the Equality Act 2010, employers may wish to consider if they have equipment designed to accommodate larger people and if they are able to make alternative arrangements within the workplace so that work spaces can accommodate larger people. Employers should be sensitive to the complicated issues that contribute to a worker being obese and the effect on self-esteem that obesity may have on a worker and should support workers who are trying to lose weight.

References

1 Equality Act 2010. (<http://www.legislation.gov.uk/ukpga/2010/15/contents>)

2 Wyke RJ, Aw TC, Allan RN, *et al*. Employment prospects for patients with intestinal stomas: the attitude of occupational physicians. *J Soc Occup Med* 1989; **39**: 19–24.

3 Saito YA, Schoenfeld P, Locke GR 3rd. The epidemiology of IBS in North America: a systematic review. *Am J Gastroenterol* 2002: **97**(8): 1910–5.

4 Statutory Notifications of Infectious Diseases (Noids) England and Wales. (<http://www.hpa.org.uk/webc/HPAwebFile/HPAweb_C/1251473364307>)

5 Food Standards Agency. *Food handlers: fitness to work—a practical guide for food business operators.* [Online] (<http://www.food.gov.uk/foodindustry/guidancenotes/hygguid/foodhandlersguide>)

6 Health Protection Agency. *HPA—topics A–Z.* [Online] (<http://www.hpa.org.uk/Topics/TopicsAZ/>)

7 The Health Protection (Notification) Regulations 2010. (<http://www.legislation.gov.uk/uksi/2010/659/contents/made>)

8 Health Protection Agency. *Vero cytotoxin-producing Escherichia coli (VTEC).* [Online] (<http://www.hpa.org.uk/Topics/InfectiousDiseases/InfectionsAZ/EscherichiaColiO157/>)

9 Health Protection Agency. *Guidance for the prevention and control of hepatitis A infection.* (<http://www.hpa.org.uk>)

10 Salisbury D, Ramsey M, Noakes K. *Immunisation against infectious disease* ('the Green Book'). London: Department of Health, 2006. (<http://www.dh.gov.uk/prod_consum_dh/groups/dh_digitalassets/@dh/@en/documents/digitalasset/dh_063665.pdf>)

11 Department of Health. *Hepatitis B infected health care workers and antiviral therapy*, 2007. [Online] (<http://www.dh.gov.uk/en/Publicationsandstatistics/Publications/PublicationsPolicyAndGuidance/DH_073164>)

12 Health and Safety at Work etc. Act 1974. (<http://www.legislation.gov.uk/ukpga/1974/37>)

13 The Management of Health and Safety at Work Regulations 1999. (<http://www.legislation.gov.uk/uksi/1999/3242/contents/made>)

14 The Control of Substances Hazardous to Health Regulations 2002. (<http://www.legislation.gov.uk/uksi/2002/2677/contents/made>)

15 Department of Health. *HSC 2000/020; Hepatitis B infected Healthcare workers*, 2000. [Online] (<http://www.dh.gov.uk/prod_consum_dh/groups/dh_digitalassets/@dh/@en/documents/digitalasset/dh_4012257.pdf>)

16 Department of Health. *Hepatitis B infected health care workers: Guidance on implementation of Health Service Circular 2000/020*, 2000. [Online] (<http://www.dh.gov.uk/en/Publicationsandstatistics/Publications/PublicationsPolicyAndGuidance/DH_4008156>)

17 Department of Health. *Health clearance for tuberculosis, hepatitis B, hepatitis C, and HIV: new health-care workers*, March 2007. [Online] (<http://www.dh.gov.uk/en/Publicationsandstatistics/Publications/PublicationsPolicyAndGuidance/DH_073132>)

18 Department of Health. *Good practice guidelines for renal dialysis/transplantation units; prevention and control of blood borne virus infection*, 2002. [Online] (<http://www.dh.gov.uk/assetRoot/04/05/95/11/04059511.pdf>)

19 Department of Health. *HSC 2002/010; hepatitis C infected health care workers*, August 2002. [Online] (<http://www.dh.gov.uk/prod_consum_dh/groups/dh_digitalassets/@dh/@en/documents/digitalasset/dh_4012217.pdf>)

20 Department of Health. *Hepatitis C infected health care workers: implementing getting ahead of the curve: action on blood-borne viruses*, August 2002. [Online] (<http://www.dh.gov.uk/prod_consum_dh/groups/dh_digitalassets/@dh/@en/documents/digitalasset/dh_4059544.pdf>)

21 Driver Medical Group. *At a glance guide to the current medical standards of fitness to drive*. Swansea: Driver and Vehicle Licensing Agency, 2011. (<http://www.dft.gov.uk/dvla/medical/ataglance.aspx>)

22 British Liver Trust website: <http://www.britishlivertrust.org.uk>

23 Vanness DJ, Kim WR, Malinchoc M. Factors Associated with Long-run Employment after Receiving a Liver Transplant. Academy for Health Services Research and Health Policy. Meeting. *Abstr Acad Health Serv Res Health Policy Meet* 2002; **19**: 44.

24 National Institute for Health and Clinical Excellence. *Obesity: the prevention, identification, assessment and management of overweight and obesity in adults and children* (CG43). London: NICE, 2006. (<http://www.nice.org.uk/nicemedia/pdf/CG43NICEGuideline.pdf>)

25 Harvey SB, Glozier N, Carlton O, *et al.* Obesity and sickness absence: results from the CHAP study. *Occup Med* 2010; **60**: 362–8.

Chapter 15

Diabetes mellitus and other endocrine disorders

Eugene R. Waclawski and Geoff Gill

Classification

The two major subtypes of diabetes mellitus remain types 1 and 2:

- *Type 1 diabetes*: this can occur at any age but usually presents abruptly in the teens or twenties. In recent years, more patients are presenting at a particularly young age (<5 years), for uncertain reasons. The disease has a genetic predisposition, and is also related to auto-immune beta cell destruction, possibly triggered by viral infection. Absolute insulin deficiency results, and insulin treatment is needed for life.

- *Type 2 diabetes*: in Western countries, type 2 diabetes accounts for 85–90 per cent of the total diabetic population and is the predominant type. Though partial insulin deficiency occurs, insulin resistance is a major feature. Lifestyle issues are strongly causative, in particular obesity and reduced exercise. Rates of type 2 diabetes are rapidly increasing. Presentation is usually between 50–70 years but it is now presenting at much earlier ages (usually obesity related).

Other types of diabetes include 'gestational diabetes' (appearing in pregnancy and usually remitting afterwards), and 'secondary diabetes' (pancreatic disease, steroids, endocrine conditions such as thyrotoxicosis). There are also rare genetically determined forms of type 2 diabetes which present at young ages—known as 'maturity-onset diabetes of the young' (MODY).

Most patients at presentation can be readily classified into type 1 or type 2, but in recent years (with younger presentation of type 2 diabetes) classification of some patients can be difficult. As well as the occasional MODY patient, true type 2 diabetes is now occurring in the teens or twenties.[1] Such problems can lead to misclassification in a small but important number of patients.[2]

Recent advances in diabetes

Significant changes and advances in diabetes therapy have continued over the last few years, affecting both types of diabetes. Important advances are as follows:

Insulin-infusion therapy ('insulin-pumps')

The technique of continuous subcutaneous insulin infusion (CSCII) has been available for many years, but its use has increased in recent years. This has also been stimulated by the publication of specific guidelines by the National Institute for Health and Clinical Excellence (NICE) in 2008.[3] These guidelines recommend consideration of pump treatment for type 1 (not insulin-treated type 2) patients who have either recurrent disabling hypoglycaemia or sustained poor glycaemic control (HbA_{1c} >8.5 per cent) despite intensified (four times daily) subcutaneous insulin injections. Insulin pump treatment requires initiation and surveillance by an expert experienced team. Major educational input is needed, including training in 'carbohydrate counting'. This encourages patients to adjust their insulin meal boluses to the amount of carbohydrate food eaten.[4] With appropriate support and motivation insulin pump therapy can offer sustained glycaemic improvement without significant hypoglycaemia.[5]

Islet cell transplantation

The technique of transplanting donor pancreatic islet cells as a potential cure for type 1 diabetes is not new, but techniques have been refined and success rates improved. The system is now available, on a limited basis, in a number of countries including the UK. Recovered donor islets are infused into the liver, and for a successful graft, two donor pancreas glands are usually needed. Success rates are reasonably good and independence from insulin injections often achieved for some years. Some milder degrees of glucose intolerance may remain, and sometimes insulin treatment may be temporarily needed, for example, during intercurrent infections. Lifelong immunosuppressant therapy is needed. The main current indication for islet cell transplantation is recurrent severe hypoglycaemia in type 1 diabetes. Even if insulin is required some time after transplant, there is less chance of recurrent severe hypoglycaemia returning.[6]

Diabetes diagnosis by HbA$_{1c}$

Now that glycated haemoglobin (HbA$_{1c}$) assays are accurate and standardized, interest has increased in the use of HbA$_{1c}$ (which reflects recent mean glycaemia) for the diagnosis of type 2 diabetes. Fasting is not required, and the test is easier than a glucose tolerance test (GTT), though it is relatively expensive. The World Health Organization (WHO) in 2011 advocated that an HbA$_{1c}$ level over 6.5 per cent could be used to diagnose type 2 diabetes (type 1 and gestational diabetes were excluded), in addition to current standard glucose-based test criteria.[7] Interest is now focusing on HbA$_{1c}$ equivalents of the borderline states of impaired glucose tolerance (IGT) and impaired fasting glycaemia (IFG). IGT is a 2-hour plasma glucose level on GTT of 7.8–11.1 mmol/L, and IFG is a fasting plasma glucose of 6.0–6.9 mmol/L. Both states represent an increased risk of later type 2 diabetes, and are independent risk factors for macroangiopathy (large vessel disease). An HbA$_{1c}$ between 5.7 per cent and 6.4 per cent may be equivalent in risk to IGT and IFG diagnosed by more standard techniques.[8]

Type 2 diabetes and the incretin system

Exenatide and liraglutide are now in widespread use for the management of obese type 2 diabetes. They are synthetic 'GLP-1 agonists' and act similarly to the naturally occurring gut hormones such as glucagon-like-peptide 1 (GLP-1)—often known collectively as the 'incretins'. The effect of these hormones (and exenatide and liraglutide) is to stimulate pancreatic insulin production (in a glucose-mediated fashion, so that hypoglycaemia does not result), reduce pancreatic glucagon secretion, and delay gastric emptying. These actions collectively lead to lowered blood glucose levels without hypoglycaemic risk, and weight loss (which is often quite significant).[9] Exenatide and liraglutide have to be given by subcutaneous injection and are relatively expensive, but can be combined with other oral agents. They can be associated with upper gastrointestinal side effects (e.g. bloating and nausea). Related drugs are the 'gliptins' (e.g. sitagliptin, vildagliptin, and saxagliptin). They inhibit the enzyme dipeptidyl peptidase 4 (DPP-4) which breaks down endogenous incretins, thus raising their levels and increasing their effect. They can be given orally, but are less potent than exenatide and liraglutide.[9]

Diabetes and employment

Equality legislation and the legal protection of individuals with health problems such as diabetes have led to higher awareness of diabetes and ability to work.[10] This has been supported actively by Diabetes UK which provides some valuable guidance on employment issues.[11]

Previous evidence indicated that having diabetes did not decrease the chance of employment or result in higher unemployment in young people with type 1 diabetes.[12,13] A recent report highlighted an unemployment rate twice that of the general population studied prior to the recent recession.[14] This is an area that merits further study given the changes in management of diabetes since the earlier papers were published.

The previously identified under-representation of diabetes in the workforce[15] may have indicated prejudice against their employment, or a failure always to declare their diabetes to their employer or occupational health service. The risk of hypoglycaemia and complications such as visual impairment and peripheral neuropathy may legitimately debar those with poorly controlled type 1 diabetes from jobs where safety is an important factor, but people with diabetes should not be assumed to be invalids and most can work normally and should not be unjustifiably discriminated against in job selection. Severe late complications can lead to lower employment rates, even in young people with diabetes, and lead to reduced income.[16] Accommodations focused on abilities may allow continuing employment.

The Equality Act 2010 provides that where an impairment is being treated or corrected, the impairment is to be treated as having the effect it would have had without the measures in question. This applies even if treatment results in the effects of disease being completely controlled and masked. In addition, the Act provides for a person with a progressive condition to be regarded as having an impairment which has a substantial adverse effect on their ability to carry out normal day-to-day activities before it actually does so. The effect need not be continuous and need not be substantial.

Within the meaning of the Equality Act type 1 diabetes must be regarded as a disability. Type 2 may be different, as people with this type of diabetes may be asymptomatic and have no complications. Where complications such as retinopathy exist, and such complications can be found at initial presentation in some cases, they will be covered by the Act as this gives indication of a progressive condition.

Prevalence, morbidity, and mortality

Diabetes epidemiology

Type 1 diabetes incidence varies greatly around the world and is generally higher in northern countries. In Yorkshire, UK, the incidence was 23.3/100 000/year in a cohort collected between 1999 and 2003 having increased from 16.0/100 000/year 20 years earlier.[17] This upward trend is predicted to cause near doubling of rates amongst children from 2005 to 2020.[17]

The burden of type 2 diabetes continues to rapidly increase in western countries. A recent estimate of total diabetes prevalence in the UK is 7.4 per cent[18] (type 2 prevalence, 6 per cent) and is likely to rise to 9.5 per cent by 2030. Rates are much higher in the elderly, and in some ethnic minorities, notably south Asians.

Mortality and morbidity

Type 2 diabetes is a major vascular risk factor, and the disease doubles mortality risk compared to those without the disease.[19] It is likely that this risk will reduce in the future, with the more vigorous risk factor management practised over the last decade. Outcome for type 1 diabetes has improved, but mortality risk remains in excess of non-diabetic rates (by a factor of five to six).[20] However, most deaths are vascular or renal (or combined 'renovascular'), and recent evidence shows that in the absence of renal disease, 20-year mortality for type 1 diabetes is equivalent to that of the general population.[21]

The complications of diabetes lead to significant morbidity. The prevalence of painful symptoms and painful diabetic neuropathy was 34 per cent and 21 per cent, respectively in a recent community based study in the North West of England.[22] In a study from Pittsburgh l, after 30 years of diabetes, the cumulative incidences of proliferative retinopathy, nephropathy, and cardiovascular disease were 50 per cent, 25 per cent, and 14 per cent, respectively, in a conventionally treated group but only 21 per cent, 9 per cent, and 9 per cent in an intensive treatment group, and fewer than 1 per cent became blind, required kidney replacement, or had an amputation because of diabetes during that time.[23] Better control of diabetes reduces the rate of complications. A recent report on subjects with impaired hypoglycaemic awareness indicated that two-thirds were in employment, indicating that being in employment is common despite the presence of a significant complication.[24]

The major implications diabetes has in regard to employment are associated disability and treatment-induced hypoglycaemia (see 'Diabetic hypoglycaemia'). Diabetes is associated with an excess of sickness absence, though this is more often due to comorbid conditions such as depression, rheumatological disorders, and asthma rather than vascular disease.[25]

Diabetes treatment

Type 2 diabetes

Lifestyle modification (by diet and exercise) can be very effective, particularly at or close to diagnosis.[26] However, type 2 diabetes is a progressive disease and drug treatment is usually inevitable. Indeed, some current guidelines advise initiating metformin at diagnosis.[27] Current available drugs for type 2 diabetes are as follows:[9,27]

♦ *Biguanides*: The one remaining prescribed member of this group is metformin. This has been available for many decades, and has a strong evidence-base. It improves insulin sensitivity and increases peripheral glucose uptake, without causing hypoglycaemia. Weight loss may occur making them particularly suitable for the obese. The well-documented side effect of lactic acidosis is very rare, particularly if the drug is avoided in significant renal dysfunction. Diarrhoea and/or upper gastrointestinal symptoms can be problematic in some patients, but less common with the modified-release preparation.

♦ *Sulphonylureas*: These are well-established drugs, of which there are several (e.g. gliclazide, glipizide, glibenclamide). They stimulate pancreatic insulin production, and therefore can cause hypoglycaemia, and also weight gain. Sulphonylureas are particularly suitable for normal weight patients. They tend to lose effect over time.

♦ *Glinides*: These are similar to sulphonylureas, but bind to different channels on the beta cell, and are shorter-acting. Examples are repaglinide and netaglinide, and they have a similar side effect profile to sulphonylureas, though hypoglycaemia may be less frequent. They are not in common use.

♦ *Glucosidase inhibitors*: The only member of this group, acarbose, inhibits the intestinal mucosal enzyme alpha-glucosidase, reducing carbohydrate absorption. Side effects of flatulence and diarrhoea limit the drug's usage.

◆ *Glitazones* (thiazolidinediones): These drugs increase insulin receptor sensitivity, and therefore augment the effect of endogenous insulin. Until recently there were two members in this group—rosiglitazone and pioglitazone—but rosiglitazone has been recently withdrawn due to concerns over long-term cardiovascular safety. The glitazones are moderately effective glucose-lowering drugs, and are able to maintain effect longer than sulphonylureas. Side effects include fluid retention and weight gain (which then can be significant). Occasionally, heart failure can be precipitated. Some recent evidence suggests a slight increase in bladder cancer risk with pioglitazone treatment, and use may become restricted.[28]

◆ *GLP agonist*: The GLP agonist drugs exenatide and liraglutide have established a place as effective agents in obese (body mass index >35.0 kg/m^2) type 2 diabetic patients (see 'Recent advances in diabetes').

◆ *Gliptins*: The gliptins (or DDP-4 inhibitors) include sitagliptin, vildagliptin, and saxagliptin (see 'Recent advances in diabetes'). Their use does not have to be confined to obese patients, and they are generally 'weight-neutral', rather than causing weight loss. Gastrointestinal side effects can occur, but are usually mild.

◆ *Insulin*: Many patients with type 2 diabetes come to need insulin. These patients are usually on treatment which includes maximal doses of a sulphonylurea and metformin. These drugs are normally continued, and bedtime isophane insulin begun and titrated upwards to normalize the fasting blood glucose level. If this does not succeed, a once-daily, long-acting analogue insulin can be tried, or beyond that a twice-daily biphasic insulin, or even four-times daily insulin (see 'Type 1 diabetes management').

The modern treatment of type 2 diabetes is complex. The most relevant employment issue is drug-related hypoglycaemia due to sulphonylureas. Significant hypoglycaemia due to these drugs is less common than with insulin but it is still a significant, if small, problem.[29] Other treatments for type 2 diabetes, such as metformin, GLP-agonists, gliptins and glitazones do not themselves cause hypoglycaemia but if added to sulphonylurea therapy may increase the risk of sulphonylurea-induced hypoglycaemia.

Type 1 diabetes

Though diet and lifestyle play a part in the management of type 1 diabetes, the major treatment is insulin. Insulins can be divided by duration of action—short, intermediate, long, and biphasic (the latter containing mixtures of short and intermediate-acting insulins). In the past insulins were beef, pork, and human but beef and pork insulins are now little used, and 'analogue' insulins are currently in common use. These insulins have no species, as they are human insulins in which the molecule has been altered slightly to give absorption which is closer to endogenous insulin release ('short-acting analogues'), or which have sustained release suitable for once-daily injections ('long-acting analogues'). In trials, long-acting analogues can reduce hypoglycaemic episodes, particularly at night.[30] Analogues are significantly more expensive than human insulins, and their cost-effectiveness has been questioned.[31] Examples of types of insulin (classified by duration of action) are as follows:

◆ *Short-acting*: these typically have action for about 4–6 hours. Examples are Actrapid® and Humulin S® (human), and Aspart® and Lispro® (analogue). Bovine and porcine preparations are also available.

◆ *Intermediat-acting*: these are the traditional 'isophane' or 'lente' insulins, with a duration of action about 8–12 hours. They include Insulatard® and Humulin I® (human), with bovine and porcine preparations available.

- *Biphasic*: these are fixed combinations of short- and intermediate-acting insulins, usually 30 per cent short and 70 per cent intermediate. Examples are Humulin M_3® (human) and NovoMix 30® (analogue). An analogue 25:75 preparation is available (Humalog Mix 25®).

- *Long-acting*: these (at least theoretically) last for 24 hours. They are exclusively analogue insulins, and two are available—glargine and detemir. In individual patients, their effective action may be less than 24 hours, and detemir in particular may need to be given twice daily.

Twice-daily biphasic insulin regimens remain simple and popular, though many patients are now on 'intensified' insulin systems i.e. four injections daily—usually either human or analogue short-acting insulin with each meal, and either human intermediate-acting or analogue long-acting insulin at night. There is evidence that addition of metformin to insulin can be beneficial in some type 1 patients. The role of insulin pumps and pancreas transplantation has been discussed in the earlier 'Recent advances in diabetes' section.

Hypoglycaemia is, of course, the most important work-related complication of insulin treatment in type 1 diabetes. If hypoglycaemia is a problem, intensive input by a secondary care diabetes team can be effective. Appropriate education on diet, hypoglycaemia avoidance, and glucose monitoring is useful, as well as dose adjustments as necessary. Movement from two to four injections daily may help, as may also a change from human to analogue insulins.

Control monitoring

The gold standard laboratory control test is glycated haemoglobin or HbA_{1c}, which reflects mean glycaemia over the previous 8–10 weeks. Self-glucose monitoring is a supplementary and important additional control system, which can be important in increasing safety in the workplace of diabetic persons. Glucose monitoring should be routine in type 1 and insulin-treated type 2 diabetes. It is also advisable for those on sulphonylureas, particularly those who drive, have busy and variable lifestyles, or work in potentially hazardous environments.

Glycaemic and risk factor control

Glycaemic targets

Targets of mean glycaemia (measured by HbA_{1c}) have for many years been based on the landmark studies examining the outcome of 'intensive' and 'routine' blood glucose control in type 1 (DCCT Study)[32] and type 2 (UKPDS Study) diabetes.[33] In both these studies the intensive control arms achieved mean HbA_{1c} levels of approximately 7.0 per cent, with clear evidence of benefit in terms of complication occurrence and progression (though this was mainly microvascular rather than macrovascular). In type 1 diabetes, microvascular risk can probably be reduced by further HbA_{1c} reductions below 7.0 per cent, but this has to be balanced against increasing hypoglycaemic risk. Generally, therefore, an appropriate type 1 target HbA_{1c} is regarded as 7.0 per cent. However, it is sensible to vary this individually, and in some (e.g. those with early retinopathy or microalbuminuria) a lower target may be appropriate, whereas with others 'looser' control may be advisable (for example, in those who are especially hypoglycaemic-prone and live alone, or those with short-life expectancy).

The situation in type 2 diabetes is, however, different. Two recent trials ('ACCORD'[34] and 'ADVANCE'[35]) have examined the effect of very tight (HbA_{1c} 6.5 per cent or below) control in type 2 diabetes. Neither trial showed significant macrovascular benefit, and the ACCORD trial[34] showed increased mortality in the tightly controlled group. In addition, a more recent large UK primary care study compared survival and HbA_{1c} in type 2 diabetes.[36] A 'U'-shaped curve of survival was found, with HbA_{1c} levels below 6.5 per cent having an increased mortality similar to those with HbA$_{1c}$ levels over 10.0 per cent. The highest survival was with an HbA$_{1c}$ of approximately 7.5 per cent. All of these studies[35,36] have some design problems, and the findings of ACCORD in particular have been hotly debated.[37] Nevertheless, there are concerns of over-vigorous glucose-lowering in type 2 diabetes, particularly in those of high cardiovascular risk, who may perhaps be especially susceptible to hypoglycaemia-induced cardiac events.[38] Overall, a general glycaemic target HbA$_{1c}$ of 7.0 per cent in type 2 diabetes therefore seems sensible, though as with type 1 disease,[39] this should be varied as necessary on an individual basis.

Risk factor targets

The described debate has led to a reappraisal of priorities in type 2 diabetes care, and it has been pointed out that hyperglycaemia is a relatively weak risk factor for cardiovascular disease (the major cause of mortality in type 2 diabetes), compared with hypertension and hyperlipidaemia,[40] and that vigorous treatment of these risk factors will have greater long-term benefit. There is good evidence of significant outcome benefits from blood pressure lowering,[33,41] and lipid-lowering therapy with statins.[42] Most trials have been in type 2 diabetes, and targets for type 1 patients are not as strongly evidence-based, though the Heart Protection Study (HPS),[42] using simvastatin 40 mg daily, did include a type 1 cohort.

Current major risk factor targets in type 2 diabetes are generally as follows:

♦ *Blood pressure*: <140/80 if there are no renal complications (microalbuminuria or nephropathy) or <130/80 if these are present.

♦ *Lipids*: total cholesterol <4.0 mmol/L and low-density lipoprotein cholesterol <2.0 mmol/L, using simvastatin 40 mg daily as first-line treatment to achieve this.

♦ *Aspirin* (or clopidogrel if contraindicated): for all with established large vessel disease, and for high-risk patients without such problems.

A variety of 'risk calculators' are available to guide statin and antiplatelet drug use, but increasingly, the majority of type 2 patients are on at least one antihypertensive drug (with angiotensin-converting enzyme inhibitors as primary treatment), a statin, and aspirin. From an employment point of view, such 'polypharmacy' does not indicate greater severity of disease; rather it is stand-ard and evidence-based preventive therapy.

Special work problems caused by diabetes

The work record of people with diabetes

Awareness of diabetes has improved. Employers are less likely to operate overall bans for diabetic persons, while diabetic employees are better able to manage and less inclined to conceal their condition. Occupations closed to those with insulin-treated diabetes are usually those in which hypoglycaemia could be highly dangerous, e.g. airline pilots. The risk here comes not from the diabetes itself but from its treatment.

For drivers with diabetes in the UK the Driver and Vehicle Licensing Agency (DVLA) apply criteria which are detailed in the document *At A Glance Guide to the current Medical Standards of Fitness to Drive*.[43] Drivers treated with insulin or tablets which carry a risk of hypoglycaemia should be provided with leaflet INF188/2. Those on insulin must notify the DVLA; those on tab-lets need not provided they meet certain criteria. From October 2011 insulin treated drivers can apply for Group 2 licences but must meet strict criteria regarding hypoglycaemia, have full aware-ness of it and understand its risks. Impaired awareness of hypoglycaemia has been defined by the

Secretary of State's Honorary Medical Advisory Panel on Driving and Diabetes as, 'an inability to detect the onset of hypoglycaemia because of a total absence of warning symptoms'. DVLA will arrange an examination by an independent hospital consultant who specializes in the treatment of diabetes every 12 months. At the examination, the consultant will require sight of their blood glucose records for the previous 3 months. Drivers will be required to sign an undertaking to comply with the directions of doctor(s) treating the diabetes and to report immediately to DVLA any significant change in their condition.

It has traditionally been considered unwise for those taking insulin to work in potentially hazardous environments, e.g. with moving machinery, in foundries, on scaffolding, and fighting fires. But even here there is room for latitude. Much depends on the exact nature of the work, the adequacy of diabetic control (in particular the frequency and warnings of hypoglycaemia), and the good sense of the patient.

Previously, in the UK applicants with existing type 1 diabetes to firefighting and the other emergency services were not accepted for employment. The Disability Discrimination Act was modified to apply to emergency services and recruitment of those with type 1 diabetes now occurs. Those who develop diabetes that requires insulin while in service are assessed and accommodations applied on an individual basis. Criteria such as those mentioned earlier are used, and considered jointly by an occupational physician and a diabetologist. This situation seems sensible as it takes into account the great variability of control, education, and motivation among those with insulin-treated diabetes, as well as the potential for employment-related risk assessment. This approach may be applicable to other potentially dangerous occupations; for further information please visit Diabetes UK (<http://www.diabetes.org.uk>).[44]

Restrictions on the employment of those with diabetes treated without insulin are much less stringent. Although hypoglycaemic episodes can occur with sulphonylurea tablets (and may be serious and prolonged[45]), they are less common. If the physician is satisfied with treatment over a period of time, and especially if the patient monitors his or her own blood glucose levels, the risk of hypoglycaemia is remote and will rarely be a bar to employment. There are exceptions, for example, in air crew and train drivers.

The suitability of a diabetic person for employment also depends on their general health. In the case of diabetes this means freedom from sight-threatening retinopathy, severe peripheral or autonomic neuropathy, advanced ischaemic heart disease, serious renal failure, or disabling cerebrovascular or peripheral vascular disease.

Previous research has suggested that diabetics are likely to have 1.5–2 times as much time off work, but in well-controlled cases the excess is small or nil.[46–51] With recent improvements in treatment and control it is not known whether this situation has changed.

Working patterns and diabetic treatment

There is, in general, no reason why a diabetic person on insulin should not undertake shift work, though diabetic workers do experience more problems with shift work than non-diabetic workers.[46] Most sensible and well-motivated diabetic shift workers can rapidly learn how to adjust their treatment, especially if they are measuring their own blood glucose levels and using multiple insulin injection techniques, particularly with long-acting insulin analogues such as glargine or detemir. However, more rapidly rotating shift cycles where day, evening, and night shifts follow each other at 2-day intervals may be more difficult. The use of long-acting analogues can help, with short-acting insulin given with meals, whatever time that may be. The Working Time Regulations[52] includes the offer of a health assessment to identify if a person can perform night work. In some instances where a person with diabetes has difficulty controlling the condition as a result of such work a medical exclusion can be supported. The employer has to accommodate the restriction or pay the worker when not working such shifts if no other work is available.[52] A recent report indicated that shift work significantly affected control of diabetes (as measured by HbA$_{1C}$) in a regression analysis.[14] People with type 2 diabetes can normally undertake shift work though it is generally less well tolerated in the older workforce where most of the cases of type 2 diabetes will occur.

Complications of diabetes

Chronic complications

These include the specific problems of retinopathy, cataract, neuropathy, and nephropathy (including its earlier stage, microalbuminuria). In addition, macroangiopathy, though not specific to diabetes, occurs more frequently and more seriously. Advanced complications can of course interfere with ability to work—including visual loss, amputation, severe CAD, stroke, and end-stage renal disease (ESRD) requiring dialysis. In such circumstances employers require to consider making reasonable adjustments to maintain employment. Some neuropathic syndromes can be particularly debilitating also—for example, chronic painful neuropathy or autonomic neuropathy (causing, for example, vomiting, diarrhoea and/or postural hypotension). It should be emphasized that few adults of working age develop such severe complications and some treatments can be highly effective; notably renal transplantation for ESRD, and laser treatment and/or vitrectomy for advanced proliferative retinopathy although one particular type of laser treatment ('pan-retinal photocoagulation' or PRP) can sometimes restrict peripheral vision sufficiently enough to interfere with driving capacity. Even with complications those with diabetes will tolerate them and wish to continue working if possible.

Acute complications

These are either hyperglycaemic or hypoglycaemic. The most common hyperglycaemic acute complication is diabetic ketoacidosis (DKA). This mostly (but not exclusively) occurs in type 1 patients and is usually related to insulin omission or intercurrent infection. Dehydration and ketosis results, and hospital treatment is needed. With modern management, DKA mortality is now very low. Unless DKA is recurrent, there should be no particular work implications. The second acute hyperglycaemic emergency was formerly known as 'hyperosmolar non-ketotic coma' (HNK), but the term 'hyperosmolar hyperglycaemic state' (HHS) is now preferred. It usually occurs in older type 2 patients, and may be initiated by infection or diuretic treatment. Patients become severely dehydrated but not ketotic, and vigorous fluid replacement is needed. HHS is relatively uncommon, but has a higher potential mortality than DKA, usually due to thrombotic complications.

Diabetic hypoglycaemia

Hypoglycaemia can result from both insulin and sulphonylurea drugs, though insulin is the major cause.[29,53] Symptoms include sweating, tremor, nausea, palpitations, confusion and clouded consciousness. Symptoms begin usually as levels fall below 3.5 mmol/L, and if unrecognized and untreated, coma may result as blood glucose falls below 2.0 mmol/L. Most hypoglycaemic events are 'mild', in that they are recognized and reversed by the patient. 'Severe' episodes require external (third-party) help, and make up less than 5 per cent of all hypoglycaemic events.[53] A particular risk factor for severe hypoglycaemia is 'hypoglycaemic unawareness', which means a lack of, or significant reduction in symptoms of impending hypoglycaemia.[54] This can occur with advanced duration of disease in type 1 diabetes, or when autonomic neuropathy exists. Also, a series of hypoglycaemic attacks can lead to reduced warnings, though this can be treated by temporarily relaxing control (and abolishing hypoglycaemia) for a while, following which warnings usually return.

Hypoglycaemia clearly has implications for safe working, particularly if work involves potentially hazardous situations, for example, driving, working with machinery, emergency or armed services. For driving in the UK, the DVLA runs its own surveillance system for insulin-treated diabetic drivers, with a 3-yearly licence renewal system. Though clearly of importance in the workplace, there is evidence that hypoglycaemia in the workplace is uncommon,[55] and most attacks occur out of work, rather than in work.

Diabetes, pregnancy, and employment

Pregnancy and diabetes occur in three different contexts:

- ◆ Pregnancy in a woman with pre-existing type 1 diabetes.
- ◆ Pregnancy in a woman with pre-existing type 2 diabetes.
- ◆ Diabetes diagnosed during pregnancy, and usually remitting afterwards ('gestational diabetes').

With the continuing occurrence of type 2 diabetes at younger ages, the second of the list is occurring more frequently. Though insulin treatment in type 2 and gestational diabetic pregnancies remains common, there is now good evidence that some oral agents can be safely used in pregnancy—notably metformin.[56] Regardless of treatment modality, there is well-established evidence that tight glycaemic control reduces pregnancy-associated complications to both the mother and child. Care is normally by a joint diabetes/obstetric team, frequent self-monitoring of blood glucose is required, and intensive (four times daily) insulin regimens are generally used.

Pregnant diabetic women are generally young, well-motivated, and usually free of comorbidity and present few employment problems. However, their tight glucose control means that there is an increased hypoglycaemic risk, though this is rarely a major problem because of the intensive support, education and surveillance received and their compliance and motivation.

Women with gestational diabetes who are treated with insulin for the first time need particular education and support, and (in the UK), if they hold a driving licence they must inform the DVLA. This may occasionally have employment implications.

Pensions, insurance, advisory services, etc.

Intensive insulin therapy is often associated with an increase in hypoglycaemic episodes, and this may have employment implications, depending on the occupation. Such 'hypos', however, are usually mild (i.e. self-correctable). In a study of diabetic patients treated with either two or four daily insulin injections, there was no significant difference between those on two or four insulin injections and the occurrence of severe hypoglycaemia (needing third-party assistance for correction).[57]

Pension schemes

In the past, difficulty in arranging associated life insurance had sometimes been given as a reason for not employing those with diabetes. The attitude of different insurance companies to diabetes has varied considerably.[58] Diabetes UK can give useful advice on insurance matters. An employer must not discriminate against a disabled person in the opportunities it affords him for receiving pension or insurance-related benefits, or by refusing him, or deliberately not affording him, any such opportunity. Pension scheme trustees and insurance providers also have responsibilities under the Equality Act 2010.

Diabetes in employer-sponsored health insurance

Healthcare expenditure has been shown to be higher for those with diabetes when compared to all healthcare consumers. Such reports require to be carefully interpreted, as when compared with individuals with other chronic diseases (heart disease, HIV/AIDS, cancer, and asthma) people with diabetes were not more expensive for employers' insurance plans.[59]

Advisory services

The diabetic specialist, family practitioner, and occupational health service should be able to give advice in cases of employment difficulty. The diabetes specialist and/or family practitioner can provide detailed medical information, while the occupational physician is best placed to assess the suitability for a particular occupation. For especially difficult decisions, the combined opinions of specialists in diabetes and occupational medicine are particularly useful.

Disability employment advisers based at Department for Work and Pensions Job Centres can advise and help anyone with diabetes and disabilities affecting their work to find or keep suitable employment. Careers officers and teachers should also be able to advise diabetic school leavers. Diabetes UK is a comprehensive source of information.

Guidelines for employment

Diabetes UK and the American Diabetes Association publish guidance for employers and occupational health services.[60]

Guidelines on recruiting insulin-treated diabetic applicants to occupations are usually fairly clear; but the situation is often unclear when someone already in employment develops insulin-requiring diabetes. The case with fire fighters has already been mentioned and the approach of individual assessment is increasingly being applied elsewhere (e.g. police, armed forces, etc.). However, though employment may be continued, the nature of the job may alter; for example, in the police force new diabetic personnel on insulin treatment may not necessarily lose their jobs but there will be restrictions (e.g. driving at high speed and membership of armed response units may be allowed based on individual assessment).

Conclusions and recommendations

A few studies of employment and diabetes in the UK[47,49,50] indicate some increase in sickness absence. Recent research on the impact of hypoglycaemia at work indicated that severe hypoglycaemia was uncommon. Serious morbidity including accidents or injuries associated with hypoglycaemia at work was very uncommon. Information is still needed on the impact of particular work activities on diabetic control, especially shift work and vocational driving. Because of the paucity of definitive information, the advice given to diabetic workers is often arbitrary and employment decisions are taken with little supporting evidence. Physicians should take care to inform employers and potential employers factually about diabetes and to dispel any prejudice that might exist.

The introduction of self-testing and modern systems of treatment have enabled those with diabetes to cope more easily with irregular work patterns. Careers officers and teachers need to know more about diabetes, so that they can give school-leavers accurate advice and enable them to make sensible career plans. A sustained effort is required to educate employers and persuade them to take a more objective view of diabetic workers.

It is essential that each individual case be assessed on its own merits with full consultation between all medical advisers. Diabetes per se should not limit employment prospects, for the majority with diabetes have few, if any, problems arising from the condition and make perfectly satisfactory employees in a wide variety of occupations.

Considerable improvements in the treatment of people with type 1 and type 2 diabetes have occurred in the past few years. These improvements are associated with better quality of life and reductions in the incidence of long-term complications. Over time these will lead to longer, healthier working lives for people with diabetes. There is also evidence that those with severe renal complications can benefit from advances in transplant surgery and have improved quality of life and ability to work. Finally, rapidly progressing transplant technology (notably islet cell transplants) may begin to deliver a true 'cure' for diabetes (at least type 1) in the not too distant future.

Endocrine disorders

Other endocrine diseases are less common than diabetes, and have less potential impact on employment. Decisions on this should be made on an individual basis. Once the specific endocrine disorder is either cured, or is stable on treatment, there are not usually any work-related issues. If the condition has caused an impairment it will be considered a disability even if treatment cures or stabilizes the condition. Where a cure occurs surgically, this may be considered a past disability, time limited from the start of impairment to the curative surgery.

Hyperthyroidism

This is usually auto-immune mediated (Grave's disease) and is more common in young or middle-aged women. Presenting symptoms include sweating, tremor, weight loss, palpitations, and diarrhoea. In older patients, there may be little or no symptoms ('apathetic thyrotoxicosis'). Treatment is with either antithyroid drugs (usually carbimazole), radioiodine or thyroidectomy. A period off work at presentation may be needed, but there are usually no long-term implications.

Hypothyroidism

Underactivity (usually autoimmune) of the thyroid gland is common, and as biochemical thyroid function tests are now very frequently undertaken, hypothyroidism is often picked up at an early or even asymptomatic phase. Established symptoms include fatigue, lethargy, weight gain, depression, constipation, dry skin and dry hair. Treatment is with long-term thyroxine replacement.

Thyroid eye disease

Dysthyroid eye disease is most commonly associated with toxic Grave's disease, but it can occur with hypothyroidism, or even in the euthyroid state. Clinical features can vary from mild conjunctivitis and/or periorbital oedema, to severe strabismus or sight-threatening proptosis. Specialist treatment is required, which may require drugs, radiotherapy, or surgery. In its severe forms, dysthyroid eye disease can have employment implications, depending on the particular occupation.[61]

Pituitary disease

There is a wide spectrum of pituitary disease, which can be classified as follows:

- *Overproduction syndromes*: usually due to functioning adenomas producing, for example, adrenocorticotropic hormone (ACTH; Cushing's syndrome), growth hormone (GH; acromegaly), and prolactin (prolactinoma).

- *Underproduction syndromes*: which can affect any hormone but follicle-stimulating hormone (FSH)/luteinizing hormone (LH), ACTH, and GH are the most common.

- *Posterior pituitary syndromes*: usually antidiuretic hormone deficiency (diabetes insipidus), which can be idiopathic or related to tumours or head injury.

- *Non-functioning adenomas*: which are usually discovered incidentally, and investigations show normal pituitary hormonal function. They may though present with intracranial pressure symptoms causing visual field defects.

Symptomatology can vary enormously, and include the skeletal abnormalities of acromegaly, dramatic weight gain and myopathy in Cushing's syndrome, amenorrhoea and galactorrhoea in prolactinoma, and extreme polyuria in diabetes insipidus. Patients with non-functioning adenomas usually have no symptoms at all. Underproduction of pituitary hormones cause symptoms dependent on the hormone(s) involved; for example, FSH/LH deficiency may cause reduced libido and erectile dysfunction in men, and cause amenorrhoea or oligomenorrhoea in women. ACTH deficiency will cause features similar to Addison's disease. Deficiency of GH is increasingly being diagnosed and is no longer regarded as untreatable. Criteria for treatment are now well accepted,[62] and response to treatment can vary.

Employment implications with pituitary disease depend on the type of problem, severity of clinical features, and type of occupation. Most patients are able to work normally, but individual assessments may need to be made.[63] Visual function (in particular fields of vision) may need to be taken into account in patients with pituitary tumours, as if these extend supratentorially, they can compress the optic chiasm. This is usually recognized early, and treated before significant visual problems occur.

References

1 Alberti KGMM, Kaufman F, Zimmet P, *et al.* Type 2 diabetes in the young: the evolving epidemic. The International Diabetes Federation Consensus Workshop. *Diabetes Care* 2004; **27**: 1798–811.

2 Farmer A, Fox R. Diagnosis, classification and treatment of diabetes. *BMJ* 2011; **342**: d3319.

3 National Institute for Clinical Excellence (NICE). *Insulin pump therapy: guidance.* NICE Guidelines TA151. London: NICE, 2008.

4 Lawton J, Rankin D, Cooke DD, *et al.* Dose adjustment for normal eating (DAFNE): a qualitative longitudinal exploration of the food and eating practices of type 1 diabetes patients converted to flexible intensive insulin therapy in the UK. *Diab Res Clin Pract* 2011; **91**: 87–93.

5 Pickup J. Insulin pumps. *Int J Clin Pract* 2010; **166**(Suppl): 16–19.

6 Press M. The current status of pancreatic islet transplantation in Britain. *Pract Diab Int* 2008; **25**: 218–20.

7 World Health Organization (WHO). *Use of glycated haemoglobin (HbA$_{1c}$) in the diagnosis of diabetes.* Geneva: WHO, 2011.

8 Heianza Y, Hara S, Arase Y, *et al.* HbA$_{1c}$ 5.7–6.4% and impaired fasting plasma glucose for diagnosis of pre-diabetes and risk of progression to diabetes in Japan (TOPIC 3): a longitudinal cohort study. *Lancet* 2011; **378**: 147–55.

9 Tahrani AA, Bailey CJ, Prato SD, *et al.* Management of type 2 diabetes: new and future developments in treatment. *Lancet* 2011; **378**: 182–97.

10   The Equality Act 2010. (<http://www.legislation.gov.uk/ukpga/2010/15/contents>)

11   Diabetes UK. *Employment and diabetes. Your rights at work.* London: Diabetes UK, 2010 (<http://www.diabetes.org.uk/How_we_help/Advocacy/Advocacy-packs/Your-rights-at-work—discrimination-and-how-to-resolve-it/9>)

12   Ardran M, MacFarlane I, Robinson C. Educational achievements, employment and social class of insulin-dependent diabetics: a survey of a young adult clinic in Liverpool. *Diabet Med* 1987; **4**: 546–8.

13   Bergers J, Nijhuis F, Janssen M, *et al.* Employment careers of young type 1 diabetic patients in the Netherlands. *J Occup Environ Med* 1999; **41**(11): 1005–10.

14   Young J. *Diabetes shift work and employment.* MFOM dissertation, 2009.

15   Waclawski ER. Employment and diabetes: a survey of the prevalence of diabetic workers known by occupational physicians, and the restrictions placed on diabetic workers in employment. *Diabet Med* 1989; **6**: 16–19.

16   Ingberg CM, Palmer M, Aman J, *et al.* Social consequences of insulin-dependent diabetes mellitus are limited: a population-based comparison of young adult patients vs healthy controls. *Diabet Med* 1996; **13**(8): 729–33.

17   Patterson CC, Dahlquist GG, Gyurus E, *et al.* Incidence trends for childhood type 1 diabetes in Europe during 1989-2003 and predicted new cases 2005-20: a multicentre prospective registration study. *Lancet* 2009; **373**: 2027–33.

18   Holman N, Forouhi NG, Goyder E, *et al.* The Association of Public Health Observatories (APHO) diabetes prevalence model: estimates of total diabetes prevalence for England 2010-30. *Diabet Med* 2011; **28**: 575–82.

19   Mulnier HE, Seamen HE, Raleigh VS, *et al.* Mortality in people with type 2 diabetes in the UK. *Diabet Med* 2006; **23**: 516–21.

20   Secrest AM, LaPorte RE, Becker DJ, *et al.* All-cause mortality trends in a large population-based cohort with long-standing childhood type 1 diabetes. The Alleghenny County type 1 diabetes registry. *Diabetes Care* 2010; **33**: 2573–9.

21   Orchard TJ, Secrest AM, Miller RG, *et al.* In the absence of renal disease, 20 year mortality risk in type 1 diabetes is comparable to that of the general population: a report from the Pittsburgh Epidemiology of Diabetes Complications Study. *Diabetologia* 2010; **53**: 2312–19.

22   Abbott CA, Malik RA, van Ross ERE, *et al.* Prevalence and characteristics of painful diabetic neuropathy in a large community-based diabetes population in the UK. *Diabetes Care* **34**(10): 2220–2224.

23   Nathan DM, Zinman B, Cleary PA, *et al.* Modern-day clinical course of type 1 diabetes mellitus after 30 years' duration. The diabetes control and complications trial/epidemiology of diabetes interventions and complications and Pittsburgh epidemiology of diabetes complications experience (1983–2005). *Arch Intern Med* 2009; **169**: 1307–16.

24   Ogundipe OO, Geddes J, Leckie AM, *et al.* Impaired hypoglycaemia awareness and employment in people with type 1 diabetes. *Occup Med* 2011; **61**(4): 241–6.

25   Kivimaki M, Vahtera J, Pentti J, *et al.* Increased sickness absence in diabetic employees: what is the role of co-morbid conditions? *Diabet Med* 2007; **24**: 1043–8.

26   Andrews AC, Cooper AR, Montgmery AA, *et al.* Diet or diet plus physical activity versus usual care in patients with newly diagnosed type 2 diabetes: the early ACTID randomised controlled trial. *Lancet* 2011; **378**: 129–39.

27   Nathan DM, Buse JB, Davidson MB, *et al.* Medical management of hyperglycaemia in type 2 diabetes mellitus: a consensus algorithm for the initiation and adjustment of therapy. A consensus statement from the American Diabetes Association and the European Association for the Study of Diabetes. *Diabetologia* 2009; **52**: 17–30.

28   Kenny C. Pioglitazone—balancing risks and benefits. *Diabet Primary Care* 2011; **13**: 199–200.

29   Amiel SA, Dixon T, Mann R, *et al.* Hypoglycaemia in type 2 diabetes. *Diabet Med* 2008; **25**: 245–54.

30 Ashwell SG, Amiel SA, Bilous RW, *et al.* Improved glycaemic control with insulin glargine plus insulin lispro: multicentre, randomised, cross-over trial in people with type 1 diabetes. *Diabet Med* 2006; **23**: 285–92.

31 Holleman F, Gale EAM. Nice insulins, pity about the evidence. *Diabetologia* 2007; **50**: 1783–90.

32 Diabetes Control and Complications Trial (DCCT) Research Group. The effect of intensive treatment of diabetes on the development and progression of long-term complications in insulin-dependent diabetes mellitus. *New Engl J Med* 1993; **329**: 977–86.

33 United Kingdom Prospective Diabetes Study (UKPDS) Group. Intensive blood glucose control with sulphonylureas or insulin compared with conventional treatment and risk of complications in patients with type 2 diabetes (UKPDS 33). *Lancet* 1998; **352**: 854–65.

34 The Action to Control Cardiovascular Risk in Diabetes (ACCORD) Study Group. Effect of intensive glucose lowering in type 2 diabetes. *N Engl J Med* 2008; **358**: 2545–59.

35 The ADVANCE Collaborative Group. Intensive blood glucose control and vascular outcome in patients with type 2 diabetes. *N Engl J Med* 2008; **358**: 2560–72.

36 Currie CJ, Peters JR, Tynan A, *et al.* Survival as a function of HbA$_{1c}$ in people with type 2 diabetes: a retrospective cohort study. *Lancet* 2010; **375**: 481–9.

37 Lachim JM. Intensive glycaemic control and mortality in ACCORD—a chance finding? *Diabetes Care* 2010; **33**: 2719–21.

38 Frier BM, Schernthaner G, Heller SR. Hypoglycaemia and cardiovascular risks. *Diabetes Care* 2011; **34**: S132–S137.

39 National Institute for Clinical Excellence (NICE). *Type 2 diabetes: the management of type 2 diabetes.* NICE clinical guideline 87. London: NICE, 2009.

40 Yudkin JS, Richter B, Gale EAM. Intensified glucose lowering in type 2 diabetes: time for a reappraisal. *Diabetologia* 2010: **53**: 2079–85.

41 Parati G, Bilo G, Ochoa JE. Benefits of tight blood pressure control in diabetic patients with hypertension. *Diabetes Care* 2011; **34**: S297–S303.

42 Collins R, Armitage J, Parish S, *et al.* for the Heart Protection Study (HPS) Collaboration Group. MRC/BHF Heart Protection Study of cholesterol-lowering with simvastatin in 5963 people with diabetes: a randomised placebo-controlled trial. *Lancet* 2003; **361**: 2005–16.

43 Drivers Medical Group. *At a glance guide to the current medical standards of fitness to drive.* Swansea: DVLA, 2011.

44 Diabetes UK. *Employment and diabetes.* London: Diabetes UK, 2010. (<https://www.diabetes.org.uk/upload/How%20we%20help/catalogue/Employment%20and%20diabetes_FINAL_171110.pdf>)

45 Stahl M, Berger W. Higher incidence of severe hypoglycaemia leading to hospital admission in type 2 diabetic patients treated with long-acting versus short-acting sulphonylureas. *Diabet Med* 1999; **16**: 586–90.

46 Waclawski ER. *Diabetes and employment.* MFOM Thesis, Faculty of Occupational Medicine, Royal College of Physicians, 1989.

47 Robinson N, Yateman NA, Protopapa LE, *et al.* Employment problems and diabetes. *Diabet Med* 1990; **7**: 16–22.

48 Griffiths RD, Moses RG. Diabetes in the workplace. Employment experience of young people with diabetes mellitus. *Med J Aust* 1993; **158**: 169–71.

49 Poole CJ, Gibbons D, Calvert IA. Sickness absence in diabetic employees at a large engineering factory. *Occup Environ Med* 1994; **51**: 299–301.

50 Waclawski ER. Sickness absence among insulin-treated diabetic employees. *Diabet Med* 1990; **7**: 41–4.

51 Skerjanc A. Sickness absence in diabetic employees. *Occup Environ Med* 2001; **58**(7): 432–6.

52 The Working Time Regulations 1998, No. 1833. (<http://www.legislation.gov.uk/uksi/1998/1833/contents/made>)

53 Donnelly LA, Morris AD, Frier BM, *et al.* Frequency and predictors of hypoglycaemia in type 1 and insulin-treated type 2 diabetes in a population-based study. *Diabet Med* 2005; **22**: 749–55.

54 Elliott J, Heller S. Hypoglycaemia unawareness. *Practical Diabetes* 2011; **28**: 227–32.

55 Leckie AM, Ritchie PJ, Graham MK, *et al.* Frequency, severity and morbidity of hypoglycaemia in the workplace in people with insulin-treated diabetes. *Diabetes Care* 2005; **28**: 1333–8.

56 Bolani J, Hyer SL, Rodin DA, *et al.* Pregnancy outcomes in women with gestational diabetes treated with metformin or insulin: a case-control study. *Diabet Med* 2009; **26**: 798–802.

57 Nachum Z, Ben-Shlomo I, Weiner E, *et al.* Twice daily versus four times daily insulin dose regimens for diabetes in pregnancy: randomised controlled trial. *BMJ* 1999; **319**: 1223–7.

58 Jones KE, Gill GV. Insurance company attitudes to diabetes. *Pract Diabetes* 1989; **6**: 230–1.

59 Peele PB, Lave JR, Songer TJ. Diabetes in employer-sponsored health insurance. *Diabetes Care* 2002; **25**(11): 1964–8.

60 American Diabetes Association. Hypoglycaemia and employment/licensure. *Diabetes Care* 2011; **34**(Suppl. 1): S82–S86.

61 Ponto KA, Pitz S, Pfeiffer N, *et al.* Quality of life and occupational disability in endocrine orbitopathy. *Dtsch Arztebl Int* 2009; **106**: 283–9.

62 National Institute for Clinical Excellence (NICE). *Human growth hormone (somatotropin) in adults with growth hormone deficiency.* NICE Technology Appraisal 64. London: NICE, 2003.

63 Milosevic P, Waclawski E, Sainsbury C. *Shift work and endocrine conditions—pilot feasibility study.* Annual Scientific Meeting, Society of Occupational Medicine, Edinburgh, June 2010.

Chapter 16

Haematological disorders

Julia Smedley and Richard S. Kaczmarski

Introduction

Few haematological disorders are caused or exacerbated by work. However, they may affect an employee's capacity to work. Mild haematological derangements (e.g. iron deficiency anaemia, anticoagulant treatment) are common, but have only minor implications for employment. Conversely, genetic and malignant haematological diseases, although comparatively uncommon, are complex and affect young people of working age. Malignant disease has a profound impact on work capability during the treatment and early recovery phases. However, advances in clinical management achieve a much greater potential for return to work during treatment, and a growing population of survivors in whom it is important to address employment issues.

The evidence base contains little research about fitness for work related to haematological disease, functional rehabilitation, or prevalence rates for specific disorders in the working population. The likelihood of an occupational physician encountering haematological disease in fitness for work assessments is therefore based on occurrence in the general population and this chapter relies primarily on traditional textbook teaching, and recent reviews of advances in clinical management.

It contains brief summaries of the more common haematological disorders that an occupational physician might encounter when advising about fitness for work. The major determinants of functional capacity are similar for many haematological conditions. In order to avoid repetition the common treatments, complications and symptoms are covered under 'Generic issues'.

Haemoglobinopathies

Sickle cell disease

Epidemiology and clinical features

Sickle cell disease (SCD) is a collection of inherited disorders characterized by the presence of abnormal haemoglobin (HbS).[1] Homozygous sickle cell anaemia (HbSS) is the most common, but the doubly heterozygote conditions with haemoglobin C and beta thalassaemia respectively (HbSC and HbSβthal) also cause sickling disease. The disorders are common in West Africa, the Middle East, and parts of the Indian subcontinent, and have become established through migration in northern Europe and North America. It has been estimated that 12 000 people in the UK have SCD. Occupational physicians working in London, the West Midlands, and Yorkshire might see a few cases annually. However, outside these areas the condition will be encountered rarely. The clinical features arise from the sickle-shaped deformation of red blood cells, due to crystallization of HbS at low oxygen concentrations. This causes chronic anaemia through reduced red

Box 16.1 Organs and systems affected by sickle cell disease

- Spleen (splenic infarcts leading to auto-splenectomy).
- Bones and joints (bone infarcts, avascular necrosis particularly of the hip and shoulders, osteomyelitis, and arthritis).
- Kidney (renal acidosis and glomerular sclerosis leading to renal failure).
- Brain and spinal cord (stroke and cognitive impairment).
- Eye (retinal infarcts and haemorrhages, retinal detachment, and central retinal artery occlusion).
- Lungs (acute lung syndrome, interstitial fibrosis, and pulmonary hypertension).
- Skin (leg ulcers).
- Gall bladder (pigment gall stones).
- Blood (anaemia).

cell survival (haemoglobin 7–9 g/dL) and episodes of vascular and microvascular obstruction. Patients develop both acute 'crises' (vaso-occlusive/painful, aplastic or haemolytic) and insidious multisystem damage from repeated infarction. Box 16.1 shows the wide range of end-organ effects.

Recent advances

Modern management of SCD has dramatically increased life and work expectancy (from 14 years in the early 1970s to 50 years in 2003). Consequently more SCD patients are likely to be working than in previous decades. Newer treatments include hydroxyurea, which increases the production of foetal haemoglobin which inhibits HbS polymerization. Patients are monitored regularly to detect end-organ damage and facilitate early intervention. Transfusion therapy may be indicated where continuing organ damage is detected. Laser therapy reduces the complications of proliferative retinopathy. Joint replacement may be indicated for patients with severe joint disease. Allogeneic (from the bone marrow of a matched donor) stem cell transplantation (SCT) is undertaken for the most severely affected individuals and this offers a definitive cure, but has long-term consequences.

Functional limitations in sickle cell disease

Fitness for work varies markedly, and adjustments must be based on an individual functional assessment. Severely affected patients are unlikely to be fit for work, but moderately and mildly affected individuals should have reasonable work capacity. The main functional issues are listed in Box 16.2. Anaemia is usually well tolerated by SCD patients at low haemoglobin levels (down to 7 g/dL) compared with other causes of anaemia. Poor performance at work might be due to a number of factors, including cerebral infarctions or untreated depression which is common in patients with moderate to severe disease. Therefore, it is particularly important to make a careful assessment, liaising with the treating clinician to arrange cognitive screening, magnetic resonance imaging, and therapeutic review where appropriate. The effects of chronic transfusion are considered under 'Generic issues'. Despite the need for opiate analgesia in severe painful crises, the incidence of drug dependence is very low.

Box 16.2 Potential functional and occupational restrictions in sickle cell disease

- Impaired exercise tolerance (anaemia, pulmonary hypertension).
- Reduced mobility (bone/joint disease, stroke).
- Impaired visual acuity (retinopathy).
- Decreased performance (cognitive impairment due to cerebrovascular events, depression, chronic pain).
- Susceptibility to infection (impaired white cell function, hyposplenism, post bone marrow transplant).
- Infectious carriage of blood-borne viruses.
- Frequent absence from work (painful crises, complications of chronic organ failure).

Adjustments to work

Employees must avoid working environments with extremes of temperature and have access to drinking water to manage hydration. If mobility or exercise tolerance is seriously impaired consideration is required over improved access to work (ramps or lifts) and reducing physically demanding work. Adjustments for visually impaired employees are covered in Chapter 9. Particular care should be taken in jobs that expose the individual to risk of infection, to ensure that prophylactic antibiotics and pneumococcal vaccine are given. Travel requirements should be carefully considered, including access to medical care and safe blood for transfusion in the event of a sickle crisis abroad. Commercial air passenger travel is safe, but special care should be taken to ensure adequate hydration on long haul flights. During pregnancy there is a higher incidence of gestational hypertension, pre-term birth and small for gestational age infants. A lower threshold for recommending abstention from work during pregnancy should be adopted, but close liaison with the responsible clinicians is strongly recommended. Some occupations are contraindicated for individuals with HbSS. Jobs that are physically demanding, or which have a risk of exposure to severe extremes of heat, cold, dehydration or hypoxia (e.g. foundry work, diving, compressed air work, armed forces) are unsuitable. Joint Aviation Authority (JAA) standards on fitness for work exclude individuals with SCD from certification as flight crew on civil aircraft.[2]

Pre-employment assessment

Pre-employment assessment raises important questions about the disclosure of a tendency for high rates of absence. The possibility of frequent absence should be based on clinical history and previous absence record. An individual with homozygous SCD is likely to fulfil the definition of disability under the Equality Act, and the prospective employer should consider reasonable adjustments such as allowing a higher level of absence and attendance for healthcare appointments etc.

Sickle cell trait

Heterozygotes for sickle haemoglobin (HbAS) have no clinical anaemia. There are no employment consequences other than restriction of activities that are associated with a risk of severe hypoxia (diving, compressed air work, or work at altitude above 12 000 feet). Certification for civil air-crew would be granted.

Thalassaemia

Epidemiology and clinical features

The thalassaemias are a heterogeneous group of genetic disorders of haemoglobin synthesis. They are most common in the Mediterranean countries, the Middle East, India, and South-east Asia, but occur sporadically in all populations. Thalassaemia is rare in the UK (800 cases). The common features are anaemia and splenomegaly. Individuals with homozygous beta thalassaemia (thalassaemia major) have severe transfusion-dependent anaemia. They can develop complications of iron overload (cardiomyopathy, liver failure, and endocrine failure including diabetes mellitus) by teenage years. Even with careful management of iron over-load with chelation therapy, life expectancy in thalassaemia major is 20–30 years. However, milder forms of the disease (thalassaemia intermedia) require transfusion less frequently. In heterozygous beta thalassaemia (β thalassaemia trait) anaemia is asymptomatic (haemoglobin levels usually >9 g/dl).

Recent advances

Genetic screening has reduced the overall incidence of thalassaemia in the UK, so fewer cases are encountered in the workplace. SCT offers a cure, but introduces other implications for work.

Functional limitations in thalassaemia

With good medical management patients with thalassaemia major are able to function normally in education and employment with allowance for hospital attendance but when complications arise there are likely to be severe limitations for work. Other variants of thalassaemia and interactions with other structural haemoglobin abnormalities (e.g. haemoglobin E/β thalassaemia) cause a range of clinical manifestations. Functional impairment is related to the degree of anaemia and haemoglobin levels are usually kept at 9–10 g/dL in transfusion dependent patients. A checklist of the limitations on fitness for work is shown in Box 16.3.

Adjustments to work in thalassaemia

The main aim is to match the physical job requirements to fatigue and impaired exercise toler-ance. Care should be taken in jobs that might expose individuals to infection due to increased susceptibility. Infection with blood-borne viruses secondary to treatment is important only

---

Box 16.3 Potential functional and occupational limitations in thalassaemia

- Reduced capacity for physical work (impaired exercise tolerance due to anaemia, cardiac failure, small stature due to endocrine complications, hypothyroidism, osteoporosis bone pain, and fractures due to hypoparathyroidism).
- Increased susceptibility to infection (splenectomy, diabetes mellitus, bone marrow trans-plantation).
- Infectious carriage of blood-borne viruses (secondary to transfusion).
- Requirement for iron chelation.

where infection might be passed to others because of the nature of the work, for example, health-care workers undertaking exposure prone procedures. Adjustments for those on chelation therapy are covered in 'Repeated transfusion'. Thalassaemia major would disqualify patients from work as commercial air-crew, but those with thalassaemia minor would be considered on an individual basis, provided full functional capacity is demonstrated.

Immune cytopaenias (AIHA, ITP)

Immune-related cytopenias, autoimmune haemolytic anaemia (AIHA), idiopathic thrombocy-topenia (ITP), and more rarely autoimmune neutropenia can occur as primary haematological disorders, secondary to infections, drugs or underlying malignancies, or in association with other autoimmune conditions (systemic lupus erythematosus, rheumatoid arthritis, etc.). These conditions occur at all ages and may be an isolated event or run a chronic or relapsing—remitting course. Mild cases are asymptomatic, often picked up during health screening.

AIHA presents with anaemia and jaundice. Chronic cases are prone to gall stones. Management is supportive, with blood transfusion and folic acid. Severe ITP presents with bruising and mucosal bleeding. Despite platelet counts less than 10×10^9/L, the risk of haemorrhagic death is very low. Treatment is rarely indicated with platelet count greater than 50×10^9/L. Treatments for ITP and AIHA include steroids and intravenous immunoglobulin (IVIG) in acute conditions. However, the monoclonal antibody rituximab, other immune suppression and splenectomy may be indicated in refractory, chronic, and frequently relapsing cases. A new class of thrombopoietic stimulating agents (thrombopoietin receptor agonists) have become available to treat patients with refractory ITP.

Coagulation disorders

Therapeutic anticoagulation

Treatment with coumarin anticoagulants and antiplatelet drugs is common and it is estimated that 500 000 people in the UK take warfarin. Overall functional impairment is more likely to relate to the underlying disorder than anticoagulant therapy. Increased bleeding tendency varies between individuals, but is proportional to the anticoagulant effect, measured by the international normalized ratio (INR). For most indications (venous thromboembolism, atrial fibrillation, cardiac mural thrombosis, cardiomyopathy, and prior to cardioversion) the target INR is 2.5, but for mechanical heart valve prostheses, antiphospholipid syndrome and recurrent venous thromboembolism while on warfarin, the target INR may be up to 3.5. The majority of patients with bioprosthetic valves do not require lifelong anticoagulation. Advances in treatment include self-management of anticoagulant therapy using near patient devices (portable coagulometers). New direct thrombin inhibitors eliminate the need for anticoagulant monitoring and are currently licensed for thromboprophylaxis post hip and knee surgery and selected risk groups of patients with atrial fibrillation. The risk of bleeding while on oral anticoagulants increases significantly with INR greater than 4.5; however, bleeding risk is low in well-controlled patients. Therefore employees on therapeutic anticoagulation can work normally and adjustments are not necessary unless anticoagulant control is erratic. *Extremely* heavy physical work or work where there is an *extremely* high risk of cuts or trauma should be avoided. Warfarin treatment currently excludes firefighters from active duty and non-marine crew from working in an offshore environment, due to the risk of injury and serious bleeds.

Antiplatelet therapy with aspirin has no important implications for work fitness.

Inherited clotting disorders: haemophilia and von Willebrand's disease

Epidemiology and clinical features

Haemophilia A is the most common of the hereditary clotting factor deficiencies (prevalence 30–100 per million). This sex-linked disorder results in deficiency of factor VIII (FVIII) of the clotting cascade. FVIII levels below 1 per cent (0.01U/mL) are associated with severe bleeding tendency, but above 5 per cent FVIII the clinical syndrome is mild. Symptoms include haemarthrosis, usually in the large weight-bearing joints (knees, ankles, and hips), muscle haematomas, less commonly haematuria, and rarely intracranial bleeds. Parenteral FVIII is indicated for prophylaxis and management of bleeding episodes. A FVIII level of 30 per cent of normal activity is required for haemostasis, but spontaneous bleeding is usually prevented at levels over 20 per cent. Long-term sequelae include the development of FVIII antibodies (inhibitors) in 10–15 per cent of patients, and degenerative joint disease resulting from repeated haemarthrosis.

Haemophilia B (hereditary Factor IX deficiency) is clinically similar to haemophilia A, but is treated with FIX replacement. Von Willebrand's disease differs from classical haemophilia in its autosomal inheritance, and bleeding tends to be mucocutaneous (epistaxis, gastrointestinal, cutaneous bruising) rather than into joints and muscle. Treatment of von Willebrand's disease is with desmopressin (DDAVP) or concentrates of von Willebrand factor (blood glycoprotein involved in hemostasis) and FVIII.

Recent advances

Improvements in blood products safety, in particular the production of recombinant clotting factors (see 'Multiple transfusion'), has removed the risk of HIV and hepatitis C although the uncertainty of new variant Creutzfeld–Jakob disease (nvCJD) with plasma products remains a concern. Consequently, young haemophiliacs currently entering higher education and employment are rarely infected with blood-borne viruses. It is hoped that gene therapy will cure these conditions in the future.

Functional limitations in haemophilia

Limitations (Box 16.4) relate mainly to the risk of acute joint bleeds, and longer-term degenerative joint disease. The former precludes physically strenuous work, although the risk of bleeding can usually be controlled in all but the most severe cases by regular factor replacement.

Adjustments to work in haemophilia

Adjustments (Box 16.5) will depend entirely on the severity of the bleeding disorder. Patients with mild haemophilia can work normally in any job. Even with severe FVIII deficiency (below 1 per cent) some patients have very infrequent bleeds, and few if any adjustments to work will be required. Work that is very heavy physically or associated with a high risk of injury is

---

Box 16.4 Potential functional limitations in haemophilia

- Impaired tolerance of extremely heavy physical work (risk of bleeding into muscles or weight-bearing joints).
- Impaired mobility (degenerative joint disease).
- Infectious carriage of blood-borne viruses.

Box 16.5 Adjustments to work in haemophilia

◆ Provide facilities for self-treatment.

◆ Avoidance of extremely heavy physical work or work with a high risk of injury.

◆ Improved access to work and sedentary work if mobility restricted.

◆ Extreme care with foreign travel. Avoid remote areas with poor medical facilities.

contraindicated in those with frequent large joint bleeds. Examples include mining, heavy construction, armed forces, firefighting, and the police service. Healthcare workers who undertake exposure prone procedures should be screened for blood-borne viruses. Special care is needed if an individual is required to travel for work, or to work in isolation. Arrangements for the safe storage of factor replacement, and access to sterile distilled water (diluent), needles, syringes, and other equipment for administration are needed. Some freeze-dried concentrates of factors VIII and IX can be stored at room temperature (up to 25°C or 77°F) for up to 6 months, but general advice is to keep all products in a refrigerator at 2–8°C (36–46° F). Documentation may be required by customs to carry medical equipment, and it is essential that appropriate insurance covers haemophilia-related complications. Work in very remote areas with poor hygiene arrangements or medical facilities, is contraindicated, except for very mild cases that are unlikely to require replacement therapy. Significantly affected haemophiliacs would be excluded from certification as commercial air crew, but very mildly affected cases might be considered on an individual basis provided there was no history of significant bleeding.[3]

Thrombophilia

The annual incidence of venous thromboembolic disease (VTE) is 1–3 per 1000. Deep vein thrombosis (DVT) and pulmonary embolism (PE) are most common, but other sites (upper limbs, liver, cerebral sinus, retina, and mesenteric veins) are affected infrequently. VTE causes significant mortality and morbidity: 1–2 per cent of patients will die of PE and up to 20 per cent of patients are debilitated by post-thrombotic syndrome (chronic leg oedema, varicose veins, and venous ulceration). Risk factors include inherited and acquired medical conditions, and external factors (Table 16.1).

The pathogenesis and risk factors for VTE and arterial thrombosis are distinctly different. In VTE age is the greatest risk factor, and stasis, immobilization, and prothrombotic abnormalities are common. Atheroma, smoking, hypertension, or hypercholesterolaemia do not increase the risk of VTE.[4,5]

The majority of cases of VTE are managed initially with low-molecular-weight heparin (LMWH) followed by warfarin. LMWH can be administered out of hospital without the need for blood monitoring. The duration of anticoagulation (3 months to lifelong) depends on severity of the event and predisposing factors. Asymptomatic family members who carry genetic mutations that confer an increased thrombotic risk require counselling about risk factors, especially enforced immobility, and advice on appropriate preventive measures. VTE is associated with long-haul (>3000 miles) air travel. This risk is likely to be significantly increased in patients with a thrombophilic tendency. It is good practice for all long-haul passengers to exercise during flight, walk around, maintain a good fluid intake, and limit alcohol consumption. Graduated compression stockings may also be worn. For 'high-risk' patients, a single prophylactic dose of LMWH may be given.

Table 16.1 Risk factors for venous thromboembolic disease

Inherited	Acquired	External
• Antithrombin deficiency (ATIII)	• Age	• Immobilization
• Protein C (PC) deficiency	• Previous venous thromboembolism	• Surgery and trauma
• Protein S (PS) deficiency		• Oral contraceptives
• Factor V Leiden (FVL)	• Malignancy	• Hormone replacement therapy
• Prothrombin 20210A	• Polycythaemia	
• Dysfibrinogenaemia	• Essential thrombocytosis	
• Elevated FVIII, IX, XI	• Paroxysmal nocturnal haemoglobinuria (PNH)	
	• Pregnancy	
	• Antiphospholipid syndrome	

There are significant issues for employment in thrombophilic patients. Patients who have suffered DVT or PE may have reduced exercise capacity, mobility and pain. Post-phlebitic limb and cardiac problems due to pulmonary hypertension may develop many years following the original event. Patients, and known carriers of risk factors, in sedentary jobs should be encouraged to mobilize frequently. Appropriate precautions should be taken during long-haul travel. Thrombophilias associated with a significant history of clotting would exclude certification as civil air crew. Because of the low incidence of a genetic predisposition to VTE, screening of frequent long-haul occupational travellers is not indicated.

Malignant haematological disorders

Epidemiology

Haematological malignancies, although individually rare, comprise 8–10 per cent of all cancers in the UK (Table 16.2).

This heterogeneous group ranges from acute leukaemias, which may be rapidly fatal, to chronic conditions for which no intervention is required. They are characterized by impairment of bone marrow (BM) function and immunity. Although many are aggressive, some have the highest cure rates among all malignant disorders.

Clinical features and recent advances

Acute leukaemias

Acute lymphoblastic leukaemia (ALL) is the commonest malignancy in children. Cure rates are above 80 per cent. Craniospinal radiotherapy is given only to poor-risk patients rather than routinely, and boys are now treated for 3 years to prevent testicular relapse. BM transplantation (BMT) would only be considered for children with poor risk or relapsed disease. Children treated with standard chemotherapy regimens, who did not receive radiotherapy, are considered cured after 10 years. Thus the majority of long-term survivors of childhood ALL entering working life will not require continuing medical care. For those who received radiation, follow up would

Table 16.2 Epidemiology of haematological malignancies

Disease	Number of cases/year (UK)	Median age at onset
Childhood acute lymphoblastic leukaemia	450	3–7
Adult acute lymphoblastic leukaemia	200	55
Childhood acute myeloblastic leukaemia	50	2
Adult acute myeloblastic leukaemia	1950	65
Non-Hodgkin lymphoma	8450	65
Hodgkin disease	1400	30
Chronic lymphocytic leukaemia	2750	66
Chronic myeloid leukaemia	750	50
Myelodysplastic syndrome	3250	70
Myeloma	3300	65

continue in view of late side-effects. For ALL presenting in adulthood, the prognosis is markedly worse (5-year survival 30–35 per cent). Transplantation is therefore a first-line option for many patients. Because craniospinal radiotherapy is integral to the regimen, adult survivors of ALL are more likely to have co-morbidities such as cognitive impairment, leucoencephalopathy, cataracts and secondary tumours and will require long-term follow-up.

Acute myeloid leukaemia (AML) is predominantly a disease of adults. A steady improvement in survival in patients up to age 60 has occurred with intensification of treatment over the last 25 years. Transplantation is reserved for intermediate/poor risk patients (see 'Stem cell transplantation' below). Overall 5-year survival is 40 per cent (range 17–73 per cent) in adults and 67 per cent in children. Standard treatment involves 4-5 courses of intensive multidrug chemotherapy with prolonged hospitalization. Patients are unable to work during this period, which usually lasts 6–8 months and full recovery from the effects of treatment can take up to 1 year. When the disease is in remission patients are able to return to work and lead normal lives. Some have residual treatment-related problems, including incomplete recovery of blood counts with consequent anaemia, infection or bleeding risk, and respiratory, cardiac, or renal dysfunction.

Chronic leukaemias

The incidence of *chronic lymphocytic leukaemia* (CLL) appears to be increasing, with involvement of younger patients. However, the increased availability of blood counts (e.g. health screening) has promoted earlier diagnosis. The disease often runs a benign course, and no survival advantage is gained from earlier intervention. Indications for treatment include symptoms of sweating, fever, weight loss, anaemia or thrombocytopenia, or rapidly rising lymphocyte count. Patients with CLL require long-term follow-up. All are immunocompromised and require influenza and pneumococcal vaccines. Some patients, particularly those with underlying chronic pulmonary disease, may benefit from immunoglobulin therapy. CLL remains incurable with conventional treatment. Standard regimes combine fludarabine and cyclophosphamide with the monoclonal antibody rituximab. Alternative combination chemotherapy and transplantation are available for patients with relapsed or poor-prognostic disease. Purine analogues and alemtuzumab produce profound immunosuppression through loss of T-cell-mediated immunity. Patients are susceptible to opportunistic infection including reactivation of cytomegalovirus and *Pneumocystis* (*carinii*) *jiroveci* pneumonia (PCP), and current guidelines recommend prophylaxis against *Pneumocystis jiroveci* for a year post treatment.

Chronic myeloid leukaemia (CML) occurs at all ages. Patients present with elevated white blood cell counts and splenomegaly. A new generation of drugs, tyrosine kinase inhibitors administered orally are now the treatment of choice in patients with chronic phase CML. Patients require outpatient monitoring during treatment but usually lead a normal life. Allogeneic transplantation which offers a cure is undertaken in patients intolerant or unresponsive to treatment.

The *myelodysplastic syndromes* (MDS) predominantly affect the elderly, but do occur in adults of working age, particularly where there has been prior exposure to chemo/radiotherapy. They are characterized by peripheral blood cytopenias and a risk of transformation to acute leukaemia. The only curative treatment is SCT (see 'Stem cell transplantation'). However, supportive care (blood transfusion and antibiotics for intercurrent infections) remains the treatment of choice for the majority. Transformation to acute leukaemia may be treated with intensive chemotherapy, but has a poor prognosis. The prognosis for MDS is very variable. Median survival varies from 67 (low risk) to 4 months (high risk). Low-risk patients may remain well, continue in work and require only occasional follow-up. However, those who are transfusion dependent require more frequent and prolonged hospital attendance and are unlikely to tolerate work. In older patients comorbidity, particularly chronic cardiac or respiratory disorders, may compound functional incapacity.

Myeloproliferative disorders: essential thrombocytosis (ET) and polycythaemia rubra Vera (PRV)

These conditions are characterized by increased production of one or more cell lines. It is important to rule out secondary causes of elevated platelet count or haemoglobin as this has a bearing on management. The main clinical consequences are related to the increased cardio- and cerebrovascular risks of elevated blood counts. Longer-term risks are related to marrow fibrosis, marrow failure and risk of leukaemic transformation.

Management of ET adopts a risk-stratified approach, taking into account age, level of platelet count and additional thrombotic risk factors. Patients may require antiplatelet drugs alone or in combination with cytoreductive therapy. PRV can be managed with periodic venesection to maintain haematocrit at less than 45 per cent or require cytoreductive therapy. The most commonly used drug is hydroxycarbamide. Patients require regular hospital attendance for monitoring, but most remain well and the conditions are unlikely to impact on work.

Lymphomas

Hodgkin's disease predominantly affects young adults. Modern treatment achieves cure rates of 90 per cent. Multidrug chemotherapy, radiotherapy, or combination protocols result in significant impairment of ability to work. Treatment lasts 6–8 months and transplantation is indicated for non-response or relapse. On recovery (6–12 months post-treatment) the majority of patients would be expected to return to a full and active life.

Non-Hodgkin's lymphomas (NHL) comprise the largest group of haematological malignancies and their incidence is increasing in Western societies. They are classified as aggressive (high grade, 30–40 per cent) or indolent (low grade). Standard treatment comprises combination chemo-immunotherapy (6–8 courses over 4–6 months). The addition of the monoclonal antibody rituximab has improved complete remission rates to 70–80 per cent. Response rates vary according to a prognostic index that includes disease stage at presentation and performance status. Overall the 5-year survival rates are 55–80 per cent. Thus more long-term survivors of high-grade NHL now return to employment. Low-grade NHL often runs an indolent course (median >10 years) and is incurable with standard treatment regimens. Increasingly patients are diagnosed on routine health screening and blood tests. Others present with lymphadenopathy, fevers, sweats, weight loss, BM failure, or disease involvement of other organs (gut, lungs, central nervous system). Many patients can be managed conservatively and will be able to continue with their daily lives. Treatment is only required if the patient becomes symptomatic. Progressive and symptomatic disease requires drug treatment and transplantation may be considered in selected patients (see later). Many cases can be well controlled with oral chemotherapy, which produces few side effects and allows patients to continue with normal daily activities and employment. Fitness to work depends on individual functional assessment.

Multiple myeloma

Although myeloma is predominantly a disease of the elderly, many working adults are affected. Haematological and immunological effects include anaemia and immuneparesis. Biochemical effects include chronic renal failure, hypercalcaemia, hyperviscosity (due to high paraprotein levels), and gout. Lytic bone lesions can cause bone pain, pathological fractures, and vertebral involvement with cord compression and paralysis. Myeloma is incurable for the majority of patients, and the principles of treatment are tumour reduction with multi-agent chemotherapy, followed (in younger patients only) by high-dose chemotherapy and autologous SCT (see 'Stem cell transplantation'). Current treatments combine chemotherapy with immunomodulatory drugs including thalidomide. Skeletal disease is treated with radiotherapy, and bisphosphonates are effective in treating hypercalcaemia, bone pain and preventing fractures. The availability of newer agents is improving the outcomes of treatment for relapsed disease. Median survival is 5 years, with 20 per cent of patients living over this.

The ability to continue to work during or after treatment for myeloma may be severely affected. Anaemia and fatigue are common. Thalidomide treatment may contribute to somnolence, and is associated with a significant risk of venous thromboembolism and neuropathy. Heavy manual or lifting work may exacerbate skeletal symptoms and risk of fractures.

Adjustments to work in malignant haematological diseases

Patients are usually absent from work during the acute phase of treatment, which can last up to a year depending on the condition. Once disease is controlled or in remission, short-term adjustments may be needed for rehabilitation of patients who have impaired marrow function. Long-term alterations are needed in some jobs to manage the life-long susceptibility to infection. Possible adjustments for generic issues are summarized in the sections that follow.

JAA standards on fitness for aircrew recommend exclusion for acute leukaemia and for initial applicants with chronic leukaemia. Certification would be considered for individuals with treated lymphoma or acute leukaemia that was in full remission. Re-certification for an established aircrew member would be considered for CLL stages O, I (and possibly II) without anaemia and minimal treatment, or 'hairy cell' leukaemia provided haemoglobin and platelet levels are normal; although regular follow-up would be required by the JAA. If anthracycline has been included in chemotherapy regimens, cardiological review would be required for certification.

Generic issues

Immunity and infection risk

Lympho-haematological malignancies and their treatment have a profound effect on the immune system, with consequent increased infection risk. This is most severe in patients undergoing

Table 16.3 Recommended vaccinations in patients with stem cell transplantation

Vaccine	Allo SCT	Auto SCT	Timing post-SCT
Tetanus toxoid	All	All	6–12 months
Diphtheria	All	All	6–12 months
Inactivated poliovirus	All	All	6–12 months
Pneumococcus	All	All	6–12 months
H. influenzae B	All	All	6–12 months
Influenza virus	All	All	Season-dependent
Measles	Individual recommendation based on risk/benefit assessment		>24 months postallogeneic stem cell transplant

myelosuppressive chemotherapy, but for the majority of patients, susceptibility to infection recovers on completion of chemotherapy and normalization of blood counts. However some patients remain immunocompromised for many years, depending on the underlying condition, previous treatment (e.g. Purine analogues, allo-SCT) or ongoing medication (e.g. immunosuppressants, steroids). The spectrum of infection risk will also depend on this; while bacterial infections are most common, patients remain vulnerable to opportunistic infections (PCP, fungal disease), CMV-reactivation and herpetic infections. Treatment-specific guidelines recommend anti-microbial prophylaxis in the relevant settings, most commonly Septrin® (PCP prophylaxis), aciclovir, penicillin V, and antifungals. Patients with hypogammaglobulinaemia and recurrent infections may benefit from IVIG. All patients should have an annual flu vaccine and, where appropriate, the post-transplant vaccination schedule (Table 16.3). In assessing a patient for return to work following treatment, account needs to be taken of recovery in blood counts (neutropenia and infection risk, platelet count, and bleeding risk) and ongoing medication.

Stem cell transplantation

SCT carries significant risks of major morbidity and mortality. The principles behind SCT differ between autologous and allogeneic procedures. Autologous SCT, where the patient is the donor, allows intensification of chemo/radiotherapy to treat the underlying condition, thereby functioning as a 'rescue' and allowing reconstitution of marrow function. Standard allogeneic (family or volunteer donor) transplantation transplants the donor's immune system. The donor (graft) immune response to the recipient (host) accounts for the graft versus host disease (GvHD), which is the major complication of allogeneic transplantation. However, the same immune response is also directed at the underlying disease (leukaemia) creating a graft versus leukaemia (GvL) effect. It is clear that the GvL effect plays a major role in the long-term cure achieved by allogeneic SCT.

Indications for stem cell transplantation and survival

The indications for SCT and number of procedures performed in the UK are shown in Table 16.4.

Many factors influence the outcome of SCT, including type of transplant, age, underlying disease, and stage at time of transplant. During the transplant and in the early post-transplant period the patient would be unable to perform work. Recovery from treatment may take months or years and will depend on the success of the procedure in curing the underlying condition and any long-term side effects (see 'Fitness for work in stem cell donors').

Table 16.4 Numbers and reasons for bone marrow transplantation in the UK, 2009

Conditions	Transplants performed	
	Allograft	**Autograft**
Acute leukaemias	508	8
Chronic leukaemias	108	2
Myelodysplastic syndrome/MPD	176	1
Plasma cell disease	36	919
Bone marrow failure	52	0
Lymphomas	204	584
Haemoglobinopathy	20	0
Primary immunodeficiency	58	0
Inherited disorders of metabolism	15	1
Autoimmune disorders	5	5
Solid tumours	8	103
Others	10	0
Total	1200	1623

Data from the British Society of Blood and Marrow Transplantation 2009.

Fitness for work in stem cell donors

Haemopoietic stem cells can be derived from bone marrow (BM) or peripheral blood (PB). Collecting stem cells involves either a BM harvest or PB stem cell (PBSC) collection. Marrow (1000–1200 mL) is harvested under general anaesthesia from the posterior iliac crests. Donors usually recover fully from the procedure within 1–2 weeks, during which time they are advised to refrain from work. Occasionally, a BM harvest can cause or exacerbate back problems. The principle of PBSC collection depends on giving a course of the haemopoietic growth factor, granulocyte colony stimulating factor (G-CSF). Transient side effects include flu-like symptoms and bone pain due to the G-CSF injections, and hypocalcaemia during the apheresis process (Table 16.5).

Splenectomy and hyposplenism

The spleen is the largest lymphoid organ and contains 25 per cent of the T-lymphocyte and 10–15 per cent of the B-lymphocyte pool. It fulfils a major role in protecting against bacterial, viral, and parasitic infections.

The causes of splenic insufficiency are summarized in Table 16.6. Patients are at risk of overwhelming bacterial infections particularly involving encapsulated organisms, *Streptococcus pneumoniae* (pneumococcus), *Haemophilus influenzae*, and *Neisseria meningitidis*.

Guidelines recommend immunization for splenectomized or hyposplenic patients (Table 16.7). Those undergoing elective splenectomy should be vaccinated at least 2 weeks prior to surgery and receive lifelong antibiotic prophylaxis with penicillin (erythromycin if allergic to penicillin). Despite these measures severe infections still occur, and patients should carry a 'Splenectomy

Table 16.5 Late effects of chemo/radiotherapy and stem cell transplantation for haematological disease

System	Complications	Treatment
Cardiovascular	Cardiomyopathy, pericarditis, arrhythmias, coronary artery disease, pulmonary hypertension	Avoid or limit radiation field
Respiratory	Pneumonitis, pulmonary fibrosis, infections, opportunistic infections secondary to immune suppression (PCP, CMV, TB)	Lung shielding and fractionation of radiotherapy reduces lung damage. Antimicrobial prophylaxis and vaccination
Immunodeficiency	Bacterial, viral, and fungal infection. Re-activation of TB, shingles. Secondary malignancies and autoimmune disorders	The immunodeficiency post treatment is related to the disease process, treatment or ongoing immunosuppressive therapy. Antimicrobial prophylaxis, vaccination, and intravenous immunoglobulin may be used.
Endocrine, neurological, and ophthalmological complications	Hypothyroidism post radiotherapy. Learning difficulties in children treated with craniospinal radiotherapy. Leucoencephalopathy, cerebral atrophy. Drug-related neurotoxicity (e.g. peripheral neuropathy from vinca alkaloids, thalidomide). Cataract post steroids and radiotherapy	Monitor thyroid function and replacement as necessary
Secondary malignancies	The overall relative risk of developing cancer post SCT is 6.4 compared with the general population	Smoking cessation. Avoid or limit environmental and occupational exposure to carcinogens (e.g. sun) Health screening (e.g. cervical and breast screening programmes)
Chronic GvHD	This is a multisystem complication of SCT causing: immune suppression and infections, skin involvement (scleroderma-type picture), gut involvement (affecting nutrition, bowel and liver function). Marrow dysfunction and cytopenias	Prophylaxis and early treatment of infections. Immunosuppressive drugs (steroids and cyclosporine A)

Card' and wear a 'MedicAlert' bracelet. Infection should be treated with a broad-spectrum penicillin and it may be advisable for patients to carry an emergency supply when away from home. During travel to affected areas, patients should be advised of the increased risk of severe malaria and must adhere scrupulously to antimalarial prophylaxis.

There are no guidelines or data on which to base recommendations for employment. The adjustments in Box 16.6 are based on traditional textbook teaching about increased risk of infection. Hyposplenic or splenectomized employees should be able to undertake almost any kind of work, and restrictions are very few. The exception is work that carries a risk of exposure to encapsulated pathogens, potentially infective biological material, and foreign travel. Individual susceptibility must be considered in addition to generic risk assessment.

Table 16.6 Indications for splenectomy and causes of splenic insufficiency

Indications for splenectomy	Causes of hyposplenism
• Trauma	• Congenital aplasia
• Malignancy	• Haematological disorders
• Autoimmune conditions (immune thrombocytopenic purpura, auto-immune haemolytic anaemia)	• Sickle cell disease
	• Myelofibrosis
• Diagnostic	• Lymphomas
• Hereditary haemolytic anaemias (e.g. hereditary spherocytosis pyruvate kinase deficiency)	• Autoimmune disorders
	• Coeliac disease
	• Inflammatory bowel disease
• Hypersplenism	• Splenic infiltration
	• Splenic irradiation
	• Splenic embolization

Table 16.7 Recommended vaccination schedule for splenectomy patients

Vaccine	Schedule
Pneumococcus	Re-immunization recommended every 5 years or based on antibody levels
Haemophilus influenza B (HiB)	Included as part of routine childhood vaccinations since 1993
Meningococcal C	Now part of routine childhood vaccinations
Conjugate vaccine	Older and non-immune patients should receive single dose
Influenza vaccine	Annual vaccination recommended

Box 16.6 Adjustments to work for hyposplenic/splenectomized employees

- ◆ Ensure immunizations up to date, and on prophylactic antibiotics.
- ◆ Avoid exposure to bacterial pathogens.
- ◆ Care with travel, carry antibiotics, and fastidious compliance with antimalarial prophylaxis.
- ◆ Avoid working in remote areas with poor medical facilities.

Repeated transfusion

Repeated transfusion, used in the management of haemoglobinopathies, bleeding disorders, and haematological malignancies, can give rise to a number of clinical problems (Box 16.7), including iron overload and cardiac, endocrine, and liver damage. The treatment of choice for iron overload is parenteral chelation with desferrioxamine usually administered by subcutaneous infusion three to five times a week. Oral iron chelators (deferasirox, deferiprone) are available as second-line treatment.

Transmission of infection is much less of a problem since the introduction of rigorous measures to reduce infection in blood products. UK blood donors are routinely screened for syphilis, hepatitis B and C, HIV1, HIV2, HTLV I, and HTLVII. In addition, selective screening includes CMV (where patients are susceptible), malaria, and *Treponema cruzi* (where donors have a risk of exposure). Pooled plasma products such as clotting factor concentrates undergo viral inactivation processes and some products are produced using recombinant technology, removing the risk of infection completely. Table 16.8 shows the risk of transfusion related infection in 2000. Four cases of transfusion-related transmission of nvCJD have been recorded. Since 1999 all UK blood cellular products have had 99.9 per cent of the white cells removed in order to reduce the risk of vCJD, and since 2004 plasma for children born after 1996 (the year in which UK meat was deemed to be safe) has come from non-vCJD endemic areas (North America).

Fitness for work resulting from infection with blood-borne viruses is covered in Chapters 14 and 23. Infectivity is only an issue where others in the workplace might be exposed to blood or body fluids from the infected employee (mainly in healthcare or dentistry). However, the risk of acquiring a transfusion-related infection is extremely low, and regular screening for infection for employment purposes is usually inappropriate.

Box 16.7 Complications of multiple treatment with blood products

+ Iron overload:
  • Cardiomyopathy
  • Liver failure
  • Endocrine failure.
+ Infection with blood-borne viruses:
  • Chronic hepatitis
  • HIV infection
  • Infectious carriage of blood borne viruses (relevant for healthcare employees).

Table 16.8 Estimated risks of transfusion-related viral infection in the UK in 2000

Viral pathogen	Estimated risk per unit of blood screened in UK
Hepatitis B	1/50 000–1/170 000
Hepatitis C	1/200 000
Human immunodeficiency virus	1/2 000 000

Anaemia

The main symptoms of chronic anaemia relevant to fitness for work are fatigue, breathlessness, and impaired exercise tolerance. These symptoms vary according to age, level of fitness, and comorbidity. In general, chronic anaemia is better tolerated than acute anaemia because of adaptive mechanisms. Measurable physiological changes do not occur until the haemoglobin falls below 7 g/dL. However, haemoglobin concentrations above 12 g/dL are associated with less fatigue and a better quality of life. Advances in the treatment of chronic anaemia include the use of recombinant erythropoietin. Individuals who have anaemia with haematocrit less than 32 per cent would be disqualified as aircrew.

Fatigue

Fatigue is commonly experienced by patients with haematological disorders and is the most prevalent and functionally debilitating symptom of cancer and its treatment. It is related to multiple factors including disease activity, treatment, anaemia, and sleep disturbance, although the specific aetiology is poorly understood. Reduced energy levels are often disproportionate to physical effort. Moreover, fatigue has emotional, behavioural, and cognitive elements. Fatigue that is sufficiently severe to threaten employment has serious psychosocial consequences for the individual, and it is important to ensure that employers are aware of the effect of fatigue on workability. The main difficulties with assessing the impact of fatigue on fitness for work are the subjective nature of the symptom and the variability between individuals. Several instruments have been developed to measure fatigue in clinical settings, either through self-report scales (e.g. Piper Fatigue Scale, Functional Assessment of Cancer Therapy Scale) or fatigue diaries. In theory these might be useful for repeated measurements prior to return to work and regular monitoring during a work rehabilitation programme. However, most of the available literature focuses on fatigue as a measure of treatment outcome rather than functional assessment for work, and these instruments have not been validated in the workplace setting.

Fatigue can last for months (or even more than a year) after treatment for malignancy. It is important to identify chronic fatigue symptoms, as adjustments to work may enable a productive return. Strategies for managing cancer-related fatigue include promotion of acceptance, positive thinking, and education about treatment and prognosis. Energy conservation strategies include increasing sleep time, pacing and restriction of activities, restoring attention and concentration (by pleasant diversionary activities), and physical exercise. The literature in this field comes from the treatment and early post-treatment phase of malignant diseases. Findings suggest that practical adjustments to allow pacing of work activities with rest and graded exercise are beneficial for the individual and allow earlier return to work. There are no studies that specifically assess interventions for the workplace management of fatigue and the evidence for recommendations in Box 16.8 for rehabilitation back to work is indirect, based on intervention studies in cancer patients. Macmillan Cancer Support provide useful information about coping with fatigue associated with cancer.[6]

Bleeding

Many haematological disorders and their treatments affect bleeding tendency through the failure of thrombopoiesis. In patients with thrombocytopenia, bleeding tendency is typically manifested as spontaneous skin purpura, mucosal haemorrhage, and prolonged bleeding after trauma. Prophylactic platelet transfusion is indicated at counts below 10×10^9/L. Bleeding in haemophilia is discussed in 'Inherited clotting disorders: haemophilia and von Willebrand's disease'.

Box 16.8 Suggested adjustments to work in employees with chronic anaemia- or cancer-related fatigue

- Flexible working arrangements.
- Part-time work.
- Late starts and early finishes.
- Minimize night work or shift work.
- Encourage frequent breaks and job variety to help maintain attention.
- Support from manager and peers to encourage positive attitude and progression towards normality.
- Reducing very heavy physical work.
- Arrangements to allow working from home.

Box 16.9 Markers of significantly high risk of bleeding in haematological conditions (threshold for advising restriction from heavy physical work or work associated with risk of injury)

- Haemophilia: Factor VIII activity below 5 per cent.
- Therapeutic anticoagulation: INR >4.5.
- Marrow suppression due to chemotherapy, radiotherapy; marrow failure due to leukaemia, myelodysplasia, aplastic anaemia—platelet count $<20 \times 10^9$/L.

Therapeutic anticoagulation, if managed carefully, is unlikely to cause bleeding that is relevant for work. Adjustments to work in bleeding disorders are indicated by the risk of haemorrhage due to physical activities. There are no specific evidence-based guidelines, but clinical markers for increased risk of bleeding are listed in Box 16.9.

Psychosocial aspects

Haematological disease may have a considerable impact on psychosocial function. Many are life threatening and chronic in nature. The high incidence of associated psychological morbidity must be taken into account in planning rehabilitation in the workplace. Depression is more prevalent among patients with haematological disease including cancers, haemoglobinopathies, and haemophilia. Surveys in cancer survivors have shown that 35 per cent had symptoms of psychological distress. Even patients in long-standing remission have a high rate of psychiatric disorders (37 per cent), including depression in 13 per cent. It is important to be aware of psychosocial morbidity when returning to work, as treatment can usefully be facilitated. Support at home and at work improves the outcome of psychological problems.

Conclusions

In recent years there have been major advances in the management of many haematological conditions. As a result there have been real improvements in long-term survival and workability, particularly among patients with haematological malignancies. More of these patients will return to the employment market than previously and, with the exception of a few jobs that are contraindicted, adjustments to work will enable them to work efficiently and safely.

References

1 Serjeant GR, Serjeant BE (eds). *Sickle cell disease*, 3rd edn. Oxford: Oxford University Press, 2001.
2 Joint Aviation Authority. *Manual of Civil Aviation Medicine*, 2005. Haematology, Chapter 6. [Online] (<http://www.jaa.nl/licensing/manual/06%20%Haematologypdf>)
3 Jones P. *Living with haemophilia*, 5th edn. Oxford: Oxford University Press, 2002.
4 Samama MM, Dahl, OE, Quinlan, DJ, *et al.* Quantification of risk factors for venous thromboembolism: a preliminary study for the development of a risk assessment tool. *Haematologica* 2003; **88**: 1410–21.
5 Glynn, RJ, Ridker PM, Goldhaber SZ, *et al.* Effect of low-dose aspirin on the occurrence of venous thromboembolism: a randomized trial. *Ann Intern Med* 2007; **147**: 525–33
6 Macmillan. *Coping with fatigue*. [Online] (<http://www.macmillan.org.uk/Cancerinformation/Livingwithandaftercancer/Symptomssideeffects/Fatigue/Fatigue.aspx>)

Further reading

Hoffbrand AV, Catovsky D, Tuddenham EGD (eds). *Postgraduate haematology*, 5th edn. Oxford: Blackwell Publishing, 2005.

Chapter 17

Cardiovascular disorders

Anne E. Price and Michael C. Petch

Introduction

Cardiovascular disorders remain one of the commonest causes of ill health and death but their incidence in Western society has been declining and there have also been significant reductions in death rates due to major advances in treatment over the last 20 years. Cardiovascular disease (CVD) affects working-age people and occupational physicians will see it regularly in the clinic. It affects fitness to work in two ways. First, an individual may suffer from symptoms on effort that limit their working capacity. Such disability is quantifiable and can often be alleviated by effective treatment. The second less common but more difficult problem is the risk of sudden incapacity, especially in individuals who appear well. This may occur for a variety of reasons including the risk of sudden cardiac death following ventricular fibrillation and whilst the instantaneous risk of sudden incapacity is very small, the consequences can be unacceptable. Assessment of this risk and its impact is possible in populations but explaining this concept to a bus driver who has lost his job is not easy.

Limitation of working capacity and the risk of sudden incapacity can be well judged in populations by specialist opinion. For the individual this must be backed up by objective data, usually derived from the results of non-invasive tests such as electrocardiography (ECG) and exercise testing. Whilst disease progression can be unpredictable the use of objective data can ensure the individual is not unfairly excluded from work they can safely do.

Sometimes cardiovascular symptoms are out of all proportion to the objective evidence of disease. This may arise from psychological disturbance following the development of CVD which in itself is associated with a high rate of common mental health problems. A heart attack proves devastating and the patient never returns to work despite prompt treatment, a full cardiac recovery, and only modest residual disease. The occupational physician needs to recognize the mental health problems associated with CVD and ensure that all treatment options are considered to facilitate rehabilitation to the workplace.

Epidemiology

Heart disease is common both in the population at large and in those of working age. CVD, including stroke and high blood pressure (BP), is very costly. CVD is the main cause of death in the UK, responsible for 190 857 deaths in 2008. The main forms of CVD are coronary heart disease (CHD) and stroke. CVD accounts for 28 per cent of premature deaths before retirement age in men and 20 per cent of premature deaths in women. CHD was responsible for 88 236 deaths in the UK in 2008 and is responsible for 23 per cent of deaths before age 65 years in men and 13 per cent in women. Significant advances in acute medical care have brought reductions in mortality from CHD over the last 10 years. Morbidity rates have not seen the same fall and there has been some increase, especially in older individuals over the last 20 years. Two million people in the UK suffer from angina, 177 000 people have heart failure, and 124 000 suffer a heart attack each year.[1]

A recent study of self-reported work-related illness suggests a prevalence for CVD caused or made worse by work of 80 000 individuals during the study year, with each illness case taking an average of 23 days of sick leave in the year.[2] This equates to 1.84 million days lost to work-related CVD, with cost to industry of approximately £120 million.

Death from CHD may be sudden if for instance ventricular fibrillation occurs. In the World Health Organization (WHO) Tower Hamlets study,[3] 40 per cent of heart attacks (defined as myocardial infarction (MI) or sudden death from CHD) were fatal, 60 per cent of deaths occurring within 1 hour of the onset of symptoms. This early high mortality has been confirmed by more recent studies, and persists despite advances in treatment. Heart attacks tend to occur more frequently in the morning or towards the beginning of shift-work, as compared with other times of the day.[4] Their onset may be associated with unaccustomed vigorous effort and acute psychosocial stress.[5]

Clinical features

CHD usually presents as chest pain, either MI or angina; it may also present with symptoms resulting from arrhythmia or heart failure, or be detected incidentally by ECG. Anyone with chest pain suspected of suffering from MI or an acute coronary syndrome should summon help urgently because prompt treatment can save lives. After recovery the risk of further cardiac events (sudden death, recurrent MI, or need for myocardial revascularization) is assessed by clinical history and simple investigations.

Assessment

Cardiologists grade symptom limitation from angina and heart failure using the Canadian Cardiovascular Society (CCS) and the New York Heart Association (NYHA) systems respectively (Tables 17.1 and 17.2). The sensitivity of exertional dyspnoea in respect of heart failure is 66 per cent with a specificity for heart failure of 52 per cent. In addition symptom-limited exercise tolerance carries an adverse prognosis, helping to identify high-risk patient subgroups.

The risk of sudden disability and death through ventricular fibrillation is the major factor affecting work capacity among victims of CHD. The risk is greatest in the early days following an acute coronary event. Those with severe myocardial damage and/or continuing ischaemia form a high-risk group. The extent of ventricular damage may be judged by the presence of heart failure, gallop rhythm, and poor left ventricular function on ECG. Residual myocardial ischaemia may be judged by a recurrence of cardiac pain or the development of angina pectoris and may be confirmed by exercise testing. An exercise test may also reveal cardiovascular incapacity in other

Table 17.1 Canadian Cardiovascular Society (CCS) grading of angina

CCS	Symptoms
I	Angina only during strenuous or prolonged physical activity
II	Slight limitation with angina only during vigorous physical activity
III	Symptoms with everyday living activities (ie moderate limitation)
IV	Inability to perform any activity without angina or angina at rest (ie severe limitation)

Reprinted with permission, Copyright © 2012 Canadian Cardiovascular Society.

Table 17.2 New York Heart Association (NYHA) grading of heart failure

NYHA	Symptoms
I	No limitation of physical activities and no shortness of breath when walking or climbing stairs
II	Mild symptoms of shortness or breath and slight limitation during ordinary activity
III	Marked symptoms and shortness of breath during less than ordinary activity (eg walking 20–100 yards). Comfortable only at rest
IV	Severe limitation of activity with symptoms at rest

ways, namely exhaustion, inappropriate heart rate, and blood pressure responses, arrhythmia, and ECG change, especially ST segment shift. In practice, the exercise test and the opinion of an accredited specialist are generally sufficient to assess fitness for work. This is reflected in the guidance material for vocational drivers (see Chapter 28). Individuals who are free of symptoms and signs of cardiac dysfunction and who can achieve a good workload with no adverse features have a very low risk of further cardiac events. This applies particularly to younger individuals and employers need have little hesitation in taking them back to work.

An individual who reaches stage 4 of the Bruce protocol on a treadmill is at such low risk of further cardiac events that vocational driving may be permitted. The carefully considered DVLA guidelines are now being applied more widely to other groups of workers whose occupation involves an element of risk to themselves and others in the event of cardiovascular collapse. Most employees, however, are not required to demonstrate such high levels of cardiovascular fitness.

Those whose early investigations are inconclusive will require further tests, often including *radionuclide imaging* to assess ventricular function and myocardial perfusion. Those who have continuing symptoms, or whose non-invasive investigations are unsatisfactory will be recommended to undergo *coronary angiography* with a view to myocardial revascularization. This is mildly unpleasant and hazardous with a risk of local complication of one in 500, and of catastrophe (including stroke and death) of one in 1000. Facilities for angiography are now widely available. Most angiograms are undertaken as day case procedures.

Management strategies: medical

Lifestyle management and drug therapy have transformed the management of CHD. Employers should support and reinforce community measures by discouraging smoking, encouraging healthy activities, and by providing a healthy diet at work.

The prognosis of patients following MI is improved by intervention and drug treatment. Aspirin improves prognosis in all patients with CHD. Nitrates, beta-adrenergic antagonists, and calcium antagonists alleviate the symptoms of myocardial ischaemia. Diuretics and angiotensin-converting enzyme (ACE) inhibitors improve symptoms and survival in patients with heart failure. Statins also improve prognosis and reduce the risk of subsequent events in all groups of patients with CHD. These and other cardiovascular drugs are generally well tolerated and remarkably free from long-term side effects. Many owe their efficacy to their vasodilating action; hence hypotension and faintness are possible complications. All patients will require lifelong medication, with aspirin and a statin as a minimum.

Coronary angioplasty and stenting (percutaneous coronary intervention)

For years balloon angioplasty was bedevilled by a high recurrence rate. The development of the coronary stent led to a substantial reduction in the restenosis rate. A stent is a tubular metal mesh that is delivered on the balloon in a collapsed state, down the artery, and subsequently deployed at high pressure (e.g. 16 atmospheres) into the arterial wall. The angiographic results are remarkable and relief of symptoms can be equally dramatic. Complex, distal, and multiple stenoses can be safely treated. The introduction of drug eluting stents for selected cases—usually smaller arteries and long lesions—has reduced the restenosis risk to almost zero.

Primary percutaneous coronary intervention (PCI) has replaced thrombolysis as the treatment of choice for MI with ST segment elevation, thrombolysis being reserved for patients who cannot reach a heart attack centre quickly (within 2 hours). Almost invariably the blocked artery can be opened up and stented. Those who receive this treatment make a speedy and dramatic recovery, often returning home after 3 days in hospital. Some people doubt that they have had a heart attack. Rehabilitation with early ECG and exercise testing is becoming the norm; return to work may be accelerated.

Urgent angiography proceeding to PCI has become a standard approach for most confirmed acute coronary syndromes. Elective PCIs constitute the minority of cases in cardiac centres. Success rates are of the order of 97 per cent. Disasters necessitating surgery occur in about one in 700 procedures. Groin haematomas are an unusual but well-recognized complication, which has led to more cases being performed via the radial artery. Return to work within 1 week is commonplace after elective PCI. However, unlike surgery, it has not yet been shown in a randomized controlled trial to improve the long-term survival of patients with CHD.

Coronary artery bypass grafting

Coronary artery bypass grafting (CABG) is a more complex method of achieving myocardial revascularization and nowadays is undertaken less commonly than PCI. It is also remarkably safe, with mortality rates of about 1 per cent for elective operations. Recovery is rapid and most patients resume work within 2–3 months and most are relieved of their angina. Patients who were working before surgery generally do so afterwards, and restrictions that may have been appropriate previously should no longer be relevant. Unfortunately, surgery constitutes a dramatic event that can prompt overprotective attitudes among family members, friends, employers, and even medical advisers. Many individuals who could and should return to work fail to do so for this reason, rather than because of continuing incapacity. However, delays in receiving coronary angiography and bypass surgery have led to many patients losing their jobs. In one study, job loss was greater in those who had been off work for more than 6 months before surgery than in those receiving an early operation.[6] This situation is changing because many people who would have had CABG are rapidly and successfully treated by coronary stenting. No special restrictions are necessary after return to work. Coronary graft stenosis and occlusion leads to a recurrence rate of angina of about 4 per cent/year. This is generally less severe than previously but may affect long-term job placement. CABG for left main stem or three-vessel disease improves prognosis. Rehabilitation programmes are now well established in many hospitals. These enable many patients to make a full recovery following a cardiac event such as MI or CABG.

Return to work after developing coronary heart disease

Studies on return to work after the onset of heart disease have shown that several different considerations apply.

The nature of the original cardiovascular event that led to the individual stopping work. Whichever form CHD takes, the important factors influencing return to work include the persistence of chest pain during exercise, the risk of arrhythmia and the level of left ventricular function. Additionally, the possibility of silent ischaemia needs consideration for high-risk individuals. While angioplasty ensures a speedier return to work than CABG, long-term employment prospects are similar in both treatment groups.[7]

The residual loss of function following the cardiac event. The individual's functional capacity should be assessed prior to return to work. For cardiac disease an exercise stress test will give the required information, while those with cardiac failure may need further investigation. Cardiac failure formerly meant that a return to work was unlikely, but improvements in treatment of the underlying cause mean now that more people with heart failure can return to work. Using the NYHA criteria for heart failure, individuals with functional capacity I and II are likely to return to their previous role. Those with NYHA functional capacity III and IV or those returning to a very strenuous job may require additional functional testing and cardiological opinion.

The prognosis of the causative CVD. Prognostic indicators are well documented for most cardiovascular problems. Where the prognosis is poor and the risk of recurrence high, return to work may be unrealistic. Where there are other comorbid conditions, the impact of these conditions will affect function and return to work. A recent occupational study found that comorbid conditions like depression, migraine and chronic bronchitis are common in those with angina; comorbidity strongly predicts functional status, mortality, hospitalization, number of days in hospital, and medical care costs.[8]

Table 17.3 Factors reducing likelihood of return to work

Individual factors	Increasing duration of absence independent of the prognosis of the CVD
	If the cardiac event happened at work
	Increasing age
	Fear of recurrence
	Poor motivation
	Poor understanding of the condition
	Secondary gain from the 'sick role'
	Where the job is perceived as unrewarding, dangerous or damaging to health
	When redeployment/retraining is difficult to achieve due to certain individual factors such as education, adaptability, or even personality
Employment factors	Employer's fear of further illness at work and subsequent litigation
	Reluctance to consider redeployment
	Demanding work environment
Other factors	Sickness benefits
	Over-cautious standards
	Low acceptability of risk by regulatory authorities

Individual factors. Psychological factors may play a bigger part in whether an individual returns to work than physical factors. Some factors which make return to work less likely following a cardiac event are summarized in Table 17.3.

Cardiac rehabilitation

Cardiac rehabilitation programmes are successful at facilitating return to normal life including work. They are structured in three phases (see Figure 17.1). The aim of the programme is to develop a functional capacity of 8 METS (metabolic equivalents). However this level is only rarely reached as heavy work is defined as activity requiring 6–8 METS and maximal work includes any activity that requires >9 METS (see Table 17.4).

Return to work

It is estimated that up to 80 per cent of patients with uncomplicated MI will return to work. When work is resumed, the levels and duration of activity should be increased progressively. In general, physical activity is good for the heart but the degree of physical activity must take into account previous fitness and the results of exercise testing. Patients with stable angina can safely work within their limitations of fitness but should not be put in situations where their angina may be readily provoked. Patients with persistent angina or an abnormal exercise test should be assessed for myocardial revascularization. Following an acute coronary event, those with no complications and good exercise tolerance may return to work in 4–6 weeks.

Not everyone will be able to go back to their previous work after a coronary event. In light engineering it has been observed that after 1 year about half those returning were fully fit, requiring no job change. The remainder had some limitations of fitness and required a job change.[9] About one-tenth of those returning to work had severe fitness limitations requiring redeployment. Fatigue usually resolves over time. It may be helpful to arrange reduced hours or other temporary restrictions, but these should be defined and not left open-ended.

Psychological factors

Psychological difficulties may be experienced even by those with no signs of cardiac damage and has a significant impact on morbidity and mortality. Half may have some anxiety or depression and of those half may have severe persisting symptoms a year later if untreated.[10] Anxieties of both the patient and partner have been shown to affect the likelihood that men who survive an MI will return to work and depression in post-MI patients increases the risk of mortality from

PHASE	AIMS
1: Acute/in-patient	• Determine exercise capacity
	• Provide patient education about necessary supervision
	• Start exercise programme under medical supervision
2: Reconditioning outpatient supervised	• Improve exercise capacity and strengthen
	• Continue lifestyle changes
	• Monitor exercise programme as an outpatient in a supervised fashion
3: Maintenance outpatient unsupervised	• Emphasise long term lifestyle changes
	• Exercise programmes three to five times per week without medical supervision
	• Monitoring in outpatient setting

Figure 17.1 Phases of cardiac rehabilitation.

Table 17.4 Some metabolic equivalents (METS)

1–2 METS
Doing seated ADLs (eating, performing facial hygiene, resting)
Doing seated recreation (sewing, playing cards, painting)
Doing seated occupational activities (writing, typing, doing clerical work)
2–3 METS
Standing ADLs (dressing, showering, shaving, doing light housework)
Standing occupation (mechanic, bartender, autorepair)
Standing recreation (fishing, playing billiards, shuffleboard)
Walking (2.5 mph)
4–5 METS
Doing heavy housework (scrubbing floor, hanging out washing)
Canoeing, golfing, playing softball, tennis (doubles)
Social dancing, cross country hiking
Swimming (20 yards/min)
Walking 4 mph (level), 3 mph (5% gradient)
Bike ride 10 mph
6–7 METS
Heavy gardening (digging, manual lawn mowing, hoeing)
Skating, water skiing, playing tennis (singles)
Stair climbing (<27 ft/min)
Swimming (25 yards/min)
Jogging 5 mph (level), 3.5 mph (5% gradient)
8–9 METS
Active occupation (sawing wood, digging ditches, shovelling snow)
Active recreation (downhill skiing, playing ice hockey, paddleball)
Bike riding (12–14 mph)
Stair climbing (more than 27 ft/min)
Swimming 35 yards/min
Running 10 mph (level), 3 mph (15% gradient)

ADL = activity of daily living.

two to seven times. Evidence links anxiety disorders to sudden cardiac death from ventricular arrhythmias consequent on altered autonomic tone.[11,12]

Friedman et al. suggested that modification of hectic work patterns marked by long hours, competitiveness, time urgency, and aggression (so-called type A behaviour) as part of other stress reduction measures, may be beneficial.[13] However, evidence on whether personality influences the aetiology of CHD and survival following MI is conflicting.

Guidance about the psychological stresses of work must be individually tailored.

Screening for coronary disease

Those populations at high risk of sudden incapacity can be identified once their disease has become manifest. But silent coronary disease is extremely common. For example, disease has been found in about one-third of patients investigated by coronary angiography before heart valve replacement.[14] Sudden death may be the first manifestation of coronary disease. Many cardiac events will therefore occur in those who appear to be fit—approximately one-quarter in studies of road traffic accidents, for example. One solution to this problem may be to screen employees by clinical examination and exercise testing for 'silent' myocardial ischaemia. This may be justifiable in certain groups and has been adopted by the US Air Force. Exercise-induced electrocardiographic ST segment change in an asymptomatic individual has several causes; using the criterion of 1-mm ST segment depression, however, only about one-third will turn out to have coronary disease on angiography.[15] Screening for asymptomatic CHD in this way cannot therefore be recommended routinely because of the high incidence of false-positive results. Simple clinical features such as age, male sex, history of chest pain, smoking habit, or a strong family history of premature CHD, and physical examination are better methods of assessing seemingly healthy individuals. The development of fast multislice CT scanners has encouraged commercial screening organizations to offer this as a means of detecting silent coronary disease. Two methods are advertised—a coronary calcium score, which is cheap and easy, and CT angiography. The former commonly leads to the latter, which carries a small radiation risk and requires careful interpretation by an experienced specialist. The place of this investigation in screening is uncertain, mainly because there are no long-term follow-up studies of prognosis by lesion type. Coronary CT can be very helpful in cardiac centres in two particular circumstances—to rule out coronary disease in patients with acute chest pain, where it has the merit of enabling other diagnoses such as aortic dissection and pulmonary embolism to be made; and in patients with complex coronary anatomy, particularly after CABG. Other applications may follow as this is a fast developing technology.

Congenital and valvular disease

Accurate anatomical and physiological diagnosis of congenital heart disease and acquired heart disease in young people can now be carried out by non-invasive methods such as ECG and magnetic resonance imaging (MRI). Often the condition and its prognosis will be established by the time an individual reaches working age and they may seek career advice. This will be most necessary for careers with defined pre-employment medical standards, such as service in the armed forces and safety critical work. Early counselling can help patients to develop appropriate and informed career expectations.

Employers should not be deterred from taking on young people who have undergone cardiac surgery for the correction of congenital defects in childhood; many lead a normal life and are capable of full-time employment. Acquired valvular disease—usually degenerative aortic stenosis or mitral regurgitation—is mostly seen now in those beyond working age, but mitral valve prolapse deserves emphasis as it affects some 2 per cent of the population and carries an excellent prognosis. It often presents as an auscultatory finding at a pre-employment medical examination, may be associated with electrocardiographic change, and may sometimes lead to a false diagnosis of significant heart disease.

The satisfactory results of valve surgery have led to the practice of early operation, before left ventricular function declines. Many mitral valves can be repaired nowadays, leading to a full functional drug-free recovery. Percutaneous balloon valvotomy is now the treatment of choice for pulmonary stenosis in rheumatic mitral stenosis and children, and occlusion devices are used to close the smaller atrial septal defects. Transcutaneous aortic valve replacement is possible although it is generally reserved for elderly patients deemed at too high risk for surgery.

Following replacement of the aortic or mitral valves by mechanical or biological prostheses patients generally recover rapidly and resume work fully 2–3 months after surgery. Those with mechanical valves need to take anticoagulants indefinitely and are therefore at slightly increased risk of bleeding, serious events occurring at a rate of about 2 per cent per annum. Biological valves undergo slow deterioration, can fail suddenly some years after implantation, and are rarely used in people of working age. However, in specific roles such as fire fighters, their use may be considered to avoid the need for ongoing anticoagulants.

Cardiac arrhythmias

Transient cardiac arrhythmias (e.g. extrasystoles) are common and do not usually indicate heart disease. They may be provoked by alcohol and coffee. Assessment by a specialist is recommended if symptoms persist. A few individuals suffer recurrent arrhythmias. The commonest is atrial fibrillation (AF), which affects 2 per cent of the population at some time in their lives and tends to be paroxysmal (PAF) in individuals of working age. Drug treatment is sometimes required and individuals need to withdraw from work and rest for a short period. AF may complicate CHD or valve disease; for those with no apparent underlying heart disease, research has shown that the focus for the arrhythmia lies in the sleeves of muscle that extend from the left atrium backwards into the pulmonary veins. This has led to the development of an increasingly popular and successful ablation technique known as pulmonary vein isolation (PVI) which can be offered where PAF is seriously troublesome. Further types of supraventricular tachycardia including atrial flutter can be cured by catheter ablation of the accessory electrical pathway that subserves the re-entrant tachycardia.

Ventricular arrhythmias are more problematic. Isolated ventricular extrasystoles in otherwise healthy hearts can be ignored. More complex ventricular ectopy can also occur in normal hearts but inherited conditions (channelopathies) such as the long QT syndrome, and subtle myocardial disorders detectable on MRI are being increasingly recognized and are a cause of sudden death in young people. Therefore, patients with an abnormal ECG or a family history of cardiac death in the absence of overt CHD should be referred for more detailed assessment. The prognosis for individuals with ventricular arrhythmias occurring because of heart muscle disease depends on the underlying pathology, which is often myocardial scarring from CHD. Continued employment for these individuals may be inadvisable.

Complete heart block generally requires permanent pacing (see 'Pacemakers and implantable devices') but first- and second-degree block may be incidental findings in otherwise healthy people; generally no further action is required. Similarly sino-atrial disorder carries a good prognosis, although pacing may be helpful in alleviating symptoms.

Syncope

Syncope, other than a simple faint, requires specialist evaluation, which may include neurological as well as cardiovascular review. Following unexplained syncope, provocation testing and investigation for arrhythmia must be undertaken. If no major problem is found return to work is recommended, including re-licensing for vocational drivers after 3 months. Careful follow-up is essential.

Pacemakers and implantable devices

Pacemakers

The presence of an implanted cardiac pacemaker to maintain regular heart action is entirely compatible with normal life, including strenuous work. The underlying heart condition for which the pacemaker was implanted may, however, impose its own restrictions.

The indications for cardiac pacing have broadened, given the sophistication of modern pacemaker technology (which allows pacing of atria and ventricles, variation in the output of the generator and facilities for telemetry).

Virtually all pacemakers have the capacity to sense and be inhibited by the patient's own heart rhythm. Somatic muscle action potentials and electromagnetic fields can in theory interfere with the pacemaker, causing temporary cessation of pacing. Usually the interference will be brief and the pacemaker will revert to a fixed-rate mode so that symptoms will be minimal.

Biventricular pacing (cardiac resynchronization therapy or CRT) involves the insertion of leads into both ventricles; this can be extremely helpful in patients with refractory heart failure and a desynchronous cardiac contraction which is usually manifest as a prolonged QRS complex. Generally the severity of the underlying heart failure precludes work.

Implantable cardioverter defibrillators

The implantable cardioverter defibrillator (ICD) is now the preferred treatment for individuals with ventricular tachycardia and/or fibrillation whose arrhythmia is refractory to drugs or myocardial revascularization; the ICD device often has CRT capacity. Generally, the individual will have experienced at least one cardiac arrest. The device is implanted by a cardiologist under local anaesthetic but is tested under general anaesthetic. Both ventricular tachycardia and fibrillation can be detected and treated, for the former by anti-tachycardia pacing and the latter by a DC shock. In either event transient impairment of consciousness is possible, so jobs like vocational driving are not permitted.

Hypertension

There are few contraindications to employment in the hypertensive person. Powerful drug regimens may carry the risk of hypotension with resultant giddiness and fatigue. Central nervous system side effects may affect judgement and the performance of skilled tasks. However, modern therapy with beta-adrenergic and calcium antagonists, diuretics, and ACE inhibitors is generally free from side effects.

Patients with controlled hypertension can expect to manage most work. Occasionally, frequent postural changes prove troublesome, owing to altered central and peripheral vascular responses. Very heavy physical work and exposure to very hot conditions with high humidity may result in postural hypotension. However, Group 2 vehicle driving is allowed provided that the blood pressure is maintained under satisfactory control and checked regularly.

The presence of resistant hypertension may be first noted as part of health surveillance or on routine medical examination (Box 17.1). This needs communicating to the primary care provider.

Those with hypertensive crisis are not fit to work and should not be considered so until the underlying cause has been treated and the blood pressure controlled. Untreated hypertensive crisis can lead to encephalopathy, left ventricular failure, MI, unstable angina, or dissection of the aorta. Rare causes of crisis include phaeochromocytoma, severe preeclampsia/eclampsia, and

Box 17.1 Causes of resistant hypertension

- Poor adherence to therapeutic plan/non-compliance with medication
- Failure to modify lifestyle—weight gain, alcohol misuse (especially binge drinking)
- Continued use of medication that increase blood pressure—liquorice, cocaine, steroids, NSAIDs
- Obstructive sleep apnoea syndrome
- Unsuspected secondary cause
- Irreversible end organ damage
- Volume overload due to inadequate diuretic therapy
- Progressive renal insufficiency
- High sodium intake
- Hyperaldosteronism
- 'Spurious' resistant hypertension—failure to use large cuff on large arm
- White coat hypertension.

severe hypertension associated with subarachnoid haemorrhage or cerebrovascular accident. Hypertensive emergencies can also be associated with recreational drugs.

Other circulatory disorders

Peripheral vascular disease may cause intermittent claudication that limits the patient's mobility. Medical treatment is relatively unsatisfactory; but surgical/interventional treatment can be very successful. The prognosis depends upon any associated coronary disease. The presence of an aortic aneurysm also indicates arterial disease and a liability to vascular catastrophe. Cerebrovascular disease is commonly accompanied by CHD, to the extent that most stroke victims die a cardiac death. All these patients should be carefully assessed, both clinically and by non-invasive investigations, with particular attention paid to the likelihood of cardiac involvement.

Raynaud's phenomenon, on the other hand, is a benign, albeit distressing, complaint. Underlying causes such as hand-arm vibration syndrome should be excluded (see Appendix 6). Ideally, sufferers should work in a warm environment or be allowed to wear gloves if indicated.

Special work issues

Physical activity

As a general rule activities that cause no symptoms can be undertaken safely. Careful history taking will identify what activities are possible, initially by eliciting activities of daily living (ADLs) then matching these with equivalent work activities (see Table 17.4). A useful model to quantify what individual workers are capable of in terms of physical activity is that of metabolic equivalents or METS. This can also be compared with the results of exercise testing in that: Stage 1 of the Bruce Protocol approximates to 4.6 METS, Stage 2 is 7.0, Stage 3 is 10.1, and Stage 4 is 12.9 METS. Jobs that may require extreme physical effort, for example, those in the emergency services, may be unsuitable for workers with CHD. Each case must be judged on its individual merits, however, and specialist advice taken as required.

Lifting weights

Only the very fit might reasonably attempt heavy work, when defined as lifting 23–45 kg (40–100 lb). Many employees quite comfortably manage medium work, such as lifting 11–23 kg (25–50 lb) at the rate of once a minute, providing they do not have other physical limitations. If weights are supported or kept at waist height, the effort is considerably reduced, and if the task only requires them to be slid along benches or roller tracks, then the effective strain will be reduced by some 50 per cent. Those with continuing symptoms as defined by NYHA class II or CCS class III may need more specific assessment including exercise testing to confirm fitness for the proposed roles. Symptoms will help define capability.

Driving

Ordinary driving (Group 1) may be resumed 1 month after a cardiac event provided that the driver does not suffer from angina that may be provoked at the wheel. Group 1 licence holders do not need to notify the DVLA, if they have made a good recovery and have no continuing disability. Vocational drivers (Group 2) must notify the DVLA and driving may be permitted at 6 weeks, subject to a satisfactory outcome from non-invasive testing. Insurance companies vary in their requirements but most policies are temporarily invalidated by illness (see Chapter 28.)

Work stress

There is considerable evidence to support the role of job strain (a combination of high work demands and low job control) as a risk factor for heart disease[16–19] despite negative previous studies from the USA[20,21] and Japan.[22] Observational data suggest an average 50 per cent excess cardiovascular risk among employees with work stress[17] and particularly in younger male populations (19–55 years), job strain causes a 1.8 times higher age adjusted risk of incident ischaemic heart disease.[23] Where an individual reports the feeling of being dealt with unfairly at work recent research suggest that this is an independent risk factor of increased coronary events and impaired health.[24]

The presence of work stress cannot be completely removed but utilization of the Health and Safety Executive Stress Management Standards for work-related stress is a helpful tool to address such issues objectively and consider risk minimization strategies.[25] In most individuals the presence of stress will not prevent return to work after a cardiovascular event. However risk reduction strategies in relation to the source of stress are likely to make a return to work more successful and help the individual adopt lifestyle strategies to prevent recurrence of the underlying cardiac problem, thereby maintaining attendance and performance at work.

The INTERHEART case–control study included 11 119 cases from 52 different countries and examined the link between psychosocial risk factors and risk of acute MI.[26] Stress at home or at work and the incidence of major life events in the preceding year showed a significant correlation with the risk of MI. A third more cases experienced several periods of work stress than controls (odds ratio (OR) 1.38; 99 per cent confidence interval 1.19–1.61), while the exposure OR for permanent work stress was doubled (OR 2.14; 1.73–2.64). The population attributable risk (i.e. the proportion of all cases in the population attributable to the relevant risk factor if causality were proven) was calculated as 9 per cent for both stress at work and depression, 11 per cent for financial stress, and 16 per cent for low locus of control. If this effect is truly causal then psychosocial factors are much more important than commonly recognized. A caveat is that exposures were self-reported in retrospect, with the potential that cases may have relatively over-reported exposures widely supposed to aggravate heart disease.

Shift work

Shift work is increasing throughout the world with approximately 22 per cent of the population in industrialized nations undertaking some type of shift work.[27] In addition there are growing number of workers with more than one job. Shift work may affect the cardiovascular system through the desynchronization of cardiovascular rhythms due to altered sleep patterns, which predisposes to heart disease by provoking hypertension, dyslipidaemia, insulin resistance, and obesity.[28] Shift working may thus confer a risk of CVD, but assessment of this is complicated because shift workers tend to differ from non-shift workers in their general risk profile for CVD (e.g. smoking habits, diet, weight, alcohol intake, uptake of preventive medical services). Having said this, a substantial body of studies in different countries using different methodologies suggest that risks of CVD in shift workers, if increased, are elevated only slightly.[29]

Shift work may need to be restricted on the basis of specific clinical features such as severe night/early morning chest pain in an otherwise stable clinical situation, but this is advice to minimize continuing symptoms not to prevent recurrence. The potential effects of shift work can be counteracted through health promotion for shift workers from the occupational health team to look at risk minimization strategies and early identification of reversible risk factors, in particular the metabolic syndrome, hypertension, and dyslipidaemia.

Hazardous substances

Work involving exposure to certain hazardous substances may aggravate pre-existing CHD and careful consideration should be given to patients who are returning to work involving exposure to chemical, gases, and pollutants. Methylene chloride, an ingredient of many commonly used paint removers, is rapidly metabolized to carbon monoxide in the body; in poorly ventilated areas, blood levels of carboxyhaemoglobin can become high enough to precipitate angina or even MI (impairment of cardiovascular function begins at a blood carboxyhaemoglobin level of 2–4 per cent). Careful assessment taking account of the total exposure to carbon monoxide (active/passive smoking, air pollutants/chemicals) and correlation against symptoms of chest pain will allow a pragmatic approach to risk assessment in these rare cases.

Smokers, especially pipe smokers, will have an elevated blood carboxyhaemoglobin, which is additive to carbon monoxide in the workplace potentially increasing their risk of adverse cardiac events.

WHO recommends a maximum carboxyhaemoglobin level of 5 per cent for healthy industrial workers and a maximum of 2.5 per cent for susceptible persons in the general population exposed to ambient air pollution.[30] This level may also be applied to workers whose jobs entail exposure to carbon monoxide (e.g. car park attendants, furnace workers). There is good correlation between carbon monoxide levels in air and blood carboxyhaemoglobin, in accordance with the Coburn equation,[31] and the WHO guideline level of 2.5 per cent implies an 8-hour occupational exposure average, well below the current occupational exposure standard of 50 ppm. In fact, to ensure that the 2.5 per cent carboxyhaemoglobin level is not exceeded, the ambient carbon monoxide concentration should not be higher than 10 ppm. over an 8-hour working day— equivalent to exposure at 50 ppm for no more than 30 minutes. Occupational exposure to carbon disulphide in the viscose rayon manufacturing industry is a recognized causal factor of CHD but the mechanism remains unclear.

Solvents, such as trichloroethylene or 1,1,1-trichloroethane, may sensitize the myocardium to the action of endogenous catecholamines resulting in ventricular fibrillation and sudden death in workers with high exposure.[32] Chlorofluorocarbons (CFCs) are still widely used as propellants in aerosol cans and as refrigerants—CFC-113 has been implicated in sudden cardiac deaths and CFC-22 has been reported to cause arrhythmias in laboratory workers using aerosols. Where an individual has poorly controlled arrhythmia and is awaiting more definitive treatment such as ablation therapy, exclusion from work where there is known exposure to solvents/CFCs may be appropriate.

There are no formal medical standards for workers who have to enter confined spaces where there may be hazards of oxygen deficiency or a build-up of toxic gases. However, workers with heart disease or severe hypertension may need to be excluded. Certain occupations may require the use of special breathing apparatus either routinely (e.g. asbestos removal workers), or in emergencies (e.g. water workers handling chlorine cylinders). The additional cardiorespiratory effort required while wearing a respirator, combined with the general physical exertion that may be required should be factored in to any risk assessment undertaken and may require specialized input from the treating cardiologist to confirm exercise capability appropriate to the demands of the role.

Hot conditions

Work in hot conditions may prove difficult for some patients with heart disease. High ambient temperatures or significant heat radiation from hot surfaces or liquid metal, added to the physical strain of heavy work, will produce profound vasodilatation of muscle and skin vessels. Compensatory vascular and cardiac reactions to maintain central BP may be inadequate and lead to reduced cerebral or coronary artery blood flow. The resulting weakness or giddiness could prove dangerous. As many cardioactive drugs have vasodilating and negative inotropic actions, some reduction in dosage may be necessary. Careful risk assessment will be required, taking account of the work conditions, the nature of the cardiac condition, how well it is managed and the impact of medication side effects.

Cold conditions

Cold is a notorious trigger of myocardial ischaemia and caution must therefore be exercised in placing individuals with CHD in cold working environments. Impaired circulation to the limbs will result in an increased risk of claudication, risk of damage to skin (frostbite), and poor recovery from accidental injury to skin and deeper structures. Clear work procedures that include short periods spent in the cold, provision of appropriate cold weather clothing/regular hot drinks, coupled with clear safety guidelines may reduce risk sufficiently to allow the individual to continue working in those conditions.

Travel

Following a cardiac event, individuals should convalesce at home and not travel. They should then be assessed by a specialist at 4–6 weeks. Those with no evidence of continuing myocardial ischaemia or cardiac pump failure can then travel freely within the UK for pleasure. Business and overseas travel is more problematical because the physical and psychological demands are greater. Additional difficulties for the overseas traveller include the uncertain provision of coronary care facilities in some countries and the reluctance of insurance companies to provide health cover.

Such travel is best deferred until 3 months have elapsed and any necessary further investigations and treatment have been carried out to ensure cardiovascular fitness.

Overseas travel for those with continuing cardiovascular symptoms need not be ruled out. Clear guidelines exist regarding fitness to fly for commercial travellers (see Table 17.5). Airport services for disabled travellers can ease the journey and modern aircraft can be very comfortable.

Table 17.5 Fitness to fly for passengers with cardiovascular disease.[41]

Condition	Functional status	Restriction/guidance
Angina	CCS angina I–II	No restriction
	CCS angina III	Consider airport assistance and possible in-flight oxygen
	CCS angina IV	Defer travel until stable or travel with medical escort and in-flight oxygen available
Post-STEMI and NSTEMI	Low risk: age <65, first event, successful reperfusion, EF >45%, no complications, no planned investigations or interventions	Fly after 3 days
	Medium risk: EF >40%, no symptoms of heart failure, no evidence of inducible ischaemic or arrhythmia, no planned investigations or interventions	Fly after 10 days
	High risk: EF <40%, signs and symptoms of heart failure, those pending further investigation, revascularization or device therapy	Delay travel until condition stable
Elective PCI uncomplicated		Fly after 2 days
Elective CABG uncomplicated	Allow for intrathoracic gas resorption. If complicated so symptomatic, *see* heart failure	Fly after 10 days if no complications. If symptomatic, follow guidance for specific symptoms
Acute heart failure		Fly after 6 weeks if stabilised (*see* chronic heart failure)
Chronic heart failure	NYHA I AND II	No restrictions
	NYHA III	May require in-flight oxygen
	NYHA IV	Advised not to fly without in-flight oxygen and medical assistance
Cyanotic congenital heart disease	NYHA I AND II	May require in-flight oxygen[a]
	NYHA III	Consider airport assistance and may require in-flight oxygen advisable[a]
	NYHA IV	Advised not to fly without in-flight oxygen and airport assistance available[a]

Table 17.5 (continued) Fitness to fly for passengers with cardiovascular disease.[41]

Condition	Functional status	Restriction/guidance
Valve disease (*see* heart failure) Following pacemaker implantation		Fly after 2 days if no pneumothorax. In the event of a pneumothorax, flying should be deferred for 2 weeks following complete resolution
Following ICD implantation		The same advice as for pacemakers but, in addition, rhythm instability should be treated.
Arrhythmia	Stable	No restrictions
Ablation therapy		Fly after 2 days[a]

[a] Consider at high risk of DVT

CABG, coronary artery bypass graft; CCS, Canadian Cardiac Society; DVT, deep vein thrombosis; EF, ejection fraction; ICD, implantation cardioverter defibrillator; NSTEMI, non-ST elevation myocardial infarction; NYHA, New York Heart Association; PCI, percutaneous coronary intervention; STEMI, ST elevation myocardial infarction; VTE, venous thromboembolism.

Adapted with permission of the British Cardiovascular Society from Fitness To Fly For Passengers With Cardiovascular Disease. The report of a working group of the British Cardiovascular Society. <http://www.bcs.com/documents/BCS_FITNESS_TO_FLY_REPORT.pdf>

The cabins are kept at a pressure equivalent to 6000 feet (2000 metres) so that those with angina are not likely to experience symptoms; most developed countries have an excellent coronary care service. Business people with continuing cardiac disorders may therefore fly to Europe and North America with very little risk. Flights in unpressurized aircraft, work in undeveloped countries or in remote areas of the world, and work in a hostile environment (both climatic and political) is best avoided. Aircrew are subject to CAA guidelines whose advice should always be sought (see also Appendix 1). Continuing medication is key for individuals with cardiac conditions. The traveller should ensure access to their medications for the whole of their trip.

Cardiac deaths are uncommon in trekkers or workers at high altitude (8000–15000 ft/ 2440–4570 m). The increase in cardiac output at altitude will exacerbate symptoms in those who already experience symptoms at sea level, but asymptomatic individuals with CHD are unlikely to be at special risk.

Cosmic radiation can disrupt the function of electronic devices even at sea level.[33] Although evidence is minimal ICD follow-up has shown electrical resets of ICDs during air travel.[34] The reset can trigger an audible alert to the patient but effects are unlikely to affect the functioning of the ICD. A sensible approach is to warn the patient with an ICD of the possible effects of cosmic radiation on the device but to reassure them that it is unlikely to affect the ability of the device to detect and treat life-threatening arrhythmias.

Vibration can affect pacemakers and ICDs (used to match pacing rate to activity levels). In fixed wing aircraft this is not problematic but in helicopters vibration levels are high throughout the flight and sustained raised levels of pacing rates are seen, which may cause problems for some individuals. Specific advice from the pacemaker clinic may be needed where helicopter travel is required.

Deep vein thrombosis and venous thromboembolism in long distance travellers

The association between long distance travel and deep vein thrombosis (DVT) and venous thromboembolism (VTE) is well recognized. Clear evidence exists as to the risks (see Table 17.6).

Table 17.6 Guidance for the avoidance of deep vein thrombosis and venous thromboembolism

Blood clots (DVT and VTE)	Risk criteria	Risk reduction advice for passengers
Low risk	No history of DVT/VTE No recent surgery (4 weeks) No other known risk factors	Keep mobile, drink plenty of non-alcoholic drinks. Do not smoke. Avoid caffeine and sedative drugs
Moderate risk	History of DVT/VTE Surgery lasting >30 min 4–8 weeks ago Known clotting tendency Pregnancy Obesity (BMI >30kg/m²)	As for 'low risk' with the addition of compression stockings
High risk	Previous DVT with known additional risk including known cancer Surgery lasting >30 min within the last 4 weeks	As for 'moderate risk' but subcutaneous injections of enoxoparin 40 mg before the flight and on the following day

Travelling for more than 4 hours doubles the risk of VTE compared with not travelling. The risk is highest in the first week following travel but persists for 2 months. The risk is similar whether the travelling is by car, bus or train over a similar period. Factor V Leiden mutation, height (>1.9m <1.6m), obesity (body mass index > 30 kg/m²), and use of the oral contraceptive pill increase the risk of VTE.

Electromagnetic fields

Industrial electrical sources such as arc welding, faulty domestic equipment, engines, antitheft devices, airport weapon detectors, radar, and citizen-band radio, all generate electromagnetic fields that can, in theory, affect pacemakers and ICDs; but the patient has to be very close to the power source before any interference can be demonstrated. Any pacemaker abnormality is usually confined to one or two missed beats or reversion to the fixed mode. The number of documented cases of interference in the UK is less than three a year.[35, 36] ICD discharges are equally rare.

If pacemaker patients are expected to work in the vicinity of high-energy electric or magnetic fields capable of producing signals at a rate and pattern similar to a QRS complex (e.g. on some electrical generating and transmission equipment and welding) then formal testing is recommended. The cardiac centre responsible for implanting the pacemaker will usually provide a technical service for this purpose, enabling the risk of interference to be defined precisely. Persons with implanted devices are generally advised to avoid work that may bring them into close contact with strong magnetic fields and this includes MRI machines as found in many hospital radiological departments and certain chemical laboratories. If patients experience untoward symptoms or collapse while near electrical apparatus then they should move or be moved away, but the likely cause of the symptoms will be unrelated to the device. Patients with implanted devices carry cards that identify the type of pacemaker and the supervising cardiac centre.

There has been one report of a patient who collapsed in the vicinity of an electronic antitheft surveillance system in a bookstore and who was shown to have ICD malfunction.[37] The advice for patients with these devices is to explain that they have an ICD or pacemaker so that they do not need to remain in the vicinity of shop doors or airport detector gates. Further advice is available from the British Pacing and Electrophysiology Group.

There has been interest in the possibility that mobile telephones might interfere with pacemakers and ICDs. Studies have shown that this is a theoretical possibility and that re-programming of a pacemaker can be achieved under exceptional circumstances if the telephone is held close (less than 20 cm) to the pacemaker. In practice no clinically significant interference has yet been reported, but individuals are advised to use the hand and ear furthest from the pacemaker, not to dial with the telephone near to the pacemaker or keep the phone in a pocket near the device.

Physical hazards

Workers requiring long term anticoagulation may need careful risk assessment in terms of potential injuries at work and also access to regular monitoring to ensure adequate anticoagulation. In certain occupations, e.g. firefighting, use of anticoagulants is considered a contraindication to operational roles.

Anticoagulation near patient testing and self-monitoring is increasing in use, particularly for the person at work. Further information including home testing kits is available from <http://www.anticoagulationeurope.org>. Newer oral anticoagulants are being developed that may have an improved risk profile. At present these are not readily available for use.

Cuts and bruises from accidental contact with furniture, machinery, and dropped objects, may not heal well in the presence of circulatory restriction. Varicose veins of the legs present similar problems; accidental injury may lead to blood loss and protection is essential; prolonged standing may aggravate symptoms. Sitting for long uninterrupted periods may aggravate ankle swelling and, if the hip and knee are awkwardly flexed, increase the risk of vascular thrombosis. (See also Chapter 16.)

The future of work

The nature of work continues to change. Downsizing and high levels of overtime can negatively affect workers' health, and act as a barrier to return to work after illness. Organizational changes contribute to increased risk of CVD, particularly in lower socio-economic groups.[38]

More women now work but still spend about three to four times as many hours per week in child care and housework as men.[39] In the Framingham Study,[40] employed women with three or more children had a higher incidence of CVD than employed women with no children, or housewives with three or more children. Women who work shifts or long hours appear to have an increased risk of hospitalization for MI, whereas moderate overtime may be protective for men. This gender difference may arise because women combine family responsibilities with irregular or long working hours.

By 2020 the UK population will include 19 million people over 60 years of age and many individuals will continue to work beyond the traditional retirement age of 65. CVD is more common in an ageing population and these demographic changes will increase the prevalence of heart disease at work, making the assessment of cardiovascular fitness all the more important.

Legal aspects

It has been established that work can be 'cardionoxious' for chemical, physical, and psychosocial reasons. In the UK the level of cardiotoxicity is subject to various regulations designed to ensure that all work is assessed in terms of its impact on health. The Management of Health and Safety at Work Regulations (1999) imposes this duty on employers and is backed up by more specific legislation, which, for example, considers chemical hazards (Control of Substances Hazardous to Health (COSHH) Regulations 2002). The Working Time Regulations 1998 aim to limit excessive working hours but will not necessarily alter shift patterns, which may, over time, impact adversely on cardiovascular health. The Equality Act 2010 will obviously apply to many cardiovascular conditions but in others it may not. Although it is difficult to give definitive advice regarding cases in which the Equality Act will apply, some useful pointers include conditions where activities of daily living are unlikely to be affected. These include angina which is defined as CCS grade I or II, heart failure defined as NYHA grade I or II, cardiac arrhythmias with minimal impact and conditions that relate to incidental findings or investigations, for example, ECG or ultrasound scan findings that do not translate into current symptoms. Importantly, assessment of whether an individual is legally disabled should be done after discounting the benefit of any treatment they are receiving or have received (including angioplasty or surgery).

References

1 British Heart Foundation Health Promotion Research Group. *Coronary heart disease statistics*. London: British Heart Foundation, 2010.

2 Jones JR, Huxtable S, Hodgson JT, *et al*. *Self reported work-related illness in Great Britain 2001–2002. Results from a household survey*. London: National Statistics HSE.

3 Tunstall-Pedoe H, Clayton D, Morris JN, *et al*. Coronary heart attack in East London. *Lancet* 1975; **ii**: 833–8.

4 Muller JE, Stone PH, Turi ZG, *et al*. Circadian variation in the frequency of onset of myocardial infarction. *N Engl J Med* 1985; **313**: 1315–22.

5 Mittleman MA, Maclure M, Tofler GH, *et al*. Triggering of acute myocardial infarction by heavy physical exertion. *N Engl J Med* 1993; **329**: 1677–83.

6 Nagle R, Gangola R, Picton-Robinson I. Factors influencing return to work after myocardial infarction. *Lancet* 1971; **2**: 454–6.

7 Hlatky MA, Boothroyd D, Harine S, *et al*. Employment after coronary angioplasty or coronary bypass surgery in patients employed at the time of revascularisation. *Ann Intern Med* 1998; **129**: 543–7.

8 Hemingway H, Valitera J, Virtanen M, *et al*. Outcome of stable angina in a working population 'the burden of sickness absence'. *Eur J Cardiovasc Prev Rehabil* 2005; **14**: 373–9.

9 Clark DB, Edward FC, Williams WG. Cardiac surgery and return to work in the West Midlands. Cardiac rehabilitation. In: *Proceedings of the Society of Occupational Medicine Research Panel Symposium*, pp. 61–70, London, 1983.

10 Glassman AH, Shapiro PA. Depression and the course of coronary artery disease. *Ann J Psychiatry* 1998: **155**: 4–11.

11 Haines AP, Imeson JD, Meade TW. Phobic anxiety and ischaemic heart disease. *BMJ* 1987; **295**: 297–9.

12 Kawichi I, Colditz GA, Ascherio A, *et al*. Prospective study of phobic anxiety and risk of coronary heart disease in men. *Circulation* 1994; **89**: 1992–7.

13 Friedman M, Thorensen CE, Gill JJ. Alteration of type A behaviour and its effect on cardiac recurrence in post myocardial infarction patients. Summary results of the recurrent coronary prevention project. *Am Heart J* 1986; **112**: 653–5.

14 Enriques-Sarano M, Klodus F, Garratt KN, *et al*. Secular trends in coronary atherosclerosis—analysis in patients with valvular regurgitation. *N Engl J Med* 1996; **335**: 316–22.

15 Froelicher VF, Thompson AJ, Wolthuis R, *et al.* Angiographic findings in asymptomatic aircrew with electrocardiographic abnormalities. *Am J Cardiol* 1977; **39**: 31–8.

16 Belvic L, Landsbergis PA, Schnall PL, *et al.* Is job strain a major cause of cardiovascular disease risk? *Scand J Work Environ Health* 2004; **30**: 85–128.

17 Kivimaki M, Virtanen M, Elovainio M, *et al.* Work stress in the etiology of coronary heart disease—a meta analysis. *Scand J Work Environ Health* 2006; **32**: 431–42.

18 Kuper H, Marmot M. Job strain, Job demands, decision latitude and risk of coronary heart disease within the Whitehall II Study. *J Epidemiol Community Health* 2003; **57**: 147–53.

19 Chandola T, Britton A, Brunner E, *et al.* Work stress and coronary heart disease: What are the mechanisms? *Eur Heart J* 2008; **29**: 640–8.

20 Eaker ED, Sullivan LM, Kelly–Hays M, *et al.* Does job strain increase the risk for coronary heart disease or death in men and women? The Framingham Offspring Study. *Am J Epidemiol* 2004; **159**: 950–8.

21 Lee S, Colditz G, Berkman L, *et al.* A prospective study of job strain and coronary heart disease in US women. *Int J Epidermiol* 2002; **31**: 1147–53.

22 Kobyaslin Y, Hirose T, Tada Y, *et al.* Relationship between two job stress models and coronary risk factors among Japanese female, part-time employees of a retail company. *J Occup Health* 2005; **47**: 2001–10.

23 Kivimalki M, Theorell T, Westerland H, *et al.* Job strain and ischaemic heart disease: does the inclusion of older employees in the cohort dilute the association? The WOLF Stockholm Study. *J Epidermiol Community Health* 2008; **62**: 372–4.

24 De Vogli R, Ferrie JE, Chandola T, *et al.* Unfairness and health: evidence from the Whitehall II Study. *Diabetologia* 2008; **51**: 1980–8.

25 Health and Safety Executive. *HSE Management Standards Indicator Tool.* [Online] (<http://www.hse.gov.uk/stress/standards/pdfs/indicatortool.pdf>)

26 Rosengren A, Hawker S, Ounpuu S, *et al.* Assocation of psychosocial risk factors with risk of acute myocardial infarction in 11,119 cases and 13,648 controls from 52 countries (the INTERHEART Study): case-control study. *Lancet* 2004; **364**: 953–62.

27 Wedderburn A. *Statistics and News: BEST 6.* Luxembourg: European Foundation for the improvement of Living and Working Conditions, 1993.

28 Mosendane T, Mosendane T, Raal FJ. Shift work and its effects on the cardiovascular system. *Cardiovasc J Afr* 2008; **19**: 210–15.

29 The Industrial Injuries Advisory Council. *Position paper 25. The Association between shift working and (i) breast cancer (ii) ischaemic heart disease.* London: The Industrial Injuries Advisory Council, 2009.

30 World Health Organization (WHO). *Carbon monoxide. Environmental health criteria, No. 13.* Geneva: WHO, 1979.

31 Coburn F, Forster R, Kane P. Consideration of the physiological variables that determine the blood carboxyhaemoglobin concentration in man. *J Clin Invest* 1965; **44**: 1899–910.

32 Boon NA (editorial). Solvent abuse of the heart. *Br Med J* 1987; **294**: 722.

33 Zeigler JF, Curtis HW, Muhfield HP, *et al.* IBM experiments in soft fails in computer electronics 1978–1994. *IBM J Res Develop* 1996; **40**: 3–18.

34 Bhakta D, Forseman LD. Cosmic radiation not science fiction but clinical reality. *Heart Rhythm* 2008; **5**: 1204–5.

35 Gold RG. Interference to cardiac pacemakers—how often is it a problem? *Prescribers J* 1984; **24**: 115–23.

36 Sowton, E. Environmental hazards and pacemaker patients. *J R Coll Phys* 1982; **16**: 159–64.

37 Santucci PA, Haw J, Trohman RG, *et al.* Interference with an implantable defibrillator by an electronic anti-theft surveillance device. *N Engl J Med* 1998; **339**: 1371–4.

38 US Departments of Labor and Commerce: Fact finding report. *Commission on the Future of Worker Management Relations.* Washington, DC: Departments of Labor and Commerce, 1994.

39 Belkić K, Schnall P, Landsbergis P, *et al.* The workplace and cardiovascular health: conclusions and thoughts for a future agenda. *Occup Med* 2000; **15**: 307–21.

40 Haynes SG, Fernlieb M. Women, work and coronary heart disease: prospective findings of the Framingham heart study. *Am J Public Health* 1980; **70**: 133–41.

41 *Fitness to fly for passengers with cardiovascular disease.* The report of a working group of the British Cardiovascular Society. (<http://www.bcs.com/documents/BCS_FITNESS_TO_FLY_REPORT.pdf>)

Chapter 18

Respiratory disorders

Keith T. Palmer and Paul Cullinan

Introduction

Respiratory illnesses commonly cause sickness absence, unemployment, medical attendance, illness, and handicap.[1] Collectively these disorders cause 19 million days/year of certified sickness absence in men and 9 million days/year in women (with substantial additional lost time from self-certified illness) and, among adults of working age, a general practitioner consultation rate of 48.5 per 100/year with more than 240 000 hospital admissions/year. Prescriptions for bronchodilator inhalers run at some 24 million/year, and mortality from respiratory disease causes an estimated loss of 164 000 working years by age 64 and an estimated annual production loss of £1.6 billion (at prices in 2000).

Respiratory disease may be caused, and pre-existing disease may be exacerbated, by the occupational environment. More commonly, respiratory disease limits work capacity and the ability to undertake particular duties. Finally, individual respiratory fitness in 'safety critical' jobs can have implications for work colleagues and the public. Within this broad picture, different clinical illnesses pose different problems. For example, acute respiratory illness commonly causes short-term sickness absence, whereas chronic respiratory disease has a greater impact on long-term absence and work limitation; and the fitness implications of respiratory sensitization at work are very different from non-specific asthma aggravated by workplace irritants.

Occupational causes of respiratory disease represent a small proportion of the burden, except in some specialized work settings where particular exposures give rise to particular disease excesses. The corollary is that the common fitness decisions on placement, return to work, and rehabilitation more often involve non-occupational illnesses than occupational ones. By contrast, statutory programmes of health surveillance focus on specific occupational risks (e.g. baking) and specific occupational health outcomes (e.g. occupational asthma). In assessing the individual it is important to remember that respiratory problems are often aggravated by other illnesses, particularly disorders of the cardiovascular and musculoskeletal systems.

Methods of assessing respiratory disability

General considerations

Respiratory fitness needs to be assessed in the context of the intended employment and its particular elements and demands. However, a number of general questions will influence the decision-making:

1 Does the combination of work and respiratory fitness result in an immediate foreseeable risk to the individual's health and safety, or that of others?

2 If so, how great are the risks likely to be?

3 Is the work in the 'safety critical' category, in which the worker has substantial responsibility for the safety of colleagues or members of the public?

4 Can the work be discharged effectively, and can reasonable levels of attendance be anticipated?

5 Are there special considerations in placement, health review, or workplace adaptation?

6 Are particular policies required in placement, control, and monitoring?

7 Are there relevant legal standards and other codes of good practice?

These questions are not particular to respiratory fitness assessments, but commonly occur in people with respiratory illness, e.g. the importance of aerobic capacity in the emergency rescue worker or the manual labourer; the risk posed to the public by tuberculosis in a healthcare worker, or pneumothorax in an airline pilot; the potential for life-threatening asthma following occupational sensitization.

Physicians in the UK have responsibilities under the Health and Safety at Work etc. Act 1974 (to place people in safe employment) and the Equality Act 2010 (to ensure that disabled workers are not discriminated against unfairly on health grounds). The dual requirements of these Acts challenge physicians to weigh matters carefully. They need to consider the likely duration of illness and its prognosis; the weight of evidence for incapacity on the one hand and risk on the other; and the scope for reasonable accommodation by the employer. These points are touched on elsewhere, but here we emphasize the need to avoid blanket judgements:

♦ Many aspects of lung function can be measured objectively but, except at the extremes, a poor correlation exists between measurements and symptoms (general fitness and motivation may be more important).

♦ Assessment of workplace demands and risks quite often vary according to individual circumstances.

♦ Many conditions improve given sufficient time, appropriate treatment, proper environmental control, or work modification.

Fitness assessment should be made in this light. An employer's failure to control potentially modifiable respiratory hazards (dusts, fumes, etc.) may be construed not only as a failure of control (under Regulation 6 of the Control of Substances Hazardous to Health Regulations 1994), but a failure to make a reasonable accommodation under the Equality Act.

Historically, some organizations and public services have applied pre-defined fitness standards; many others have conducted routine measures of respiratory function, and applied predetermined protocols and decision algorithms. However, the provisions of the Equality Act make it increasingly appropriate to tailor risk assessments to each individual's needs.

Measurements of lung function

Respiratory disease produces impairment in lung function which, if severe enough, will impair the ability to perform some work tasks. Whether a given loss of lung function causes difficulty at work depends on the nature of the job and the presence or absence of coexisting disease. The duration, intensity, and pattern of work, the environmental conditions (e.g. temperature, humidity, dust and fume content), and the attitude and personality of the individual all play a part. Pulmonary function testing is, therefore, only one component in the process of assessing fitness for work.

In an occupational setting lung function tests are used routinely in one of two ways. First, as a single set of measurements performed at a point in time (typically the pre-placement assessment, or during or following illness) to assess lung function in relation to accepted norms; and second, as serial measurements over time, to detect adverse occupational effects at an early stage or monitor disease control or progression. Used serially, the diagnostic value of the testing is probably higher.

Standard lung function tests are conveniently classified into measurements of airway function, static lung volume, and gas exchange. Measurements of *airway function* (e.g. spirometry and peak expiratory flow) should be routinely available in occupational healthcare, and can be augmented, under medical supervision, by trials of response to bronchodilator medication; the other tests, as well as measurements of bronchial responsiveness to inhaled histamine or methacholine, require specialist facilities, and are generally employed in secondary care and research settings.

Spirometry is performed by taking a maximal inspiration and then blowing as hard as possible into the machine, and continuing to blow until the lungs are empty. Modern spirometers produce a short list of measurements including: FEV_1, the volume of gas expired in the first second as a measure of the speed of airflow through larger airways; forced vital capacity (FVC), the total volume of expired gas; and a set of measurements at different points of exhalation (variously described as $FEF_{25/50/75}$ or $MEF_{25/50/75}$) indicative of flow through smaller airways. Measurements of peak flow are recorded but are unreliable when made during forced spirometry. The absolute volumes obtained depend upon age, height, sex, and racial origin, and values need to be compared with appropriate 'predicted normal values' of which several are available.

Most spirometers will also produce two graphical depictions of the forced manoeuvre (Figure 18.1). The first, a spirogram, is a plot of the volume of gas expired against time. The trace should be a smooth curve. The second, the expiratory flow–volume curve or 'loop', plots flow against expired volume between maximal inspiration (total lung capacity) and maximal expiration (residual volume). A normal 'loop' has a steep up-curve, a sharp angle, and a flat downward slope to the end of expiration.

A number of basic points of technique need to be observed to minimize measurement errors.[2] Spirometry equipment needs to be calibrated regularly, and checked for leaks, wear and tear, and blockages. Spuriously low results can occur if inspiration is incomplete, if partial leakage occurs (around the mouthpiece or in the tubing), or if expiratory effort is submaximal. The FVC is commonly underestimated because the blow is finished early, as is apparent in tracings that fail to attain a plateau. Variable effort is indicated by wobbly curves and poor reproducibility. Subjects should be encouraged to repeat the procedure until three acceptable manoeuvres are achieved (the best two FVCs should be within 5 per cent or 0.1 L of one another). The documented values should be the highest values from *any* of the three chosen curves. Benchmark standards and a

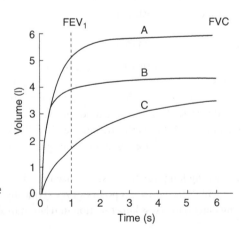

Figure 18.1 Spirograms illustrating normal (A) restrictive (B) and obstructive (C) patterns of abnormal ventilation.

more detailed account of these techniques have been provided by the European Respiratory and American Thoracic Societies in a consecutive series of published articles, the first of which[3] refers to general considerations; briefer summaries are also available.[4,5] Other factors that need to be considered include variation between observers and between machines, and recent infections, irritant exposures (including smoking) and exercise.

Sometimes, despite encouragement and multiple attempts, subjects are unable to produce acceptable tracings. This commonly results from an inability to master the technique, but in some of these cases so-called 'test failure' is a marker of incipient health problems.[6]

Two main patterns of ventilatory abnormality can generally be defined, namely obstructive and restrictive.[5] Obstruction is evident in some cases of asthma and is intergral to the diagnosis of chronic obstructive pulmonary disease (COPD), producing a diminution in FEV_1 greater than that in FVC. The ratio of FEV_1 to FVC should normally be greater than 0.7 (70 per cent), but in airflow obstruction lower values arise accompanied by a reduction in FEV_1. Early obstruction may be evident in measures of low flow (such as FEF_{25-75}), although these measurements are less reproducible than FEV_1 and their reference ranges less precise. Restrictive lung changes are uncommon and caused by diffuse inflammatory and fibrotic diseases of the lung parenchyma, such as fibrosing alveolitis and asbestosis, by pleural disease and by respiratory muscle weakness. In this case FEV_1 is reduced but so too is FVC, so that the ratio of FEV_1 to FVC is preserved and often increased.

When interpreting lung function tests it is helpful to consider the pre-test probability of disease. In most healthy non-smokers this probability is low and abnormal spirometry is usually attributable to poor technique. In addition, it needs to be remembered that the range of normal values is large, two standard deviations being approximately 20 per cent of the average value. This means that a healthy individual can appear to have deficient lung function simply because their lung function lies in the lower tail of the normal Gaussian distribution; or that an individual with impaired lung function can still produce values within the normal range. In the latter case, if measurements have moved from the top of the predicted normal range for a particular parameter to the bottom, the fall will represent 40 per cent of the population mean. Hence, serial patterns are more informative than a single snap-shot.

Measurements of airflow such as FEV_1 and peak expiratory flow are influenced most by disease in the larger airways, where most of the resistance to flow lies. The cross-sectional area of the bronchial tree increases exponentially with distance from the trachea as the bronchi divide, and resistance to flow falls concomitantly. Narrowing in the peripheral airways of less than 2 mm in diameter has little effect on FEV_1 and peak expiratory flow (PEF) unless damage is extensive. This means that early disease in small airways, such as that caused by smoking and toxic fume damage, is poorly reflected in these measurements.

PEF measures the highest flow recorded during a forced expiratory manoeuvre and is measured with a peak flow meter. The subject must perform a short, sharp, hard blow into the meter. The best of three attempts is taken, providing the readings are reproducible. As with simple spirometry, a number of errors are possible, particularly variable subject effort, errors in reading PEFs and transcribing them to a diary, and incomplete returns. A great deal of instruction and encouragement are required to obtain adequate data. Self-treatment with bronchodilators and corticosteroids may affect the record, but the influence of the first of these factors can be minimized by recording PEFs before drug delivery.

PEF measurements are usually made serially over time, and used in one of two ways: to assess the degree of control achieved in patients with established asthma; and to look for work-related changes in situations where occupational asthma is suspected (the later section on asthma describes this last application more fully).

Measurements of *static lung volumes*, such as total lung capacity (TLC) and residual volume (RV), involve advanced techniques including inert gas dilution and body plethysmography; they require a specialized pulmonary function laboratory, but may be useful in clarifying diagnoses. Thus, in airflow obstruction, all static lung volumes are increased, but the increase in RV is proportionately greater than in TLC because of gas trapping; while in restrictive lung disease all lung volumes are reduced.

Measurements of gas exchange such as oxygen consumption (VO_2) during incremental exercise, CO_2 production (VCO_2), and arterial blood gases, may be useful in assessing disability, especially in those with interstitial lung disease or emphysema. However, the findings reflect total cardiorespiratory function as well as peripheral muscle deconditioning, require sophisticated equipment, and are time-consuming to perform. Simpler tests of exercise capacity such as shuttle walk tests, step tests, and 6- or 12-minute walks are easier to use in the field, but still require skilled technical help and time.[7] Carbon monoxide diffusion, expressed as transfer factor (TLCO), or gas transfer coefficient (KCO), measures the uptake of carbon monoxide from the lung to the blood. Carbon monoxide is of similar molecular weight to oxygen, and is bound to haemoglobin, so its uptake provides a measure of oxygen diffusion. It is reduced in interstitial lung disease and in emphysema, but it is also affected by other factors such as smoking habits, haemoglobin levels, and resting cardiac output. Again its measurement requires a dedicated lung function laboratory. In the clinical setting the portable pulse oximeter provides a simple inexpensive guide to diffusion, and can be used to detect desaturation of haemoglobin at rest and during exercise.

Several other tests are used as adjuncts to diagnosis. Asthma in an occupational setting is sometimes investigated by *serology, skin prick tests*, or by *bronchial provocation challenge*. Immunological responsiveness (sensitization) to workplace agents may be detected by the serological identification of specific IgE antibodies, or by the response to a specific challenge to the skin or airways. The usefulness of these investigations varies from one agent to another. They also depend on identification of the suspected agent, and in the case of skin prick and provocation tests may depend on obtaining a correct formulation of the material, or achieving a representative challenge. The subject is more fully discussed later.

Screening questionnaires

In occupational health practice, screening questionnaires are commonly used. The best known respiratory questionnaire is the Medical Research Council (MRC) standardized questionnaire on respiratory symptoms.[8] This was devised for the epidemiological investigation of chronic bronchitis, but has since been adapted to assess respiratory symptoms and risk factors in working groups. The original questions on sputum production had a high sensitivity and specificity in relation to measured sputum production, but such questions are of limited interest today. Several other versions have been tried, including the European Community for Coal and Steel (ECSC) questionnaire, the American Thoracic Society and the Division of Lung Disease (ATS-DLD-78) questionnaire, and the International Union Against Tuberculosis and Lung Disease (IUATLD) questionnaire. (For sample questions and an assessment of their validity see Toren et al.[9]) Venables et al.[10] have proposed a simple nine-item panel of questions for use in asthma epidemiology that correlate well with bronchial hyper-responsiveness, and a simple extension to cover work-related symptoms (Table 18.1). Work limitation arises commonly from the sensation of breathlessness, and for monitoring and documentary purposes this can be graded on a clinical scale, such as the one proposed by the MRC (Table 18.2).

Table 18.1 Screening questions used in the epidemiological investigation of asthma

Current health (during the last 4 weeks)	
If you run, or climb stairs fast do you ever:	
Cough?	Yes/No
Wheeze?	Yes/No
Get tight in the chest?	Yes/No
Is your sleep ever broken by:	
Wheeze?	Yes/No
Difficulty with breathing?	Yes/No
Do you ever wake up in the morning (or from your sleep if a shift worker) with:	
Wheeze?	Yes/No
Difficulty with breathing?	Yes/No
Do you ever wheeze:	
If you are in a smoky room?	Yes/No
If you are in a very dusty place?	Yes/No

Answers of 'Yes' to 3 of the 9 questions correspond to a sensitivity of 91 per cent and a specificity of 96 per cent for current bronchial hyper-responsiveness.

Reproduced from Respiratory symptoms questionnaire for asthma epidemiology: validity and reproducibility. Venables KM et al. *Thorax*, Volume 48, Issue 3, pp. 214–19, Copyright © 1993 with permission from BMJ Publishing Group Ltd.

Table 18.2 The MRC breathlessness scale

1	Troublesome shortness of breath when hurrying on level ground or walking up a slight hill
2	Short of breath when walking with other people of own age on level ground
3	Have to stop for breath when walking at own pace on level ground

Chest radiography

Chest radiography plays a role in assessing those exposed to fibrogenic dusts such as asbestos and silica[11] (see 'Interstitial lung disease') and may be valuable in the assessment of workers exposed to tuberculosis who develop persistent respiratory symptoms.

However, the routine application of chest radiography in most employment situations has fallen into disfavour. For example, a former requirement for routine radiography in commercial divers has been lifted, with investigation dictated rather by clinical need. Radiography it is no longer considered helpful in routine surveillance of asymptomatic healthcare workers with potential tuberculosis exposure; likewise, the yield in asymptomatic workers who work with lung fibrogens or carcinogens is generally considered too low to justify the cost or radiation risk. Indeed, for the common round of health problems (upper respiratory tract infections, asthma and COPD), decisions on fitness for work seldom rest upon the outcome of radiography.

In the detection of pleural and interstitial lung disease more information is obtained by computed tomography (CT) scanning than radiography, but the procedure is expensive and its routine application for screening cannot presently be justified.

Clinical conditions and capacity for work

Asthma

Asthma affects about 5 per cent of the adult population. It is a condition of variable airflow limitation associated with bronchial hyper-responsiveness and symptoms of cough, breathlessness, and chest tightness. The predominant physical sign is wheeze. Onset in childhood or early adult life is frequently associated with the syndrome of atopy, characterized by elevated immunoglobulin (Ig) E antibody levels, positive skin prick tests to common inhaled antigens, and an increased incidence of eczema and allergic rhinitis. Childhood symptoms often remit in early adult life, but may recur in middle age. New-onset disease in middle life is not usually associated with manifestations of atopy, and the condition tends to be more persistent and more likely to progress in severity with time.

There are some difficulties in defining asthma. Wheeze is a highly prevalent symptom in the community, and many people with occasional wheeze do not have asthma. Conversely, subjects with bronchoconstriction do not recognize the symptom as often as might be supposed.[12] A further difficulty, in middle-aged employees, arises in distinguishing between chronic asthma and COPD, as there may be overlap between the classical features of asthma (wheeze and reversibility) and those of COPD (sputum, dyspnoea and irreversible airflow obstruction). It is important for doctors making a fitness assessment to decide whether the diagnosis is truly asthma and whether some response to treatment is likely. A more detailed history, including smoking habits, periodicity, currency and remission of symptoms, and precipitating factors is essential. Ideally the history should be supported by diurnal measurements of PEF and evidence of responsiveness to bronchodilators. Because of asthma's variable nature, simple screening questions and a single measurement of lung function and bronchodilator responsiveness may prove misleading. The most usual pattern on spirometry is to observe an obstructive deficit (low FEV_1 with an abnormal FEV_1/FVC ratio), but these measurements, though specific, have a relatively low sensitivity[13] in a disorder characterized by variable airflow limitation. Another common mistake is to confuse asthma with recurrent chest infection, especially in those who smoke. One unfortunate consequence of this mislabelling is to undertreat asthma and to limit employment opportunities thereby.

In the worker with established asthma, fitness and placement judgements may hinge on a number of important questions:

How severe is the condition?

Hyper-responsive airways represent a biological continuum. Asthma varies from mild disease with intermittent symptoms, through mild-to-moderate persistent disease requiring regular prophylactic treatment, to severe disease requiring regular high-dose inhaled steroids, or more rarely, continuous oral steroids.

In the common situation where asthma is mild, infrequent, or amenable to simple treatment, job placement decisions are straightforward. Adequate control may require only occasional use of a bronchodilator at times of unusual exertion or intercurrent infection. The anticipatory use of an inhaler (before exertion, and in the early stages of respiratory infection) will further ameliorate any problem, though short-term work modification may be helpful, and brief spells of sickness absence can arise. Under these circumstances the label 'asthmatic' may be unhelpful, leading simply to misinformed and prejudicial decisions on work fitness. Disease at the moderate to severe end of the spectrum poses more concern and at the extreme end, asthma may be severe and life threatening. A particular worry arises if the workplace is far removed from medical care facilities and emergency transfer is expensive, disruptive, or technically difficult but it is worth noting that serious, unexpected attacks are rare.

A broad indication of disease activity can be gained from the frequency of bronchodilator use and the degree of sleep disturbance. In more severe disease it is essential to know whether, when, and how often a patient has been admitted to hospital with asthma; whether or not they have required ventilation because of asthma; or received emergency intravenous therapy; or have been prescribed oral steroid medication. A number of guidelines on assessing disease severity have been produced by specialist societies, such as those regularly published by the British Thoracic Society and Scottish Intercollegiate Guidelines Network.[14]

An alternative approach, particularly in physically demanding jobs, is to measure changes in lung function during representative work tasks. Exercise tests are difficult to standardize and seldom specific enough to be used routinely in pre-placement screening, but in subjects with active troublesome disease a fall in FEV_1 greater than 15 per cent may indicate current work handicap.

Are there any work factors that are liable to aggravate constitutional asthma?

Asthmatic airways can be hyper-responsive to a wide range of non-specific irritants that are commonly encountered at work, as well as many highly prevalent environmental irritants and allergens. Extremes of temperature or humidity, irritant dusts or fumes, pollens, and house dust or pet allergens may all provoke or aggravate constitutional asthma, as may heavy physical exertion. These can pose temporary or enduring employment problems to employees with asthma in a wide range of occupations, from cold store workers in refrigeration plants through to outdoor workers in construction and farming. A useful summary of the available literature has been published by the American Thoracic Society.[15]

In practice, however, it is not easy to predict the sensitivity of a sufferer to irritant conditions since the degree of susceptibility to different stimuli varies considerably between individuals; for example, airways that bronchoconstrict in response to cold air may be less sensitive to dusts, and vice versa. In general, individuals with severe disease tend to be most vulnerable to irritant conditions, but not to the point where generalized judgements can be applied. Thus, severe asthmatics with a significant component of fixed airways obstruction may be less susceptible to non-specific irritants than those with severe labile asthma.

Can the principal aggravating factors be removed or limited?

Can irritant fumes or dusts be better controlled by exhaust ventilation or different work practices? Can less irritating materials be used? Can the process be enclosed? Can respiratory protection be used to limit exposure? If physical exertion is a limiting factor, can the effort of the work be reduced (e.g. by providing a lifting aid)? These are areas in which occupational health practitioners need to be particularly influential.

Has optimum treatment been offered, or could disease control be improved?

Asthma is often undertreated, with insufficient use made of long-term prophylactic treatment. Regular use of inhaled corticosteroids has a beneficial effect on attack frequency, sleep disturbance and hospital admission rates. The well-informed patient should be able to self-monitor, self-medicate, and self-refer. Deteriorating serial peak flow and worsening nocturnal symptoms should trigger an increase in medication and early medical consultation attendance; while in severe asthma, a home supply of oral steroids has enabled earlier treatment in those most in need.

Current UK guidelines[14] provide a detailed stepwise approach to the treatment of asthma and it is important to determine whether better control is possible at an early stage.

Might the patient have occupational (sensitization) asthma?

This is an important question to consider when asthma begins or recurs in adulthood, and a vital question in industries from which most case reports arise (Table 18.3).[16] The possibility is suggested if symptoms are worse at work or on work days, are better when away from work (at weekends and on holiday), and deteriorate upon return to work; and when work-related eye and nose symptoms are also present. A similar asthmatic picture can arise from a non-specific response to irritant conditions, as described earlier, and the distinction between these possibilities is important. Sensitized workers may react to amounts of material so tiny that workplace controls cannot be guaranteed to afford reliable protection; and occupational asthma may (rarely) result in severe bronchospasm. By contrast, it is more realistic to achieve the control measures that ease the problems of aggravated ('work-exacerbated') non-occupational asthma, so the prospects for continued healthy employment are correspondingly brighter.

In practice, it may be difficult to distinguish between the two diagnoses: irritant industrial exposures often coexist with the presence of a workplace sensitizer, and workers with pre-existing asthma are not immune to occupational sensitization. A separate diagnostic problem arises in sensitized workers who manifest late asthmatic reactions, rather than immediate ones. Symptoms often arise at night-time, and thereby mimic the pattern of constitutional asthma. In difficult cases, assistance in diagnosis from a respiratory specialist with an interest in occupational lung disease is recommended.

FEV_1 is an insensitive indicator of occupational asthma and alternative investigations are required to secure a diagnosis. Agents that cause occupational asthma can be classified broadly into those that sensitize with the induction of specific IgE antibodies, and those like diisocyanates, colophony and some wood dusts that sensitize by other poorly understood means, and have mute or inconsistent antibody responses. Hence, for some causes of occupational asthma the detection of specific IgE antibodies may serve as an indicator of sensitization, as may a positive skin prick test. Examples include sensitivity to flour and enzymes in bakery workers, to animal products in exposed workers, or to latex in those who wear (powdered) latex gloves. These specific tests can

Table 18.3 Agents frequently reported to cause occupational asthma and occupations that often give rise to such reports

Agents	Occupations
Diisocyanates	Paint spraying, foam manufacture, industrial gluing, other chemical processing
Flour and grain dust	Baking, pastry making, dockworks
Colophony and fluxes	Electronic assembly
Animal proteins	Laboratory animal work, animal handling
Wood dusts (some)	Woodwork, timber handling
Enzymes	Baking, food processing, detergent manufacture
Persulphate salts	Hairdressing, circuit board manufacture
Complex platinum salts	Precious metal refining

Data from Nicholson et al. *Occupational asthma: Prevention, identification, and management: Systematic review and recommendations*. Copyright © 2010 The British Occupational Health Research Foundation (BOHRF).

be relatively sensitive for some agents[16] and can be used in case investigation. In some settings, such as the detergent industry, they are used in routine surveillance as an adjunct to exposure controls but the predictive value of a test depends not only on its sensitivity and specificity, but also on the prevalence of the disorder in the population tested, so in general tests of sensitization are unhelpful in screening. The distinction between sensitization and frank occupational asthma is an important one to draw; skin prick and serological tests do not in themselves indicate work-limiting disease and corroborative evidence is required before making placement decisions.

It is rarely necessary for an employee to be removed from their work while undergoing investigation for occupational asthma. If they are still exposed, and fit for further exposure, the standard investigative tool is serial measurement of PEF.[17] A pattern is sought of exaggerated PEF variability and a fall in mean PEF level around times of exposure. Normally, several readings a day (at work and away) will be required over a 3–4-week period—at least four per day to ensure adequate sensitivity and specificity.[16] Care is needed in the execution and interpretation of the test, and the variability of occupational asthma needs to be differentiated from normal diurnal changes in PEF and other determinants of airways responsiveness (exercise, infection etc.). The record must cover a period in which the potential for exposure exists, and this may require some pre-planning if exposures are intermittent. It is important to keep to the same pattern of measurement at work and on rest days.

Different PEF patterns can arise in affected workers, dependent on their response and recovery times. An immediate response and a short recovery interval will generate obvious PEF dips related in time to work, but late responses will produce dips at home, and those that occur at night can readily be confused with constitutional asthma. Slower recovery times may result in a day on day decline in the working week, with recovery at weekends. If recovery is protracted, ordinary work breaks may be insufficient for recovery, and a week on week decline ensues, leading to a nadir of persistently low values. Recovery may take weeks or months away from exposure and thus be difficult to determine from a relatively short period of monitoring. Diagnosis has traditionally been based on pattern recognition by an experienced physician, but rule-based quantitative approaches have been suggested and computerized diagnostic algorithms have been developed with some success.[18] Serial PEF measurement, if conducted correctly, is dependable with good agreement on interpretation between experts and few false positive results, but it may miss about 20 per cent of cases.[16] Questionnaires and history-taking display the obverse pattern, of relatively poor specificity but good sensitivity.

The 'gold standard' for diagnosis is a specific bronchial provocation (or inhalation) challenge test (BPT) with the suspected sensitizer: a simulated industrial exposure conducted under controlled conditions, with FEV_1 and responsiveness to histamine or methacholine measured serially. A late response, in particular, is taken as evidence of an allergic response; bronchial hyper-reactivity can also be demonstrated for 2–3 days after the challenge. The procedure entails a small risk of severe bronchospasm, and needs to be undertaken as an inpatient in a specialist hospital unit. Because of its risk and cost, BPT is usually reserved for special circumstances, which include the investigation of mixed exposures and novel agents, and situations of significant diagnostic uncertainty. Although it is often assumed that BPT is always correct, false negatives can arise if testing is conducted with the wrong material or too low an exposure or the patient has been unexposed to the sensitizing agent for a long period.

Occupational asthma is important and comparatively common; over 400 causal agents have been identified and several hundred new cases are diagnosed annually by UK specialists. It can result in acute severe bronchospasm in the workplace and chronic ill-health during employment. For some sensitizing agents, such as isocyanates, non-specific bronchial hyper-responsiveness is known to persistent for several years after leaving employment. There is reasonable research evidence that early re-deployment away from exposure can mitigate against the risk of continuing symptoms, and thus improve the long-term prognosis.[16,19] A comprehensive systematic review of this and other issues in occupational asthma, undertaken by Nicholson et al. on behalf of the British Occupational Health Research Foundation and the Faculty of Occupational Medicine, draws attention to the benefits of early withdrawal from exposure (Box 18.1).[16]

In the UK, the Control of Substances Hazardous to Health (COSHH) Regulations require health surveillance programmes to be conducted where there is a risk of occupational asthma. Guidance on the ingredients of suitable programmes is available through the UK Health and Safety Executive.[20] Periodic symptom enquiries (including nasal symptoms, an important precursor of occupational asthma), measurements of lung function and review of sickness absence reports are advised, the exact schedule being based on an assessment of risk. The effectiveness of health surveillance, in detecting early reversible disease, has not been rigorously established so far, and the ingredients that have the most impact are not well defined.[16] Nonetheless, screening, early detection of symptoms and prompt action are seen as vital ingredients in fitness assessment of workers from high-risk industries. The strong presumption is that those with occupational asthma should be re-deployed, and removed from further exposure to the sensitizing agent that caused their asthma, a policy for which there is persuasive evidence.[16,19]

Box 18.1 Evidence-based guidelines relating to the need to withdraw from causal exposures in subjects with occupational asthma

Statements and strength of evidence

The likelihood of improvement or resolution of symptoms or of preventing deterioration is greater in workers who:

- Avoid further exposure to the causative agent (2+).
- Have relatively normal lung function at the time of diagnosis (2+).
- Have a shorter duration of symptoms prior to diagnosis (2+).
- Have a shorter duration of symptoms prior to removal from exposure (2+).

Redeployment to a low exposure area may lead to improvement or resolution of symptoms or prevent deterioration in some workers, but is not always effective (3).

Where clinical considerations permit, reduction of exposure may be a useful alternative associated with fewer socioeconomic consequences to complete removal from exposure (2+).

Air-fed helmet respirators may improve or prevent symptoms but not for all workers who continue to be exposed to the causative agent (3).

2+: evidence from well-conducted case-control or cohort studies with a low risk of confounding or bias and a moderate chance of causality.
3: evidence only from non-analytic studies (e.g. case reports).

Data from Nicholson et al. *Occupational asthma: prevention, identification, and management: systematic review and recommendations,* Copyright © 2010 The British Occupational Health Research Foundation (BOHRF).

Nonetheless some doctors perceive a difficulty with employees who develop mild occupational asthma with normal pulmonary function when exposures are low or occasional. The pressure to continue in work (and preserve earning power) has to be balanced against the longer-term risks of deterioration, chronicity of symptoms and fixed airflow limitation. With respiratory protection, modification of their job to reduce exposure and effective treatment, many workers with occupational asthma have continued to work successfully. Under these circumstances close supervision is essential, and the ever-present risk of control failures should be borne in mind. Every effort should be made to explore work and process modifications that minimize the risk. Ideally patients should withdraw permanently from all further exposures; but if not, they should be aware that progression of symptoms can and sometimes does occur despite great care and redeployment to work areas of lower exposure.[21]

Some authorities have recommended policies that restrict the placement of workers perceived to be at greater risk of developing occupational asthma. Atopic individuals appear to be at increased relative risk when working with agents that induce specific IgE such as animal or bakery proteins, while smokers are at greater risk of asthma from diisocyanates, complex platinum salts and seafood proteins. In general, these risk factors are too common and too poorly discriminating to form a rational basis for health-based pre-placement selection. However, prudence dictates that persons with poorly controlled asthma should not be newly placed in environments known to contain respiratory sensitizers, since supervening occupational asthma will be more troublesome than in normal people.

Chronic obstructive pulmonary disease

Chronic obstructive pulmonary disease (COPD) is a common diagnosis, made in about 900 000 adults in the UK although it is estimated that a further 2 million (10 per cent of those aged 18–65) have the condition unrecognized.[22] Smoking leads to a syndrome of chronic mucus production with goblet cell hyperplasia (simple chronic bronchitis), and also to chronic airflow limitation with airways narrowing and emphysema. Exposure to industrial dust and fumes may contribute to both syndromes, although smoking tobacco is a more important cause. COPD often coexists with other diseases that share tobacco smoking as a risk factor, of which the most common are heart disease and lung cancer.

The principal symptoms in COPD are cough, sputum, and breathlessness on effort. Frequently, however, the symptoms and signs are non-specific and detection of latent airflow limitation is delayed until disease is more advanced. There have been several guidelines published for the diagnosis and management of COPD over the years, of which the most recent and most comprehensive is that commissioned by the National Institute for Health and Clinical Excellence (NICE) in 2010.[22]

In assessing the fitness for work of a person with COPD for employment, a number of matters need to be considered:

Is the problem primarily one of mucus hypersecretion or of airflow limitation?

Mucus hypersecretion by itself does not limit capacity to work, and in the absence of airflow limitation simple chronic bronchitis is compatible with a wide range of normal employment. Infective exacerbations and sickness absence may be more frequent, although a programme of winter influenza vaccinations may ameliorate the problem. In these circumstances a medical label may be unhelpful and prejudicial to employment prospects. Frequently, however, mucus hypersecretion coexists with airflow limitation, which can be a real cause of disability.

If airflow limitation is present, how severe is it and what is its functional effect?

Emphysema and airflow limitation are defined, respectively, in pathological and functional terms but their presence can be presumed when there is an obstructive pattern on spirometry with evidence of increased static lung volumes (TLC), gas trapping (disproportionate increase in RV with reduced RV/TLC ratio), and impaired gas transfer (TLCO). Although FEV_1 may be normal despite significant small airways disease, there is a broad correlation in COPD between FEV_1 and breathlessness, and it provides a better guide to disability than PEF. Spirometry predicts prognosis in COPD; for example, ventilatory failure (hypercapnia) is unusual if the FEV_1 is more than 1.5 L. More comprehensive measures, such as the 'BODE' index (comprising BMI, FEV_1, dyspnoea, and exercise tolerance) may provide better prognostic value than FEV_1, a reflection probably that breathlessness in COPD is multifactorial.[23] This potential advantage is offset by the additional inconvenience of making the various component measurements.

Measurements of lung function should, in principle, provide a fair guide to work capability in patients with airflow limitation, and spirometric findings can be banded according to their likely impact on function (see Table 18.4). However, the energy demands of work vary through time as the component activities of a task vary; individuals also vary in their oxygen requirements for a given task, because of personal and job-related factors; and resting lung function tests explain only a small part of the variance in VO_{2max}. The subjective appreciation of breathlessness usually proves to be the limiting factor. Hence, 'objective' measurements of disability provide no more than a rough guide to work capacity.[24,25] Crudely speaking, those with 'mild' impairment (Table 18.4) can manage most ordinary work, whereas those with 'moderate' impairment fail to meet the physical demands of many jobs, and those with 'severe' or 'very severe' impairment do not cope in most jobs. However, given wide individual variation and scope for job modification, fitness decisions still depend on subjective medical judgements.

Has optimum treatment been offered, or could disease control be improved?

In individuals with airflow limitation due to COPD there is limited scope for therapeutic improvement, and certainly less than for asthma. Detailed guidance on the stepped treatment of COPD is to be found in recent evidence-based guidelines.[22] Inhaled β-agonists, both short and long acting, are less effective than in asthma, and need to be used in doses that often provoke tremors. Anticholinergic agents, such as ipratropium bromide or the longer-acting tiotropium, may be more effective, and in disease of moderate severity either or both may be employed on a regular basis

Table 18.4 Spirometric criteria for the diagnosis of chronic obstructive pulmonary disease (COPD)

Post bronchodilator measurements		NICE	GOLD
FEV$_1$/FVC ratio	FEV$_1$% predicted		
<0.7	≥80	Mild[a]	Mild
<0.7	50–79	Moderate	Moderate
<0.7	30–49	Severe	Severe
<0.7	<30	Very severe	Very severe

[a] Symptoms should be present to diagnose COPD in people with mild airflow obstruction

GOLD: Global Initiative for Chronic Obstructive Lung Disease (2008); NICE: National Institute for Clinical Excellence UK (2010).

or long-acting beta-agonists substituted for shorter-acting ones. Bronchodilators may improve breathlessness and exercise tolerance, even in the absence of measurable bronchodilation.

The inflammation of COPD tends to be less responsive to steroids than in asthma, but there is evidence in patients with more severe COPD (FEV_1 <50 per cent predicted) or in those with persistent breathlessness that regular use of inhaled corticosteroids will reduce the number of exacerbations and slow the rate of decline in health status despite little improvement in lung function.

Theophyllines have only a modest bronchodilatory effect, but may modify small airways function and gas trapping and can be used in combination with other bronchodilators. Beneficial effects on exercise tolerance have been reported, but not consistently. Plasma theophylline levels should be monitored in view of their narrow therapeutic range and propensity to cause side effects and drug interactions. Mucolytic drugs have no effect on lung function, but may reduce the volume of expectorated sputum, the number of exacerbations and the number of days of COPD illness.

Formal exercise programmes ('pulmonary rehabilitation') increase functional and maximal exercise tolerance in symptomatic patients with moderately severe COPD. Programmes of rehabilitation should be tailored to individual needs; ingredients include disease education, including smoking cessation, and a review of medication and an assessment of psychological and nutritional needs. Patients should be encouraged to commit to an ongoing exercise programme.

It is essential to encourage COPD sufferers to stop smoking. In people with smoking-induced COPD the rate of decline in FEV_1 is increased from the average value of 20–30 mL per year seen in non-smokers to a value of around 60–80 mL per year or more. In smokers with moderate impairment of lung function, the rate of loss of function returns to normal upon smoking cessation, but the benefit in severe COPD and in industrial disease is less certain. Thus, an important preventive role for the occupational health service is to educate and to provide support for attempts to stop smoking, especially in employees with COPD. Guidance on smoking cessation in workplaces has been published by NICE.[26]

Finally, intercurrent infections require prompt treatment to prevent acute deteriorations and chronic airways damage. Annual vaccination against influenza (and one-off vaccination against pneumococcal infection) is generally recommended.

Are there any work factors that are liable to aggravate COPD?

In workers who develop troublesome progressive airflow limitation, continuing employment may still be possible in more sedentary work, or under a modified work schedule. One possible strategy may be to conduct less arduous work spread over a longer time period. Better process control (dust and fume control at source, assisted mechanical lifting, etc.) may also extend the range of employment possibilities and these measures should all be considered before declaring the worker unfit.

Are there special work problems for COPD sufferers?

The wearing of respiratory protective equipment (RPE) may increase the effort of work. Some RPE, like self-contained breathing apparatus (SCBA), can be bulky, heavy or awkward; while some RPE systems, such as canister respirators and half-face masks increase the work of breathing, requiring the wearer to inspire air against the resistance of a filter. It may be possible, instead, to provide a filter free 'active' system (air fed respirators blow a stream of fresh air across the face behind a visor, the positive pressure generated preventing the ingress of hazardous fumes), but even these require extra weight to be carried around whilst physically active; and the choice of system may be limited by the circumstances (e.g. the need to attain very high degrees of protection may necessitate SCBA, and work in oxygen deficient atmospheres may necessitate the carriage of gas cylinders). Fitness decisions need to be made in the light of residual lung capacity, the work in question and the options for process control over and above RPE use.

The presence of emphysema, particularly bullous disease, increases the risk of spontaneous pneumothorax and is thus a bar to employment in certain occupations that involve changes in barometric pressure (such as diving and air flight—see 'Special work problems and restrictions').

Interstitial lung disease

The important diseases in this group include interstitial fibrosis, chronic pulmonary sarcoidosis, and extrinsic allergic alveolitis. All these conditions can produce pulmonary fibrosis. In functional terms they reduce pulmonary compliance, reduce static lung volumes and impair gas transfer. $FEV_1/FVC\%$ is usually preserved, but airflow limitation may be present in addition to fibrosis. These conditions are all associated with radiological abnormalities; high-resolution CT scanning is more sensitive than plain radiography in assessing the extent of disease.

Pulmonary fibrosis may be cryptogenic, secondary to other clinical disorders (such as rheumatoid arthritis, systemic sclerosis, inflammatory bowel disease, sarcoidosis and chronic allergic alveolitis), or due to occupational contact with fibrogenic dusts. A number of professional groups, including miners and quarrymen, stone dressers, foundry fettlers and construction workers, are at special risk, although this fact may go unrecognized.[27]

Established fibrosis from whatever cause frequently progresses, although the rate of progression can be very variable. In the case of fibrogenic dust disease, progression may occur despite removal from the industry,[28,29] and early identification and withdrawal from exposure may result in a better long-term outcome. It seems prudent therefore to identify this disorder at an early stage and to recommend avoidance of further exposure. Unfortunately, there are no unique symptoms or signs and disease onset is insidious (over a decade or longer). Gradually progressive dyspnoea may be erroneously attributed to ageing or smoking, particularly when the potential for exposure is overlooked. A programme of regular surveillance in high risk professions obviates this problem. Tests of pulmonary function are not diagnostically specific, so plain radiography is the preferred approach. Radiography is considered to be about 80 per cent sensitive in asbestosis and silicosis, and other diagnostic methods such as high-resolution CT are often used in preference.

Table 18.5 details two model surveillance programmes advocated by the World Health Organization.[30] These include radiography, symptom enquiry and spirometry. In the UK, guidance has been provided by the HSE, though this is somewhat different in its content[31] and currently subject to review, given international variations in approach to surveillance in silica-exposed workers.[32] A surveillance programme must be instituted if the risk assessment indicates a reasonable likelihood of silicosis developing. It may include symptom inquiry, functional assessment, and regular chest x-rays but (for now) decisions about precise content are at the discretion of a doctor or nurse who must be engaged for the purpose.[31] Old tuberculosis may become reactivated in silica-exposed workers, so a history of earlier respiratory tuberculosis should also be sought. For health surveillance in asbestos workers, the HSE provides guidance for its Appointed Doctors.[33]

X-rays may be scored against a standard set of ILO films, based on the presence, profusion, size, and shape of opacities.[34] Category 1 changes can occur without evidence of impaired lung function. Category 2 change and above is associated with increasing impairment of lung function, and warrants removal from contact with fibrogenic dust, as does simple silicosis and asbestosis.

Table 18.5 WHO recommendations for health screening of workers exposed to asbestos or silica[27]

Agent	Surveillance procedure	Interval/frequency[a]
Silica (crystalline quartz) dust	• Chest radiograph	• At baseline, after 2–3 years of exposure, then every 2–5 years
	• Spirometry/symptom questionnaire	• At baseline, then annually, or at the same frequency as CXR
Asbestos	• Chest radiograph	• At baseline, then: – Every 3–5 years if less than 10 years since first exposed – Every 1–2 years if longer than 10 years but less than 20 years – Annually if longer than 20 years since first exposure
	• Spirometry/symptom questionnaire/physical examination	• Annually, or at the same frequency as the CXR

[a]In both cases, surveillance should be life-long.

Adapted from *The Lancet*, Volume 349, Issue 9061, Gregory R Wagner, Asbestosis and silicosis, pp. 1311–15, Copyright ©1997, with permission from Elsevier.

Established fibrotic lung disease is irreversible, and presently untreatable. Oral corticosteroids and other forms of immunosuppression such as cyclophosphamide or azathioprine, have been tried, but the results are generally disappointing. The principal disability is breathlessness on effort, which is often accompanied by significant falls in arterial oxygen levels. Spirometry and measurements of oxygen saturation during representative exercise provide a basis for fitness assessment; the general considerations are the same as those for COPD with airflow limitation. Affected workers may remain gainfully employed in less manual work, but disability tends to progress with time, and a periodic medical review is appropriate. Many forms of pulmonary fibrosis are associated with an increased risk of bronchogenic carcinoma.

Extrinsic allergic alveolitis (EAA) is a hypersensitivity pneumonitis, provoked principally by occupational allergens such as moulds or bird excreta. In its acute form it produces a mild systemic flu-like illness, with fever, aches and pains, malaise, weight loss, and dry cough. Symptoms develop within a few hours of exposure. Mild attacks resolve spontaneously, but severe attacks may require corticosteroid therapy. The condition is self-limiting if contact with the offending protein ceases, or if adequate respiratory protection is provided but chronic exposure can cause pulmonary fibrosis and permanent respiratory disability. Established fibrosis is unresponsive to treatment, so regular surveillance (through symptoms questionnaire and lung function testing, with chest radiography as clinically indicated) is appropriate for those with continuing potential for exposure.

Respiratory infections

Respiratory tract infections

These are very common. Occupational environments which are enclosed with little natural ventilation favour the spread of prevalent upper respiratory infections, particularly viral ones. These contribute importantly to short-term sickness absence, but are self-limiting and pose no special difficulties in fitness assessment.

More serious are a range of viral upper respiratory tract infections that may be complicated by chest problems or protracted debility. *Influenza* is a highly infectious condition that involves a longer period of sickness and a greater risk of complicating illness (tracheobronchitis, pneumonia, exacerbated COPD). Some occupational groups such as healthcare workers and teachers, are at particular risk, and may benefit from prophylaxis with influenza vaccine. Vaccination in these worker groups is also important in limiting risk to clients. It is recommended in those with pre-existing lung diseases such as asthma and COPD, irrespective of occupation.

Glandular fever and the other infectious mononucleoses are relatively common in young adults. Although these diseases are self-limiting, it is not uncommon to feel tired and fatigued for 3–6 months after the acute stage of illness. Sufferers who lack their normal stamina are often signed off as unfit to attend work, although a modified work programme with phased rehabilitation is a more constructive approach. Ideally this would encourage the individual to work their normal duties, but only for a part of the week to begin with, the hours gradually increasing as their stamina increases.

Some respiratory infections may be occupationally acquired (e.g. Q fever in slaughterhouse workers and veterinary surgeons and *Legionella* pneumonia in industries using humidification and water cooling plants), but these are uncommon occurrences. Occasionally respiratory infection may be transmitted from workers to members of the public, the most important example being tuberculosis (TB) in healthcare workers. Welders have an increased risk of contracting pneumococcal pneumonia and it is advisable to offer them specific vaccination.

Tuberculosis

TB is a respiratory infection spread by infected droplets from person to person. In the UK after 1950 the number of cases fell tenfold from around 50 000 per year, but this decline has reversed and the number of annual cases has risen to about 9000; the rise has been especially steep since 2000 and most prominent in English cities, in particular in parts of London. Worldwide, 9 million new cases occur each year, 95 per cent of which arise in low-income countries. Migrants from these countries bring with them an increased risk of tuberculosis. Among people born in the UK the annual incidence of TB is about 4/100 000 but rates in those born in other parts of the world, and especially Africa or the Indian subcontinent, are over 20 times higher so that 75 per cent of new cases reported in the UK occur in immigrants. In countries with a high prevalence of TB, the advent of human immunodeficiency virus (HIV) disease is promoting the disease in working-aged people. In the UK, where the reservoir of tuberculous infection has traditionally been in elderly people, HIV has been less of a factor but this is now changing with increasing numbers of HIV-positive cases of TB being diagnosed in patients arriving from high-risk countries. Worldwide about 2 million people die from tuberculosis each year of whom one in seven have HIV infection. Rates of TB are also high in other vulnerable groups such as homeless people, asylum seekers, prisoners, and substance misusers.

Cross-infectivity in TB arises principally in the close (domestic) contacts of patients with smear positive sputum. A survey of patients in the UK[35] found that 9–13 per cent of close contacts of smear-positive index cases developed disease. In casual contacts the risk was 0.3 per cent, and in close contacts of smear-negative index cases only 0.5 per cent of non-Asian and 2.8 per cent of Asian subjects developed TB. The risk of cross-infection with non-respiratory TB is very low. The principal risk, therefore, lies with close contacts of sputum smear-positive cases. Most occupational contacts are considered to be 'casual' rather than 'close'. Screening of workplace contacts is only necessary if the index case is smear positive and contacts are unusually susceptible—for example, immunocompromised adults—or the index case is considered highly infectious as shown by transmission to more than 10 per cent of close contacts. In the UK, cases of TB must be notified by the physician making or suspecting the diagnosis to the Health Protection Agency, which will institute screening of people at risk.

While it is uncommon for healthcare staff to acquire TB from patients, there is a duty of care to reduce the risks of transmission from staff to patients. Figure 18.2 displays an algorithm summarizing the advice provided by the 2011 NICE guidelines for the pre-placement screening of new NHS employees.[36] The recommended procedures depend on whether the employee is from a country of high or low (including the UK) TB incidence; and whether or not they will have contact with patients or clinical specimens. There is a strong emphasis on documented evidence and a reminder that students, locums, agency staff, and contract ancillary workers may easily be overlooked but should not be. NHS Trusts arranging care for NHS patients in non-NHS settings should ensure that healthcare workers there undergo the same screening.

At the pre-placement stage, details should be sought of any symptoms suggestive of TB, and of previous Bacillus Calmette–Guérin (BCG) vaccination (or the presence of a BCG scar confirmed by an occupational health professional), TB skin testing, or interferon gamma assay. The last of these should be offered to employees who are new to the NHS and from countries of high TB incidence, or who have had contact with patients in settings with a high TB prevalence. The test is a sensitive marker of infection and unlike skin tests is unaffected by prior BCG vaccination. If negative, as with a negative Mantoux result, BCG should be offered. If positive, the employee should be referred for clinical assessment for diagnosis and possible treatment of latent infection or active disease.

Vaccination has been shown to reduce the risk of active tuberculosis by 70–80 per cent. It is not necessary to inspect the site after the vaccination unless as a means of quality control of the technique of administering BCG. BCG vaccination is contraindicated in HIV-positive individuals. Potential employees from countries or groups with a high prevalence of HIV infection who are Mantoux negative (<6 mm) should be considered for HIV testing before BCG vaccination.

Healthcare workers who are found to be HIV positive during employment should have medical and occupational assessments of TB risk, and may need to modify their work to reduce exposure; HIV-positive healthcare workers should not be employed in areas where there is a risk of contacting active TB.

Similar guidance is provided for healthcare workers who care for prisoners and remand centre detainees; and for prison service staff and others who have regular contact with prisoners, for example, probation officers and education and social workers. Routine pre-placement screening is no longer required for schoolteachers and others working with children but it is important that these groups are aware of how TB presents.

During employment, routine periodic chest radiography is neither necessary, nor effective in screening. Awareness and early reporting of suspicious symptoms is the mainstay of detection.

If a worker contracts TB, treatment will usually comprise the *6-month, four-drug initial regimen* of 2 months of isoniazid, rifampicin, pyrazinamide, and ethambutol, followed by 4 months of isoniazid and rifampicin. Treatment should be supervised by a physician experienced in the management of TB. In fully sensitive infections (the majority in the UK), the patient is non-infectious after 2 weeks of treatment, and it is not usually necessary to restrict work after 2–3 weeks of treatment. Caution may be appropriate, however, where there is reason to suspect drug resistance, and in healthcare workers who deal with vulnerable patient groups (such as the immunosuppressed and young children). An infectious risk should be assumed until drug sensitivities are known or the sputum is known to be negative on culture. Drug resistance should be suspected in patients who have relapsed from earlier treatment, and those who come from areas where drug resistance

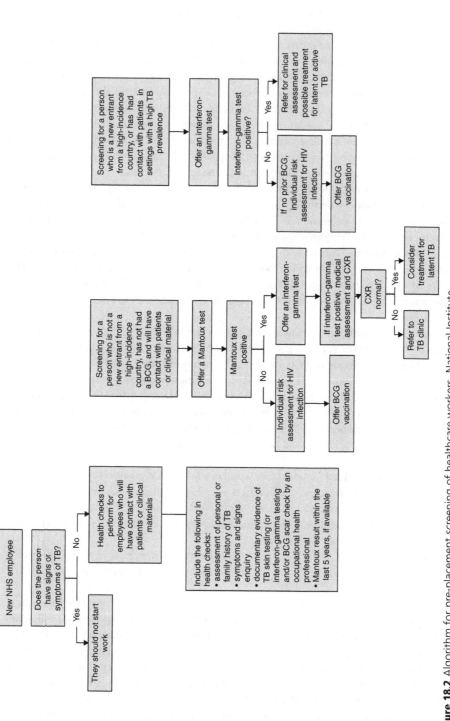

Figure 18.2 Algorithm for pre-placement screening of healthcare workers. National Institute for Health and Clinical Excellence (2012). Adapted from 'NICE Tuberculosis Pathway'. London: NICE (<http://pathways.nice.org.uk/pathways/tuberculosis>). Reproduced with permission. Information accurate at time of publication, for up-to-date information please visit <http://www.nice.org.uk>.

is common (e.g. Africa and the Indian subcontinent). HIV infection is a risk factor for drug-resistant TB. Problems may also arise in patients who comply poorly with treatment.

Neoplastic disease

Lung cancer

The most important risk factor for lung cancer is smoking. A number of occupational risk factors are also well recognized, asbestos exposure being numerically the most important. For asbestos-induced lung cancer, the risks multiply with those of smoking. Occupationally-related lung cancers may also arise in the extraction of chromium from its ore, the manufacture of chromates, nickel refining, and exposure to polycyclic aromatic hydrocarbons, cadmium compounds, arsenic (in mining, smelting, and pesticide production) and bis-chloromethyl and chloromethyl methyl ethers.

The different histological types of lung cancer vary in their growth rate. In the absence of treatment, a patient with adenocarcinoma is likely to survive for about 2 years from diagnosis, a patient with a squamous cell tumour for about 1 year, and a patient with a small cell tumour for about 4 months. Small cell tumours metastasize early, and are rarely amenable to surgical cure but 85 per cent respond to combination chemotherapy. The median survival is thus extended to about 8 months in patients with extensive disease, and to about 14 months in patients with limited disease; but a minority survive longer (10 per cent for 2 years, 4 per cent for 5 years). During this period, patients often enjoy a good quality of life and can sometimes continue in light work.

For non-small cell lung cancer (adenocarcinoma, squamous carcinoma, and undifferentiated tumours), chemotherapy is much less successful, and the preferred treatment is surgical resection. Radiotherapy is usually used as an adjunct to surgery, or for the palliation of specific problems, such as haemoptysis and localized bone pain. Unfortunately, most tumours present when advanced, and other smoking-related lung disease often limits resectability. About 25 per cent of patients are suitable for surgery. Of these, about a third survive for 5 years (65–85 per cent in the absence of lymph node, chest wall, and metastatic involvement; but only around 25–35 per cent when there is ipsilateral mediastinal lymph node involvement). Patients below retirement age who undergo successful resection may well be able to return to work, though the choice of employment will depend on the physical demands of the job and their residual lung function.

Mesothelioma

Mesothelioma is a rare tumour in the absence of asbestos exposure. It is a malignant condition affecting the pleura, or less often the peritoneum. The tumour arises after a long latent period—rarely less than 20 years from first exposure, and typically 35–40 years. Thus, most cases arise after retirement.

The incidence of the tumour continues to rise in the UK, reflecting the greater use of asbestos after the 1960s. Currently there are about 2000 cases/year, 80 per cent of them in men, and the great majority attributable to occupational asbestos exposure, but there has been a shift from those employed in industries with primary exposure such as asbestos manufacture and lagging to those with secondary exposures such as plumbers, builders, and other crafts trades. Amphibole fibre types (crocidolite and amosite) pose a far higher risk than chrysotile although this is seldom relevant in the UK where fibre mixtures were widely used. Rates of mesothelioma in the UK are as high as anywhere in the world and are expected to increase until 2015/2020.

Mesothelioma often presents with chest wall pain, breathlessness, and pleural effusion. It progresses mainly by local invasion, although distant metastases can sometimes occur. Involvement of the chest wall, diaphragm, mediastinum, and neck root is common, and results in local pain, restricted chest movement, dysphagia, obstruction of the great veins, and pericardial involvement. The condition is incurable and most patients die within 2 years of presentation. It is rare for a patient with mesothelioma to be able to continue for long in active employment.

Other diseases of the pleura

A common manifestation of pleural disease is *pleural effusion*. Effusions that result from inflammatory processes are exudates, with a high protein content (>30 g/L). Underlying causes include infection, collagen vascular disease, malignancy, and pulmonary infarction. Pleural malignancy, pulmonary infarction, and asbestotic pleurisy can also produce blood-stained effusions. Effusions of low protein content (transudates, protein <25 g/L) may arise in cardiac failure and low protein states such as nephrotic syndrome and cirrhosis of the liver.

Fitness decisions require accurate information on the cause of the effusion and its prognosis. Investigation by aspiration, examination and culture of the fluid, and closed pleural biopsy normally enable the various possibilities to be distinguished, but otherwise thoracoscopy with biopsy, or open pleural biopsy are necessary.

When inflammatory effusions resolve, they frequently leave behind an area of pleural thickening, and adhesions that obliterate the pleural space. If extensive, this thickening can restrict lung movement and produce chest discomfort and breathlessness on exertion.

A *pneumothorax* may be a primary, 'spontaneous' event or a complication of trauma or of other, serious lung disease such as emphysema, pulmonary fibrosis, or cystic fibrosis. Its incidence is five times higher in men than in women. It characteristically afflicts young, tall men and causes symptoms of breathlessness and chest pain commensurate with its size; a tension pneumothorax is potentially lethal. Treatment depends on the extent of the air leak and ranges from simple observation to intrapleural drainage. The natural incidence of recurrence after spontaneous pneumothorax is about 50 per cent over 4 years; but is virtually eliminated by surgical pleurodesis. The occurrence (and recurrence) of pneumothorax is of concern in certain occupations where sudden changes in ambient air pressure are expected; specific guidance is available (see 'Special work problems and restrictions').

At work, asbestos exposure frequently causes *pleural plaques*, which are circumscribed areas of thickening on the parietal pleura that may gradually calcify. They are composed of areas of hyaline fibrosis, a few millimetres up to one centimetre in thickness. Plaques are discovered radiographically, (and seldom become evident within 15 years of first exposure), but they do not obliterate the pleural space, and produce no impairment of lung function or other disability. Their presence does not correlate well with that of pulmonary fibrosis (asbestosis), nor do they predicate the occurrence of mesothelioma (which is related to levels of exposure, but no more common in those who develop plaques than in those who do not). They tend to be discovered accidentally and do not require work restriction or re-deployment.

Asbestos exposure sometimes leads to *pleurisy* and haemorrhagic exudative pleural effusion. Effusion may also be discovered as an incidental radiographic finding. The majority occur 10–15 years after first exposure. They may persist for several months, recur after drainage, or affect both sides in sequence over a year or two. Biopsy simply shows non-specific pleural inflammation. These pleural effusions may lead on to adhesions and *diffuse, visceral pleural thickening*. This latter condition, if extensive, produces restriction of lung expansion, dyspnoea and work limitation. Bilateral pleural thickening is a prescribed disease. There is no evidence that simple pleural plaques progress to diffuse pleural thickening, which is a different entity.

Smoking

Smoking is a major cause of respiratory disability, being the principal cause of both COPD and lung cancer, the two conditions that together account for the majority of deaths from primary respiratory disease. The heavier the smoking the greater the risk. It is clearly good preventive practice to offer help and support to those who want to stop smoking and to make the workforce generally aware of the risks. The benefits of smoking cessation in COPD have already been discussed. A review of smoking cessation interventions in the workplace concluded that measures directed towards individual smokers, including counselling and pharmacological treatment of nicotine addiction, all increase the likelihood of quitting (the effects being similar to those when offered outwith the workplace). Self-help interventions and social support seem to be less effective. There is only limited evidence that participation in cessation programmes can be increased by competitions and incentives organized by the employer.

In the past, some 600 premature deaths annually in the UK could be attributed to passive workplace smoking,[37] a figure about three times higher than the annual number of deaths from industrial accidents. Legislation in the UK no longer permits smoking in any wholly or substantially enclosed workplace used by more than one person, or in any vehicle used for business purposes. Smoking rooms are not allowed except in exempted premises (e.g. prison cells, hospices, and residential homes); and employers are not obliged to provide an outside smoking area.

Special work problems and restrictions

Sometimes work is conducted in adverse environments, or in safety critical roles characterized by a requirement for high standards of respiratory fitness. Such is the case in airline pilots and cabin crew, commercial and military divers, caisson workers, and members of the armed forces, police, and rescue services. A number of these work activities involve changes in gas pressure and composition, and the use of breathing apparatus to extend the range of hostile environments in which work can be conducted; and all require a general level of fitness that transcends simple respiratory health. In some cases the fitness standards are such as to mandate assessment by approved medical examiners (e.g. HSE Approved Medical Examiners of Divers under the Diving at Work Regulations 1997).

The fitness standards of pilots and divers, and the physiological demands of their work are more fully described in Appendices 1 and 4, but reference is made here to some of the respiratory aspects of the work.

Flying and diving result in ambient gas pressure changes that pose major respiratory problems. The airways become irritated by changes in pressure and humidity and the muscles of the chest tire within minutes if transmural pressures exceed 5 kPa. At transmural pressures of about 10 kPa (one-tenth of an atmosphere) the lungs rupture. The fall in ambient pressure encountered in aeroplane ascent may thus result in pneumothorax, if gas trapping occurs in the chest (as might arise in bullous emphysema, asthma, or recent chest trauma). Similarly, ascent from a commercial or military dive may result in trapped gas at higher than ambient pressure seeking a means of escape, and causing pulmonary barotrauma or decompression sickness. Pneumothorax, peribronchial rupture, mediastinal emphysema, and air emboli are all well-recognized outcomes.

Related problems arise from altered oxygen tensions. The lowered partial pressure of oxygen at elevated altitudes may aggravate hypoxia in air crew with existing airways disease; and, in fighter pilots, the problem may be exacerbated by physiological shunting in the dependent parts of the lung during high-G turns.

High standards of respiratory fitness are required in such work, from the viewpoint of personal safety and well-being, and (especially in the case of aircrew) because of their responsibility for expensive equipment and other lives. In new entrants, a history of spontaneous pneumothorax (untreated by pleurodesis), poorly controlled asthma, or other obstructive respiratory disease may be a bar to employment.

In established workers who develop chest disease, the criteria are slightly less stringent: it may, for example, be possible for well-controlled asthmatics, or patients with a pleurectomy or pleurodesis, to continue as members of an aircrew. The standards are set down respectively by the Civil Aviation Authority and armed services for flight fitness, and the HSE in the UK for fitness to dive.[38] In each of these cases, regular assessment is required by approved medical assessors, followed by certification of continuing fitness. Assessments may include a number of subsidiary investigations, as described in Appendices 1 and 4.

Intercurrent respiratory illness is a temporary bar to diving and flying. Failure to equilibrate pressures across the eustachian tube in catarrhal illness, and air trapping in the sinuses can cause decompression trauma, so diving and flying are best avoided until natural recovery has occurred. Professional divers who have recently surfaced (decompressed) sometimes wish then to fly: this may represent a further extreme of decompression, and they should be advised to refrain from flying until a minimum of 12 hours has elapsed.

Recommended minimum fitness standards for workers in the UK *armed services* are laid down in a Joint Services System of Medical Classification (JSP 346). New applicants with active TB, chronic bronchitis, or bronchiectasis are normally rejected, but if disease appears for the first time in service, the worker is individually assessed. Current asthma, or recurrent wheeze requiring recent treatment (within the past 4 years), is treated similarly; while those with a more distant history are tested for exercise-induced decrements of FEV_1. The occurrence of pneumothorax requires individual assessment, and depends on the nature of the work and the success or otherwise of surgical treatment.

The armed services use the 'PULHHEEMS' system to rank fitness for a number of physical and mental attributes against an eight-point scale of descriptors. Respiratory fitness is not separately identified in the rubric, although the P scale (physical fitness) encompasses cardiorespiratory fitness. Between services and between jobs there may be some differences. For example, the fitness standards in RAF air crew are more stringent than for ground personnel, such as engineers and technicians. However, for many jobs the minimum standard (fit with training for heavy manual work, including lifting and climbing, but not to endure severe or prolonged strain) precludes sufferers of significant chest disease.

Firefighters are required to operate in very adverse environments, to wear breathing apparatus, and to perform physically arduous tasks. UK regulations require *fire service workers* to have their FEV_1 and FVC measured by a doctor, and to have their aerobic capacity measured in a step test prior to employment. The regulations stipulate that a duly qualified medical practitioner must be satisfied that these measurements are compatible with the fitness requirements of firefighting, but refer to these only in general terms. Guidance from central government is available,[39] but is soon to be updated. Currently it recommends regular fitness assessments and a 3-yearly health surveillance programme that involves measurement of height, weight, pulse, blood pressure, and visual acuity, as well as FEV_1 and FVC although the performance standard for spirometry is not specified.

The Fire and Rescue Services Act 2004 has permitted an individual approach to fitness assessment in fire service personnel, matching the requirements of the Equality Act. Approximate standards have evolved on the basis of careful job analysis and the separation of operational from other roles but current guidance recognizes that individuals with the same diagnosis may differ considerably in the severity of their condition, and advice on respiratory restrictions (still evolving) is less prescriptive than hitherto. Intercurrent illnesses provide no more than a temporary bar to active duties, but conditions of airflow limitation may jeopardize employment prospects. Rescue workers may encounter irritant or sensitizing fumes and many products of combustion; some of these will exacerbate asthma, and some, including products of PVC combustion, may incite new asthma (reactive airways dysfunction syndrome or RADS). Poorly controlled asthma on application often leads to rejection; if there is a prior history, or disease develops during employment, the circumstances should be individually assessed, but recurrent, severe, or refractory symptoms may precipitate medical retirement. In contrast to earlier advice, however, it is likely that most firefighters with well-controlled asthma are able to function effectively, including when wearing breathing apparatus. Severe reductions in FEV_1 and FEV_1/FVC ratio in firefighters with COPD may be incompatible with active firefighting, and close monitoring is advocated in the case, for example, of restrictive lung disease and recurrent pneumothorax. The occurrence of pneumothorax should trigger individual review, but a successful pleurodesis may enable active duties to continue. Finally, the development of lung cancer would lead to rejection or retirement, but a successfully resected benign tumour is not a definite bar.

References

1 British Thoracic Society. *The burden of lung disease: A statistics report from the British Thoracic Society.* London: British Thoracic Society 2006. (<http://www.brit-thoracic.org.uk/Portals/0/Library/BTS%20 Publications/burden_of_lung_disease.pdf>)

2 Townsend MC and the Occupational and Environmental Lung Disorders Committee. Spirometry in the occupational health setting—2011 update (ACOEM guidance statement). *J Occup Environ Med* 2011; **53**: 569–84.

3 Miller MR, Crapo R, Hankinson J, *et al.* General considerations for lung function testing. *Eur Respir J* 2005; **26**(1): 153–61.

4 De Jongh F. Lung function testing features: spirometers. *Breathe* 2008; **4**(3): 251–4.

5 Miller MR. Lung function testing features: how to interpret spirometry. *Breathe* 2008; **4**(3): 259–61.

6 Eisen EA, Dockery DW, Speizer FE, *et al.* The association between health status and the performance of excessively variable spirometry tests in a population-based study in six U.S. cities. *Am Rev Respir Dis* 1987; **136**(6): 1371–6.

7 Singh SJ, Morgan MD, Scott S, *et al.* Development of a shuttle walking test of disability in patients with chronic airways obstruction. *Thorax* 1992; **47**(12): 1019–24.

8 Medical Research Council on the Aetiology of Chronic Bronchitis. Standardized questionnaires on respiratory symptoms. *BMJ* 1960; **ii**: 665.

9 Toren K, Brisman J, Jarvholm B. Asthma and asthma-like symptoms in adults assessed by questionnaires. A literature review. *Chest* 1993; **104**(2): 600–8.

10 Venables KM, Farrer N, Sharp L, *et al.* Respiratory symptoms questionnaire for asthma epidemiology: validity and reproducibility. *Thorax* 1993; **48**(3): 214–19.

11 Wagner GR. Asbestosis and silicosis. *Lancet* 1997; **349**(9061): 1311–15.

12 Stenton SC, Beach JR, Avery AJ, *et al.* Asthmatic symptoms, airway responsiveness and recognition of bronchoconstriction. *Respir Med* 1995; **89**(3): 181–5.

13 Stenton SC, Beach JR, Avery AJ, *et al.* The value of questionnaires and spirometry in asthma surveillance programmes in the workplace. *Occup Med* 1993; **43**(4): 203–6.

14 Scottish Intercollegiate Guidelines Network and British Thoracic Society. *British guideline on the management of asthma: a national clinical guideline,* revised 2011. [Online] (<http://www.sign.ac.uk/pdf/sign101.pdf>)

15 Henneberger PK, Redlich CA, Callahan DB, *et al.* An official American Thoracic Society statement: work-exacerbated asthma. *Am J Respir Crit Care Med* 2011; **184**(3): 368–78.

16 Nicholson, PJ, Cullinan, P, Burge, PS, *et al. Occupational asthma: prevention, identification, and management: systematic review and recommendations.* London: BOHRF, 2010.

17 Moore VC, Jaakkola MS, Burge PS. A systematic review of serial peak expiratory flow measurements in the diagnosis of occupational asthma. *Ann Respir Med* 2010; 1(1): 31–44.

18 Moore VC, Jaakkola MS, Burge CB, *et al.* A new diagnostic score for occupational asthma: the area between the curves (ABC score) of peak expiratory flow on days at and away from work. *Chest* 2009; **135**(2): 307–14.

19 de Groene GJ, Pal TM, Beach J, *et al.* Workplace interventions for treatment of occupational asthma. *Cochrane Database Syst Rev* 2011; **5**: CD006308.

20 Health and Safety Executive. *Medical aspects of occupational asthma.* London: HMSO, 1991.

21 Tee RD, Gordon DJ, Hawkins ER, *et al.* Occupational allergy to locusts: an investigation of the sources of the allergen. *J Allergy Clin Immunol* 1988; **81**(3): 517–25.

22 National Institute for Health and Clinical Excellence. *Chronic obstructive pulmonary disease.* NICE clinical guideline 101. London: NICE, 2010. (<http://www.nice.org.uk/nicemedia/live/13029-49397/49397.pdf>)

23 Celli BR, Cote CG, Marin JM, *et al.* The body-mass index, airflow obstruction, dyspnea, and exercise capacity index in chronic obstructive pulmonary disease. *N Engl J Med* 2004; **350**(10): 1005–12.

24 Harber P. Respiratory disability. The uncoupling of oxygen consumption and disability. *Clin Chest Med* 1992; **13**(2): 367–76.

25 Williams SJ, Bury MR. Impairment, disability and handicap in chronic respiratory illness. *Soc Sci Med* 1989; **29**(5): 609–16.

26 National Institute for Health and Clinical Excellence. *Smoking cessation services in primary care, pharmacies, local authorities and workplaces, particularly for manual working groups, pregnant women and hard to reach communities. NICE public health guidance.* London: NICE, 2008. (<http://www.nice.org.uk/nicemedia/live/11925-39596/39596.pdf>)

27 Wagner GR. Asbestosis and silicosis. *Lancet* 1997; **349**(9061): 1311–15.

28 Steenland K, Brown D. Silicosis among gold miners: exposure—response analyses and risk assessment. *Am J Public Health* 1995; **85**(10): 1372–7.

29 Becklake MR, Liddell FD, Manfreda J, McDonald JC. Radiological changes after withdrawal from asbestos exposure. *Br J Ind Med* 1979; **36**(1): 23–8.

30 Wagner GR. *Screening and surveillance of workers exposed to mineral dusts.* Geneva: WHO, 1996.

31 Health and Safety Executive. *G404 COSHH essentials: General guidance. Health surveillance for those exposed to respirable crystalline silica (RCS).* Control approach 4 Special. Sudbury: HSE Books, 2011.

32 Bradshaw L, Bowen J, Fishwick D, et al. *Health surveillance in silica exposed workers.* Sudbury: HSE Books, 2010.

33 Health and Safety Executive. *Guidance for appointed doctors on the Control of Asbestos Regulations.* Sudbury: HSE Books, 2011. (<http://www.hse.gov.uk/pubns/ms31.pdf>)

34 International Labour Office. *Guidelines for the use of ILO international classification of radiographs of pneumoconioses.* Geneva: ILO, 1980.

35 A study of a standardised contact procedure in tuberculosis. Report by the Contact Study Sub-Committee of The Research Committee of the British Thoracic Association. *Tubercle* 1978; **59**(4): 245–59.

36 National Institute for Health and Clinical Excellence. *Tuberculosis—clinical diagnosis and management of tuberculosis, and measures for its prevention and control.* Clinical guideline 33. London: NICE, 2006.

37 Jamrozik K. Estimate of deaths attributable to passive smoking among UK adults: database analysis. *BMJ* 2005; **330**(7495): 812.

38 Health and Safety Executive. *The Medical Examination and Assessment of Divers (MA1)*, updated April 2008. [Online] (<http://www.hse.gov.uk/diving/ma1.pdf>)

39 Office of the Deputy Prime Minister. *Medical and Occupational Evidence for Recruitment and Retention in the Fire and Rescue Service.* London: TSO, 2004. (<http://www.communities.gov.uk/documents/fire/pdf/130418.pdf>)

Chapter 19

Renal and urological disease

John Hobson and Edwina A. Brown

Introduction

The kidney has the vital function of excretion, and controls acid–base, fluid, and electrolyte balance. It also acts as an endocrine organ. Renal failure, with severe impairment of these functions, results from a number of different processes, most of which are acquired, although some may be inherited. Glomerulonephritis, which presents with proteinuria, haematuria, or both, may be accompanied by hypertension and impaired renal function. Pyelonephritis with renal scarring is the end result of infective disorders. Diabetes is now the commonest cause of end-stage renal disease (ESRD) in the UK and other systemic disease such as hypertension and collagen disorders can also affect the kidney. Polycystic kidney disease is the commonest inherited disorder leading to renal failure. Chronic renal failure implies permanent renal damage, which is likely to be progressive and will eventually require renal replacement therapy.

Treatment of ESRD using haemodialysis (HD) and peritoneal dialysis (PD) can significantly improve physical and metabolic well-being and function but the proportion of those who continue to work with ESRD remains very low despite advances in treatment. Kidney transplantation enables many patients to return to normal lives including work. Reintegration of patients into the workforce following transplantation or dialysis offers an exciting and rewarding challenge to the wider health team.

Renal disease is not within the top ten of the most costly diseases for employers and accounts for less than 1 per cent of sickness absence and incapacity claims. Urinary incontinence affects significant proportions of the workforce particularly women. Better management of urinary infections and calculi, prostatic obstruction, incontinence, and other complications of urinary tract disease has significantly reduced time lost from work.

Prevalence and morbidity

The 2010 UK Renal Registry report[1] shows that the 2009 annual acceptance rate for new patients starting on renal replacement therapy (RRT) is stable at 109/million population. Acceptance ratios, standardized for age and gender of the population served, correlate significantly with both social deprivation and with ethnicity; the number of patients requiring RRT increases in areas with high numbers of ethnic minorities.

The 2010 report also shows that the number of patients on RRT in the UK in 2009 was 794/million population compared to 626/million population in 2002. The median age for HD, PD, and transplant patients, respectively, was 65.9, 61.2, and 50.8 years. Transplantation is the most common treatment modality (48 per cent).

Chronic kidney disease (CKD) is relatively common, with only a minority developing ESRD requiring RRT. The prevalence in the USA in 1999–2004 appeared to be increasing compared to the previous 5 years owing to the rising prevalence of diabetes, hypertension, and high body mass index;[2] 7.7 per cent of the population had CKD stage 3 with a glomerular filtration rate (GFR) of 30–59 mL/min per 1.73 m^2 (vs. 5.4 per cent in the earlier period) while 0.35 per cent (vs. 0.21 per cent) had CKD stage 4, with a GFR less than 15–29 mL/min per 1.73 m^2. Planning for renal replacement therapy starts when the estimated GFR (eGFR) is less than 20 mL/min per 1.73 m^2. Dialysis is not usually commenced until eGFR is less than 10 mL/min per 1.73 m^2. Increasingly, however, patients eligible for transplantation are being pre-emptively transplanted from live donors or placed on the deceased donor waiting list once eGFR has declined below 20 mL/min per 1.73 m^2.

In terms of certified sickness and claims for benefit, diseases of the genitourinary tract (International Statistical Classification of Diseases and Related Health Problems (ICD)-10 N00–N99) make up a small proportion of claimants nationally accounting for 1 per cent or less of each.

Although many *urinary tract infections* are asymptomatic, there is much morbidity from this condition. Below the age of 50 the disease only affects women but after the age of 60 it becomes more frequent in males, owing to lower urinary tract conditions, especially prostatic problems.

Urolithiasis of the upper urinary tract has a prevalence of 5 per cent in the UK with a peak incidence in males at the age of 35 years.

Benign prostatic hyperplasia (BPH) is common after the fourth decade; 50 per cent of men have BPH when they are 51–60 years old. At the age of 55, 25 per cent notice some decrease in force of their urinary stream. At age 40 (surviving to 80) years there is a cumulative incidence of 29 per cent for prostatectomy. In England and Wales *prostate cancer* (ICD-10 C61) is the most frequently registered malignancy in males accounting for over a quarter of registrations (34500) in 2009.[3] *Bladder cancer* (ICD-10 C67) is the fifth most common tumour in men (4 per cent of male cancer deaths) and the eleventh in women (2 per cent of female cancer deaths), but 90 per cent occur over the age of 65.

Mortality

The majority of patients with renal disease will die from cardiovascular disease before they require RRT. An analysis of causes of death from 1996 to 2000 in over a million adults enrolled in the Kaiser Permamente managed healthcare programme of Northern California showed that risk of death from any cause increased sharply as the estimated GFR declined, ranging from a 17 per cent increase in risk with an estimated GFR of 45–59 mL/min per 1.73 m^2 to a 343 per cent increase with an estimated GFR less than 15 mL/min per 1.73 m^2.[4] There was a similar increase in cardiovascular events and hospitalization. The age-adjusted mortality rate for an estimated GFR of 15–29 mL/min per 1.73 m^2 was strikingly high at 11.4/100 person-years, which is similar to those on RRT. The vast majority (90 per cent) of deaths from renal failure (ICD-10, N17–19)[3] occur over retirement age, although the associated morbidity is incurred during the working years. Survival rates for urological cancers are shown in Table 19.1.

Table 19.1 Five-year survival rates for England and Wales

	Bladder	Kidney	Prostate
Males	57%	49%	77%
Females	47%	49%	

Data from <http://www.cancerresearchuk.org/>

Presentation

Kidney disease is easily missed. Early disease can often be asymptomatic and present as urinary abnormalities on routine urine testing, hypertension or as biochemical abnormalities. GFR should then be estimated, as significant renal impairment can be present even when the plasma creatinine is normal. The discovery of asymptomatic haematuria, whether macroscopic or microscopic, and not related to urinary tract infection, requires further investigation. If positive, dipstick testing should always be repeated to distinguish transient from other causes of haematuria. The finding of two out of three positive (1+ or more) tests warrants further investigation for malignancy in appropriate age groups.[5]

Guidelines for identification of kidney disease

Clinical guidelines for the identification and management of chronic kidney disease were formulated by NICE (National Institute for Health and Clinical Excellence) in 2008.[6] NICE state that people should be offered testing for CKD if they have any of the following risk factors:

♦ Diabetes (types 1 and 2).

♦ Hypertension.

♦ Cardiovascular disease (ischaemic heart disease, chronic heart failure, peripheral vascular disease, and cerebral vascular disease).

♦ Structural renal tract disease, renal calculi, or prostatic hypertrophy.

♦ Multisystem diseases with potential kidney involvement (e.g. systemic lupus erythematosus).

♦ Family history of stage 5 CKD (dialysis or transplantation) or hereditary kidney disease.

The guidelines also state that reagent strips should be used rather than urine microscopy when testing for the presence of haematuria. To detect proteinuria, urine albumin:creatinine ratio (ACR) should be used as it can detect low levels of proteinuria. Urine protein:creatinine ratio (PCR) can be used for higher levels of proteinuria and to monitor urine protein excretion. As a rough guide, ACR of 30 mg/mmol is approximately equivalent to PCR of 50 mg/mmol or urinary protein excretion of 0.5 g/24 hours.

Not all patients with CKD should be referred for a specialist nephrological opinion. The guidelines include the following criteria for specialist referral: eGFR less than 30 mL/min/m²; heavy proteinuria (ACR ≥70 mg/mmol or PCR ≥100 mg/mmol) or lower levels (ACR ≥30 or PCR >50 mg/mmol) in presence of haematuria; rapidly declining eGFR (>5 mL/min/1.73 m²) in 1 year; poorly controlled hypertension.

The Renal Association and British Association of Urological Surgeons have also written guidelines regarding initial assessment of haematuria.[7] These state that all patients with visible haematuria (any age), all patients with symptomatic non-visible haematuria, and those aged 40 or older with asymptomatic non-visible haematuria (having excluded urinary infection and significant proteinuria) should be referred to urology for further investigation including ultrasonography and cystoscopy.

Diabetes

Diabetes is the commonest cause of ESRD accounting for 24 per cent of patients starting dialysis in the UK in 2009 (and up to 40–50 per cent in many countries in the developed world). The natural history is the development of microalbuminuria, progressing to overt proteinuria with hypertension and subsequent decline in renal function. In young patients with insulin-dependent diabetes, this process does not commence until at least 10 years after the onset of diabetes. This is not true for non-insulin-dependent diabetes where the onset of the disease is less clear-cut; it is not uncommon for patients to have proteinuria or even significant renal disease at the time of diagnosis. The majority of patients with renal disease associated with type 1 or 2 diabetes will also have diabetic retinopathy with its associated problems.

Complications and sequelae of renal disease

Hypertension

Most patients with renal disease will eventually develop hypertension. This needs aggressive treatment as tight blood pressure control (<125/75 mmHg in patients with proteinuria) significantly slows the progression of renal damage. This usually requires multiple drugs, which may cause side effects. Frequent monitoring of blood pressure is important and patients are encouraged to self-monitor as this correlates better with 24-hour blood pressure measurements and avoids white coat hypertension.

Cardiovascular disease

Cardiovascular disease is the major cause of death in patients with renal failure and even mild renal disease is associated with increased cardiovascular risk. Patients with cardiovascular disease have a worse outcome if they have even mild renal disease.[8]

Renal failure

The early symptoms of renal failure are fatigue with poor exercise tolerance. These can develop when the GFR is as high as 30 mL/min and can be exacerbated by the presence of anaemia, which can occur with GFRs of 30–40 mL/min. Deteriorating renal function leads to poor appetite with subsequent weight loss, fluid retention with associated ankle swelling and shortness of breath on exercise, loss of libido, and nocturia due to polyuria from osmotic diuresis. Many of these symptoms improve when the anaemia is corrected with appropriate use of erythropoietin (EPO) and iron supplements. Prior treatment with EPO has been found to be a significant factor in maintaining employment once dialysis commences.[9] The level of symptoms should determine the start of dialysis rather than blood tests or GFR measurements. It is more important that a patient remains relatively well and in employment rather than waiting to become really ill and then requiring prolonged rehabilitation.

End-stage renal disease

The aims of RRT are not simply correction of blood abnormalities and maintenance of fluid balance. Patients can live on RRT for decades so the aims are for them to live as normal a life as possible. It is important that they adopt a mode of RRT that they tolerate and comply with, that provides physical well-being, and allows social and employment rehabilitation. There are now many options for the treatment of ESRD (Box 19.1).

Dialysis

Patients with ESRD can now expect a reasonable survival and quality of life on dialysis. The 2010 UK renal registry report shows that the annual survival rate for patients younger than 65 years old is 92 per cent. For patients who can use any modality, the choice of HD or PD will depend on individual patient preference, nephrologist bias, and local resources. Approximately 28 per cent of patients younger than 65 years old start PD in the UK but this can vary between hospitals in the same city. Dialysis affects all aspects of life including work, diet, family life, holidays, and travel. From the patient's perspective, perceived quality of life is the principal reason for choosing

Box 19.1 Treatment modalities for ESRD

- ◆ **Haemodialysis (HD)**
  - Centre
  - Satellite
  - Home
- ◆ **Peritoneal dialysis (PD)**
  - CAPD (continuous ambulatory PD)
  - APD (automated PD)
- ◆ **Transplantation**
  - Cadaver
  - Living donor (related or unrelated)
- ◆ **Conservative management**
- ◆ **Best supportive care**

between dialysis modalities. As shown in Box 19.2, the main differences between PD and HD arise because PD is a home-based treatment and HD (with few exceptions) is a hospital-based treatment.

A study of patients commencing dialysis in the Netherlands showed that of the 864 patients who chose their dialysis modality, 36 per cent starting PD were employed as compared with

Box 19.2 Quality of life and modality of dialysis

Haemodialysis

- ◆ Hospital-based treatment.
- ◆ Suitable for dependent patients.
- ◆ Provides social structure for frail elderly patients.
- ◆ Requires transport time.
- ◆ Interferes with work.
- ◆ Increased hospitalization for vascular access problems.
- ◆ Difficult to travel for holiday or work.

Peritoneal dialysis

- ◆ Home-based treatment.
- ◆ Patient independence.
- ◆ Fits in with work.
- ◆ Can be done by carer at home.
- ◆ Fewer visits to hospital.
- ◆ Easier to travel and go on holiday.

16 per cent starting HD.[10] There is some evidence that automated PD with a cycling machine at night while asleep may allow patients more time for work and leisure activities.[11]

Work and dialysis

The well-being of someone on dialysis depends on many factors, both physical and psychological. The physical symptoms that some continue to experience will depend on adequacy of dialysis and compliance with treatment. Depression, anxiety, and denial of illness can contribute to poor compliance and interfere with treatment. Family and social support is important.

Half of those commencing dialysis are under the age of 65 but studies show very high rates of unemployment (>70 per cent) compared to the general population.[12] In non-diabetic renal disease, choosing PD, employer support, and EPO treatment all increase the likelihood of maintaining employment.

Some of the complexities faced in helping an individual remain at work are illustrated by the following case.

> Mr C is a 50-year-old man from Hong Kong who had a successful career as an accountant in a large firm. At age 45 he developed angina, required coronary bypass surgery, and was found to be diabetic with renal impairment. He found it hard to discuss things with his family. As his renal function declined, he found his job increasingly stressful and therefore left his firm and took on short-term contracts. He denied he had symptoms of renal failure but was eventually persuaded to start dialysis when his plasma creatinine was 950 µmol/L. He chose automated PD as this left him free during the day. He initially managed to work full-time. However, after a year he announced that he had given up work and now spent all his time at home. At a meeting with him, his wife, and members of the healthcare team, it became apparent that compliance was poor—he often failed to put himself on dialysis at night and missed EPO injections; he had lost self-esteem and felt a burden on his family. He accepted counselling, compliance improved, he felt better and was able to return to part-time work.

Many individuals do continue to work in all sorts of professions. They can be enabled to do so with the aid of the occupational health team at the place of work, or if the employer has some understanding of the flexibility required in the working day. It is important for the dialysis team caring for the patient to adapt the treatment round the needs of the patient, by, for example, arranging HD in the evening if the patient works during the day, and being flexible over the times of clinic appointments. It is often easier to fit RRT round work if treatment is carried out at home, whether HD or PD. Box 19.3 lists some of the specific work problems patients encounter on dialysis.

Transplantation

Successful transplantation not only provides the best quality of life for patients with ESRD but also prolongs life expectancy as compared with patients fit enough to be on a transplant list but who do not receive a transplant. The median wait for a cadaveric kidney in the UK has increased from 407 days in 1990–1992 to 1110 days in 2010–2011 (data from UK Transplant). Patients in blood group B have lowered chance of transplant than other blood groups. This is of particular importance for Indo-Asian patients as blood group B is more common among them than in Caucasians. Patients who are on the waiting list for cadaveric transplantation need to come to the transplant unit as soon as they receive their call. The initial inpatient stay is usually 1–2 weeks and for the first 3–4 months frequent blood tests are needed. Over a third of transplants are now from living donors. Living donor transplantation can be timed to suit the patient—for example, during the school holidays for a teacher. Increasingly, live donor transplantation is done pre-emptively before starting dialysis. This maximizes quality of life and survival.

Box 19.3 Employment and dialysis

Haemodialysis

- ◆ Rigid timing—usually 4 hours three times a week plus transport to and from dialysis unit.
- ◆ HD units usually have two to three shifts a day with little flexibility of timing for patients on shift work.
- ◆ Difficult to arrange treatments at other units, particularly at short notice, making travel difficult.
- ◆ Intermittent treatment so dietary and fluid restrictions.
- ◆ Patients often feel washed out for some hours after dialysis and can be relatively hypotensive, though this is very variable and some patients are well enough to drive to and from their dialysis sessions.
- ◆ Presence of arteriovenous fistula in arm—need to avoid heavy lifting with that arm.
- ◆ If patient opts for home HD, some weeks dialysing at hospital needed to accustom patient to dialysis, and to train patient to needle their own fistula and manage machine.

Peritoneal dialysis

- ◆ Home-based treatment allowing flexibility round work routine.
- ◆ Travel relatively easy—patient can transport own fluid for short trips or fluid can be delivered to many parts of the world.
- ◆ Can be difficult to fit in four exchanges a day if on CAPD and working, but some patients can arrange a clean and private place at work to do an exchange.
- ◆ More freedom during day if patient on APD—at most, one bag exchange is needed and this can be done at a time convenient for patient.
- ◆ Continuous treatment, so no 'swings' in well-being of patient.
- ◆ Heavy lifting should be avoided because of the increased risk of abdominal hernias and fluid leaks.
- ◆ PD usually started 2 weeks after catheter insertion with a training period of 1 week.

Patients can lead a normal life after successful transplantation, but need to continue daily immunosuppressive therapy (the actual immunosuppressive regimen will vary from unit to unit, as many different agents are now available—prednisolone, azathioprine, ciclosporin, tacrolimus, sirolimus, mycophenylate). Transplant patients are therefore at increased risk of infection. In the first few months, patients are advised to avoid people with bad colds, influenza, and chicken pox. This is particularly important for teachers working in schools and others in similar situations.

Transplant patients have a slightly increased risk of developing malignancy. Skin malignancies are among the most common, so patients should be advised to make liberal use of sunscreens when working outside. There are complications related to specific immunosuppressive drugs such as hirsutism with ciclosporin or diabetes with tacrolimus. Many patients also remain hypertensive after transplantation. Cardiovascular disease remains a major cause of morbidity and mortality but less so than in patients on dialysis.

Long-term follow-up studies in relation to work are encouraging. A study of 57 adult survivors from childhood transplantation showed a high level of employment (82 per cent) and 95 per cent reported their health as fair or good.[13] This was despite a high retransplantation rate and significant morbidity such as hypertension, bone and joint symptoms, fractures, hypercholesterolaemia, and cataracts. A study of 267 Japanese transplant recipients found patient and graft survival rates of 80 per cent and 51 per cent at 10 years and 56 per cent and 33 per cent at 20 years.[14] The main causes of death long-term were cancers and hepatic failure due to viral hepatitis. In 15 patients with grafts surviving beyond 20 years, 11 remained in full-time employment.

Renal failure and employment

In the USA differences have also been found in vocational rehabilitation in end-stage renal therapy patients.[15] Follow-up studies have found employment rates of 28 per cent (Spain), 43 per cent (USA), and 45 per cent (Canada) following transplantation, but prior employment tends to be the strongest independent predictor of employment after transplant.[16–18] Patient and physician expectation with regard to employment appear to be important in both dialysis and following transplantation, but can be modified.[17,19]

The main problems surround those on dialysis. Loss of work is an important issue in both pre-dialysis and dialysis patients. A joint study from the Manchester and Oxford renal units found that there was a sharp decline in the percentage of those working some 6–12 months after the start of CAPD (44 per cent from 73 per cent), or of HD (42 per cent from 83 per cent).[20,21] Other studies have also shown high rates of leaving full-time employment after dialysis, with 50 per cent retired within 2 years of starting HD in Croatia; employment rates of 42 per cent before the initiation of dialysis, falling to 21 per cent at initiation and below 7 per cent a year later in the US; and declines in employment rate from 31 per cent to 25 per cent (HD patients) and 48 per cent to 40 per cent (PD patients) after 1 year of dialysis in the Netherlands.[22–24] Independent risk factors for job loss were impaired physical and psychosocial functioning.

A US study of 359 chronic dialysis patients (85 employed and 274 unemployed) found education to be a significant correlate of employment but neither mode of dialysis, length of time on dialysis, number of comorbid conditions, nor cause of renal failure (e.g. diabetes) were associated with employment status.[25] Measures of functional status were positively associated with employment but patients' perceptions that their health limited the type and amount of work that they could do were negatively associated with employment. Twenty-one per cent of unemployed patients reported that they were both able to work and wanted to return to work. Other factors affecting employment in dialysis patients include selection of fitter patients for transplantation, availability of disability benefits and health insurance, education and employer attitudes.[26–28] However, pre-dialysis intervention has been shown to be of benefit in assisting workers with end-stage renal failure. In a Californian study, those who had assessment by a social worker, instruction and counselling, and renal unit orientation were 2.8 times more likely to continue work after starting HD.[29]

Renal failure and fitness for work

With flexibility, adaptation, careful planning and support, and a change of attitude on the part of employers, many more dialysis patients could work successfully. The aim should be to adapt the work to the patient's needs and the patient's treatment regimen to the work. Many employers, although sympathetic, misunderstand what can be achieved by patients with chronic renal failure, and this by itself may preclude successful employment. There is a need to educate both doctors and employers about the work capabilities of those with ESRD and to encourage a positive attitude in the patients themselves. The close cooperation of all concerned, (the patient, the renal unit, the general practitioner, occupational health staff, and the employer), is often needed to effect a successful placement. The occupational physician is usually best placed to catalyse the necessary adjustments.

Successful transplant patients should be capable of virtually any normal work. The work situation should carry no undue risk of blows or trauma to the lower abdomen and likewise the arteriovenous fistula at the wrist should be protected from injury by sharp projections or tools.

Restrictions and contraindications

The essential and relative employment contraindications for dialysis patients are shown in Table 19.2.

Patients in irreversible renal failure are ill-suited to work as firefighters, police on the beat, rescue personnel, or members of the armed forces, because these jobs have high energy demands, extended hours, and a need always to be on-call for emergencies. Similar restrictions may apply to particularly stressful jobs demanding a high degree of vigilance (e.g. air traffic controllers). Jobs combining both a high radiant heat burden and high physical activity may also be contraindicated

Table 19.2 Haemodialysis and continuous ambulatory peritoneal dialysis and types of employment

Contraindications (unsuitable)	Relative contraindications (possible)	No contraindications (suitable)
Armed Forces (active service)	Catering trades[a]	Accountancy
Chemical exposure to renal toxins	Farm labouring[a]	Clerical/secretarial
Construction/building/scaffolding	Heavy goods vehicle driving[a]	Driving
Diving	Horticultural work	Law
Firefighters	Motor repair (care with fistula in HD patients)	Light assembly
Furnace/smelting	Nursing[a]	Light maintenance/repair
Heavy labouring	Painting and decorating[a]	Light manufacturing industry
Heavy manual work	Printing[a]	Medicine
Mining	Refuse collection[a]	Middle and senior management
Police (on the beat)	Shiftwork	Packing
Work in very hot environments	Welding[a]	Receptionist
		Retail trade
		Sales
		Supervising
		Teaching

[a]Not contraindicated in HD.

For patients on HD, shiftwork and extended hours may present problems requiring greater adaptation. Some patients have learnt to dialyse while asleep using the built-in warning devices on the machine.

Should occupations in the middle column entail much heavy lifting, or manual work, they may be unsuitable.

because of the risk of fluid depletion with ensuing hypotension and worsening renal function, particularly when using angiotensin-converting enzyme inhibitors or angiotensin receptor blockers for blood pressure control. Patients in ESRD on dialysis are unfit for underground working, for diving, or other work in hyperbaric conditions such as tunnelling under pressure. They are also unlikely to meet the fitness standards required for merchant shipping, which may require lengthy periods at sea in tropical and subtropical climates.[30] Additionally, most seafarers nowadays will need to join and leave ships by air travel.

Although air travel is not contraindicated for those undertaking continuous ambulatory PD regimens, it imposes extra difficulties and the added inconvenience of carrying supplies of the dialysate solution. Also in the context of travel abroad, the reduced dosage required for drug prophylaxis against malaria for those in renal failure should be recognized.

It is essential for those on PD to avoid work in dirty or dusty environments, and work that requires heavy lifting or constant bending. Tight or restrictive clothing should not be worn. Patients also need a clean area to perform their midday fluid exchange, as it is vital to avoid infection. The suitability, both of the type of work and of an area at the workplace for the exchange, should be assessed on site by the renal unit specialist nurse, in conjunction with the occupational health staff and the employer.

Patients on HD need to be within easy reach of a dialysis facility, so work involving much distant travel and frequent periods away from home may not be suitable.

If there are canteen facilities, it can be helpful to ensure that the necessary low salt and high/low protein foodstuffs are readily available.

Usually there are no restrictions to employment for workers with only one well-functioning kidney.

Holidays

Most patients on PD can take a holiday without restrictions, but HD patients need either to make special arrangements for a dialysis facility at the holiday centre, or arrange for the use of portable machines. Such provisions need to be planned well beforehand.

Shiftwork

Shiftworking is not contraindicated for patients with renal or urinary tract disorders or necessarily for dialysis patients if their treatment can be rescheduled to fit in with their shift rota. Rapidly rotating shift systems can be more difficult to accommodate, especially for patients on HD.

Drivers

PD and HD are not incompatible with vocational driving, but the issue of a Group 1 licence is dependent on medical enquiries. Exceptions arise where the individual is subject to symptoms that impair vehicle control, such as sudden disabling attacks of giddiness or fainting, or impaired psychomotor or cognitive function.[31] Group 2 licence holders on PD or HD are assessed individually by the Driving and Vehicle Licensing Agency. However, driving goods vehicles may be unsuitable owing to the prolonged time away from home, fatigue, and the many hours spent on the road. The physical demands of loading and unloading vehicles (e.g. removals, warehouse storage, or dockyard labouring) may preclude work in transportation.

Patients on PD can seek an exemption from wearing a seatbelt under the Motor Vehicles (Wearing of Seat Belts) Regulations 1993 if a valid medical certificate is supplied by a registered medical practitioner. However, the danger of not wearing a seat belt must be weighed against any relatively minor inconvenience and restriction. Adaptations to seat belt mountings can often solve any problems.

Urinary tract infections

Symptoms of urinary tract infection are very common, but rarely serious unless there is underlying anatomical abnormality. A minority of women suffer from recurrent infections or remain symptomatic despite antibiotic therapy. Anatomical abnormalities (such as ureterovesical reflux or obstruction) are associated with repeated infection, which can lead to chronic renal failure later in life. Tuberculous infection of the urinary tract is increasingly common, but employment can continue, as therapy is usually administered as an out-patient.

Urinary incontinence and retention

Better incontinence devices, more thorough investigation, and improved therapy with anticholinergic drugs have assisted sufferers to stay at work, although incontinence remains an underestimated problem at work. In a recent study almost 40 per cent of women reported urine loss during the preceding 30 days and those with the most severe loss reported that it had at least some negative impact on concentration, performance of physical activities, self-confidence, or the ability to complete tasks without interruption.[32] The main strategies for managing incontinence at work include frequent bathroom breaks, wearing pads and pelvic floor exercises. Incontinence nurse practitioners can help improve work attendance by giving advice, reassurance, practical help, and support. Patients should be aware of available support groups and organizations. The value of intermittent self-catheterization for helping patients with poor bladder emptying, urinary retention and incontinence, or even voiding difficulties, often associated with a neuropathic or hypotonic bladder, is underestimated.[33] Those who learn the technique can become dry, gain more social acceptance, and, by establishing effective drainage, protect their kidneys from the effects of back pressure and urinary infection. Male patients in wheelchairs who learn to catheterize themselves increase their ability to attend work. However, it is more difficult for female disabled patients to self-catheterize and urinary diversion procedures may be considered. The patient's lower disconnected ureter is brought out as a stoma above the inguinal ligament and the patient uses Lofric catheters. This may be acceptable for those who are unable to empty their bladder and get fed-up with self-administered intermittent catheterization or those who are totally incontinent and whose bladder necks are closed off surgically.

Those with incontinence, repeated urinary infections, ileal conduits, or catheterization need access to good toilet facilities at work. Ileostomy bags may be compressed by low benches, or desks, or the sides of bins or boxes. Excess bending, crouching, or poor seating may inhibit the free flow of urine in the bag, or damage it, causing leakage. A clean and private place is required to effect catheter changes or bag emptying, so dusty work environments (e.g. mines, quarries, and foundries) are likely to be unsuitable for these patients. Most working environments, however, can accommodate this requirement.

Approximately 50 per cent of men over the age of 50 will seek help for troublesome lower urinary tract symptoms. Symptoms in men with BPH are measured using the International Prostate Symptom Score, which includes seven questions measuring symptoms on an overall scale from 0 to 35, with higher scores representing more frequent symptoms. Rates of acute urinary retention range from 1–2 per cent a year. Alpha-blockers and transurethral resection of the prostate are effective treatments. Surgery does not increase the risk of erectile dysfunction or incontinence.

Transurethral incision, electrical vaporization, and visual laser ablation also appear to be effective treatments but the latter may be associated with a greater need for blood transfusion.[34]

Prostatic cancer

Prostate cancer is rare below the age of 50. The lifetime risk of developing microscopic foci is 30 per cent, with a 10 per cent risk of clinical disease and a 3 per cent risk of dying from the disease. There is insufficient evidence to warrant screening for prostate cancer using either digital rectal examination or prostate specific antigen or both in combination.

Urinary tract calculi

Kidney stones affect up to 5 per cent of the population, with a lifetime risk of passing a kidney stone of about 8–10 per cent.[35] The predominant composition of idiopathic renal calculi is calcium oxalate. Increased incidence of kidney stones in the industrialized world is associated with improved standards of living and is strongly associated with race or ethnicity and region of residence. Seasonal variation is also seen, with high urinary calcium oxalate saturation in men during summer and in women during early winter. Stones form twice as often in men as women. The peak age in men is 30 years; women have a bimodal age distribution, with peaks at 35 and 55 years. Once a kidney stone forms, the probability that a second stone will form within 3 years is approximately 40 per cent. Stone formers will all form stones again within 25 years and should be investigated metabolically. Risk factors include family history, insulin-resistant states, hypertension, primary hyperparathyroidism, gout, chronic metabolic acidosis, surgical menopause, and anatomical abnormality leading to urinary stasis. Occupational factors such as a high ambient temperature, chronic dehydration, and physical inactivity because of sedentary work, are also implicated.

Stone formation is more frequent in male marathon runners, lifeguards in Israel, hot metal workers, and some British navy personnel. An Italian study of machinists at a glass plant found a prevalence of renal stones of 8.5 per cent in those exposed to heat stress against 2.4 per cent in controls working in normal temperature.[36] In those exposed to heat stress, 39 per cent of stones were composed of uric acid and associated with significantly raised serum concentrations.

Those with a strong history of stone formation, if accepting overseas postings in tropical climates and undertaking strenuous outdoor work, should be encouraged to increase their fluid intake. Fitness for furnace or other very hot work must be carefully assessed because of the increased tendency for stone recurrence.[37] Patients need to be warned about becoming dehydrated on long-haul flights (over 4 hours) and should aim to drink 600 mL/hour while airborne.

About 10–20 per cent of all kidney stones need intervention to remove the stone. For proximal ureteric stones, extracorporeal shock wave lithotripsy (ESWL) is useful if the stone is less than 1 cm in size, and ureteroscopy is more successful for stones larger than 1 cm. ESWL, ureteroscopy, and percutaneous nephrolithotomy have replaced open surgery for treating urolithiasis.[38] Most simple renal calculi (80–85 per cent) can be treated with ESWL as an out-patient procedure, with minimal postoperative discomfort and a resumption of normal activity within a day or so; but recurrence rates can be up to 50 per cent. Ureteroscopy achieves a higher cure rate but with a longer hospital stay and a higher risk of complications.[39] Medical prophylaxis is effective in up to 80 per cent of patients with recurrent calcium stones.

Tumours of the renal tract

Adenocarcinoma of the kidney is the commonest adult renal tumour. In the bladder more than 95 per cent of tumours are urothelial in origin. It is estimated that 7.1 per cent of male and 1.9 per cent of female bladder cancer deaths are occupational within the UK which equated to 550 total registrations in 2004 and 245 attributable deaths in 2005. This is the fifth most common occupational cancer after lung, non-melanotic skin cancer, breast cancer and mesothelioma. Bladder cancer registrations have been attributed to diesel exhaust and mineral oil exposure and work as a painter.

Bladder cancer arising from exposure to various compounds during chemical manufacturing or processing(1-naphthylamine, 2-naphthylamine, benzidine, auramine, magenta, 4-aminobiphenyl, MbOCA, orthotoluidine, 4-chloro-2-methylaniline, and coal tar pitch volatiles produced in aluminium smelting) is a prescribed disease and reportable under Reporting of Injuries, Diseases and Dangerous Occurrences Regulations 1995 (C23). Between 1990/1991 and 2008/2009 there were 525 cases of compensated bladder cancer or about 28 cases per annum.[40]

Employees in certain industries with historic exposure to known bladder carcinogens may be required to provide regular samples for urine cytology. This is usually every 6 months and can be carried out by post if employees leave or retire. Routine urine cytology is also suggested for those exposed to 4,4′-methylene *bis*(2-chloroaniline) (MbOCA). In those who have had tumours an early warning of cytological change can herald recurrence and thus allow early treatment.

Existing legislation: seafarers

Restrictions on the employment of persons suffering from diseases of the genitourinary tract are imposed by the Merchant Shipping (Medical Examination Regulations) 2010 Statutory Instrument 2002 No. 2055, which requires a statutory examination for fitness to work (see Appendix 2). The medical standards are not met by those with acute urinary tract infections or urinary incontinence if recurrent or with an untreatable underlying cause, recurrent stone formation (less than 5 years), prostatic enlargement with urinary obstruction if irremediable, or for new entrants in distant water or tropics with only one kidney.

Conclusions and recommendations

Because of the great advances in dialysis and the good results of renal transplantation, most people with renal failure can now achieve significant rehabilitation, and often a degree of independence and quality of life sufficient to allow useful, gainful, and active employment.

Employment is predicted by being in employment before onset of renal failure and by preconceptions of the patient and their doctor. Renal failure will be considered a disabling condition as defined by the Equality Act 2010 and so employers will need to consider reasonable adjustments to enable someone to work around their dialysis schedule or catheterize when at work or to make allowances for frequent short absences from work. Occasionally patients will experience difficulty in arranging associated life insurance cover, or joining superannuation schemes and this may be given as the reason for not employing someone in end-stage renal failure but a successful transplant restores the recipient to full health with the same capability as their contemporaries.

References

1 UK Renal Registry. *Report 2010*. Bristol: UK Renal Registry, 2010. (<http://www.renalreg.com/Reports/2010.html>)

2 Coresh J, Selvin E, Stevens LA, *et al*. Prevalence of chronic kidney disease in the United States. *JAMA* 2007; **298**: 2038–47.

3 Office for National Statistics. *Cancer statistics registrations*, 2009. [Online] (<http://www.ons.gov.uk>)

4 Go AS, Chertow GM, Fan D, *et al*. ET Chronic kidney disease and the risks of death, cardiovascular events, and hospitalisation. *N Engl J Med* 2004; **351**: 1296–305.

5 NICE. *Chronic kidney disease*. NICE clinical guideline 73. London: NICE, 2008.

6 National Collaborating Centre for Chronic Conditions. *Chronic kidney disease: national clinical guideline for early identification and management in adults in primary and secondary care*. London: Royal College of Physicians. September 2008.

7 Joint Consensus Statement on the Initial Assessment of Haematuria Prepared on behalf of the Renal Association and British Association of Urological Surgeons, 2008. [Online] (<http://www.renal.org/Libraries/Other_Guidlines/Haematuria_-_RA-BAUS_consensus_guideline_2008.sflb.ashx>)

8 Anavekar NS, McMurray JJV, Velazquez EJ, *et al.* Relation between renal dysfunction and cardiovascular outcomes after myocardial infarction. *N Engl J Med* 2004; **351**: 1285–95.

9 Rebecca J, Muehrer RJ, Schatell D, *et al.* Factors affecting employment at initiation of dialysis. *Clin J Am Soc Nephrol* 2011; **6**: 489–96.

10 Jager KJ, Korevaar JC, Dekker FW, *et al.* The effect of contraindications and patient preference on dialysis modality selection in ESRD patients in The Netherlands. *Am J Kidney Dis* 2004; **43**: 891–9.

11 Rabindranath KS, Adams J, Ali TZ, *et al.* Automated vs continuous ambulatory peritoneal dialysis: a systematic review of randomized controlled trials. *Nephrol Dial Transplant* 2007; **22**(10): 2991–8.

12 Sandhu GS, Khattak M, Rout P, *et al.* Social Adaptability Index: application and outcomes in a dialysis population. *Nephrol Dial Transplant* 2010; **26**: 2667–74.

13 Bartosh SM, Leverson G, Robillard D, *et al.* Long-term outcomes in pediatric renal transplant recipients who survive into adulthood. *Transplantation* 2003; **76**: 1195–200.

14 Yasumura T, Oka T, Nakane Y, *et al.* Long-term prognosis of renal transplant surviving for over 10yr, and clinical, renal and rehabilitation features of 20-yr successes. *Clin Transplant* 1997; **11**: 387–94.

15 Simmonds RG, Anderson CR, *et al.* Quality of life and rehabilitation differences among four ESRD therapy groups. *Scand J Urol Nephrol* (Suppl.) 1990; **131**: 7–22.

16 Pertusa Pena C, Llarena Ibarguren R, Lecumberri Castanos D, *et al.* Relation between renal transplantation and work situation. *Arch EspUrol* 1997; **50**(5): 489–94.

17 Markell MS, DiBenedetto A, Maursky V, *et al.* Unemployment in inner-city renal transplant recipients: predictive and sociodemo-graphic factors. *Am J Kidney Dis* 1997; **29**(6): 881–7.

18 Laupacis A, Keown P, Pus N, *et al.* A study of the quality of life and cost-utility of renal transplantation. *Kidney Int* 1996; **50**: 235–42.

19 Newton SE. Renal transplant recipients' and their physicians' expectations regarding return to work post-transplant. *ANNA J* 1999; **26**(2): 227–32; discussion 234.

20 Auer J, Gokal R, Stout JP, *et al.* The Oxford–Manchester study of dialysis patients. *Scand J Urol Nephrol* 1990; **131**(Suppl.): 31–7.

21 Gokal R. Quality of life in patients undergoing renal replacement therapy. *Kidney Int* 1993; **38**(Suppl. 40): S23–7.

22 Orlic L, Matic-Glazar D, SladojeMartinovic B, *et al.* Work capacity in patients on hemodialysis. *Acta Med Croatica* 2004; **58**: 67–71.

23 Tappe K, Turkelson C, Doggett D, *et al.* Disability under Social Security for patients with ESRD: an evidence-based review. *Disabil Rehabil* 2001; **23**(5): 177–85.

24 van Manen JG, Korevaar JC, Dekker FW, *et al.* including NECOSAD Study Group. Netherlands Cooperative Study on Adequacy of Dialysis. Changes in employment status in end-stage renal disease patients during their first year of dialysis. *Perit Dial Int* 2001; **21**(6): 595–601.

25 Curtin RB, Oberley ET, Sacksteder P, *et al.* Differences between employed and non-employed dialysis patients. *Am J Kidney Dis* 1996; **27**(4): 533–40.

26 Raiz L. The transplant trap: The impact of health policy on employment status following renal transplantation. *J Nephrol Social Work* 1997; **17**: 79–94.

27 Friedman N, Rogers TF. Dialysis and the world of work. *Contemp Dial Nephrol* 1988; **19**: 16–19.

28 King K. Vocational rehabilitation in maintenance dialysis patients. *Adv Renal Replace Ther* 1994; **1**: 228–39.

29 Rasgon S, Schwankovsky L, James-Rogers A, *et al.* An intervention for Maintenance among blue-collar workers with end-stage renal disease. *Am J Kidney Dis* 1993; **22**: 403–12.

30 Maritime and Coastguard Agency. *Merchant Shipping Notice MSN 1822 (M). Seafarer medical examination system and medical and eyesight standards; Application of the Merchant Shipping (Maritime Labour Convention) (Medical Certification) Regulations* 2010. Southampton: Maritime and Coastguard Agency, 2010.

31 Drivers Medical Group. *At a glance guide to the current medical standards of fitness to drive.* Swansea: DVLA, 2011.

32 Fultz N, Girts T, Kinchen K, *et al.* Prevalence, management and impact of urinary incontinence in the workplace *Occup Med* 2005; **55**(7): 552–7

33 Nursing Standard. Intermittent self catheterisation. Patient guide. *Nurs Stand* 2002; **16**(29).

34 Interventions in benign prostatic hyperplasia. In: *Clinical evidence from the British Medical Journal.* [Online] (<http://www.clinicalevidence.com>)

35 Parmar MS. Kidney stones. *BMJ* 2004; **328**: 1420–4.

36 Borghi L, Meschi T, Amato F, *et al.* Hot occupation and nephrolithiasis. *J Urol* 1993; **150**(6): 1757–60.

37 Pin NT, Ling NY, Siang LH. Dehydration from outdoor work and urinary stones in a tropical environment. *Occup Med* 1992; **42**: 30–2.

38 Miller NL, Lingeman JE. Clinical review management of kidney stones. *BMJ* 2007; **334**: 468.

39 Nabi G, Downey P, Keeley F, *et al.* Extra-corporeal shock wave lithotripsy (ESWL) versus ureteroscopic management for ureteric calculi. *Cochrane Database Syst Rev* 2007; **1**: CD006029.

40 HSE. *Health and safety statistics.* [Online] (<http://www.hse.gov.uk/statistics>)

Chapter 20

Women at work

Sally E. L. Coomber and Peter A. Harris

Introduction

Although nearly half the UK workforce is female, they differ from men in the jobs they do, the hours and patterns of work, and even their rates of pay. These factors impact on women's health and fitness for work. This chapter considers fertility to conception, childbirth through to post-natal health, menstruation to the menopause and gynaecological surgery and ergonomics.

The Royal College of Obstetrics and Gynaecology (RCOG) publishes a wide range of guidance documents which can be accessed on their website.[1] This includes the 'Green-top Guidelines' which are systematically developed recommendations, written to assist clinicians and patients in making decisions about appropriate treatment for specific conditions. Green-top guidelines are concise documents, providing specific practice recommendations on focused areas of clinical practice and produced under the direction of the Guidelines Committee of the RCOG. Many of them are referenced in this chapter. The RCOG also produces the *Return to Fitness: Recovering Well* series of patient information leaflets with clear expectations of recovery and return to work times.[2]

Demographics

The Office for National Statistics (ONS) in the UK is a rich source of online information. Table 20.1 shows work patterns and gender in the 3 months to January 2012.

In April 2011 the ONS reported that median gross weekly earnings for full-time employees were £498. For men, full-time earnings were £538, compared with £440 for women. The gender pay gap is still between 12 per cent and 22 per cent, depending on how it is calculated.[3] Since 1996, the employment rate of mothers has shown a steady rise prior to the recession of 2009 (Figure 20.1). The rate is highest in the age group 35–49, as women have their babies later in life. Employment for women aged 16–24 years without children in particular has fallen sharply since the recession.

Sickness absence rates, reported by ONS, also differ between the sexes (Figure 20.2). In the final quarter of 2010, 2.9 per cent of all female versus 2.1 per cent of male employees were absent from work. For men, the top reason was musculoskeletal problems followed by back pain, while for women, the top reason was stress, depression, and anxiety followed by musculoskeletal problems.

The working woman has considerable legal protection against discrimination and complicated rights during and after pregnancy. These are covered elsewhere (see Chapter 2). Fitness to return to work following breast surgery and gynaecological procedures is covered in Chapter 21, but return to work times are given in Table 20.1.

Table 20.1 Return to work times following gynaecological procedures

	Some women are fit to RTW by	Most women are fit to RTW by
Endometrial ablation	–	2–5 days
Surgical management of miscarriage	1–2 days	1 week (Note: emotional recovery may take longer)
Diagnostic laparoscopy	2 days	1 week
Laparoscopic procedure	1 week	2–3 weeks
Mid-urethral sling operation for stress urinary incontinence	3–4 days	3 weeks
Vaginal hysterectomy	2–3 weeks	4–6 weeks
Laparoscopic hysterectomy	2–3 weeks	4–6 weeks
Abdominal hysterectomy	3–4 weeks	6–8 weeks

Data from Royal College of Obstetricians 'Return to Fitness: Recovering Well' series of patient information leaflets.

Figure 20.1 UK employment rates of mothers and women without children, 1996–2010. Note: Recession period shaded. Reproduced from Office of National Statistics, *Mothers in the Labour Market* 2011 © Crown copyright 2011.

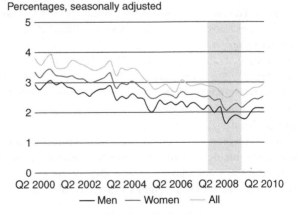

Percentages, seasonally adjusted

Figure 20.2 UK sickness absence rates of employees, 2000–2010. Data from Labour Market Statistics, February 2011 © Crown Copyright 2011.

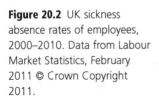

Conception and fertility issues

Early diagnosis of pregnancy

Home pregnancy urine testing kits which detect human chorionic gonadotrophin (hCG) release can now confirm pregnancy as early as 7 days post ovulation, before a period is even missed. A positive test is rarely wrong. False negatives may result from testing too early, depending on the sensitivity of the test (20–100 mIU/mL) and the interaction of some drugs. Errors can result from poor technique, out-of-date testing kit, and if hCG is given as part of *in vitro* fertilization (IVF) treatment.

Miscarriage

Miscarriage is a common experience (see Box 20.1). It is defined as pregnancy loss before 24 weeks, although late second trimester miscarriages may be referred to as an intrauterine death (IUD). Miscarriage is known to have significant psychological sequelae, and timing of return to work is based more on emotional than physical recovery.

The RCOG specifies the terminology for different types of miscarriage, and the term 'abortion' is no longer in clinical use.[4]

Miscarriage rates also increase with maternal age with rates of 10 per cent for under 30s; 20 per cent for 35–40-year-olds and 50 per cent for women over 45.

Historically, the majority of miscarriages required surgical evacuation of retained products of conception (ERPC). Gradually this has changed, and Early Pregnancy Assessment Units (EPAUs) can diagnose, treat, and support women with early pregnancy of unknown viability and suspected ectopic pregnancy. More detailed investigations including transvaginal ultrasound scans (TVS) and serial hCG levels greatly enhance differential diagnosis. Conservative and medical management (with prostaglandin analogues) are options now available in the first trimester.

Miscarriage and work

In 2009, a comprehensive literature review identified work factors and jobs associated with increased miscarriage rates and the possible mechanisms.[5] Prolonged standing variously defined as standing for greater than 3, 5, or 6 hours/day represented a *moderately increased risk* for miscarriage. Long working hours (>40 hours per week), heavy physical work, manual handling, and lifting had a *small increased risk* for miscarriage. The same study reported that radiology technicians, operating room nurses, those working in agriculture and horticulture, nursing assistants and attendants, and food and beverage servers all had evidence of increased rates of miscarriage.

Box 20.1 Miscarriage rates depend on the stage at which pregnancy is diagnosed

- From conception: probably 50 per cent.
- From positive urine test: 30 per cent.
- Once foetal heart seen on ultrasound scan: 5 per cent.
- After 12 weeks since last menstrual period: 2 per cent.
- After 16 weeks since last menstrual period: 1 per cent.

Recurrent miscarriage

Recurrent miscarriage is defined as the loss of three or more pregnancies. The incidence is 1 per cent and rises with maternal age and previous number of miscarriages.[6]

In clinical practice, the gynaecologist assessing a woman with recurrent miscarriages may not enquire about work, and the RCOG guidelines give no reason to do so. A biochemical or physical cause is only found in a small number of cases (e.g. polycystic ovary syndrome, antiphospholipid syndrome, and congenital abnormalities of the uterus).

However, one study found that standing at work for more than 7 hours per day was associated with a significantly increased risk of a further miscarriage in women who had already had two or more spontaneous miscarriages.[7] Based on this evidence, a woman with a history of recurrent miscarriage whose work is physically demanding and/or requires long periods of standing could benefit from a short-term change in her duties.

Declaration of pregnancy to employer

Declaration is often after the first ultrasound scan, the 12th week when the risk of miscarriage reduces or following Down's syndrome screening by nuchal fold thickness from 11 weeks. Declaration may be delayed if there is a perception that job offers and promotion may be adversely affected, although this is unlawful. (See Chapter 2.)

There is no legal requirement for a worker to declare pregnancy until 15 weeks before the due date. Once aware, the employer legally only need revisit the existing risk assessment (RA) and apply it to the pregnant worker.[8] Guidance regarding this is provided on the Health and Safety Executive (HSE) website.[9] In practice, often a specific RA is undertaken, though it still does not take account of an individual woman's pregnancy risks.

The timing of informing the employer will vary with individual circumstances, including perception of the associated risks, obvious symptoms, perceived financial disadvantage to stopping certain duties/shifts, and motivation. Nonetheless, occupational physicians will see jockeys not wanting to stop riding, air hostesses not wanting to be grounded, research laboratory staff who wish to continue working with novel compounds, and pharmacy staff rotating to cytotoxic drug reconstitution duties when known to be trying for a baby.

Workplace hazards to the pregnant worker

Medical assessment takes place within an employer's legal framework of risk assessment for 'new and expectant mothers' i.e. those who are pregnant, have given birth within 6 months or are breastfeeding. As with any risk assessment, there is a need to consider systematically the workplace hazards and the likelihood of their causing harm to the health or safety of the mother and/or foetus. The HSE provides a useful guide for employers on this that considers in turn physical, chemical, and biological agents.[9]

Ionizing radiation

Ionizing radiation is a relatively well understood foetal risk. It is known to interfere with cell proliferation and the embryo and foetus are therefore highly radiosensitive. Natural radiation can account for, on average, 1 mSv to the foetus during pregnancy. The Ionising Radiation Regulations 1999 restricts exposure for declared duration of pregnancy and also for breastfeeding to an effective dose limit of 1 mSv for the foetus.[10] Non-pregnant woman have the same limits as men. Cosmic radiation can account for 0.3 mSv per year at ground level but 2.4 mSv to aircrew and as high as 5–6 mSV for some aircrew working on long-range flights although the International

Commission for Radiological Protection has determined that the weighting factor can be reduced.[11] Many airlines, however, ground pilots on declaration of pregnancy to minimize any potential exposure of the foetus to solar radiation (see Appendix 1).

Non-ionizing radiation

Electromagnetic radiation at lower, non-ionizing frequencies has been less vigorously studied but there is no current evidence of any significant reproductive hazard and there are no gender-specific occupational limits.[12]

Computer work/display screen equipment

A 2006 review of available evidence suggested that exposure to contemporary visual display terminals was suspected to have only a slight association with a slight increase in the risk of miscarriage (10–20 per cent).[13] It was unclear whether this was attributable to electromagnetic radiation or to other work-related conditions such as ergonomic factors, work stress, and long working hours.

Extreme heat

Pregnant women are normally advised to avoid saunas and prolonged hot baths as a core temperature of over 38.9°C presents a theoretical teratogenic risk. Few jobs pose a risk of hyperthermia, but environments hot enough to cause fainting need consideration.[14]

Violence in the workplace

The few studies of violence and trauma in pregnancy tend to be non-work related but some duties, notably in health and social care, may expose the pregnant woman to risk of assault.[15,16]

Road traffic collisions

Deceleration during a road traffic accident can cause foetal death even in the absence of major abdominal injury.[17]

Electric shock

An electric shock to the foetus could theoretically be fatal, but few case reports exist to assess the risk.[18]

Chemical hazards

When assessing risk from chemicals, existing occupational exposure standards take into account information available on reproductive toxicity. Similarly, risk phrases required on a safety data sheet may identify a specific reproductive concern: R60 and R62 (fertility); R61 and R63 (development); R64 (may cause harm to breast-fed babies); or a more general carcinogenic hazard: R40, R45, R49, R68. Where information is not available on a substance, absence of these identifiers provides no guarantee that the substance is safe for the fertile female.

Lead

Lead has been extensively studied. It is known to cross the placenta and have adverse effects on the foetus, including miscarriage, neural tube defects, and low birth weight.

The Control Of Lead at Work Regulations (CLAW) place work restrictions on 'women of reproductive capacity', e.g. in lead smelting/refining processes and lead battery manufacture and they have lower blood lead limits for 'action' (25 µg/dL) or 'suspension' from work (30 µg/dL).[19] Once pregnancy is declared, CLAW guidance states that the woman should be removed from any work where exposure to lead is 'liable to be significant'.

Anaesthetic gases

Common anaesthetic agents (e.g. halothane, isoflurane, nitrous oxide) currently carry workplace exposure standards, but no risk phrases. Historically, they have been associated with concerns about miscarriage, although more recent studies have not supported this: the advent of active scavenging systems has reduced the exposure in operating theatres. However, in paediatric anaesthesia the anaesthetist may be less well protected: more gaseous induction is used, higher flow rates may be required, and scavenging is technically more difficult. A small American study showed a higher prevalence of spontaneous abortion in anaesthetists doing more than 75 per cent paediatric (as opposed to adult) anaesthesia.[20] Nitrous oxide may be used in environments less well ventilated than operating theatres, e.g. delivery rooms, accident & emergency, and dental surgeries. There is some evidence that this may cause impaired fertility,[21] increased spontaneous abortion,[22] and low birth weight[23] although no other evidence of teratogenicity. Ventilation, scavenging, and/or air monitoring should be considered where exposure may be prolonged.

Carbon monoxide

Carbon monoxide binds strongly with haemoglobin and acts as a chemical asphyxiant. It crosses the placenta and acute exposure can cause foetal death or malformations. In acute exposure, foetal outcome is related to both maternal carboxyhaemoglobin level and maternal toxicity.[24] Dichloromethane, a solvent used for paint removal, is readily absorbed through the skin and lungs producing carbon monoxide as a metabolite and presents a similar risk to the pregnant worker.

Organic solvents

Workers exposed to organic solvents in laboratories, electronics production and dry cleaning work have all been shown to have a higher risk of miscarriage.[13] A case control study of mixed organic solvent exposure in a pharmaceutical factory showed more than double miscarriage rates (odds ration (OR) = 2.68) and increased time to pregnancy (TTP) over 1 year (OR = 2.2) in those exposed.[25] A case series from the Lyon Poison Centre studied 206 pregnant workers exposed to solvents.[26] Based on comprehensive occupational and toxicological risk assessment, 22 per cent were considered to have hazardous exposures and withdrawal from the workplace recommended. Half were assessed as low/very low dose exposure or low risk solvent (e.g. acetone) and remained in the same role. For the remainder, restricted duties and increased personal protective measures were advised. Prospective follow-up with matched controls showed no adverse outcomes (no increased risk of malformations, pregnancy loss and no change in birth weight or gestational age at delivery).

Cytotoxic drugs

In therapeutic doses, the health risks of these drugs are well known and it is reasonable to assume that workplace exposure is not safe in pregnancy. The exposure can occur in women who manufacture, reconstitute, administer cytotoxic drugs to patients and subsequently handle their body fluids.

Biological hazards

Pregnant women are, theoretically, in an immunocompromised state, but in practice they are not more likely to become infected and the risk to the mother is not significantly increased for most agents except chickenpox (varicella zoster) and malaria. However, many infections cross the placenta and therefore have important implications for the foetus.[27]

Significant contact: occupational health practitioners are often asked for advice about the safety of pregnant women who might come into contact with infectious diseases at work, for instance, from other employees. The RCOG 2012 Study Group Statement on Infection and Pregnancy defines *significant contact* for rubella and parvovirus ('slapped cheek disease') as '15 minutes in the same room or face to face contact'.[28] Pregnant women who develop a rash or have known exposure to parvovirus B19 should be seen promptly by their midwife to assess serological status.

For *chickenpox*, the RCOG also includes contact in an open ward as *significant exposure*: VZV is highly infectious for 48 hours before the rash appears and until the vesicles have crusted over.[29] Regarding *shingles*, the RCOG guideline states:

> The risk of acquiring infection from an immunocompetent individual with herpes zoster (Shingles) in non-exposed sites (for example, thoracolumbar) is remote. However, disseminated zoster or exposed zoster (such as ophthalmic) in any individual or localized zoster in an immunosuppressed patient should be considered to be infectious.

Immunity to VZV: a history of chickenpox is adequate evidence of immunity in a woman raised in the UK but women from tropical and subtropical are less likely to be immune and a blood test is recommended. At booking of pregnancy, blood samples are routinely tested for rubella, syphilis, hepatitis B and HIV viruses and then stored, hence VZV immunity can be checked rapidly (i.e. within 48 hours) by the obstetric team, if necessary. Women susceptible to varicella, regardless of gestational age, should be given immunoglobulin (VZIG) within 10 days of significant exposure.

The RCOG Study Group Statement on Infection and Pregnancy has also now tightened the definition of rubella immunity in a clinical context, and advises on malaria:

> Non-immune pregnant women should be advised against travel to a malarious area. If travel is unavoidable, advice should be given about personal protection and chemoprophylaxis. This advice also applies to previously immune women from malaria-endemic areas who have lived in the UK for more than two years and who will therefore have lost much of their pre-existing immunity.

The *British National Formulary* (BNF) and Department of Health provide online up-to-date information and advice. All live vaccines are contraindicated in pregnancy.

Zoonoses

There are theoretical risks during pregnancy from animals harbouring infection including toxoplasmosis, chlamydiosis, brucellosis, listeriosis, and Q fever (*Coxiella burnetii*). A small number of case reports also exist regarding infection contracted from protective clothing in contact with ewes/lambs, occupational exposure to contaminated raw meat and unpasteurized dairy products, and handling cat litter or faeces.

Physical demands and shift work

While recreational physical exercise is known to be beneficial, physically demanding work may have significant adverse effects on intra-abdominal pressure, uterine blood flow, and possibly nutritional status and hormone levels.[30] The 2009 Physical and Shift Work in Pregnancy review looks at complex and conflicting evidence.[5] Its conclusions were:

- Heavy physical work carries no more than a moderate risk of low birth weight/intra-uterine growth retardation/small for gestational age babies, but there is only limited and inconsistent evidence of risk for preterm birth and pre-eclampsia.

- There is consistent evidence suggesting that lifting at work carries no more than a moderate risk of preterm birth and low birth weight, but there is limited inconsistent evidence for pre-eclampsia.
- There is consistent evidence suggesting that prolonged standing (>3 hours) carries no more than a small risk of preterm birth and low birth weight/intrauterine growth restriction/small for gestational age (SGA) foetus, and limited evidence for no effect for pre-eclampsia.
- For long working hours there is consistent evidence suggesting no more than small to moderate risk of preterm birth, and low birth weight/SGA, but there is limited inconsistent evidence for pre-eclampsia.
- For shift work there is insufficient evidence of a risk to pregnant women to make recommendations to restrict shift work, including rotating shifts or night/evening work.

On the basis of this level of evidence, the duties of a pregnant woman, especially one with a high-risk pregnancy can be individually assessed, discussed, and adjusted accordingly. The RCOG guidance on management of a SGA foetus states there is insufficient evidence to assess the impact of hospitalization and bed rest, advises these mothers to stop smoking, and does not refer to duties at work.[31] There is limited evidence elsewhere associating noise and whole-body vibration with adverse pregnancy outcomes.[13] Congenital cardiac malformations have been studied and no link has been made with physical demands or thermal stresses at work.[32] Lower social class (4 and 5) where many of these workplace hazards are more likely to occur is widely accepted as an independent risk factor for poor obstetric outcomes, e.g. low birth weight, premature labour, and miscarriage.

Stress and pregnancy

Becoming and being pregnant is a significant life event and as such is described by the HSE as a psychological stressor in itself.[33] Whilst pregnancy is often a joyful event it can also lead to uncertainty, fear, loss of control, physical discomfort, and disturbed sleep. Life events are associated with an increased risk of mental health symptoms and may impact on the ability to cope with existing workplace stressors. There is a substantial amount of literature showing associations between psychosocial stress and adverse pregnancy outcomes, whether the source of the stress is work or life events.[34] These poor outcomes include hypertension, preterm delivery and low birth weight. However, there are no data on stopping work as an intervention, and there are almost as many studies showing no adverse effect for the same outcomes. It is therefore beyond the scope of the authors to make specific recommendations, but giving time off work in pregnancy following stressful events, or during workplace stress, may reasonably be seen by the general practitioner (GP) as a safe and compassionate decision.

Pregnancy changes that affect fitness to work

A comprehensive risk assessment should consider continuing practical and safety issues as the shape, physiology, and mobility of the pregnant worker change. Assessment will vary with both the individual pregnancy and the particular job. A medical opinion may not be required in a normal pregnancy, but issues to consider include the following:

- Need to urinate more frequently/urgently.
- Nausea and need for frequent meals/snacks/increased fluid intake.
- Intolerance of strong odours.

◆ Liability to faint.

◆ Tiredness.

◆ Poor tolerance of shift work.

◆ Susceptibility to occupational stressors.

◆ Reduced ability to run: effects of heavily pregnant abdomen, joint laxity, and/or ankle oedema (especially in the third trimester).

◆ Centre of gravity changes, affecting risk of falls, work at heights.

◆ Heat intolerance.

◆ Fit and efficacy of protective clothing and equipment.

◆ Work in confined spaces, access via emergency exits.

Travel in pregnancy

Both fitness for the travel itself and the destination need to be considered. The normal discomforts of travel by car, train, or plane may be less well tolerated by a pregnant woman but there are a few specific risks to consider. The risk of deep vein thrombosis is increased in pregnancy and more so when flying. Travel to where malaria is endemic needs special consideration. In 'high-risk' pregnancies the obstetrician should be consulted about fitness to fly. Under IATA (International Air Transport Association) guidelines, pregnant women are allowed to fly in weeks 36–38 if the flying time does not exceed 4 hours. However, many airlines will not carry pregnant women after 36 weeks: the aircraft captain is responsible for passenger safety. Written confirmation from the airline is advisable and a letter from the obstetrician may be helpful.

Driving

Occupational driving in pregnancy requires a common-sense approach for the management of most pregnancy symptoms, e.g. tiredness, feeling faint, backache, and limited space behind the steering wheel in the third trimester. Seatbelt wearing is still compulsory and the Royal Society for the Prevention of Accidents provides advice on this.[35] In an accident, a seat belt reduces the risk of injury to the unborn child by up to 70 per cent.[36] Two infrequent complications require Driver and Vehicle Licensing Agency (DVLA) notification: eclamptic fits (considered a 'provoked seizure') and gestational diabetes (considered as 'temporary insulin treatment') may both be bars to Group 2 entitlement.[37] A Group 1 driver must stop driving and report it to the DVLA if experiencing disabling hypoglycaemia. Eclamptic seizures are not thought to represent continuing liability to future seizures, and are dealt with by the DVLA on an individual basis.

Time off work during pregnancy

Increased sickness absence is likely during pregnancy, and several non-medical factors may contribute to this:

◆ A public perception that pregnancy should be treated as an illness and work may be intrinsically harmful.

◆ A view that absence from work during pregnancy is short term and therefore a minor problem.

◆ A reluctance to affect patient rapport by seeming unsupportive.

◆ Ill health in the baby.

◆ Such decisions tend to go unchallenged.

The Chartered Institute of Personnel and Development (CIPD) produces guidance jointly with Acas (Advisory, Conciliation and Arbitration Service) and the HSE on the management of short-term absence.[38] It states that 'great care must be taken when dealing with sickness absence during pregnancy as the law says that a pregnant woman may not be subjected to detriment, directly or indirectly, on grounds of pregnancy. In general, any dismissal arising out of pregnancy will automatically be unfair' as it could be direct discrimination for pregnancy and maternity, which are 'Protected Characteristics' in the Equality Act 2010.

Acas guidance on the Equality Act 2010 states:

> A woman is protected against discrimination on the grounds of pregnancy and maternity during the period of her pregnancy and any statutory maternity leave to which she is entitled.[39] During this period, pregnancy and maternity discrimination cannot be treated as sex discrimination. You must not take into account an employee's period of absence due to pregnancy-related illness when making a decision about her employment.

Complications of pregnancy

'High risk' pregnancy Clinical risk assessment of the pregnancy is routinely used by the obstetric team during antenatal care. Designation of 'high' or 'low' risk depends on factors including problems identified at booking and those that develop through the pregnancy. In practice, many cofactors may be involved in a high-risk pregnancy: she may have a poor obstetric history, smoke, have a poor diet, or work in a manual job. Assessing the extent of risk associated with work is hard to separate out but ideally decisions on restriction of duties in a high-risk pregnancy should be made jointly between the obstetrician and occupational health.

Surgery and invasive investigations during pregnancy *Amniocentesis and chorionic villus sampling* are invasive tests carried out under ultrasound control. The most common indication is to carry out foetal karyotyping (chromosome analysis) following a high-risk result from a screening test. Such procedures are associated with an increased miscarriage rate of less than 1 per cent. It is a minor procedure and the woman could be expected to return to work the next day.

The *Caesarean section* rate assessed in England in 2010 remained relatively high at 23.8 per cent and varied between trusts from 14.9–32.1 per cent (adjusted rates).[40] More of the variation was in emergency, not elective C-sections. Normally this is performed through a transverse suprapubic incision. Early return to work may need to be deferred in the event of a C-section, as lifting and driving may be a problem, comparable with abdominal hysterectomy (see Table 20.1).

The 'minor disorders of pregnancy'

An obstetrician will correctly refer to many of the unpleasant symptoms of pregnancy as 'minor disorders of pregnancy' as they have a minor effect on the pregnancy outcome. However, these may have a significant effect on the pregnant employee and her ability to work. These are often worse in women with a multiple pregnancy.

Musculoskeletal problems are common. This is partly due to a rise in relaxin levels that soften connective tissue and increase joint mobility. There is an increase in body mass as well as a redistribution of the load, plus a reluctance to prescribe or to take analgesia. There are a number of braces and splints that can give symptomatic relief and seeing a physiotherapist or chiropractor is often more helpful than an obstetrician.

Up to 75 per cent of women report having *backache* at some time in pregnancy and 30 per cent find it a severe problem. It is often worse in the third trimester. It has been suggested that many of the symptoms are similar to overuse disorders and that antenatal restriction of activity is more useful than the progressive strengthening programmes used in non-pregnant back pain management.

Carpal tunnel syndrome occurs in up to 20 per cent of pregnancies particularly in the second half. Compression of the median nerve results in pain, numbness, and weakness. Initial treatment is by rest and wrist splinting.

Symphysis pubis dysfunction involves painful mobility of the symphysis pubis. It can present at any stage, gradually or suddenly (even immediately postnatally), and is common in the last trimester. Symptoms include localized pain, provoked by getting up from a chair, lifting, walking, or climbing stairs, which is relieved by rest.[41] The exact cause remains unclear, and it tends to be under-recognized. The amount of discomfort and disability is variable—some patients can barely walk, even with a Zimmer frame. Recovery following delivery is also variable: the majority improve rapidly after delivery but one-quarter still have symphysis pubis dysfunction pain up to 6 months postnatally; 85 per cent recur in a subsequent pregnancy. Referral to an obstetric physiotherapist for assessment and treatment is advised, and adjustments to work duties and working hours if necessary should be considered.

Tiredness and emotional lability may be significant in the first trimester, even before the pregnancy is declared. It may affect work performance but usually improves as pregnancy progresses.

Hyperemesis

Seventy-five per cent of all pregnant women experience nausea and in 10 per cent the condition persists beyond the first trimester. Although rest and dietary advice is common it has not been evaluated in randomized trials. Small amounts of carbohydrate may be helpful and if retained may provide some nutrition. Proven treatment includes antiemetics such as antihistamines, vitamin B6, ginger, and acupressure, e.g. wrist bands used for travel sickness, which apply pressure to the Neiguan acupuncture point.[42]

Heartburn Heartburn affects 70 per cent of all women at some stage in their pregnancy and may be aggravated by stooping or bending. Management involves avoiding fatty or spicy food and minimizing bending or lying flat after eating. Antacids are often sufficient but H_2 blockers are sometimes justified though the manufacturers' advice is to 'avoid unless essential' in pregnancy.

Hypertension A diastolic pressure of greater than 90 mmHg requires urinalysis and referral for further assessment. Rest is often recommended for non-proteinuric hypertension, though a woman with pre-school children is unlikely to be able rest without help with childcare. Despite controlled trials the value of bed rest is still not clear and time off work may not be necessary. Methyldopa is commonly used to treat hypertension in pregnant women, and can affect concentration and alertness.

Cognitive function While pregnant women frequently report impairments in memory and attention, there is sparse and conflicting evidence whether this is an objective mild cognitive impairment or only a perceived one, possibly related to low mood in pregnancy.[43] Reduced learning and retrieval in early pregnancy have been reported in a cross-sectional study of 71 pregnant women and matched controls.[44] There may be work situations where such subtle changes can be noticeable, but the woman is likely to be aware and compensate for it. Problems in late pregnancy and the immediate postnatal period have been reported but are less relevant to work.

Postnatal issues

Return to work Return to work postnatally tends to be dictated by socioeconomic issues, e.g. duration of paid or unpaid maternity leave, childcare arrangements. Medical reasons for delayed return to work include:

♦ Complications of wound healing, usually infection (perineal or Caesarean section).

♦ Musculoskeletal problems.

♦ Psychological well-being.

♦ Ill health in the baby.

Breastfeeding and work There are few medical contraindications to return to work while breast-feeding, but there are some practicalities to consider. How often are they breastfeeding? The assessment may differ where a baby is dependent on the mother for much of its nutrition, or simply has a night-time comfort feed. What facilities are available at work if she needs to feed or express milk during working hours? It is good practice to provide facilities and there are legal requirements to support this. Are there potential hazardous substances (risk phrase R64) in the workplace that could be absorbed and secreted in breast milk? Examples include highly fat-soluble compounds such as organic solvents, organochlorine pesticides, and polychlorinated biphenyls. There have been case reports of maternal hydrogen fluoride exposure causing dental fluorosis in her children and tetrachloroethylene causing jaundice in a baby and mercury excreted in breast milk may be up to 5 per cent of blood levels.[45] Some employers take the view that breastfeeding is not compatible with certain 'front-line jobs', e.g. armed forces, fire, and police services. There may be several reasons for this: a potential for uncontrolled workplace exposures; perceived reduced physical fitness; the impact of serious injury on the dependent baby; unpredictable working hours incompatible with feeding or expressing demands.

Postnatal depression During the first 6 months after delivery, the prevalence of major depression is estimated at 12–13 per cent. Postnatal depression is thought to be generally underdiagnosed and most patients can be treated in primary care settings. There is a simple screening tool available: the 10-item Edinburgh Postnatal Depression Scale and a score of 12 or more out of 30 indicates the likelihood of depression but not its severity.[46] Several studies have reported that antidepressants can be used safely by nursing mothers of healthy full-term infants. Cognitive-behaviour therapy has been demonstrated to be comparably effective for non-psychotic depression.[47]

Gynaecological problems

This section mainly addresses the impact of gynaecological disorders on both attendance and performance at work. There is very little evidence of relevant occupational hazards.

Fertility issues

In vitro fertilization IVF involves (1) hyperstimulation of the ovaries to produce a number of eggs, (2) egg collection (usually transvaginally under ultrasound control), (3) fertilization *in vitro*, (4) incubation, before (5) embryo transfer. Additional embryos may be frozen and used in subsequent cycles. The overall success rate is 20 per cent but varies with personal factors. The duration of treatment is hard to anticipate as treatment protocols between IVF units and patients vary in their response. Predicting time off work is therefore also difficult: treatment schedules change at short notice and patients may travel considerable distances to receive it. Work performance may also be affected by emotional lability associated with the drugs, physical and emotional demands. Complications can include ovarian hyper-stimulation syndrome where hospital admission may be required.

What interferes with conception? Patients with subfertility (failure to conceive after a year) may be concerned about the impact of occupational stress and night work. There is some evidence these can increase prolactin levels, which in turn may inhibit ovulation.[48] A Danish study of 297 couples found reduced fertility in women with high-strain jobs.[49] Occupational health should consult the woman's gynaecologist before making individual recommendations about significant changes at work.

Menstrual disorders

Troublesome symptoms of the menstrual cycle include heavy bleeding, pain, and mood changes. A few days each month of absence and/or reduced performance can easily cause a considerable impact on work. Medical management in primary care should be able to control many of the symptoms although there may be a reluctance by the patient to take hormonal treatment, e.g. a combined pill for non-contraceptive reasons.

Menorrhagia is a common problem: each year 5 per cent of women aged 30–49 years consult their GP describing heavy periods that may disrupt work and home life (dysfunctional uterine bleeding). A range of medical management can be offered before specialist referral. Surgical treatment includes endometrial ablation (with heat, microwaves, or cryotherapy) and hysterectomy.

Dysmenorrhoea can be associated with menorrhagia, fibroids, or endometriosis, which may require treatment of the underlying cause. Pain management includes simple analgesia and non-steroidal anti-inflammatory drugs such as mefenamic acid.

Premenstrual syndrome (PMS): the RCOG defines PMS as 'a condition which manifests with distressing physical, behavioural and psychological symptoms, in the absence of organic or underlying psychiatric disease, which regularly recurs during the luteal phase of each menstrual (ovarian) cycle and which disappears or significantly regresses by the end of menstruation'. The variety of attributed symptoms is enormous (up to 88 have been described), and the luteal phase is 7–10 days before a period, though other patterns occur. Many women will have self-diagnosed premenstrual syndrome and as there is no quantifiable assessment tool, a detailed history of significant symptoms should be documented. A wide range of self-help and some medical treatments can be tried, but none are universally effective.[50] The RCOG provide a comprehensive guide to the management of PMS.

Endometriosis, where the presence of endometrial-like tissue outside the uterus, induces a chronic, inflammatory reaction most commonly in the pelvic organs and peritoneum is another highly variable condition. Symptoms are primarily of pain, plus fatigue and infertility. The amount of disease visible at laparoscopy (the main diagnostic test) does not correlate with the level of symptoms. A serum CA125 level may be raised but this is not a diagnostic test. Classically, the pain is cyclical but may be continuous. Treatment includes controlling pain, suppression of ovarian function, and surgery.[51]

Menopause

In the UK, 70 per cent of women between 45 and 59 are employed, potentially working through and beyond the menopause. The average age of the menopause is 51 and up to 75 symptoms have been attributed to it. A high follicle stimulating hormone level may support the diagnosis of menopause but is not helpful in predicting when the symptoms will stop. Whilst occupational health practitioners may not see it as a major fitness for work issue, a 2003 TUC survey reported that over a third of workers felt embarrassment or difficulties in discussing the menopause with their employers and that hot flushes, headaches, tiredness, and lack of energy were the symptoms most likely to be perceived to be made worse by work.[52] Work may be affected by sleep deprivation, hot flushes, mood alteration, memory, or concentration difficulties. Vasomotor instability may be helped by clonidine. Hormone replacement therapy may help some symptoms but needs careful assessment of the risks and benefits by the GP or gynaecologist.

Gynaecological cancers

Historically, association has been shown between ovarian cancer and asbestos exposure,[53] but in general, gynaecological cancers are not occupational in origin. Anticipating time off work is difficult to predict as the management depends on the staging of the disease. This may not be clear with the initial diagnosis but may depend on operative findings, imaging, or histology. Management may include radical surgery, radiotherapy, chemotherapy, or a combination of these approaches.

Urogynaecology (see also Chapter 19)

Urinary problems are common in women but often unreported. In practice patients often have mixed symptoms of stress incontinence and overactive bladder symptoms. In cases where diagnostic studies have been performed, the nomenclature has recently been changed by the International Continence Society to 'urodynamically proven stress incontinence' or 'detrusor overactivity'. Urodynamic assessment is not essential in the initial management. Work that entails lifting, bending and even brisk walking may exacerbate *stress incontinence* symptoms but will not alter the course of the condition. Initial management should include pelvic floor physiotherapy with a 40 per cent reported cure rate. The drug duloxetine was licensed in 2004 for stress incontinence, though is also used as a treatment for depression. Open surgery such as a Burch colposuspension or sling involves a suprapubic or Pfannenstiel incision and has an 80–90 per cent cure rate with a return to work date of 6–12 weeks. The tension-free vaginal tape (TVT™) is a popular minimal access operation with similar cure rate to open surgery and in practice has a return to work date of 3–4 weeks.[54]

Overactive bladder symptoms vary from frequency and urgency to urge incontinence all of which may interrupt work, and make some jobs very difficult to do. A urinary tract infection should be excluded. The GP should have access to a continence advisor who has a lot to offer, including teaching bladder drill. Some effective anticholinergic medications used have centrally-acting side effects such as drowsiness.

Gynaecological surgery and work

The RCOG have produced an excellent series of patient information guides, including advice on return to normal activities at home, driving, and return-to-work (RTW) intervals for common gynaecological surgery.[2] Early RTW is not usually associated with adverse wound outcomes and pain and tiredness are more limiting than wound integrity. Where a significant wound infection has involved dehiscence and/or cellulitis, RTW intervals may need to be extended. See Table 20.1.

Major abdominal surgery Most open gynaecological surgery is performed though a transverse suprapubic incision. This includes abdominal hysterectomy, myomectomy, salpingo-oopherectomy, and Burch colposuspension. Mid-line incisions are performed for ovarian malignancy or when better access is required such as removing a large fibroid. Patients with mid-line incisions take longer to recover and are more prone to complications.

Hysteroscopic procedures Diagnostic hysteroscopy is now routinely done as an outpatient procedure. There is a risk of fainting from vagal stimulation that can last beyond the procedure, and most units do not advise driving immediately afterwards. Hysteroscopic surgery, e.g. resection of fibroids, usually requires a general anaesthetic and return to work after a few days.

Termination of pregnancy As a procedure this can be done medically or surgically and the patient should normally be physically fit almost immediately. Medical termination usually involves oral mifepristone followed 48 hours later by oral or vaginal misoprostol. Psychological fitness may be less predictable, as for miscarriage. Complications include retained products of conception that may require further intervention.

Colposcopic treatment Colposcopic assessment of the cervix varies from examination only to loop excision but rarely require more than a day or so off work unless complications arise.

Working women: other issues

Work–life balance

As well as working, women often have significant additional commitments and responsibilities in the home and outside of work. There is evidence that differences in sickness absence rates between men and women reflect the need to manage other, immediate and domestic respon-sibilities (Figure 20.2). The 2000 UK Time Use Survey studied 6400 households between June 2000 and July 2001.[55] Research was based on an interview and a diary of 10-minute time slots throughout the week and weekend, plus a weekly timetable. The amount of childcare varies with the age of the youngest dependent child. See Figure 20.3. For parents of under-fives, on a weekday, non-working mothers spent 5 hours 50 minutes/day on 'childcare activities'; full-time working mothers spent 3 hours/day, and working fathers spent 1 hour and 20 minutes/day (2 hours 30 minutes at weekends). 'Childcare activities' were broadly defined as including physical care and supervision, teaching the child, reading, playing and talking with the child, accompanying the child, and travel escorting to/from education or other activity.

Understanding the work–life balance is particularly important in planning a successful return to work after major illness. Domestic responsibilities rarely reduce on return to work and a phased start can be highly successful, e.g. working mornings only at first and increasing back to full duties within 4–6 weeks. This allows for increased rest and pacing of work while rehabilitation contin-ues, physically and/or psychologically.

Ergonomic issues

It is obvious that not only are there male–female differences in body size and function but that there is considerable variation and overlap. For example, women on average have 61 per cent of

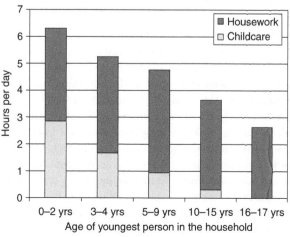

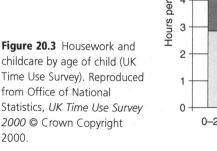

Figure 20.3 Housework and childcare by age of child (UK Time Use Survey). Reproduced from Office of National Statistics, *UK Time Use Survey 2000* © Crown Copyright 2000.

Table 20.2 Comparison of historical RAF recruitment standards and Pheasant's anthropometric data. Examples of gender difference for sitting height and arm length

Anthropometric measurements	RAF aircrew entry standards (57)		5th centile	50th centile	95th centile
Sitting height	Minimum 865 mm	Males	850 mm	910 mm	965 mm
		Females	795 mm	850 mm	910 mm
Arm length:	Minimum 720 mm	Males	720 mm	780 mm	840 mm
		Females	655 mm	705 mm	760 mm

Data from Pheasant S. *Bodyspace. Anthropometry, ergonomics and the design of work*, Taylor & Francis, London, UK Copyright © 2006.

male muscle strength, but there is still a 10 per cent 'chance encounter of female exceeding male' strength.[56] Joint flexibility has been shown to be 5–15 per cent greater in females. On average, women are smaller in all dimensions except hip breadth: 13 cm shorter in stature, 5 cm lower eye height when sitting. Grip reach is 15 cm less when standing, 10 cm sitting, and 7 cm less for forward reach. These anthropometric differences affect women's ability to use equipment designed or set up for men and vice versa, either where there is a mechanical advantage from both height and strength (e.g. pushing and pulling) or when 'hot desking' requires frequent adjustment of office equipment. The Royal Air Force provides a well-worked example. The aircrew entry standard anthropometric limits for a pilot require, for example, a minimum sitting height of 865 mm and functional reach (or arm length) of 720 mm in order that aircrew can fly a wide range of aircraft.[57] Using standard anthropometric data it can be shown that typically fewer women than men meet these criteria, illustrated in Table 20.2. RAF air crew standards are gender-free: each aircraft has authorized limits with the rationale justified for critical control of cockpit equipment. So, for example, the Chinook Mark 2 cargo helicopter requires a functional reach (FR) of 710 mm: for critical control of brake steering. A Sea King Mark 3 or 3a 'search and rescue' helicopter requires a FR of only 660 mm minimum: for critical control of the winch (data from Dr David McLaughlin, 2012).

Physical fitness and injury

In a role requiring a high level of physical fitness (e.g. armed forces or fire service) physiological differences can present at extremes of activity. The British Armed Forces published data from 1985 to 2000 showing that female medical discharge rates for musculoskeletal disease were more than three times that for males.[58] Undertaking the army phase 1 basic fitness training (which was designed as 'gender free') males were typically exercising at 30–40 per cent of capacity and females at 80–90 per cent. Females were less likely to complete the training and were known to be more prone to stress fractures. Continuous high-impact exercise with inadequate recovery disturbs bone remodelling: resorption is accelerated faster than bone formation. It is thought that female recruits' inadequate diet and the popularity of depot medroxyprogesterone contraception (DMPA) may both have reduced bone density and increased the risk of stress fracture in this particular occupational group.[59] Gender-specific army fitness training was therefore put in place to accommodate the typical male/female physiological differences.

Conclusion

When considering fitness to work of a female worker, there may be more to consider than the duties of the job and declared medical history. Some relevant clinical problems may not be raised without skilful, direct enquiry e.g. postnatal depression, stress incontinence. In addition to the role at work, women still tend to undertake the lion's share of the childcare and family commitments: this should be considered when planning for a successful phased return to work.

References

1 Royal College of Obstetricians and Gynaecologists website: <http://www.rcog.org.uk>

2 RCOG 'Return to Fitness: Recovering Well' leaflets: <http://www.rcog.org.uk/recovering-well>

3 ONS. *Annual survey of hours and earnings, 2010 revised results*. [Online] (<http://www.ons.gov.uk/ons/rel/ashe/annual-survey-of-hours-and-earnings/2010-revised-results/index.html>)

4 RCOG. Green-top guideline no 25: early pregnancy loss, management. London: RCOG, 2006.

5 NHS Plus, Royal College of Physicians, Faculty of Occupational Medicine. *Physical and shift work in pregnancy: occupational aspects of management. A national guideline*. London: RCP, 2009.

6 RCOG. Green-top guideline no 17: the investigation and treatment of couples with recurrent miscarriage. London: RCOG, 2011.

7 Fenster L, Hubbard AE, Windham GC, *et al*. A prospective study of work related physiological exertion and spontaneous abortion. *Epidemiology* 1997; **8**: 66–74.

8 HSE. *Management of health and safety at work regulations 1999*. Sudbury: HSE Books, 1999. (<http://books.hse.gov.uk>)

9 HSE. *New and expectant mothers at work. A guide for employers*. Sudbury: HSE Books, 1997 (<http://books.hse.gov.uk>)

10 HSE. *Ionising Radiations Regulations 1999. Approved code of practice and guidance*. Sudbury: HSE Books, 2000. (<http://books.hse.gov.uk>)

11 International Commission on Radiological Protection. 2007 Recommendations of the International Commission on Radiological Protection. Publication 103. *Ann ICRP* 2007; **37**: 2–4.

12 Kheifets L, Mezei G. Extremely low frequency electric and magnetic fields. In: Baxter PJ, Aw T-C, Cockroft A, *et al*. (eds), *Hunter's diseases of occupations*, 10th edn, pp. 668–9. London: Hodder Arnold, 2010.

13 Figà-Talamanca I.Occupational risk factors and reproductive health of women. *Occup Med* 2006; **56**(8): 521–31.

14 Office of The Deputy Prime Minister. Medical and occupational evidence for recruitment and retention in the fire and rescue service. London: HMSO, 2004.

15 Rachana C, Suraiya K, Hisham AS, *et al*. Prevalence and complications of physical violence during pregnancy. *Eur J Obstet Gynaecol Reprod Biol* 2002; **103**: 26–9.

16 Peterson R, Gazmararian JA, Spitz AM, *et al*. Violence and adverse pregnancy outcomes: a review of the literature and directions for future research. *Am J Prevent Med* 1997; **13**(5): 366–73.

17 Theodorou DA, Velmahos GC, Souter I, *et al*. Foetal death after trauma in pregnancy. *Am Surg* 2000; **66**(9): 809–12.

18 Einarson ARN, Bailey B, Inocencion G, *et al*. Accidental electric shock in pregnancy: a prospective cohort study. *Am J Obstet Gynaecol* 1997; **176**(3): 768–81.

19 HSE. *Control of Lead at Work Regulations 2002. Approved code of practice and guidance*, 3rd edn. Sudbury: HSE Books, 2002. (<http://books.hse.gov.uk>)

20 Gauger VT, Voepel-Lewis T, Rubin P, *et al*. A survey of obstetric complications and pregnancy outcomes in paediatric and non-paediatric anaesthesiologists. *Paediatr Anaesth* 2003; **13**(6): 490–5.

21 Rowland AS, Baird DD, Weinberg CR, *et al*. Reduced among women employed as dental assistants exposed to high levels of nitrous oxide. *N Engl J Med* 1992; **327**: 993–7.

22 Rowland AS, Baird DD, Shore DL, *et al.* Nitrous oxide and spontaneous abortion in female dental assistants. *Am J Epidemiol* 1995; **141**(6): 531–8.

23 Bodin L. The association of shift work and nitrous oxide exposure in pregnancy with birth weight and gestational age. *Epidemiology* 1999; **10**(4): 429–36.

24 Norman CA, Halton DM. Is carbon monoxide a workplace teratogen? A review and evaluation of the literature. *Ann Occup Hyg* 1990; **34**(4): 335–47.

25 Attarchi MS, Ahouri M, Labbafinejad Y, *et al.* Assessment of time to pregnancy and spontaneous abortion status following occupational exposure to organic solvents mixture. *Int Arch Occup Environ Health* 2012; **85**: 295–303

26 Testud F, D'Amico A, Lambert-Chhum R, *et al.* Pregnancy outcome after risk assessment of occupational exposure to organic solvent: a prospective cohort study. *Reprod Toxicol* 2010; **30**: 409–13.

27 HSE. *Infection risks to new and expectant mothers in the workplace: a guide for employers.* Sudbury: HSE Books, 1997. (<http://books.hse.gov.uk>)

28 RCOG. *Infection and Pregnancy – study group statement*, 2001. [Online] (<http://www.rcog.org.uk/womens-health/clinical-guidance/infection-and-pregnancy-study-group-statement>)

29 RCOG. *Green-top guideline no 13: chickenpox in pregnancy.* London: RCOG, 2007.

30 Ahlborg G. Physical work load and pregnancy outcome. *J Occup Environ Med* 1995; **37**(8): 941–4.

31 RCOG. Green-top guideline no 31: small-for-gestational-age fetus, investigation and management. London: RCOG, 2002.

32 Judge CM. Physical exposures during pregnancy and congenital cardiovascular malformations. *Paediatr Perinat Epidemiol* 2004; **18**(5): 352–60.

33 HSE. *What about stress at home?* [Online] (<http://www.hse.gov.uk/stress/furtheradvice/stressathome.htm>)

34 Hobel CJ, Goldstein A, Barrett ES. Psychosocial stress and pregnancy. *Clin Obstet Gynecol* 2008; **51**(2): 333–48.

35 The Royal Society for the Prevention of Accidents. *Seat belts: advice and information.* [Online] (<http://www.rospa.com/roadsafety/adviceandinformation/vehiclesafety/in-carsafetycrash-worthiness/seat-belt-advice.aspx>)

36 Directgov. *Using a seatbelt.* [Online] (<http://www.direct.gov.uk/en/TravelAndTransport/Roadsafetyadvice/DG_4022064>)

37 Driver Medical Group. *At a glance guide to the current medical standards of fitness to drive.* Swansea: DVLA, 2011. (<http://www.dvla.uk/at_a_glance>)

38 CIPD. *Absence management. 3 How do you deal with short-term recurrent absence?* [Online] (<http://www.cipd.co.uk/binaries/3862Absencemanagement3.pdf>)

39 Acas guide. *The Equality Act 2010: What's new for employers?* [Online] (<http://www.acas.org.uk/>)

40 Bragg F, Cromwell DA, Edozein LC, *et al.* Variation in rates of caesarean section among English NHS trusts after accounting for maternal and clinical risk: cross sectional study. *BMJ* 2010; **341**: c5065

41 Leadbetter RE, Mawer D, Lindow SW.Symphysis pubis dysfunction: a review of the literature. *J Matern Foetal Neonat Med* 2004; **16**: 349–54.

42 Rosen T, de Veciana M, Miller HS, *et al.* A randomized controlled trial of nerve stimulation for relief of nausea and vomiting in pregnancy. *Obstet Gynaecol* 2003; **102**: 129–35.

43 Crawley RA, Dennison K, Carter C. Cognition in pregnancy and the first year post-partum. *Psychol Psychother* 2003; **76**: 69–85.

44 De Groot RHM, Hornstra G, Roozendaal N, *et al.* Memory performance, but not processing speed, may be reduced during early pregnancy. *J Clin Exp Neuropsychol* 2003; **25**(4): 482–8.

45 Baxter P, Igisu H. Mercury. In: Baxter PJ, Aw T-C, Cockroft A, *et al.* (eds), *Hunter's diseases of occupations*, 10th edn, p. 324. London: Hodder Arnold, 2010.

46 Cox JL, Holden JM, Sagovsky R. Detection of postnatal depression. Development of the 10-item Edinburgh Postnatal Depression Scale. *Br J Psychiatry* 1987; **150**: 782–6.

47 Hendrick V. Treatment of postnatal depression. *BMJ* 2003; **327**: 1003–4.

48 Wallace M. *National Occupational Health & Safety Commission. Review: The effects of shiftwork on health.* [Online] (<www.nohsc.gov.au/ResearchCoordination/researchreports>)

49 Hjollund NHI, Kold Jensen T, Bonde JP, *et al.* Job strain and time to pregnancy. *Scand J Work Environ Health* 1998; **24**(5): 344–50.

50 RCOG. *Green-top guideline no 48: premenstrual syndrome, management.* London: RCOG, 2007.

51 RCOG. Green-top guideline no 24: endometriosis, investigation and management. London: RCOG, 2008.

52 Paul J. *Working though the change.* London: TUC Publication, 2003.

53 Wignall BK, Fox AJ. Mortality of female gas mask assemblers. *Br J Ind Med* 1982; **39**: 34–38.

54 Ward K, Hilton P. Prospective multicentre randomised trial of tension-free vaginal tape and colposuspension as primary treatment for stress incontinence. *BMJ* 2002; **325**: 67–74.

55 ONS. *Time use,* 2000. [Online] (<http://www.statistics.gov.uk/timeuse/summary_results/>)

56 Pheasant S. *Bodyspace. Anthropometry, ergonomics and the design of work.* London: Taylor & Francis, 1996.

57 AP1269A. *Royal Air Force manual of medical fitness,* Section 5, (3rd edn). 1998.

58 Geary KG, Irvine D, Croft AM. Does military service damage females? An analysis of medical discharge data in the British Armed Forces. *Occup Med* 2002; **52**(2): 85–90.

59 Greeves JP, Bishop A, Morgan CK. *The effect of depot-medroxyprogesterone acetate on bone health and stress fracture risk during British Army Phase-1 Training.* QinetiQ report for the MoD QinetiQ/K1/CHS/TR0315359 December 2003). Farnborough: QinetiQ Ltd, 2003.

Chapter 21

Fitness for work after surgery or critical illness

Tony Williams and Bill Thomas

Introduction

Occupational health practitioners are frequently asked for advice on fitness to return to work after surgery. Providing the best answer is not always clear cut, as there is little evidence and a great deal of misunderstanding among patients and clinicians. One patient may be back at work within a week of a hysterectomy while another insists she is not fit to return after 5 months. There are medical issues here, but these are often confounded by inappropriate beliefs, unhelpful motivators, and uneducated advice.

Perhaps the problem is best illustrated in a simple study published in the *British Medical Journal* in 1995. Majeed et al.[1] asked 100 general surgeons and 90 GPs to recommend time off work for patients aged 25 or 55 years in sedentary, light manual, and heavy manual roles. The answers varied so widely that it was apparent that those giving advice had no full understanding of the issues. For example, after unilateral inguinal hernia repair in a 25-year-old returning to heavy manual work, surgeons' recommendations varied from 1 to 12 weeks, and GP recommendations varied from 2 to 13 weeks.

Often, however, there is a limitation in the evidence base. An expert working group, attempting to develop guidelines for the Royal College of Obstetricians and Gynaecologists (RCOG), found it easy to agree that a woman who had a vaginal hysterectomy would probably be at risk from heavy lifting within the first 4 weeks because of the nature of the surgery undertaken, but found no empirical evidence to support this. It is therefore difficult to quantify the actual risk and the advice finally given by the group was to adapt a 4-week cut off point. This represented a substantial shift from the 12 weeks not uncommonly recommended but in the absence of evidence to the contrary, it was considered that this was the best advice that could be provided.

What do patients do in the absence of any advice?

What do patients themselves believe about return to work after surgery, and what do they do in the absence of medical advice? A good example of a procedure where there is no obvious reason for a delay in return to work is a simple discectomy. The result is a stable spine with minimal disruption to surrounding tissues. Many practitioners advise months off before returning to work, but without any objective justification. Carragee et al.[2] studied a group of 45 worker volunteers undergoing discectomies, and urged them to return to full activities as soon as possible. The patients worked in various roles from sedentary work to heavy manual labour. Eleven patients returned to work on the next available working day. Many returned to adjusted duties initially, and the mean time to return to full duties involving light manual work was 2.5 weeks, and 5.8 weeks for heavy manual work.

The results of this small study suggest that most clinicians are giving over-cautious advice and that patients who are motivated can return faster than clinicians expect. Factors such as sick pay schemes have a major impact on return to work times (see Chapter 4).

Does advice from clinicians have an impact on patients' beliefs and behaviours?

Carpal tunnel release is a commonly performed procedure, from which some patients return to work very quickly with others remaining off sick for many weeks. Ratzon et al.[3] followed up 50 consecutive patients operated on by five surgeons, assessing them before and after for severity of symptoms. They found that the surgeons' recommendations for return to work varied from 1 to 36 days, and the time to return to work varied from 1 to 88 days. The surgeons appeared to relate their advice to the type of work done but this was not highly predictive. The duration of sickness absence was not related to the severity of symptoms before or after surgery. The surgeon's recommendation had the strongest influence on duration of absence.

The fact that patients follow their surgeon's advice is not surprising. It becomes a problem if the surgeon's advice is not evidence-based and a much longer period of absence than necessary is recommended. This is particularly a problem if long rest periods are recommended, as this can lead to substantial deconditioning with possible associated weight gain. In middle-aged and older patients it can be extremely difficult to regain fitness and pre-surgery weight.

The evidence base

There is substantial evidence for long-term recovery from various surgical procedures, but almost none for the relatively brief recovery period between the operation and a return to work. So while it is possible to predict what someone might be able to do when they have fully recovered from a total hip replacement, there is little or no documented evidence on how long it will be before they can safely squat, walk a mile, or lift a bag of shopping or cement.

There is, however, a substantial evidence base concerning the principles of surgical recovery. A great deal is known about wound healing, complications that may arise during the recovery period, and the impact of concurrent factors such as diabetes, age, and smoking. Until good studies produce direct evidence, we should rely on our knowledge of the principles of healing and recovery to assess scope for return to work after surgery.

What do we mean by 'fit for work'?

There are three main fitness issues to consider after an operation. The first is simple capability: can the person get out of bed and get to work, can they physically cope with any or some work? The second is safety: will they be harmed or potentially cause harm to others by going to work, and by doing any particular activity at work? The third is motivation: how well do they cope with pain, do they want to return or are they seeking time away from work? All are relevant.

A person may be safe returning to heavy lifting within a few hours of a mesh repair of an inguinal hernia, but as the anaesthetic wears off they may experience substantial pain. Is it reasonable to expect them to return if they will be in pain? How much pain or discomfort is it reasonable to expect an employee to endure? How can their account of pain be verified, or its severity adjudged?

Beliefs about the safety of work will also play a major part, as will workers' specific occupational responsibilities. If driving is involved, can the patient safely execute an emergency stop? Does the patient trust the hernia repair or the new hip? Do they trust their employer to make adjustments for them at work? Do they trust the occupational health practitioner who advises them that they will not be harmed?

These issues need to be explored with each patient to determine what they can do and what they believe they can do, and what they want to do. Each patient will be different; one may return after a carpal tunnel release within 3 days with no adjustments, another may not return for 2 weeks, and on reduced hours and workload to help them regain confidence. Care should be taken not to be judgemental in this process, but there is a need to address obvious motivational barriers.

Evidence from wound healing studies

The rate at which wounds heal inevitably plays a part in the decision regarding a patient's return to work. Wound healing depends on the reparative ability of the tissue involved and is dependent on growth factors known as cytokines. The process can be delayed by infection, ischaemia, malignancy, poor nutrition and the presence of a haematoma or foreign body. Intercurrent illnesses and treatments may also delay healing, including diabetes mellitus, jaundice, uraemia, use of irradiation and treatment with oral steroids, immunosuppressive drugs and chemotherapeutic agents. Malnutrition, with deficiencies of protein, vitamins, and trace elements such as zinc and manganese, can also delay healing.

The time course for healing will depend on the tissue involved. For skin and mucosal lined organs, the stages of wound healing are relatively constant. Six stages can be recognized:

- Within minutes blood clots form within the wound, the surface starts to dehydrate and a scab starts to form.
- Within 24 hours the first phases of inflammation are seen with neutrophil infiltration, the epidermal edges start to thicken, and there is increased mitotic activity.
- Within 3 days granulation tissue has formed and is covered by epidermal cells, the neutrophils are replaced by macrophages, and collagen fibres start to grow into the wound at its edges.
- By 5 days the epidermal lining becomes multilayered, new vessels start to proliferate, and collagen fibres start to bridge the wound.
- After 2 weeks remodelling has started while fibroblasts continue to proliferate and the vessels start to diminish.
- By 4–6 weeks the wound has strengthened, the inflammatory response disappeared, the collagen is remodelled, and the wound appears healed, although the scar may still be pink.

This sequence of events needs to be considered when advising patients when to return to work. The process and timescale is slightly different for bone where healing is dependent on osteoblast activity producing woven bone. Mesenchymal cells in the soft tissues around a fracture also become activated and start to secrete both fibrocartilage and hyaline cartilage. After 3 weeks the mass of healing tissue is maximal but has little strength and is unsuitable for weight bearing, but the newly formed cartilage starts to ossify and new bone starts to bridge the fracture gap. The remodelling process can take many weeks but eventually the bone may be remodelled to the effect that it may resemble the original bone shape as long as reduction of any fracture displacement was accurate.

Evidence from use of different closure methods and internal support

How a wound is closed and the technique and materials used may also influence recovery. Choice of suture material is crucial to maximize healing rates. A balance needs to be struck between absorbable sutures that minimize the foreign body irritation and of non-absorbable sutures that can provide permanent strength to a wound. For abdominal closure many surgeons now use a long-lasting absorbable suture material such as PDS (polydioxanone) that maintains its tensile strength for about 8 weeks. Mass absorption takes about 6 months. Thus, the suture materials provide stability for the wound but eventually disappear, circumventing long-term wound irritation. Where prolonged approximation of tissues is required (e.g. the repair of an incisional hernia), a non-absorbable suture material or mesh of such material as polypropylene may be used. Skin closure adds very little to a wound's strength, but whether sutures, skin clips, steristrips, or glue is used, the attending clinician needs to pay attention to the nature, the site and the method of closure of any wound in making the recommendation for return to work. There is no reason why a patient may not return to sedentary work even with skin sutures still *in situ*, but it would be unwise for a patient to undertake heavy manual labour or for the wound to be exposed to water, dust, or abrasive contact.

Diabetes

Significant postoperative complications are seen in patients with diabetes, reflecting a variety of specific physiological problems. Nitric oxide is a key mediator for many functions at cellular level including the mobilization of endothelial progenitor cells. Elevated glucose leads to an uncoupling of endothelial nitric oxide synthase to produce the superoxide anion (O_2^-) instead of nitric oxide.[4,5] Failure of mobilization of the endothelial cells leads to failure of revascularization which is essential in successful wound healing. Clearance of dead cells (efferocytosis) within wound sites is an essential part of resolution of inflammation and successful healing. This role should be carried out by macrophages but they are dysfunctional in diabetes. The result is continued exposure of the healing wound to the toxic contents of dead and dying cells, resulting in persistent inflammation and delayed wound healing.[6]

Obesity

There is evidence that obesity is associated with a state of chronic low-level inflammation with overexpression of the cytokine tumour necrosis factor (TNF)-α by adipose tissue (which in turn contributes to insulin resistance). Adipocytes produce adiponectin, resistin and visfatin, all molecules with immunological activity, and there is a close relationship between adipocytes and macrophages accumulation.[7] There is also evidence of impaired antibody responses in overweight individuals[8] and an increased risk of chest infections with delayed mobilization.

Smoking

Smoking has two particular effects on wound healing. Inhaled carbon monoxide and hydrogen cyanide reduce available oxygen in the blood, and therefore available oxygen at the wound site. High nicotine levels impair angiogenesis and therefore reduce the blood supply available to the healing wound. Smoking may also impair collagen production and maintenance, weakening any scar formation. The result is a significant delay in healing and a weaker scar.

One study looked at the effects of smoking on wound healing following laparotomy for sterilization. Out of 120 women, 69 were smokers and the width of their midline scars measured on average 7.4 mm compared to 2.7 mm in non-smokers, with the smokers having significantly worse cosmetic results.[9]

Another study looked at smoking cessation prior to head and neck surgery among 188 patients who had either never smoked or had stopped smoking. Quitters had either stopped 8–21 days (late), 22–42 days (intermediate), or more than 42 days (early), before surgery. Impaired wound healing was found in 68 per cent of late quitters, 55 per cent of intermediate quitters, 59 per cent of early quitters against 48 per cent of non-smokers. After controlling for other factors, the odds ratios of developing impaired wound healing were 0.31 for late quitters, 0.17 for intermediate and early quitters, and 0.11 for non-smokers (p = 0.001).[10]

The risk of incisional hernia is substantially increased in those who smoke. In a series of 310 laparotomies with an incidence of incisional hernia of 26 per cent, smokers had an odds ratio of 3.93 for developing incisional hernia when compared with non-smokers.[11]

Smoking is also a major factor in delayed fracture healing, perhaps because of reduced blood supply, high levels of circulating reactive oxygen species, low levels of antioxidants and vitamins, and the attenuating effect of nicotine on endothelial nitric oxide synthase.[12] In one study vertebral fusion failed in 40 per cent of smokers but only 8 per cent of non-smokers.[13]

Age

It is generally assumed that age affects recovery time, and that older patients take longer to return to work. There is limited evidence on this however. Holt et al. showed that the effect of age alone was minimal, with patients over 65 taking on average 1.9 days longer to heal than those aged under 65.[14] The much longer recovery times anticipated by clinicians reflect comorbidities that are more likely to be seen in the older patient.

The nature of the operation

It is important that the occupational physician understands the exact nature of the surgical procedure carried out before giving advice. Two procedures seen frequently in occupational health clinics—subacromial decompression and bunion surgery—illustrate how the nature of the procedure is influential.

Subacromial decompression may involve just debridement of excess acromial bone with an expected return to work within a week, and only minor discomfort. More frequently the thickened synovium will need to be excised leaving a very sore joint taking 4–6 weeks to recover sufficiently for light manual handling. If the rotator cuff needs repair, although the patient may be able to return to light administrative duties wearing an abductor brace after a couple of weeks, they are unlikely to be able to use the arm for any significant light manual handling duties for around 12 weeks and may not be able to return to heavy manual handling for 6 months. This is a particular problem if there is a poor vascular supply to the healing muscle, delaying recovery.

Bunions may represent just a little extra bone over the medial aspect of the first metatarsal head, or significant lateral displacement of the proximal phalanx with substantial degenerative changes in the metatarsophalangeal joint. Surgery may involve distal osteotomy of the metatarsal, proximal osteotomy of the metatarsal, or even surgery to the adjacent tarsal bones. Distal surgery is usually managed with a walking plaster at 2 weeks and early mobilization to avoid stiffening while proximal surgery may require non-weight bearing for 6 weeks. So some patients may be fit to return to most duties within a few weeks and may even be running after a couple of months while others will take substantially longer to recover. While sedentary duties may be an option for some, care needs to be taken to find out exactly what procedure was undertaken before advising on a suitable return to work date and work duties.

Psychology and surgery

Any surgical procedure is likely to be a significant event in someone's life and different people will have different expectations and beliefs about their recovery and what activity is safe and not safe.

Unfortunately these beliefs can be reinforced as a result of medical advice but in general patients can be reassured following most surgical procedures that normal activity will be safe and they should be encouraged to carry out exercise activity such as walking and return to normal activity as quickly as possible. Occupational physicians should be alert for yellow flags as these can be an important indicator of outcome and whether someone is at risk of extended absence and subsequent deconditioning which can make return to work more difficult.

Time to return to work following surgery

This and the next main section provide guidelines on how long someone will typically need to return to work following common surgical procedures. In the absence of direct evidence on optimal return to work times after surgery, the next best approach is to achieve consensus among clinicians. Consensus guidelines should prevent large variation in recommendations and can help achieve standardization. They should also help employers predict the amount of time off, allowing them to make alternative arrangements for cover if necessary. The main sources of consensus advice have been used as a source of guidance for this chapter but it should be noted that few are based on firm evidence and that a range of views sometimes exists. Where this is so, the text and tables attempt to capture the existing range of expert opinion. The Royal College of Surgeons of England (RCS), and RCOG have both recently developed consensus-based guidelines for a number of common procedures.

The RCS identified a small number of surgeons for each procedure who were asked to draft guidelines which included advice on what patients could expect at different stages in the recovery process including returning to work.[15] These were then assessed by a working group including an anaesthetist, general practitioner (GP), occupational physician, and patient representative. The result is a series of downloadable leaflets which include a 'traffic light' system indicating likely timelines for return to work of various types. These guidelines are based on consensual opinion and some patients may be able to return significantly sooner than suggested without coming to harm, while others may develop complications or may just take longer to adjust to recovery. They are useful tools, however, for the occupational physician, assisting discussion with patients who may lack confidence to return or who may be reluctant to increase their physical activity.

The RCOG has likewise developed a series of downloadable leaflets on common procedures.[16] Each guideline was drafted by a small number of gynaecologists and then discussed in detail by a working group that included the same anaesthetist, GP, and occupational physician as the RCS working group, and nursing and patient representatives. These leaflets give advice to patients on the recovery process, activity levels that are safe during recovery and likely timelines for a return to work. In preparing the RCOG guidelines it was recognized that many women undergoing gynaecological procedures will be middle aged and may have been relatively inactive for several years, often because of the underlying health problem. Emphasis was therefore placed on the value of early activity, particularly walking. Walking immediately after these procedures will not be harmful and it should be encouraged. This is particularly important for conditions where traditionally many patients have been encouraged to rest. Such an approach can result in substantial loss of fitness and substantial weight gain, perhaps never to be reversed. Employers may allow employees several months off to recover, but the employee should be encouraged to use this time to regain full physical fitness and if possible to adopt a new, healthier lifestyle now that their underlying problem has been treated.

In addition, the guidelines given on return to work times have been augmented with data from two unpublished studies. In 2007 a study was undertaken in The United Bristol Healthcare Trust, later extended to involve seven other NHS hospitals in the South West to examine postoperative return to work timescales for routinely performed surgical operations in six surgical specialities, (general/abdominal, orthopaedic, urology, gynaecology, vascular, and breast/endocrine) ('the Bristol study'). Estimates were made for 46 operations for sedentary workers and 38 operations for heavy manual workers based on timescales published in previous editions of this textbook, from the Department for Work and Pensions, and from a number of published papers. Forty-four surgeons completed the questionnaire about advice given, and 50 surgeons commented on timescales. Sixty per cent of surgeons stated that they always gave advice on return to work and sickness absence and 91 per cent stated that consultants would be involved in giving this advice, noting that other team members could also be involved. Most stated they gave advice preoperatively either verbally or in writing. In terms of consensus there was good agreement between orthopaedic surgeons. General surgeons, gynaecologists, and urologists had moderate agreement on return to work timescales. Amongst breast surgeons agreement was only fair.

A second similar study to that in Bristol was circulated among surgeons in NHS Greater Glasgow and Clyde ('the Glasgow study') and their estimates have also contributed to the suggested return times included below. There are many guidelines available on the Internet, often local consensus guidelines from single trusts or hospital groups. Further recommended times on return to work following surgery can be found at the Working Fit website (<http://www.workingfit.com>).

Advice to employees

Ideally employees should be advised about their procedure and shown the web-based resources from the RCS or RCOG *before* surgery, so they know what to expect and can prepare to return to work in the recommended timelines. This can be a useful role of the occupational health department and is an opportunity to reinforce the significant benefits of exercise both before surgery and during the recovery period. There may be value in directing the employer to the web-based resources too, so there is a good understanding between employee and employer over what to expect and what support will be needed when the employee returns.

Specific operation sites and procedures

Abdominal surgery

Laparoscopic surgery

Laparoscopic cholecystectomy is currently the operation of first choice for the treatment of symptomatic gallstones and is increasingly performed as a day case procedure. The role of laparoscopy has since expanded in several specialities including general surgery, gynaecology, and urology, and large painful surgical wounds have been replaced with small, relatively painless, 'keyhole' incisions, facilitating more rapid postoperative recovery for many patients. The small wounds of laparoscopic surgery are also less prone to complications such as wound infection and incisional hernia. Furthermore, the handling of the intestine and the fluid loss involved in abdominal procedures performed through laparotomy wounds is largely avoided by laparoscopic techniques. Postoperative ileus and pulmonary and thromboembolic complications are less frequent after laparoscopic surgery. Laparoscopic techniques thus promote early recovery and enable quicker return to work. Other minimally invasive procedures such as arthroscopy and thoracoscopy similarly contribute to earlier recovery after orthopaedic and chest surgery respectively.

Table 21.1 Suggested return to work times in weeks following abdominal surgery

Abdomainal		Sedentary	Light manual	Heavy manual	Ref.
Laparoscopic surgery	Cholecsytectomy	1–2		2–4	a
	Nephrectomy			6	a
	Bowel resection			6	b
Gastric banding		2–4	4–6		
Gastric bypass		2–6		<12	
Appendicectomy	Laparoscopic	1		2–3	
	Open	2		3–4	
Laparotomy		4	4–6	6–8	
Stoma			8–12		
Hernia repair	Inguinal open	1–2	2–3	6	a
	Inguinal laparoscopic		1–2		b
	Femoral		3		b
	Epigastric		4		b
	Umbilical		6		b
Surgical haemorrhoidectomy				4	b
Pilonidal sinus (primary suture)	Primary suture	1–3	3–6		b

References: a: RCS guidelines;[15] b: The 'Bristol study' (see text)

Some patients make a very quick and uneventful recovery after a laparoscopic cholecystectomy and can return to some sedentary work within a week or so (see Table 21.1). Patients should be able to return to non-manual work within 2 weeks of gastric banding surgery but may need longer after other bariatric procedures. In many cases there are significant dietary issues over the first 2 or 3 months and although a return to non-manual work in 2–4 weeks and manual work in 4–6 weeks should be expected, some patients may lack energy to cope with manual work for the first 3 months or longer after surgery.

Laparotomy

Standard open abdominal wounds are still required when a laparoscopic procedure (e.g. cholecystectomy) proves technically impossible or dangerous, and for many major abdominal operations (e.g. certain procedures on the pancreas, those for abdominal aortic aneurysms when endovascular surgery is unsuitable, and some colorectal resections). The major abdominal wound involved in laparotomy, as opposed to laparoscopy, is a cause of considerable postoperative pain and morbidity.

Most abdominal wounds are now closed with non-absorbable or slowly absorbable materials rather than the rapidly absorbed cat gut used by many surgeons in the past. As a result of improved suture techniques the incidence of wound dehiscence is reduced and early return to non-manual work should not increase the risk of the development of an incisional hernia. Heavy manual work, however, will not normally be undertaken for 6–8 weeks after a major laparotomy. The length of convalescence after laparotomy will be affected not only by the type and size of wound but also by the procedure performed, the occurrence of complications in the postoperative period and the nature of the patient's occupation. A subcostal incision for removal of the gall bladder (if laparoscopic access has been unsuccessful) is less traumatic for the patient than a full-length vertical abdominal incision, as is commonly needed for colonic or vascular procedures. Whereas the former may result in a hospital stay of 2–5 days and a quick return to work, some patients with a long vertical abdominal wound will remain in hospital for 1–2 weeks if there are no procedural or wound-related complications and thus absence from work may be longer.

Complications of laparotomy wounds include wound infection and wound dehiscence and, at a later date, the development of an incisional hernia. Occasional consequences of laparotomy, for whatever cause, include small bowel obstruction due to ileus in the immediate postoperative period or due to adhesions at a later date. Following bowel surgery, including creating a stoma, it will often take 8–12 weeks before the patient is fit to return to non-manual work, and a significant manual role will need to wait until the patient is confident in managing the stoma (see 'Stomas'). Often there are other factors involved, such as adjuvant therapy following surgery for malignancy or 'dumping' following gastrectomy. There may be difficulty swallowing solid food for up to 3 months after oesophageal or gastric surgery, but this should not delay a return to work.

Hernia repair

The methods now used for hernia repair, using tension-free mesh and sutures,[17] lead to a very strong structural repair immediately after wound closure, so the patient is normally unlikely to be harmed by any activity as soon as they recover from the anaesthetic. Although there may be slightly less discomfort, less risk of wound infection, and a smaller wound after laparoscopic repair, the overall recovery times do not vary greatly between laparoscopic and open repairs. The main issues affecting return to work are discomfort and complications such as wound infection. Where a recurrent hernia repair is undertaken there is likely to be significantly more local tissue damage with slower healing and greater discomfort for longer. The estimated timelines before returning to work are therefore maximal estimates, and most employees would be expected to return before the times suggested. Amid et al showed that open prosthetic mesh repair can withstand any degree of stress immediately[18] and Schulman et al. noted that postoperative activity need not be restricted at all.[19] Rest should be discouraged and patients should be encouraged to walk on the first day postoperatively. The RCS recommends 6 weeks to heavy manual work after inguinal hernia repair, and a return to playing football after 8 weeks and rugby after 12 weeks. These are all conservative recommendations. The key message is to allow employees to return as soon as they want to after hernia repair. There is no need to advise a willing worker to delay their return unless there are significant complications.

Haemorrhoids

There is no absolute clinical need for patients to remain off sick after thrombosed internal haemorrhoids although discomfort is likely to prevent many from working for a week or two. Surgical haemorrhoidectomy will lead to significant discomfort and initial discharge. However, there is no need to wait until full healing has taken place before returning to work. Whilst some employees may be able to return after 2–3 weeks full healing may take 5–6 weeks.

Anal fissure, pilonidal sinus, and anal fistula

Employees will be safe working at any stage after treatment for anal fissure, pilonidal sinus, or anal fistula but the discomfort and logistics of dressing changes may prevent a return until healing is near complete. Adjustments to working hours to allow dressings to be changed around working hours and the use of shaped cushions to help workers sit more comfortably at work may facilitate earlier return to work. A lateral internal sphincterotomy causes little external disruption so a return after a day or two can be expected. Where healing is delayed the employee may have no option but to wait several months until the wound has healed sufficiently to allow them to sit at work.

Stomas

Stomas may be created with ileum or colon, including an ileal conduit for a urostomy. A temporary colostomy or ileostomy may be created to allow for distal anastomotic healing before stoma closure in 3–6 months, or the stoma may be permanent. All stomas require some means to collect waste, and the design and process followed can vary significantly. Some patients with distal colostomies are able to manage the stoma by irrigation to stimulate emptying, so no collection bag is required and the stoma can be covered with a cap or plug allowing substantial freedom of movement and activity. Irrigation is a relatively prolonged affair taking 45–60 minutes and ideally is only required around once every 48 hours—otherwise patients are likely to prefer the convenience of a bag which can be easily changed. Stoma bags can be drainable or may separate from a base plate to allow changing. The base plate is generally left attached for 3–5 days. Most patients are able to undertake all physical activities, including swimming and non-contact sports, with a stoma. More vigorous activities will require the use of a protective belt or shield. However, patients have returned to work and coped well as prison and police officers whose work can involve the control and restraint of others.

There are a number of complications of stomas. In ballooning, flatus fails to escape through the integral filter, requiring early pouch change. Parastomal hernias are common, but not all are symptomatic and there is no evidence that regular exercise and heavy manual handling are more likely to cause a parastomal hernia provided that a support belt is worn. Problems may arise where the stoma is close to a scar or skin fold, affecting adhesion of the pouch plate. Leakage is unusual but may be problematic at work. Ileostomies tend to fill more often with more fluid contents and are more likely to produce odours.

Most people can return to full employment with a stoma and usually only require minimal adjustments. There are only a few roles where difficulties arise, such as employees working overseas away from normal toilet facilities, or those working outside with limited access to toilet facilities (e.g. postmen, forestry workers, linesmen). In a few cases individuals develop complications, or have significant psychological issues with their stoma that undermine their confidence or ability to cope in the workplace. All patients with stomas should be supported by a stoma nurse and should have good access to advice and support. A useful source of support is the Colostomy Association.[20]

Reconstructive bowel surgery

As an alternative to a stoma, the surgeon may be able to fashion a pouch from small bowel to replace the rectum and colon. Although the anal sphincters are retained, the patient may need to use a catheter several times a day to empty the pouch. The combination of recovery from surgery and adaptation to the new anatomy can take several months before the patient is ready to return to work. Appropriate toilet arrangements may be necessary, with a supportive phased return to work aimed initially at rebuilding confidence.

Cardiothoracic surgery

Many patients having cardiothoracic surgery will have substantial comorbidity which will affect recovery. Various access routes may be used, and choice of route will have a major effect on recovery times (see Table 21.2). Cardiothoracic surgery has seen some significant developments in minimally invasive techniques including percutaneous valve procedures and radiofrequency ablation.

Thoracoscopic procedures

Thoracoscopy has significantly reduced morbidity relative to thoracotomy, allowing a much quicker return to work. After thoracoscopy a return to non-manual work can be expected after a couple of weeks and a return to manual work after a month. Typically this method is used for cervical sympathectomy, pulmonary resection and surgery for pneumothorax.

Thoracotomy

A full thoractomy is required for major lung and heart surgery. A return to non-manual work after partial pneumonectomy can be expected after 6 weeks and to manual work after 12 weeks. After a full pneumonectomy a return to non-manual work may be possible after

Table 21.2 Suggested return to work times in weeks following cardiothoracic and vascular surgery

		Sedentary	Manual	Ref.
Cardiothoracic				
Thoracoscopy		2	4	
Open pneumonectomy	Partial	6	12	
	Total	8–12		
Spontaneous pneumothorax			4–6	
Surgery for recurrent pneumothorax		2–3	6	
Cardiac angioplasty		<1		
CABG		6	6–12	a
Oesophagectomy		6–8	8–16	a
Vascular				
Angioplasty		1	2–3	b
Aortic aneurysm	Open	16–26		c
	Percutaneous endovascular grafting	1	2–4	
Femoro-popliteal bypass		4	12	b
Carotid endarterectomy		2–5	4–8	b
Varicose veins	Stripping	1–2	2–3	c
	Foam sclerotherapy	<1	<1	

References: a: RCS guidelines;[15] b: 'The Bristol study'; c: 'The Glasgow study' (see text).

2–3 months but a return to manual work may be problematic if there is substantially reduced exercise tolerance which may be exacerbated by lifestyle issues particularly smoking. However many people, particularly if younger and fitter, can have effectively normal function despite removal of a lung.

Lifestyle change is encouraged after coronary artery bypass grafting (CABG)—more so than the 'rest, rest, rest' often encouraged after other surgical procedures. As a result recovery rates often seem substantially faster than for other less invasive surgical procedures. The RCS recommends a return to non-manual work after CABG in 6 weeks, and a return to most manual work in 6–12 weeks. The main delay in return to manual work is healing of the chest wall as rib and sternal pain may persist for several months after surgery. Heavy upper body exercise should be avoided for the first 3 months to allow full healing of the sternum. Light upper body activity is encouraged to avoid extensive scarring and restricted mobility. Patients are unlikely to be harmed by working in a manual role after 3 months, even if they get unusual sensations or discomfort in the chest wall. It is important to encourage exercise in a controlled environment, as this will help the patient regain confidence as well as fitness.

Oesophagectomy is usually only used for malignancy, and although this is the mainstay of treatment, adjuvant chemotherapy may be used before or after surgery. If chemotherapy is given prior to surgery there should be no delay to recovery from the surgery. A jejunostomy may be used for feeding, and the tube is usually removed 3–6 weeks after surgery well before returning to work. The RCS recommends a return to non-manual work after oesophagectomy in 6–8 weeks, and a return to manual work in 2–4 months. The poor prognosis in most cases often means that the patient opts for ill health retirement, and in those trying to return to a manual role, it is unusual for them to succeed.

Spontaneous pneumothorax

An employee should be safe to return after spontaneous pneumothorax to a non-manual role without significant delay once they have left hospital, but may need several weeks to enable healing before returning to a heavy manual job. A period of 4–6 weeks would be reasonable depending on the nature of the patient's employment. After surgery for recurrent pneumothorax a return to non-manual work can be expected within 2–3 weeks of surgery, but a return to most manual work is likely to take at least 6 weeks to allow for healing. Chest discomfort is common after pleurodesis and this is the main reason for the slower return to non-manual work.

Cardiac angioplasty

A quick recovery can be expected after elective angioplasty, and light exercise is usually safe immediately after the procedure although it would be reasonable to allow 3 days for stabilization of the coronary vessels and catheter access site. Care will need to be taken to avoid trauma to the catheter access site when undertaking heavy manual work. It is important to liaise with the treating cardiologist if the patient plans to return to high levels of physical activity as this should be included in a rehabilitation plan for the underlying ischaemic heart disease.

Vascular surgery

Aortic aneurysm

Healing after open abdominal surgery for aortic aneurysm grafting would be expected to enable a return to non-manual work after 2–3 months, but multiple comorbidities are likely and these could extend the recovery time significantly (see Table 21.2). Treatment by percutaneous endovascular grafting would be expected to lead to a much more rapid recovery, with return to work in 5–7 days possible for non-manual work and 2–4 weeks for manual work. Again, multiple comorbidities are likely to be the limiting factor and may well prolong recovery times.

Arterial graft and reconstructive surgery

Vascular reconstruction of the abdominal and lower limb arterial system is now generally a treatment of last resort. Patients are likely to have major comorbidities including cardiac problems and diabetes and they are more likely to be older workers if still working. These issues are likely to play a major role in any decision on fitness to return to work. Where a laparotomy is required, the usual 2–3 months to return to manual labour would apply and 1–2 months for non-manual work. Faster healing would be expected for femoro-popliteal bypass (see Table 21.2). Recovery after carotid endarterectomy can be affected by psychological issues.

Angioplasty

Peripheral angioplasty when undertaken electively, with or without stenting, allows a relatively swift return to work. A return to non-manual work should be expected in a week, and a return to manual labour can be expected in 2–3 weeks.

Varicose veins

Following traditional surgical techniques for stripping and tying varicose veins, the expected return to work time is 1–2 weeks for non-manual work and 2–4 weeks for manual work. Patients may take a little longer after bilateral vein treatment, while laser ablation should allow a faster recovery. Bandages are usually replaced with thromboembolic deterrent (TED) stockings after a day, with stockings worn for 2 weeks. Many surgeons now use foam sclerotherapy, and early activity is encouraged after this treatment as prolonged inactivity can be harmful. Patients are typically advised to walk every day from the day following surgery.

Head, neck and ENT surgery

Many head, neck, and ENT procedures are undertaken for malignancy, and there may be significant comorbidity where the thyroid or parathyroid glands are involved. This will inevitably affect return to work times. In the absence of significant additional morbidity, return to non-manual work can generally be expected in a couple of weeks and to manual work in 1–2 months (see Table 21.3).

Thyroidectomy

Hemithyroidectomy for a solitary thyroid nodule is a relatively minor procedure, and a return to non-manual work may be expected in 1–2 weeks. Subtotal or total thyroidectomy is significantly more traumatic and may be associated with alteration in thyroid function and disorders of calcium metabolism if the parathyroid glands are removed or injured.

Parotid and submandibular glands

The good vascular supply around the head and neck generally allows a quick return to work, with a return to non-manual work after 7–14 days where the submandibular gland is involved, or 2 weeks after surgery on the parotid gland. Return to manual work should take around 2–3 weeks irrespective of the site. Removal of a stone from the submandibular duct is a simple procedure and a return to work can be expected in 1–2 days.

Table 21.3 Suggested return to work times in weeks following head and neck, and urological surgery

		Sedentary	Light manual	Heavy manual	Ref.
Head and neck					
Thyroidectomy		2	4		a
Salivary gland	Surgery	1–2	2–3		
	Stone removal	<1			
Nasal septoplasty		1		6	a
Wisdom teeth extraction			<1	<1	a
Urological					
Cystoscopy		<1			
Vasectomy		<1		2	b
	Reversal	1	1	2	
Orchidectomy (via abdomen)		2			
Prostatectomy	Transurethral	2–4	4–8		b
	Radical	4	6	8	
Lithotripsy				2	b
Transplant	Laparoscopic		4–6	4–6	a
	Abdominal	6–8	6–8	6–8	b

References: a: RCS guidelines;[15] b: 'The Bristol study' (see text).

Nasal septoplasty

Nasal septoplasty is a common procedure in young fit workers. Once the packing is removed on the following day the main symptom is stuffiness and mouth breathing for up to a week. A return to non-manual work in 3–7 days will not harm the employee, but slightly longer times may be expected, with around a week suggested by the RCS. Hard physical exercise may cause nosebleeds within the first week or so, but this should not be a problem from around 10 days, and a return to manual work can be expected in the second or third week. A delay of around 6 weeks would be expected before undertaking 'control and restraint' activities at work.

Wisdom teeth extraction

This is a common procedure in young employees and there is no need for long periods of recovery after extraction. The RCS suggests that most people can expect to return to non-manual work in 1–3 days and it is reasonable to wait a day or so longer before returning to heavy physical activity. Although employees are unlikely to be harmed by an early return to work, attempting hard physical activity the day after surgery is unwise, particularly if a general anaesthetic has been used. A return to contact sports and work involving control and restraint would not be recommended in less than a week and these employees may need a second week for the inflammation and discomfort to settle.

Urological surgery

The most common urological procedures are cystoscopy and vasectomy, with prostate surgery in older men. Most patients will return to work the day after a cystoscopy and many men will return to non-manual work the day after a vasectomy although 2 weeks may be required before resuming heavy manual activity (see Table 21.3). Longer would be required after vasectomy reversal, with a week off before returning to non-manual work suggested. Two weeks off would be reasonable after an orchidectomy assuming this involves entering the abdomen to retrieve the testis. A faster return would be expected following scrotal surgery.

Prostatectomy

The main issue after prostatectomy is regaining urinary continence, rather than recovering from the surgery itself; this can be delayed after surgery via the transurethral route. Those undergoing radical prostatectomy are likely to have longer recovery times and it may be 8 weeks before return to manual work.

Renal surgery

Return to any work should be possible within 2 weeks following lithotripsy and within 6–8 weeks following renal transplant (see Table 21.3).

Breast surgery

Breast surgery is common, but the underlying reasons may have a major impact on individuals' ability and motivation to work. A return after a couple of days would be expected after a simple procedure, and a return to non-manual work within 1 week after a benign lumpectomy and a return to manual work after 2 weeks. Factors including the size of the scar, the amount of disruption caused internally, and the breast size will all affect discomfort and in turn affect return to work times (see Table 21.4).

Table 21.4 Suggested return to work times in weeks following breast and gynaecological surgery

		Sedentary	Light manual	Heavy manual	Ref.
Breast					
Benign lumpectomy		1	2		a
Cosmetic		2		4–6	
Mastectomy for malignancy		2	6		b
Gynaecological					
Laparoscopic ovarian cyst		1	2–3		
Endometrial ablation		<1	1–2		c
Hysterectomy	Laparoscopic	2–4	4–6	4–6	c
	Vaginal	2–4	4–6	4–6	c
	Abdominal	2–4	6–8	6–8	c
Mid urethral sling			3		c
Pelvic floor repair		2–3	3–4	6	c
Dilatation and curettage		<1			c

References: a: 'The Bristol study' (see text); b: RCS guidelines;[15] c: RCOG guidelines.[16]

Cosmetic breast surgery

The surrounding tissues need to settle and heal after breast enlargement surgery, and women will usually be advised to remain off work for 2 weeks and avoid significant arm or chest exercise, with no heavy lifting for 4 weeks after surgery. If the implant is placed under the muscle, up to 6 weeks may be needed before resuming full activities. Similar guidelines apply for breast reduction surgery.

Lumpectomy and mastectomy

Most breast surgery for malignancy will involve a wide local excision and sentinel node biopsy initially, and the RCS recommend a return to non-manual work in 2 weeks or to manual work in 6 weeks. There is little difference in tissue disruption or healing with wide local excision and axillary clearance as compared with mastectomy, so the RCS recommends the same timelines.

Radiotherapy typically involves daily treatment over 3–6 weeks depending on the available procedure. Some women choose to continue working part time during this period, and the main side-effect of fatigue may not arise until towards the end of treatment, typically continuing for a month or two afterwards. Chemotherapy will depend on the staging, sensitivity and grading of the tumour, and may involve a course of six or eight cycles with 3 weeks between, or weekly infusions of Herceptin® for 52 weeks. Side-effects vary depending on the treatment and fatigue may persist for several months after treatment. Many women will choose to work part time between cycles of treatment. Herceptin may cause significant flu-like symptoms, nausea and diarrhoea within a day or two of the first few treatment cycles, but these normally settle after the first two or three doses.

Gynaecological surgery

The RCOG website provides excellent patient information leaflets covering eight common procedures and sensible advice about expected timescales and activity during the recovery period. They emphasize the need to regain physical fitness and promote walking immediately after surgery as a good way to do this. Traditionally there has often been an expectation of much longer recovery periods of 3 or more months following gynaecological procedures and some websites continue to recommend prolonged periods of inactivity. This can be counterproductive and is only rarely necessary. Employers should be advised regarding this and encouraged to refer employees either pre-operatively for advice and counselling or early following surgery where there is an expectation or risk of extended absence. Some guidelines on indicative return to work times are given in the following subsections and in Table 21.4. (For further information on gynaecological surgery, see Chapter 20.)

Laparoscopy

Gynaecological laparoscopy may be exploratory with little active surgery, in which case the RCOG suggests a return to non-manual work in 2–3 days and a return to manual work within a week. Longer would be expected after procedures such as removal of an ovarian cyst, when a return to non-manual work may take a week and a return to manual work may take 2–3 weeks.

Endometrial ablation

Some cramping abdominal pain may be experienced for 48 hours after endometrial ablation, but the RCOG recommends that most women can return to work within 2–5 days. It would be reasonable to limit manual handling within the first week.

Hysterectomy

There are three different approaches to hysterectomy, the classical abdominal route (now reserved for a large bulky uterus), or the less invasive laparoscopic/vaginal hysterectomy or vaginal hysterectomy for the smaller uterus. When discussing the potential risks, the RCOG working group acknowledged the lack of research evidence but expressed a general feeling that there could be a risk to internal structures if the patient attempted heavy lifting within the first 4 weeks after hysterectomy. Accordingly, a guide time of 2–4 weeks before returning to non-manual work was recommended for all three types of operation, with 4–6 weeks before returning to manual work for the less invasive procedures and 6–8 weeks before returning to manual work after abdominal hysterectomy. Many women get back to work well within this timetable.

The main reason for delay in returning to work is obesity with wound infection. Provided the infection clears up within the first 2 weeks, little or no delay would be expected in returning to work. Many women see hysterectomy as a life-changing procedure and this may be an opportunity to consider major lifestyle changes at the same time, including stopping smoking and doing more exercise. Motivational interviewing techniques[21] can be very useful when approaching these matters, using the RCOG leaflets and guidance on early walking as part of the approach.

Mid-urethral sling

Sling or tape support for the urethra is a common procedure for stress incontinence, with the tape either running trans-vaginally with two incisions on the abdomen or through both obturators with incisions on both inner thighs. Pain may persist in the thighs for 2 weeks or more after a transobturator tape procedure and although women will not be harmed by working through this, some will not wish to do so.

Pelvic floor repair

Pelvic floor repairs may involve stitching or mesh support. Where mesh is used this may require access through the inner thighs for an anterior vaginal repair and through the buttocks for a posterior repair. Subsequent discomfort may prevent driving for at least 2 weeks, with a delay in returning to work related more to the discomfort than to any risks from working.

Dilation and curettage

A dilation and curettage (D&C) is usually a straightforward day case procedure following which there is no physical need for delay in returning to work. The RCOG suggests 1–2 days for return to any work but the psychological issues surrounding a miscarriage may require further support and advice from occupational health if it results in extended absence.

Orthopaedic surgery

There are many orthopaedic procedures carried out on people of working age often with widely varying recommendations about returning to work. With orthopaedic procedures it is particularly important to identify procedures where there is a substantial risk of harm if the person returns too soon to active work, particularly heavy manual handling. On the other hand, many individuals can return on crutches or with a sling to sedentary administrative work within a week or two of surgery without adverse effects. As noted earlier, it is important to find out exactly what procedure was undertaken and as with any other condition, motivation is an important influence on timescales to return to work.

The following subsections give some indicative return to work times after a selection of common orthopaedic operations. (Details for a full range of specialist procedures appear in Chapter 12.)

Shoulder surgery

The most common shoulder procedure is arthroscopic subacromial decompression. Patients may return to non-manual work within a week if this only involves debridement of the acromion, but where the bursa is debrided, the discomfort usually prevents significant use of the arm for 4–6 weeks although the patient won't be harmed by working at any stage after surgery.

Rotator cuff repairs often involve completely severing and reattaching the tendon using staples, so the patient must keep the arm immobilized for at least three weeks and care needs to be taken using the arm for the first 6 weeks. The tendon is often significantly damaged by prolonged wear and tear, with a compromised vascular supply and extensive scarring and this can delay healing by several months. A return to non-manual duties may be accommodated with the arm in a sling, with many patients managing to use a keyboard and mouse with the sling in place after 2 weeks but a return to manual work may take substantially longer and between 3–6 months.

Wrist surgery

Carpal tunnel release is usually a simple procedure with minimal damage to surrounding structures. There is no need to delay a return to work as the patient is unlikely to be harmed and some people return within a few days. It may be sensible to discourage heavy manual work for a week or two while the wrist heals. Around 1–3 weeks is recommended,[22] and the RCS suggests a return by 1–2 weeks to non-manual work, 2–4 weeks to light manual work, 4–6 weeks to medium manual work such as nursing or cleaning, and 6–10 weeks before returning to heavy manual work or control and restraint duties.

Total hip replacement

Better surgical technique is now allowing much earlier mobilization and weight bearing after hip replacement, with patients walking out of hospital after 3 or 4 days on a cemented prosthesis with only two sticks for support. Cementless prostheses require a period of partial weight-bearing, often 6 weeks, to allow bone ingrowth.

Some employees may wish to return to work quickly, particularly if they have administrative roles. They are unlikely to be harmed by doing so for a few hours per day after a couple of weeks. As a general guide the RCS recommends a return to non-manual work after 6–8 weeks and to manual work after 12 weeks. There is a significant risk of posterior dislocation within the first 6 weeks of surgery, particularly following a posterior approach, and patients may be advised to take care to avoid flexing beyond 90 degrees and rotating more than 45 degrees internally or externally. This does, however, affect recovery time. In one randomized study, patients who were given no advice to restrict activity early in the recovery period returned to work after an average of 6.5 weeks as compared with 9.5 weeks in those advised to restrict activity.[23]

There seems to be little evidence against early return to work, with early activity seeming beneficial, and a review found that where surgeons gave advice, this tended to delay return to work and delay recovery without apparent benefit.[24]

There is little evidence for and against particular work activities after hip replacement, but there is good guidance from the 1999 American Hip Society Survey[25] on return to sport. Activities such as stationary cycling, doubles tennis and swimming are recommended or allowed, activities such as canoeing and horse riding are allowed with experience and activities such as jogging, squash, and football are not recommended. Recommendations are also made for activity after knee replacement (see 'Knee surgery') and are similar.

After hip replacement, flying carries a substantially increased risk of DVT. Employees should avoid all flying until around 6 weeks after surgery and avoid flights exceeding 3 hours until 12 weeks after surgery.

Knee surgery

Arthroscopy does not disrupt the knee significantly so many patients can return to work within 2–3 days of surgery, although prolonged sitting may be uncomfortable in the early stages and lead to stiffness. The RCS suggests an average of 10–14 days before returning to non-manual work and 2–6 weeks for manual work after arthroscopic partial menisectomy.

Recovery times after total knee replacement can be very variable, often related more to weight and fitness rather than to the surgery itself. Some patients may do some part-time sedentary work after a couple of weeks. The RCS suggests a return to non-manual work by 6–8 weeks and manual work by 12 weeks. There is a significant risk of DVT when flying after knee surgery, and patients should avoid short flights for 6 weeks and long flights for 12 weeks.

Foot surgery

After bunion surgery a return to sedentary work can be expected within a couple of weeks, and where the extent of surgery is limited, early mobilization is encouraged, with a return to manual work in around 6 weeks. If non-weight bearing is recommended for the first few weeks, a return to manual work will not be feasible until around 12 weeks. A study of emergency brake response time after first metatarsal osteotomy found that 25 per cent of patients were fit to drive at 2 weeks and all were safe after 6 weeks.[26]

After Achilles tendon rupture return to work times are little influenced by whether the tendon is repaired surgically or treated conservatively. The patient may be able to cope with non-manual work within a few weeks while wearing a support boot, with some mobility after 3 months but no significant manual work until 6 months after rupture.

Returning to work after critical care treatment

The term 'critical care' encompasses intensive care on intensive care units (ICUs), intensive therapy units (ITUs), and high-dependency care (HDUs). Many patients are admitted to intensive care on a precautionary basis after injury or surgery for a period of observation before discharge to a general ward after 1–2 days. The time they have spent on ICU does not therefore reflect any complications in their treatment or a severe underlying pathology. Extended periods of time on intensive care are required for serious illness or serious complications of treatment. Recovery is affected both by the underlying pathology and by a period of complete inactivity often promoted by a combination of sedatives, analgesics, and physical constraints. Psychological issues are common because of the worry of the life-threatening event and there will be social issues surrounding the impact on immediate family, loss of income, and potential future changes in lifestyle. Prolonged stays on intensive care are often associated with widespread vascular and metabolic problems resulting from sepsis, shock, or systemic inflammatory response leading to organ hypoxia and organ failure. Damage may be permanent, or recovery may be very slow, leaving the patient very weak and fatigued.

The National Institute for Health and Clinical Excellence has developed a guideline for rehabilitation after critical illness[27] which emphasizes the importance of identifying patients at risk and starting rehabilitation early within a structured programme involving frequent follow-up reviews. As a result patients can expect to be referred to follow-up clinics for intensive care rehabilitation, which may include a self-directed rehabilitation manual.[28]

Physical effects

A prolonged period of complete inactivity may lead to massive loss of muscle bulk and strength through a combination of atrophy and catabolism, so a patient may leave hospital with functioning organs but so little strength that they struggle to walk more than a few steps and cannot cope with stairs. Loss of bone mass may also be seen.[29] Two months after discharge from ICU almost half of survivors still cannot manage stairs or have difficulty climbing more than a few steps, and one-third are still using a wheelchair outside the house.[30] Fatigue may persist, with 63 per cent of men and 60 per cent of women reporting fatigue at 3 months and 32 per cent of men and 38 per cent of women reporting fatigue at 1 year.[31] Acute axonal neuropathy related to sepsis may play a part in muscle atrophy, and can lead to permanent muscle weakness with quadriplegia.[32] Neurophysiological tests should help distinguish those with myopathy, who may recover strength, from those with severe neuropathy, who have a poor prognosis. Immobility and associated vascular compromise may lead to muscle contractures particularly affecting the ankles, fingers, and neck. Neck and shoulder pain are other recognized problems associated with prolonged periods of ventilation in the prone position. Joint immobility affects 5–10 per cent of patients, and immobility of the large joints, weakness, and fatigue, are common reasons for failing to return to work.[33]

Respiratory effects

Acute lung injury may be associated with widespread inflammation, leading to acute respiratory distress syndrome (ARDS). As the inflammatory process resolves there may be permanent residual fibrotic changes. In the long term the restrictive pattern seen on lung function testing is usually mild, and spirometric values are usually within 80 per cent of normal by 6 months. Persistent breathlessness is usually muscular in origin, rather than pulmonary. Only a small proportion of patients will have long term lung injury and some may require domiciliary supplemental oxygen. Tracheostomy may lead to long-term tracheal stenosis in 2–5 per cent of surviving patients, but tracheal compromise can usually be corrected surgically.

Psychological effects

The trauma of severe illness or injury commonly leads to post-traumatic stress disorder (PTSD) and associated psychiatric morbidities; the incidence of PTSD in patients following ARDS was 27 per cent.[34] Younger patients seem more vulnerable, possibly because they metabolize or clear sedative drugs more rapidly and have a better memory of distressing events during their illness. Prolonged treatment and the slow recovery may cause affective disorders, half of survivors having clinically significant anxiety and depression.[35] Physical damage to the brain, either from trauma or oxygen deficit, may lead to cognitive impairment, a common sequel to sepsis-related encephalopathy.[36] A year after hospital discharge three-quarters of survivors of ARDS have impaired memory, attention, concentration and processing speed, and a quarter still have mild cognitive impairment 6 years later. Side effects of opiate, sedative, and other medication, lack of sleep and circadian disruption can also be problematic. Substantial weight loss and the effects of trauma may affect appearance, alopecia being surprisingly common (seen in 47 per cent of women and 8 per cent of men, although normally resolved by 6 months).

Returning to work

A review by the Intensive Care National Audit and Research Council (ICNARC) found that of those who had been working prior to ICU admission, 42 per cent were still absent 6 months later, most (79 per cent) for health reasons. Of those who had returned to work, 23 per cent stated that their health was affecting their work. A recent Australian study found that only half of patients admitted to ICU for more than 48 hours had returned to work at 6 months follow-up.[37] Any patient who has spent more than 48 hours on ICU may develop the complications outlined above. Occupational physicians need to be alert to this, to check for sequelae and be prepared to recommend prolonged and comprehensive rehabilitation programmes as necessary, liaising with treating physicians to ensure that all parties are working in concert to rebuild the patient's confidence and achieve fitness to return to work.

References

1 Majeed AW, Brown S, Williams N, *et al.* Variations in medical attitudes to postoperative recovery period. *BMJ* 1995; **311**: 296.

2 Carragee EJ, Han MY, Yang B, *et al.* Are postoperative activity restrictions necessary after posterior lumbar discectomy? A prospective study of outcomes in 50 consecutive cases. *Spine* 1996; **21**: 1893–7.

3 Ratzon N, Schejter-Margalit T, Froom P. Time to return to work and surgeons' recommendations after carpal tunnel release. *Occup Med* 2006; **56**: 46–50.

4 Ken YL, Ito A, Asagami T, *et al.* Impaired nitric oxide synthase pathway in diabetes mellitus. *Circulation* 2002; **106**: 987–92.

5 Thum T, Fraccarollo D, Schultheiss M, *et al.* Endothelial nitric oxide synthase uncoupling impairs endothelial progenitor cell mobilisation and function in diabetes. *Diabetes* 2007; **56**: 666–74.

6 Khanna S, Biswas S, Shang Y, *et al.* Macrophage dysfunction impairs resolution of inflammation in the wounds of diabetic mice. *PLoS ONE* 2010; **5**: e9539.

7 Wellen KE, Gokhan SH. Inflammation, stress and diabetes. *J Clin Invest* 2005; **115**: 1111–19.

8 Marti A, Marcos A, Martinez JA. Obesity and immune function relationships. *Obes Rev* 2001; **2**: 131–40.

9 Siana JE, Rex S, Gottrup F. The effect of cigarette smoking on wound healing. *Scand J Plastic Reconstr Surg Hand Surg* 1989; **23**: 207–9.

10 Kuri M, Nakagawa M, Tanaka H, *et al.* Determination of the duration of preoperative smoking cessation to improve wound healing after head and neck surgery. *Anaesthesiology* 2005; **102**: 892–6.

11 Sorensen LT, Hemmingsen UB, Kirkeby LT, *et al.* Smoking is a risk factor for incisional hernia. *Arch Surg* 2005; **140**: 119–23.

12 Sloan A, Hussain I, Maqsood M, *et al.* The effects of smoking on fracture healing. *Surgeon* 2010; **8**: 111–16.

13 Brown CW, Orme TJ, Richardson HD. The rate of pseudarthrosis (surgical nonunion) in patients who are smokers and patients who are nonsmokers: a comparison study. *Spine* 1986; **11**: 942–3.

14 Holt DR, Kirk SJ, Regan MC, *et al.* Effect of age on wound healing in healthy human beings. *Surgery* 1992; **112**: 293–7.

15 http://www.rcseng.ac.uk/patient_information/get-well-soon

16 http://www.rcog.org.uk/recovering-well

17 Stoker DL, Spiegelhalter DJ, Wellwood JM. Laparoscopic versus open inguinal hernia repair: randomised prospective trial. *Lancet* 1994; **343**: 1243–5.

18 Amid PK, Shulman AG, Lichtenstein IL. Critical scrutiny of the open 'tension–free' hernioplasty. *Am J Surg* 1993; **165**: 369–71.

19 Schulman AG, Amid PK, Lichtenstein IL. Returning to work after herniorrhaphy. *BMJ* 1994; **309**: 216.

20 Colostomy Association website: <http://www.colostomyassociation.org.uk>.

21 Miller WR, Rollnick S. *Motivational interviewing: preparing people for change.* New York, NY: Guilford Press, 2002.

22 Ratzon N, Schetjer-Margalit T, Froom P. Time to return to work and surgeons' recommendations after carpal tunnel release. *Occup Med* 2006; **56**: 46–50.

23 Peak EL, Parvizi J, Ciminiello M, *et al.* The role of patient restrictions in reducing the prevalence of early dislocation following total hip arthroplasty. A randomized prospective study. *J Bone Joint Surg Am* 2005; **87**: 247–53.

24 Kuijer PPFM, de Beer MJPM, Houdijk JHP, *et al.* Beneficial and limiting factors affecting return to work after total knee and hip arthroplasty: a systematic review. *J Occup Rehabil* 2009; **19**: 375–81.

25 Golant A, Christoforou DC, Slover JD, *et al.* Athletic participation after hip and knee arthroplasty. *Bulletin of the NYU Hospital for Joint Diseases* 2010; **68**: 76–83.

26 Holt G, Kay M, McGrory R, *et al.* Emergency brake response time after first metatarsal osteotomy. *J Bone Joint Surg Am* 2008; **90**: 1660–4.

27 National Institute for Health and Clinical Excellence. *Rehabilitation after critical illness.* NICE clinical guideline 83. London: National Institute for Health and Clinical Excellence, 2009.

28 Jones C, Skirrow P, Griffiths RD, *et al.* Rehabilitation after critical illness: a randomized, controlled trial. *Crit Care Med* 2003; **31**: 2456–61.

29 Ferrando AA, Lane HW, Stuart CA, *et al.* Prolonged bed rest decreases skeletal muscle and whole body protein synthesis. *Am J Physiol* 1995; **270**: 627–33.

30 Jones C, Griffiths RD. Identifying post intensive care patients who may need physical rehabilitation. *Clin Intens Care* 2000; **11**: 35–8.

31 Eddleston J, White P, Guthrie E. Survival, morbidity and quality of life after discharge from intensive care. *Crit Care Med* 2000; **28**: 2293–9.

32 de Seze M, Petit H, Wiart L, *et al.* Critical illness polyneuropathy. A 2-year follow-up study of 19 severe cases. *Eur Neurol* 2000; **43**: 61–9.

33 Herridge MS, Cheung AM, Tansey CM, *et al.* One year outcomes in survivors of the acute respiratory distress syndrome. *N Engl J Med* 2003; **348**: 683–93.

34 Scheeling G, Stoll C, Haller M, *et al.* Health-related quality of life and post traumatic stress disorder in survivors of the acute respiratory syndrome. *Crit Care Med* 1998; **26**: 651–9.

35 Scragg P, Jones A, Fauvel N. Psychological problems following ICU treatment. *Anaesthesia* 2001; **56**: 9–14.

36 Gordon SM, Jackson JC, Ely EW, *et al.* Clinical identification of cognitive impairment in ICU survivors: insights for intensivists. *Intensive Care Med* 2004; **30**: 1997–2008

37 Dennis DM, Hebden-Todd TK, *et al.* How do Australian ICU survivors fare functionally 6 months after admission? *Crit Care Resusc* 2011; **13**: 9–16.

Chapter 22

Dermatological disorders

Ursula T. Ferriday and Iain S. Foulds

The skin acts as a protective barrier against a number of hazards within our environment. These hazards can be: *chemical*, e.g. acids, alkalis, solvents, cutting, or soluble oils; *biological*, e.g. bacteria, plant allergens, or raw food; or *physical*, e.g. ultraviolet light, or mechanical shearing forces. In some situations the defensive properties of the skin are exceeded resulting in cuts, grazes, inflammation, ulceration, infection, and occasionally malignant change.

The risk factors for breakdown of skin defences can be categorized as: (i) *occupational*—common at-risk groups are cleaners, food handlers, hairdressers, and workers in contact with cutting fluids; and (ii) *non-occupational*—where genetic predisposition to skin disorders is an important factor.

Workers with non-occupational skin disorders can suffer exacerbations of their underlying dermatological condition in workplaces where the environment is hot and humid or extremely cold or dry.

Prevalence

It is estimated that 23–33 per cent of the UK population suffers with some form of skin disease at a given time, with eczema and infectious disorders being the most commonly presenting complaints to general practitioners (GPs) and dermatologists. Approximately 15–20 per cent of a GP's workload and 6 per cent of hospital outpatient referrals are for skin problems.[1]

The 2009/2010 Self-reported Work-related Illness survey, part of the national Labour Force Survey, estimated that 22 000 people in the UK who worked in the last 12 months suffered skin problems that were caused or made worse by work.[2]

The Industrial Injuries Disablement Benefit Scheme, which compensates workers who have been disabled by a prescribed disease, has seen a fall in the numbers receiving benefit for occupational dermatitis from 400 in the early 1990s to 75 in 2009.[2]

In 2009 a total of 2455 cases of occupational skin disease were reported to EPIDERM, which is a voluntary surveillance scheme for dermatologists in the UK and OPRA (Occupational Physicians Reporting Activity), a similar reporting system for occupational physicians. A breakdown of these occupational dermatoses showed that contact dermatitis represented 71 per cent of the total and most of the remainder (20 per cent) were skin cancers. The majority of occupational dermatitis arises from contact irritants.

Based on reports made during 2007–2009 to the THOR (The Health and Occupation Research network) GP scheme (reports of work-related ill health by GPs), skin diseases accounted for 2.9 per cent of total days of sickness absence certified due to all occupational illnesses. For skin diseases, a sickness certificate was issued in 18.3 per cent of cases and the average length of sickness absence was 3.6 days per case.[3]

In 2007–2009 the *occupations* most commonly reported to EPIDERM and OPRA with contact dermatitis were: health professionals (i.e. nurses and health support workers), floral arrangers/florists, hairdressers and barbers, beauticians and related occupations, assemblers of vehicles and metal goods, chemical and related process operatives, and chefs.

The most common *agents* cited by dermatologists and occupational physicians as causes of work-related skin disease were wet work and soaps and detergents, followed by rubber chemicals and materials.

Occupational dermatitis can be defined as an inflammation of the skin caused by work, and is classified into allergic or irritant contact dermatitis. These two types of skin disorder may be indistinguishable by clinical history and examination alone and investigation usually requires skin patch testing. If an occupational cause is identified, a reduction in exposure to irritants or allergens in the workplace is needed to control symptoms. Medical treatment of dermatitis is with moisturizers and topical steroid preparations.

At pre-employment

In occupations where the prevalence of occupational dermatitis is high, prospective employees should be made aware of the potential risks of the work and individuals with pre-existing skin problems encouraged to seek advice from the occupational health department.

Eczema

Atopic eczema affects one in five children. In later life it can render an employee more susceptible to the effects of irritants that come in contact with the skin. If the condition was severe in childhood, and particularly if the hands were involved, then the risk for developing (non-allergic) dermatitis in employment with irritants is significant.[4] Atopics with a history only of asthma or hay fever do not have an increased susceptibility. There is no evidence that atopics are at increased risk of developing allergic contact reactions, and clinical experience suggests that they are less likely to develop sensitization to potential contact allergens than non-atopics. However, all atopics are more likely to develop contact urticaria, asthma, and anaphylaxis from natural rubber latex, and preventative measures need to be considered.[5] Many organizations, particularly those employing healthcare workers, now have policies on the wearing of gloves at work for specific tasks, including guidelines on the type of glove to select.

Several jobs should be considered unsuitable for those with a history of severe childhood atopic eczema and active hand involvement e.g. hairdressing (shampoos), catering (wet work and detergents), and machine engineering (metal-working fluids).

Caution is also needed in placing nursing and healthcare workers. Ideally, occupational health advice should begin with the parents of children who have severe atopic eczema, to avoid careers involving significant irritant exposure. The requirement for hand washing between patients has increased, to reduce methicillin-resistant *Staphylococcus aureus* infections, and this has increased the risk of flare-ups of dermatitis in atopics with a past history of hand eczema. The situation is worsened by demands for alcohol cleansers at every hospital bedside in the UK; alcoholic preparations are poorly tolerated by those with a history of atopic skin disease, and up to 15 per cent of all nurses experience intolerance of such products. On balance, this suggests a need to discourage those with active skin involvement or a past history of severe eczema from training as a healthcare worker. Those who do proceed should receive a carefully supervised programme of hand care and should be followed-up in case of further difficulty.

Other occupations that carry a significant risk from irritant contact exposure are domestic cleaning, bar work, construction work, motor vehicle maintenance, horticulture and agriculture. Extremes of temperature and low humidity can also aggravate atopic eczema.

In certain occupations, hand involvement can also pose a risk of bacterial contamination. Eczematous skin is more prone than normal skin to be colonized with *Staphylococcus aureus*, and sometimes with *Streptococcus pyogenes*. Densities of *S. aureus* may exceed $10^6/cm^2$, leading to clinically apparent infection (impetigo); non-involved skin is colonized in up to 90 per cent of individuals.[6] Any organism that colonizes or contaminates the skin surface is dispersed into the environment during the natural shedding of skin scales. This can have serious implications in healthcare (risk of patient infection), catering (food poisoning), and the pharmaceutical industry (product contamination). Active eczema in these occupations therefore carries a risk of infective spread and requires individual assessment.

It has been shown[7] that, even where the occupation provides no apparently recognizable hazard to the skin, around half of those with a previous history of atopic eczema may develop hand eczema *de novo* or exacerbations of pre-existing hand eczema. When hand eczema develops in an atopic person exposed to a skin irritant, it is often difficult for the patient, their trade union, and insurers to accept that the condition may not be occupational. In claims for compensation, industrial injury assessors and expert witnesses will often allow patients the benefit of the doubt.

Seborrhoeic eczema may be aggravated by exposure to chemical irritants, but hot environments will contribute most to potential flare-ups of the disease. As the hands are unaffected, restrictions for occupations involving wet work are not required. The main problem is shedding of scales from the skin with risks of bacterial contamination similar to those found in atopics.

Stasis (varicose) eczema, which may be associated with varicose ulceration, can be aggravated by prolonged standing. Clinical management requires extra support compression for the legs and encouragement to walk regularly, to increase venous return. Leg elevation may be required during rest periods.

Discoid (nummular) eczema carries few implications for employment, as it is treatable with appropriate topical therapies and rarely aggravated by the work environment. Sometimes it can present as a feature of chromate dermatitis and soluble oil dermatitis, but in this situation it is usually associated with coexisting hand dermatitis.

Asteototic eczema (eczema craquelé) is a type of eczema that is caused by drying out of the skin. It commonly affects the lower limbs. Low humidity (air conditioning, car and lorry heaters), frequent showering, and use of degreasing chemicals (soaps, shampoos) will cause the skin to dry and crack. It can be prevented or treated by minimizing the causative factors.

Other non-cancerous skin disorders

Chronic urticaria can be aggravated by temperature (heat and rarely cold) and emotional stresses. Cholinergic urticaria is specifically triggered by exercise. Most forms of urticaria can be controlled by adequate doses (sometimes greater than the licensed amount) of non-sedating antihistamines during the daytime, and may also require the addition of sedative antihistamines at night. If sedative antihistamines are used then short-acting ones should be considered (e.g. chlorpheniramine) at night to avoid sedative after-effects. Sedative antihistamines are contraindicated where alertness is required, particularly when operating machinery or driving. Where urticaria is associated with natural rubber latex, the provision of a latex-free environment will be needed to prevent anaphylaxis.

Photosensitive dermatoses and, to a lesser extent, *vitiligo* may make outdoor work inadvisable. Up to 80 per cent of available ultraviolet light penetrates through cloud cover. Sufficient protection in the form of clothing and high-factor sunscreens will be needed. The latter should be applied frequently around the middle of the day (e.g. 10 a.m., noon, and 2 p.m.). Many medications (e.g. tetracyclines, amiodarone) can increase the risk of photosensitivity.

Acne, if severe and nodulocystic, can be a contraindication to working in hot, humid, steamy environments as severe exacerbations can occur. There is no evidence that pre-existing acne increases the risk of oil-induced acne, which is caused by occlusion and blockage of the pilosebaceous units in the skin. Acne is responsive (albeit slowly) to treatment, and even the most resistant cases can be treated with systemic isotretinoins. There is a higher prevalence of acne in the unemployed and it is suspected that unfair discrimination on the grounds of appearance may be occurring at the recruitment stage.[8]

Viral warts have a predilection for the hands and are a source of cosmetic embarrassment. Most viral warts involute spontaneously over time. They pose little risk to fellow workers as adults typically acquire immunity in childhood and become protected. In occupations involving food handling, patient care, and contact with the public, a pressure often exists to actively treat the condition. Butchers and abattoir workers are at special risk of hand warts, as the causative papillomavirus can infect meat and poultry. These occupations are associated with repeated minor trauma to the skin of the hands, so spread and cross-contamination can easily occur. Active treatment is therefore justified for these groups. Verrucas, which are also papillomaviruses, pose little risk to other people. No restrictions need to be placed upon swimming pool attendants, divers, and workers sharing showering facilities.

Fungal skin infections are common. The antifungal action of sebum in post-puberty tends to discourage fungal growth in adults. Therefore ringworm in the scalp (tinea capitis) from cats and dogs (*Microsporum canis*) is rare in adults. More aggressive fungi, as found on cattle and hedgehogs, can grow in the presence of sebum, leading to potential hair loss (alopecia) and secondary bacterial infections (kerion).

In warm and moist body locations (e.g. between the toes and in the groin) the common fungus *Trichophyton rubrum* thrives (tinea pedis, tinea cruris). It is easily spread in occupations that require communal showering or the use of occlusive footwear. Infected individuals should not be excluded from work, but diagnosis and treatment should be initiated. Athlete's foot (tinea pedis) is commonly misdiagnosed. One-third of suspected cases arise from other causes. Unresponsive cases may actually be due to occlusive maceration between the toes, with overgrowth of commensal bacteria (*Staph. pyogenes*). This disorder can be treated with appropriate footwear, wedging toes apart with cotton wool rolls, and adequate drying. Ringworm on the body (tinea corporis) is over-diagnosed and confused with other skin conditions (e.g. psoriasis, granuloma annulare).

Although *zoonoses* can be acquired by humans from animals, they cannot be transferred between humans and so no restrictions are required for infected employees.

Bacterial skin infections are potentially transmissible to other employees. Impetigo, which is the commonest, is usually caused by *Staph. aureus* and requires prompt local treatment. For widespread infections, temporary exclusion from the workplace may be required, although the risk of cross-contamination becomes minimal after 2 days of treatment. Boils (carbuncles) are also usually caused by *Staph. aureus*, but the potential for contamination is less than for impetigo. Staphylococci can grow in foods and release endotoxins that cause serious food poisoning and therefore occupations involving food handling require exclusion until clinical resolution occurs.

Hyperhidrosis that affects the hands may cause problems in engineering, as sweat can corrode ferrous metalwork pieces (these employees are known as 'rusters'). Hyperhidrosis may also be a disadvantage in public relation jobs that require frequent hand shaking. Although historically treatment was limited (aluminium salts, iontophoresis, chemical or surgical sympathectomy), the use of botulinum toxin has revolutionized treatment.

Psoriasis is present in one in 20 persons, but most cases are minor and not apparent even to the sufferer. Psoriasis may be aggravated occupationally by physical or chemical trauma (Köebner phenomenon). The commonest presentation is with psoriatic knuckle pads.

The disease can be unpredictable, with sudden active and extensive flare-ups. Rarely this can involve the entire body surface. Although psoriasis typically develops in early teens and twenties, it can start at any age. The absence of psoriasis at pre-employment assessment does not guarantee subsequent freedom from the condition. With adequate treatment it is possible to control most cases of active psoriasis, although only with adequate compliance. Psoriasis may also undergo spontaneous remission. In practice, individuals with psoriasis from early childhood and with more than 40 per cent of the surface skin affected are the most difficult to control.

Within the workplace, psoriasis that affects the palms and soles can be particularly troublesome. Affected individuals are unable to wear protective shoes and have difficulty with work involving heavy manual handling, and work in the construction and service industries. Embarrassment because of visible psoriatic patches on hands or scalp can compromise emotional and social well-being.[9,10]

Some chemicals and solvents can cause existing psoriasis to flare up. Solvents such as trichloroethylene will degrease the skin, causing drying and cracking, which then köebnerizes the psoriasis. Other everyday products such as soap, detergents, washing-up liquids, and shampoos also have a similar degreasing effect. The effect of chemicals is minimal compared with the effects of friction, which is the main perpetuating factor in the hands and feet. Demanding and stressful work has also been associated with exacerbations of the disease.

Psoriatic arthropathy can affect mobility, while the associated pain can increase sickness absence. Although infection of psoriatic lesions can occur, work in catering or nursing is generally tolerated and helped by regular monitoring by the occupational health department.

Alopecia or hair loss, particularly in women, can lead to a degree of mental anguish that makes attendance at work difficult. Treatable causes such as endocrine disorders, drugs, or iron deficiency need to be excluded. The wearing of a wig will sometimes aid return to work.

Disorders of pigmentation, particularly if on the face (vitiligo or hyperpigmentation), can cause embarrassment, especially in Asian people and individuals of African descent. Specialists in cosmetic camouflage can help such cases.

Skin cancer

There are over 100 000 new registrations for skin cancer in the UK annually, of which few arise from occupational causes. Epithelioma of the scrotum due to contact with mineral oils is hardly ever seen these days, although cases have been reported at other anatomical sites such as arms and hands. Ultraviolet radiation from excessive exposure to sunlight is one of today's main causes of skin cancer.[11] Other causes include x-rays, arsenic, tar products, and industrial burns. Ultraviolet radiation from welding is a potential risk factor for non-melanotic skin cancer among welders.[12]

Basal cell carcinoma, or rodent ulcer, is the commonest skin cancer. It is frequently found on the face and is associated with exposure to sunlight. Fair-skinned expatriates working in sunny climates are a group at particular risk. However, excess risks have not been consistently demonstrated in surveys of outdoor workers.[13,14]

Squamous cell carcinomas commonly occur on hands, ears, and lips. Sunlight, chronic trauma, and chronic inflammation are aetiological factors.

Malignant melanoma is one of the most aggressive skin cancers. Its incidence has increased dramatically over the last few decades with over 11 000 cases annually in the UK, probably due to people's greater exposure to sunlight. Some reports indicate a higher prevalence of malignant melanomas in aircrew, possibly because of cosmic radiation. A higher than average sunlight exposure may also contribute.[15]

Common primary cancers that can metastasize to skin are breast, lung, and leukaemia.

Surgical excision is the most effective and preferred treatment for primary skin cancer. A return to work is normally possible after excision and wound healing. A poor cosmetic result occasionally affects the outcome.

Skin and the psyche

There are many myths surrounding skin disorders. One of the commonest is that eczema is in some way contagious. Bacterial contamination can occur but the risk to work colleagues is small and restrictions are only relevant in selected occupations, such as food handlers or healthcare workers. However, concerns within the workplace can sometimes lead to individuals being shunned and excluded from communal and social activities. There is a need to ensure that health education is undertaken and that the supervisor or line manager understands the nature of the skin condition.

Skin ailments are sometimes a feature of sick building syndrome. Symptomatology tends to vary, ranging from dryness of the skin to skin rashes. It is important to rule out underlying causes such as infections, scabies, or irritant dermatitis from an occupational hazard. Not infrequently, however, the presenting skin conditions in the workforce are not related to the work at all.

Cases of scabies, athlete's foot, psoriasis, constitutional eczema, symptomatic dermographism, and rosacea are some of the commoner skin diseases falsely attributed to dermatitis when there is an outbreak of skin disease in the workforce. If unions are involved or new work practices have been introduced then an emotionally charged situation can develop which requires skill to resolve. Intervention by an occupational physician or a dermatologist may alleviate the concern of affected staff.

Investigations

Patch testing has a vital role to play in the investigation of persistent dermatitis, and will identify hidden causes of delayed type IV hypersensitivity. No employee should be advised to give up their work without the benefit of detailed patch test investigations at a regional centre. Patch testing will identify causes of acquired sensitization and allow avoidance and substitution of contact allergens to be planned, permitting continuing employment for the majority. However, it will not identify those individuals who are not yet sensitized but who subsequently become sensitized, so it has no role to play in pre-employment screening. A possible exception to this is when, prior to employment, a history of dermatitis (present or previous) has not been properly investigated.

Prick testing prior to employment has little value apart from confirming an atopic constitution. If an assessment into type 1 hypersensitivity is necessary, immunoglobulin E and radioallergosobent test (RAST) blood tests, (for sensitivity to specific allergens), can be used instead to confirm atopic tendency. However, as it is only people with active atopic eczema who carry a risk of developing dermatitis from irritants, these investigations really add no added benefit to a good medical history and examination. RAST tests are also not 100 per cent specific. In particular, some atopics will have a strong positive reaction to latex and yet can handle latex with impunity, whereas others who have negative antibodies develop anaphylaxis with minimal latex exposure. In this situation a prick test can be more reliable, but in view of the risk of anaphylaxis it should never be carried out without having full resuscitation measures to hand.

Rehabilitation

Rehabilitation of employees with skin ailments can usually be undertaken without too much difficulty. This is true even where the skin problem is occupational dermatitis and the employee is working with a known irritant or sensitizer. If temporary employment can be found away from the offending agent, a return to work can usually be effected prior to the complete resolution of the skin condition.

Flexible working and working from home have allowed workers with significant skin disfigurements to continue in employment while preserving their psychosocial well-being and avoiding the sense of rejection and social stigmatization.

However, some occupations with special safety needs may be considered unsuitable—for example, secondary skin infection may preclude employment in healthcare, food handling, and in the pharmaceutical industry.

Individuals with widespread skin lesions may not be suitable for work in some industries because of a heightened risk to themselves. For example, in the nuclear industry extensive skin disease could reduce the protective barrier of the skin, provide a portal of entry, and make decontamination more difficult. Likewise in the sewage or waste disposal industry, there is a greater risk of exposure to infection.

Close collaboration between the occupational physician, the dermatologist, the GP, the employer, and the employee may be needed to effect a successful rehabilitation and return to work.

Skin care

Skin care at work should be part of a positive but pragmatic managerial response to healthcare. Good housekeeping, adequate washing facilities, attention to maintenance programmes, and cleanliness within the working environment can lead to positive behaviours by individual employees (e.g. more frequent uniform changing and hand washing).

Good occupational hygiene practice provides the basis of preventative measures.

Emollients or moisturizers have now gained a place in the secondary prevention of dermatitis. Their frequent use during the working day helps to overcome excessive degreasing of the skin.

Barrier creams often contain lanolin, paraffin, silicones, or polyethylene glycols. Occasionally, these constituents can in themselves cause sensitization. Some barrier creams are also highly fragranced and may contain detergents to aid cleansing, which are potentially irritant to already damaged skin.

Studies of *alcohol handrubs* that contain skin emollients versus soap, show that healthcare workers have accepted this method of reducing hand contamination and complaints of dry skin are fewer than with other hand hygiene products.[16]

Protective clothing can be provided in the form of gloves, aprons, overalls, hats, masks, safety boots, etc. Commonly the hands and arms are most at risk. Protective gloves can be made from many different materials, and the characteristics of permeability and durability need to be considered in selecting the correct type. Further information is available from the 'British Standard' specification for industrial gloves. The Health and Safety Executive has also provided guidance for the selection of gloves.[17] However, the use of gloves should be the last solution (after elimination, substitution or control of hazardous substances), in reducing harm, as compliance is often a problem.

When powders such as cement dust or paper dust are being handled, the operator may not be aware of the possible entry of contaminants under the cuff. This can be prevented by the wearing of gauntlets or armbands, or by tucking sleeves underneath the cuff. Extract ventilation may help reduce dust exposure and subsequent irritant or allergic skin reactions. Regular washing or changing of gloves will help to reduce surface contamination.

Legal considerations

The Control of Substances Hazardous to Health and the Management of Health and Safety at Work Regulations require that all employers offer appropriate information, instruction, and training to employees with regard to substances that can damage the skin. The training should include the characteristic features of the particular dermatoses and arrangements should exist to identify new cases of skin disorder.

Employees should be encouraged to examine their own skin and report all changes.

It should also be borne in mind that the true risk of irritation or sensitization may be understated on many health and safety data sheets.

Employers have a legal duty to report cases of dermatitis under the Reporting of Injuries, Diseases and Dangerous Occurrences Regulations 1995. A case of work-related dermatitis becomes reportable only when the disease is confirmed by a medical practitioner.

Employers need to be aware that discrimination within the employment setting against individuals with chronic skin disorders or severe disfigurement, such as facial scarring, is unlawful under the Human Rights and Equality Acts (see Chapter 3).

Final comments

Most skin conditions in the workplace are neither infectious nor contagious.

Should it become necessary for an employee to change their job because of a skin condition, the opinion of a dermatologist is essential to ensure that such a decision is based on sound medical evidence.

Redeployment within a company should be the first option if job change is inevitable. Many individuals can now be kept at work despite chronic skin disorders, if appropriate workplace adjustments are implemented.

References

1 Schofield JK, Grindlay D, Williams H. *Skin conditions in the UK—a health care needs assessment.* Nottingham: Centre of Evidence Based Dermatology, University of Nottingham, 2009.

2 Health and Safety Executive. *Dermatitis and other skin disorders: trends in incidence,* 2009. [Online] (<http:www.hse.gov.uk/statistics/causdis/dermatitis/trends.htm>)

3 Health and Safety Executive. *Dermatitis and other skin disorders—working days lost,* 2009. [Online] (<http://www.hse.gov.uk/statistics/causdis/dermatitis/days-lost.htm>)

4 Rystedt I. Factors influencing the occurrence of hand eczema in adults with a history of atopic dermatitis in childhood. *Contact Dermatitis* 1985; **12**: 185–91.

5 Posch A, Chen Z, Raulf-Heimsoth M, *et al.* Latex allergens. *Clin Exp Allergy* 1998; **28**: 134–40.

6 Noble WC. *Microbiology of human skin,* p. 325. London: Lloyd Luke, 1981.

7 Rystedt I. Work related hand eczema in atopics. *Contact Dermatitis* 1985; **12**: 164–71.

8 Cunliffe WJ. Acne and unemployment. *Br J Dermatol* 1986; **115**: 386.

9 Krueger G, Koo J, Lebwohl M *et al.* The impact of psoriasis on quality of life: results of a National Psoriasis Foundation patient-membership survey. *Arch Dermatol* 2001; **137**(3): 280–4.

10 Ginsburg IH, Link BG. Psychosocial consequences of rejection and stigma feelings in psoriasis patients. *Int J Dermatol* 1993; **32**(8): 587–91.

11 Snashall D, Patel D (eds). *ABC of occupational and environmental medicine*, 2nd edn. Oxford: Wiley-Blackwell, 2003.

12 Currie CL, Monk BE. Welding and non melanoma skin cancer. *Clin Exp Dermatol* 2000; **22**: 259–67.

13 Freedman DM, Zahn SH, Dosemeci M. Residential and occupational exposure to sunlight and mortality from non-Hodgkin's lymphoma: composite (threefold) case control study. *BMJ* 1997; **314**: 1451–5.

14 Green A, Battistutta D, Hart V, *et al.* Skin cancer in a subtropical Australian population: incidence and lack of association with occupation. *Am J Epidemiol* 1996; **144**: 1034–40.

15 Rafusson V, Hrafnkelsson J, Tulinius H. Incidence of cancer among commercial airline pilots. *Scand J Work Environ Med* 2000; **57**: 175–9.

16 Ojajarvi J. Finnish experience shows that alcohol rubs are good for hands. *BMJ* 2003; **326**: 50.

17 Health and Safety Executive. *Choosing the right gloves to protect skin: a guide for employers*, 2010. [Online] (<http://www.hse.gov.uk/skin/employ/gloves.htm>)

Chapter 23

Human immunodeficiency virus

Paul Grime and Christopher Conlon

Introduction

By the end of 2010 there were an estimated 91 000 people living with human immunodeficiency virus (HIV) in the UK. The majority of these are of working age, reflecting the main mode of transmission, which is through sexual exposure. In many developing countries where antenatal testing and treatment programmes are still being developed, HIV is also a disease of infancy, transmitted vertically from mother to child during childbirth or breastfeeding.

The development in the 1990s of highly active antiretroviral treatment (HAART) with three or more antiretroviral drugs used in combination has greatly improved disease-free survival in developed countries. This has increased the potential for those of working age to remain in, or return to, work following their diagnosis. While antiretroviral treatment (ART) has increased survival, many HIV-infected people remain symptomatic, either through drug side effects, HIV-related illnesses, or the psychological morbidity associated with the diagnosis and disease. All of these factors can have a significant effect on an individual's ability to find, and remain in, work. In addition, an employer's approach to those with chronic illness, and HIV in particular, can have a major influence on the workplace support received by infected workers.

As the epidemiology, treatment, and drug resistance of HIV infection is evolving so rapidly, it is difficult to predict what the future holds for HIV-infected individuals of working age. It is likely that prognosis will continue to improve and that stigma associated with HIV will slowly disappear. Vaccines continue to be sought but remain a distant hope at present. This chapter reviews the current epidemiology and clinical picture of HIV, barriers to work, available support, legal and ethical considerations, occupational risks for HIV-infected workers and the risk of acquiring HIV through work. Particular attention is given to HIV in healthcare workers, which raises some specific issues.

Epidemiology of HIV in the UK

In 2010, approximately 6660 new cases of HIV were diagnosed in the UK. This compares with 7000 newly diagnosed cases in 2003 and 3088 new cases in 1999. Of these new cases in 2010, about two-thirds were diagnosed late, with low CD4 (cluster of designation 4) counts. Just over half of the new cases diagnosed in 2010 acquired their infection in the UK, double the proportion seen in 2001. Of these new cases, it is estimated that 14 per cent were recently acquired. It was also estimated that in 2010 around 21 000 people were living with HIV but did not know that they were infected.[1]

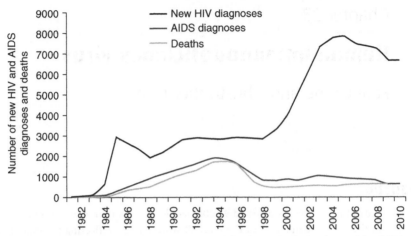

Figure 23.1 Annual new HIV and AIDS diagnoses and deaths: United Kingdom, 1981–2010. Reproduced with permission from *HIV in the United Kingdom: 2011 Report*, London, Health Protection Services, Colindale, November 2011 © Health Protection Agency 2011.

Although the incidence and particularly the prevalence, of infection continues to increase, the demography of HIV has changed substantially over the last 10 years. In the 1990s, HIV was more prevalent in males and whilst this remains the case in the UK, the greater *rise* is now in females. In some parts of the world, particularly sub-Saharan Africa, infected females now outnumber infected males.

In the UK in 2010, 45 per cent of new diagnoses were in men who have sex with men, who despite accounting for a minority of these newly diagnosed infections are still the highest risk group for acquiring HIV in the UK. Over half of newly diagnosed cases of HIV in 2010 were in heterosexual men and women. About three-quarters of these heterosexually acquired HIV infections were probably acquired in Africa.

Despite the increased incidence of HIV infection, the incidence of AIDS has decreased significantly due to effective and earlier treatment (see Figure 23.1). It is likely that the epidemiology of HIV and AIDS will continue to change in future decades, driven by the science of drug development, viral mutation, drug resistance, and socio-demographic variables such as migration and routes of transmission.

Natural history of HIV infection

Patients who are untreated will develop an AIDS-defining illness on average 10 years after acquiring HIV infection. Within 2–3 weeks of being infected, there is a burst of HIV viraemia with several million copies of virus in the plasma. This level falls over the succeeding few weeks. Within 6 months of infection, the plasma viral load settles at a relatively stable value and subsequently changes little over a number of years. Both the CD4 (a T-cell-helper subset) count at this time and the viral load are predictive factors for the rate at which the first opportunistic infection will develop. In addition the degree of activation of the immune system, measured by the levels of CD38 (an activation marker) on either CD4 or CD8 cells, provides an additional prognostic marker to determine the speed at which AIDS is likely to develop.

Factors influencing the rate of progression to AIDS

1 *Age*: this has the most marked influence on the rate of development of opportunistic infections. The rate increases with age.

2 *Social and educational factors*: the less privileged and the less well educated develop opportunistic infections at a faster rate because of poor access to medical care.

3 *Genetic factors*: two groups of genes affect the rate of progression to AIDS. Individuals with a specific HLA haplotype progress more slowly, while individuals with a specific deletion (CCR5Δ32) rarely become HIV-infected (homozygous) or progress at slower rates (heterozygous).

4 *Treatment*: the most important influence on progression rates in the 21st century is access to effective antiretroviral treatment. This has revolutionized care in the developed world. Many would now predict that patients who have developed HIV infection recently will never develop an opportunistic infection providing they take the drugs on a regular basis.

There is no evidence that means of acquisition, lifestyle issues such as smoking, nutrition, or stress-related illnesses, have any impact on the rate of progression towards AIDS. However, the life expectancy of individuals who continue intravenous drug use is reduced.

Markers of HIV infection and their clinical relevance

The CD4 count and HIV viral load have an independent prognostic value for determining the rate of progression to AIDS and are commonly used to chart the progress of individuals with HIV infection. The CD4 count has become important for determining the timing of treatment. Opportunistic infections are relatively rare with a CD4 count above 200 cells/mm^3 and reconstitution of the immune system following the introduction of HAART is relatively complete. Most international guidelines now recommend that treatment should be started once the CD4 count has fallen to about 350 cells/mm^3. The viral load is chiefly used to assess how rapidly the CD4 count is likely to fall in an individual patient. Relatively low viral loads (<50 000 copies per mL) are associated with a low annual fall rate of CD4 count of about 40 cells. A high viral load (above 100 000 copies per mL) is associated with a much more rapid annual fall of CD4 count of 80 cells or more per year. The relative importance of the CD4 count and viral load measurements are reversed following initiation of therapy. The main aim of HAART is to stop viral replication as completely as possible and thus prevent the development of viral resistance. Thus the most important monitor of success of HAART is regular measurement of the plasma viral load, which if at all possible should be kept below the detection limit of a highly sensitive assay (usually less than 20 copies per mL).

Patients' symptoms and signs are also of considerable importance both as markers of progression of known HIV infection and of alerting the physician or patient to an underlying HIV diagnosis, but late diagnosis of HIV remains a problem. Up to 50 per cent of individuals who are eventually diagnosed as HIV positive have previously come into contact with the medical profession with conditions that should have led to an earlier diagnosis. A recent audit by the British HIV Association (BHIVA) suggested that this group of patients most commonly consult doctors because of diarrhoea, weight loss, skin complaints, lymphadenopathy, or glandular fever-like illnesses. Mild blood dyscrasias, such as thrombocytopenia, are also not uncommon. These non-specific symptoms and signs, as well as the opportunistic infections detailed in 'Symptoms', should alert the clinician to the possibility of HIV. Suspicions should be further aroused if these symptoms and signs occur in high-risk individuals.

Symptoms

Symptoms in HIV-infection may be due to the disease process itself or from complications of drug treatment.[2]

Primary HIV infection

About 75 per cent of those who become HIV-infected develop an illness within 2–3 weeks. This illness is usually mild and often non-specific and rarely leads to patients seeking medical advice. Sometimes there is a macular-papular rash and there may be prominent cervical lymphadenopathy and abnormal liver function tests. Occasionally there are neurological symptoms and, very rarely, opportunistic infections may occur during this period because of a precipitous decline in the CD4 count. Patients with a symptomatic illness at the time of infection (sometimes called a seroconversion illness), progress to AIDS more rapidly. Diagnosis of primary HIV infection is important, as those patients with a high viral load are particularly likely to transmit infection to others. Although it is theoretically possible that treatment at this early stage with HAART may have an effect on long-term outcome, a recent large trial (SPARTAC) did not show a clear benefit of early versus deferred treatment for primary HIV infection. Nevertheless, identification of the recently infected patient allows appropriate counselling about safe sex and risk reduction.[3]

Latent period

Following a seroconversion illness, most patients are relatively well for a period of some years but not entirely asymptomatic and the course of their disease, if untreated, is punctuated by a number of minor ailments. Perhaps the most common of these are skin conditions caused by infections that are particularly florid in HIV-infected individuals. Examples are seborrhoeic dermatitis, bacterial skin infections, tinea pedis, and molluscum contagiosum. Of particular importance is herpes zoster infection. While shingles is a relatively common disease, multiple dermatome involvement should strongly suggest the possibility of HIV-related immunosuppression. In somebody who is known to be HIV-infected, herpes zoster infection indicates a high likelihood of AIDS development in the next 2 years. Herpes simplex is also more common in HIV-infected individuals and frequently recurrent with severe attacks. One of the most common manifestations of an underlying immune deficiency during this latent period is mucocutaneous candidiasis. Oral thrush strongly suggests the possibility of underlying immunosuppression and should lead to relevant questioning about potential risk factors for HIV and an offer of testing. In the pre-treatment era for those known to be HIV positive, 50 per cent developed full-blown AIDS within 18 months of having an episode of thrush. Another, rare, manifestation is hairy oral leucoplakia, which is thought to be a reaction to opportunistic infection with Epstein–Barr virus. Again this is strongly predictive of HIV infection. Unexplained weight loss, diarrhoea, and fever are also features of this latent period but symptoms are usually due to an opportunist infection or tumour rather than HIV itself.

Opportunistic infections

There are many opportunistic infections associated with HIV, some of which may be acquired through work. The common ones are listed in Table 23.1.

Lung manifestations

The most common AIDS-defining diagnosis, particularly in individuals previously not suspected to be HIV positive, is *Pneumocystis jiroveci* pneumonia (PCP). This is a fungal disease

Table 23.1 Common opportunistic infections associated with HIV infection

Pneumocystis jiroveci pneumonia (PCP)

Toxoplasmic encephalitis

Cryptosporidiosis

Microsporidiosis

Tuberculosis

Disseminated MAC (*Mycobacterium* avium complex) infection

Bacterial respiratory infections

Bacterial enteric infections

Candidiasis

Cryptococcosis

Histoplasmosis

Coccydioidomycosis

Cytomegalovirus disease

Herpes simplex virus disease

Varicella zoster virus disease

HHV-8 infection (Kaposi sarcoma-associated herpesvirus)

previously recognized as a rare opportunistic infection in debilitated patients in the pre-HIV era. The symptoms are predominantly those of insidious-onset breathlessness in an unwell patient which may be misdiagnosed as bad asthma or community-acquired pneumonia. Frequently, there are few if any chest signs but the typical chest x-ray appearance is of bilateral mid-zone infiltrates. Treatment is high-dose co-trimoxazole which is also used as prophylaxis or to prevent recurrent attacks. The mortality should be less than 10 per cent for a first attack. Prophylaxis can be stopped after HAART is initiated once the CD4 count has risen above 200 cells/mm^3.

Another important HIV complication is pneumococcal pneumonia and vaccination is now recommended. Infections with *Haemophilus influenza* are also increased in HIV but because these are usually caused by non-encapsulated strains, vaccination is not helpful. A number of other opportunistic infections involve the lung but are rare in the UK. These include histoplasmosis, cryptococcosis, and coccidioidomycosis. Sometimes patients present with a condition called lymphocytic interstitial pneumonitis (LIP) that can mimic PCP but responds to steroids. LIP is more common in children than in adults.

Tuberculosis

The major pandemic of tuberculosis (TB) is intimately related to the HIV epidemic and, in the UK, TB is an increasingly common presentation of HIV infection. More than 50 per cent of people with TB in the developing world are coinfected with HIV. While the lifetime risk of developing TB in an immunocompetent patient who has had a primary infection is 10 per cent, this risk rises to 10 per cent per year for those who are infected with HIV. It is also likely that HIV-infected patients are more liable to acquire TB and develop progressive disease than the general population and even those with a 'normal' CD4 count above 400 have a twofold risk of TB compared with immunocompetent HIV-negative individuals. TB in the context of HIV infection has a number of differences compared with classical infection. Cavitation in the lungs is less likely, so the chances of the patient being sputum positive on microscopy are lower. There is also a higher incidence of disseminated disease and a greater chance of mycobacterial blood cultures being positive. However, treatment of TB should be the same and recent studies show that in newly diagnosed HIV patients with TB, the TB and the HIV treatment should be given together rather than waiting for the TB to be treated first if the CD4 count is below 100 cells/mm^3.

Gastrointestinal manifestations

Oesophageal disease

Oesophageal candidiasis is a common AIDS-defining illness, which is usually implied by the presence of candida in the mouth plus symptoms of pain on swallowing. The diagnosis can be confirmed by upper gastrointestinal endoscopy. Although this is straightforward to treat with azole antifungals, it is an important marker of a severely compromised immune system. Cytomegalovirus (CMV) infection also causes an oesophagitis. Rarely, patients present with dysphagia and are found to have aphthoid ulcers in the oesophagus, which can be treated with thalidomide or intralesional steroids.

Diarrhoea

Although HIV itself affects the gut and may cause diarrhoea, there are a number of opportunistic infections that cause diarrhoea in HIV-infected patients, which are markers of severe immunodeficiency and constitute an AIDS diagnosis. The three most common of these are cryptosporidiosis, microsporidiosis, and CMV infection. Both cryptosporidiosis and microsporidiosis produce diarrhoea with dehydration and massive weight loss and the outcome is frequently fatal without effective HAART. Although not often seen in the UK, these diseases remain a problem in developing countries. CMV infection of the lower gut produces diarrhoea, which is often bloody. Untreated colonic CMV is a particularly serious condition and frequently leads to perforation, colonic dilatation, and massive bleeding. In the short term both lower and upper gut infections with CMV are treatable using antiviral agents, such as ganciclovir or cidofovir. Prevention of recurrent infection is crucially dependent upon the ability to control HIV viral replication using HAART.

Neurological presentations

Meningitis

A lymphocytic meningitis, thought to be related to HIV infection, can occur at the time of primary infection. It is often misdiagnosed as a simple viral meningitis of no significance. However, the most important cause of meningitis is that caused by *Cryptococcus neoformans*. This fungus, excreted by birds, is widespread in the environment and may be inhaled by humans. The diagnosis and treatment is straightforward providing the diagnosis is considered and made in good time. Complications include cranial nerve palsies and raised intracranial pressure from communicating hydrocephalus.

Stroke-like syndromes

Other neurological conditions usually present with stroke-like syndromes with sudden onset of focal neurological defects or, less commonly, a general decline in cognitive function.

Toxoplasma gondii is the most common of these infections and leads to the formation of cerebral and cerebellar abscesses. In most patients this is caused by reactivation of a previously acquired infection but in a few there may have been recent acquisition from a primary host (e.g. domestic cat). Computed tomography or magnetic resonance imaging (MRI) scans show fairly characteristic lesions and serology may be helpful. Because it is the most common central nervous system (CNS) infection resulting in mass lesions, the normal practice is to treat with anti-toxoplasma drugs; the diagnosis being confirmed by a clinical response. A quarter of patients, however, have residual neurological defects, caused by irreversible neuronal damage before the initiation of treatment.

Progressive multifocal leucoencephalopathy is caused by an opportunistic infection with the JC variant of the polyoma virus, which is extremely rare outside the context of HIV infection. The diagnosis is usually made by MRI scan. There is no specific treatment for this condition but with the advent of HAART at least half the cases make a good or partial recovery.

Primary cerebral lymphoma is also more common in HIV-infected patients. Epstein–Barr virus can be detected in the cerebrospinal fluid by polymerase chain reaction. In contrast to non-HIV-infected patients, primary cerebral lymphoma, even in the era of HAART, has a poor prognosis with an average survival of only 100 days.

Eye manifestations

An important AIDS-defining diagnosis that leads to loss of vision is CMV retinitis. This is rare with a CD4 count of more than 100 cells/mm^3 and is treatable but the only way to control this disease in the long term is to provide effective HAART. Another rare condition that leads to rapid blindness is progressive outer retinal necrosis, thought to be caused by a herpes virus infection. Toxoplasmosis of the eye is also more common in HIV-infected individuals.

Tumours

A variety of tumours are increased in HIV-infected individuals. Most of these result from unrestrained proliferation of opportunistic oncogenic viruses. A variety of tumours form the basis for an AIDS diagnosis but a much wider range of tumours occur more commonly in HIV disease, including Hodgkin's disease, T-cell lymphomas, carcinoma of the lung, and testicular tumours.

Kaposi's sarcoma

The hallmark tumour of the AIDS epidemic is Kaposi's sarcoma (KS), caused by a human herpesvirus-8 (HHV8) commonly known as KS-associated herpes virus (KSHV). Although this virus causes KS in non-HIV-infected people, particularly those who are elderly, in certain geographical distributions, and those who are immunosuppressed for other reasons (e.g. transplantation), it is markedly more common in those who are HIV infected. Men having sex with men are particularly likely to acquire KSHV. KS presents with classic purplish nodules, often in the flexural creases, and affects the extremities. It can also be visceral and a marker for this is KS involving the palate. Tumours of the gut are often asymptomatic but may bleed and KS involving the lung can be rapidly fatal, producing symptoms of severe cough and shortness of breath. This unusual multicentric tumour does not metastasize and is rare in people who are on appropriate treatment for HIV infection. In those who have never been treated for HIV who develop KS, the first step is the introduction of HAART, which usually stops KS progression. Chemotherapy is usually reserved for those with progressive disease despite the introduction of HAART and those with KS of the lung.

Lymphoma

Non-Hodgkin's lymphoma is a common manifestation of HIV infection and is strongly related to the patient's lowest CD4 count. If the patient's CD4 count has never fallen below 250 cells/mm^3 the incidence of this malignancy is no different to that in the general population but below this, the incidence is approximately 10-fold that in the general population. About half the cases of non-Hodgkin's lymphoma are associated with Epstein–Barr virus infection and the others with genetic abnormalities, which are commonly seen in non-Hodgkin's lymphoma unrelated to HIV disease. Two rare forms of lymphoma (primary effusion lymphoma and plasmacytoid multicentric Castleman's disease) are both thought to be associated with KSHV. The prognosis for the treatment of lymphoma has improved markedly with the introduction of HAART such that in most patients who are virologically undetectable at the time of diagnosis, the overall prognosis is not dissimilar from that in the non-HIV-infected population.

Tumours associated with the papillomavirus

Anal cancer, which is particularly common in HIV-infected homosexual men, and cervical cancer indicate AIDS. Both are treated along standard lines. It is recommended that women with HIV have annual cervical smears regardless of age.

Psychiatric morbidity

Depression is common in HIV-positive individuals, with the majority of studies reporting prevalence between 15 per cent and 40 per cent. Depression may alter the course of HIV infection by impairing immune function or influencing behaviour such as non-adherence to therapy. The signs and symptoms of depression and effectiveness of therapy are similar in HIV-infected and non-infected patients.[4]

Treatment of HIV infection[5,6]

The prognosis of HIV infection has been transformed by the use of HAART. Currently six different classes of agents are available to inhibit viral replication. All six classes take advantage of the unique aspects of the viral replication cycle.

Commonly used drugs

Nucleoside analogue reverse transcriptase inhibitors (NRTIs)

Drugs from this group act to inhibit reverse transcription, an essential step in HIV replication. Common adverse effects include peripheral neuropathy (stavudine and didanosine), pancreatitis (didanosine), and myopathy (zidovudine). Certain NRTIs, particularly when used in combination, lead to a potentially fatal complication—lactic acidosis.[2]

Non-nucleoside reverse transcriptase inhibitors (NNRTIs)

Drugs from this group also act to inhibit reverse transcription but as direct enzyme inhibitors rather than as nucleoside analogues. Two agents are currently in widespread use. Efavirenz is preferred by most clinicians but can cause central nervous system toxicity in the early stages of treatment and has been associated with teratogenicity. Nevirapine has a small recorded incidence of fatal hepatotoxicity and serious skin reactions including Stevens–Johnson syndrome.

Proteinase inhibitors (PIs)

The other agents in widespread use are PIs and the newer PIs (atazanavir, darunavir, and tipranavir) have a much longer plasma half-life, allowing once daily dosing. In modern treatment regimens the PI of choice is 'boosted' with ritonavir to prolong the half-life, allowing once or twice daily treatment.

Integrase inhibitors

HIV, when replicating, needs to insert cDNA into the host cell genome by means of an integrase enzyme. There are now drugs that inhibit this process and raltegravir is the first to be licensed. It can cause rashes and rhabdomyolysis.

Chemokine receptor antagonists

In order for HIV to bind to target cells, it needs to attach to a co-receptor in addition to the CD4 molecule. In most untreated patients this co-receptor is CCR-5, a chemokine receptor. Maraviroc is the first licensed drug in this class and shows good activity but special assays are needed to test whether the patient's virus is susceptible.

Fusion inhibitors

Enfuvirtide (T20) is an example of an agent developed as a result of basic understanding of the virology of HIV. The process by which HIV gains access to the cell, i.e. fusion, has been explored in detail and as a result a short peptide was developed that was predicted to inhibit this process. This has proved to be a relatively effective antiretroviral agent but it needs to be administered twice daily by subcutaneous injection and so is mainly used in the so-called salvage therapy (see 'Salvage therapy'). It is associated with unpleasant injection-site inflammation.

Current consensus guidelines relating to HIV treatment

There is considerable agreement in the developed world that treatment should begin for HIV-infected individuals when the CD4 count lies somewhere between 300—350 cells/mm^3. However, up to a third of patients will be treated much later than this because they first present with an opportunistic infection and a very low CD4 count. One of the ways of improving outcome is to identify such groups earlier. Standard treatment is a combination of two NRTIs and either an NNRTI or a PI (usually boosted with ritonavir). With such a wide array of drugs available, randomized controlled trials cannot be used to assess all potential combinations. Current UK treatment guidelines can be found on the BHIVA website (<http://www.bhiva.org>).[5]

Complications of HAART

All of the drugs used in HAART combinations have potential side effects but the details are beyond the scope of this chapter. However, some longer-term problems are emerging with therapy and these are outlined as follows.

Metabolic changes

There is increasing evidence that HIV treatment is associated with abnormalities in lipid and glucose metabolism. Cholesterol and triglyceride levels in plasma are often increased and some patients develop insulin resistance, which can result in overt diabetes mellitus. In addition, some patients develop clinically apparent changes in the distribution of body fat. In these cases, subcutaneous fat atrophies but visceral fat increases. Men particularly have increased intra-abdominal fat and women may have increased fat deposition in the breasts. Some patients develop a 'buffalo hump' with a thick fat pad at the back of the neck. These problems are more common in advanced disease and may be associated with PI use. Lipoatrophy is more common with stavudine and, to a lesser extent, zidovudine. The cause of these abnormalities is unclear.

Cardiovascular risks

Epidemiological studies suggest there is an increased relative risk of vascular disease in patients with HIV on HAART. Some of this may be related to the lipid abnormalities outlined earlier but it is also likely that HIV itself may affect vascular endothelium in an adverse manner. The absolute risk of cardiovascular disease is not much greater than the general population but this may increase as the cohort of people with HIV ages. Cardiovascular risk reduction has become part of the patient management.

Bone changes

There is an increased risk of avascular necrosis of the femoral head in HIV. There is also evidence that bone mineral loss is accelerated in those infected. At present there is no good evidence of an increased risk of fractures in HIV beyond the usual risk factors such as age, smoking, and alcohol consumption. Nevertheless, it is possible that in the future, osteoporosis may present at younger ages in those with HIV.

Adherence issues

Adherence is the single most important factor in determining the ability of HAART to suppress HIV replication in the long term and therefore produce a sustained improvement in prognosis. Adherence has been much studied in the context of HIV infection and there are a number of demographic factors, lifestyle issues, and belief systems that have profound effects on adherence but are difficult to modify with behavioural intervention. Other adherence issues are more amenable to pharmaceutical manipulation. These include total pill burden, frequency of dosing, freedom from strict food requirements in relationship to dosing, short-term drug toxicities, and fears of long-term toxicities. Present standard regimens of first-line therapy can usually now be given once a day with a pill burden of one or two tablets a day. Careful attention to gastrointestinal side effects is important in the initial stages of therapy giving treatment to prevent these wherever possible. Careful explanation of the evanescent nature of the CNS toxicities associated with efavirenz helps adherence in the early stages. Most clinicians now avoid stavudine as part of an initial regimen so they can reassure the patient that the regimen chosen is least likely to cause lipoatrophy.

Drug interactions

Other factors that influence the success of HAART include pharmacokinetic variability and unexpected pharmacological interactions when other drugs are given in conjunction with antiviral agents. The list of potential interactions is very long and clinicians prescribing any drugs to patients known to be taking antiretrovirals are strongly advised to consult an expert to ensure that the treatment they are proposing to give with the HAART is safe.

Second-line regimens

The choice of an optimum second-line regimen is usually straightforward and is aided by tests now available to detect drug resistance. Usually a new combination of nucleoside analogues is coupled with a boosted PI if an NNRTI has been used as part of the initial regimen.

'Salvage therapy'

This term refers to therapy where achieving complete virological undetectability is unlikely. In this group of patients the risk of death is closely related to the CD4 count and is low providing this can be kept above 50 cells/mm³. For long-term survival, these patients will be dependent on the development of new drugs, which can be combined in such a way as to completely inhibit viral replication. This is a highly specialized area of treatment and such patients need to be referred to experienced centres.

Employment status and barriers to employment

The profound effect of combination HAART on HIV-related morbidity and mortality has transformed what was once a terminal illness into a manageable, chronic condition. Health, quality of life, and life expectancy for HIV-infected individuals are now greatly improved. Ninety per cent of people living with HIV in the UK are of working age.[7] With effective treatment, HIV-infected individuals can lead productive lives.

Employment is a key determinant of physical and mental health,[8,9] reducing health inequalities and improving life chances.[10] Obtaining and retaining employment can present major challenges for people with chronic illnesses. This is as true for HIV as for other conditions. Recent changes to the UK welfare and benefits system have triggered a debate about how people with chronic conditions such as HIV can best be encouraged and supported to find and retain work, particularly in times of economic austerity and high unemployment.

One study undertaken in 2008/2009, found that 73 per cent of female HIV patients and 78 per cent of male HIV patients were working.[10] This compared with UK national employment rates of 76 per cent in women and 89 per cent in men.[11] Male HIV patients therefore had proportionately lower employment rates. Although these are comparable to some other chronic conditions such as rheumatoid arthritis,[12] they are lower than for other disabling conditions such as multiple sclerosis.[13]

Factors associated with unemployment in HIV patients include poor psychological health, more than 10 years since HIV diagnosis and a subjective assessment of health status as poor.[10] Employment status is not associated with objective measures of ill health such as CD4 count.[10] Patients with a more recent diagnosis of HIV are more likely to be in employment, which may reflect a perception that HIV has become a manageable, chronic condition.[10] Black African patients may be less likely to disclose their HIV status to their employer, possibly reflecting differential expectations of stigma in African communities.[10]

Although physical health is not a primary barrier to employment for people living with HIV, those not in work have significantly poorer psychological health.[10] Negative perceptions about work are more likely in those unemployed, who fear stigma at work and problems securing time off to attend appointments. However, most of those in work do not experience these problems. Patients diagnosed with HIV in the 1980s and early 1990s may have been told that they were terminally ill and would never be fit to work. Changing these beliefs is challenging and HIV services have a role in supporting patients to obtain and/or retain employment. This may include providing psychological support to address stigma, confidence, perceptions and negative attitudes associated with unemployment.[10]

Vocational support and rehabilitation

The UK government Department for Work and Pensions (DWP) provides support for disabled people, such as those with HIV infection, via its national network of Jobcentre Plus offices. Disability employment advisers provide advice and support to disabled people in finding and keeping a job.

Disabled job applicants and employees can apply to the 'Access to Work' scheme for advice and support with extra costs that may arise because of disability needs.[14] Access to Work advisers liaise with disabled employees or job applicants and their employers, and seek approval for agreed support packages from Jobcentre Plus. It is the employer's responsibility to arrange the agreed support and/or buy the necessary equipment. Employers can then claim repayment of approved costs from Access to Work.[15]

For the common disabilities experienced by HIV-infected workers, the type of support required might include:

- Voice-activated computer software (neuropathy).
- Installation of home office (fatigue, diarrhoea).
- Taxi to work (fatigue, diarrhoea, neuropathy).

Funding under the Access to Work scheme is available when *additional* costs are incurred because of a disability; not to provide support usually provided by employers or required under legislation for all employees. In addition it does not necessarily absolve the employer of its duties under the Equality Act 2010.[16] The employer still has to make reasonable adjustments to reduce or remove any substantial disadvantage that a physical feature of the work premises or employment arrangements causes a disabled employee or job applicant compared with a non-disabled person.

UK AIDS charities

Many charitable organizations provide specific advice and support for HIV-infected individuals. Some of these provide comprehensive advice on employment issues (Box 23.1).

Legal and ethical framework for assessing work fitness

The disability provisions of the Equality Act 2010 protect against HIV-related discrimination in the workplace.[16] Asymptomatic HIV now falls within the definition of disability from the date of diagnosis, along with multiple sclerosis and cancer. 'HIV infection means infection by a virus capable of causing the Acquired Immune Deficiency Syndrome.'

The Equality Act 2010 prohibits both direct discrimination, i.e. due to the disability itself, and disability-related discrimination, i.e. less favourable treatment for reasons related to the disability. *In High Quality Lifestyles* v. *Watts* (2006) an Employment Appeal Tribunal held that Watts' employer was liable for disability-related discrimination.[17] Watts had been dismissed

---

Box 23.1 Examples of UK HIV charities that provide employment advice

The Terrence Higgins Trust: THT, 314–320 Grays Inn Road, London WC1X 8DP. Tel.: 0808 802 1221; website: <http://www.tht.org.uk>

UK coalition of people living with HIV and AIDS (UKC): website: <http://www.ukcoalition.org>

The National AIDS Trust (NAT): NAT New City Cloisters, 196 Old Street, London EC1V 9FR. Tel: 0207 814 6767; website: <http://www.nat.org.uk>

National Aidsmap (NAM): website: <http://www.aidsmap.com>

from his job as a support worker in a residential home for people with learning difficulties and severely challenging behaviour, when he disclosed that he was HIV positive. The employer concluded from its risk assessment that if Watts was scratched or bitten by a resident, there was a risk that HIV infection could be transmitted to the resident. However, official guidance from the Department of Health[18] concluded that the risk of transmission of HIV to a patient who bites an HIV-infected healthcare worker was negligible, and therefore healthcare workers infected with blood-borne viruses should not be prevented from working in or training for specialties where there is a risk of being bitten.

Reasonable adjustments

The Equality Act 2010 requires employers to make 'reasonable adjustments' if their employment arrangements or premises place disabled people at a substantial disadvantage compared with non-disabled people. Reasonable adjustments for employees infected with HIV might be:

+ To accommodate more sickness absence than they would in someone without the illness.

+ To allow time off to attend treatment (may include psychological treatment if psychological illness is a direct result of diagnosis).

+ To make arrangements for home working where symptoms of HIV interfere with ability to attend work.

+ To make arrangements for protection from infectious diseases in the healthcare setting to which they have increased susceptibility, such as tuberculosis (TB).

Pre-employment screening, HIV testing, and the Equality Act

There are very few circumstances where an individual's HIV status is directly relevant to their employability. Section 60 of the Equality Act 2010 prohibits employers from asking questions about or screening for the health of applicants before offering work to an applicant or including an applicant in a pool of applicants from whom the employer intends to offer work in future. Under section 60,[7] employers can ask questions for the purpose of supporting disabled applicants during recruitment such as:

+ Determining whether any reasonable adjustments will be required to ensure that the applicant can participate in interviews and other forms of assessment.

+ Establishing whether the applicant is able to undertake functions intrinsic to the work. This could be relevant to HIV-infected healthcare workers applying for posts requiring exposure-prone procedures (Box 23.2). More information about HIV and healthcare workers is given later in this chapter. For those whose employment will take them to countries where an HIV test is a requirement of entry, it could be argued that pre-employment HIV testing, along with other tests required for travel, is necessary to assess fitness to work abroad.

+ Monitoring diversity among applicants.

+ Establishing the presence of a specific impairment required for the job.

+ To take positive action under section 158, to ensure that a disabled applicant can benefit from measures to improve representation of disabled people in the workforce.

It is important for recruiting employers to make clear to applicants the reason questions are asked and the purposes for which the information will be used.

Box 23.2 Definition of exposure-prone procedures

Exposure-prone procedures

Procedures in which injury to the healthcare worker could result in the worker's blood contaminating the patient's open tissue.

These procedures include those where the worker's gloved hands may be in contact with sharp instruments, needle tips or sharp tissues (spicules of bone or teeth) inside a patient's open body cavity, wound or confined anatomical space where the hands or fingertips may not be completely visible at all times.

Extract reproduced from: *HIV-infected healthcare workers: guidance on management and patient notification*, July 2005, Department of Health, UK © Crown Copyright 2005.

There are ethical and other criticisms of pre-employment HIV screening. The test may be negative for up to 3 months after infection and tested employees may become infected after employment. Occupational physicians and nurses asked to arrange such tests must satisfy themselves that there is a justifiable reason for requesting an HIV test. For testing in any circumstances, they must ensure that explicit, informed consent has been obtained and an adequate pre- and post-test discussion held.

Ethical framework

Occupational physicians, like other doctors, are bound by the General Medical Council's (GMC's) ethical code. Additionally, the Faculty of Occupational Medicine of the Royal College of Physicians publishes its interpretation of the GMC generic guidance.[19] Other healthcare professionals must follow similar guidance produced by their relevant regulatory body.

Healthcare workers

The ethical position for HIV-infected doctors is addressed by GMC guidance, *Good Medical Practice 2006*,[20] (Box 23.3). At the time of writing (2012) a revision of *Good Medical Practice* is subject to consultation.[21] A new duty at paragraph 61 is relevant to the care of HIV-infected patients (Box 23.4).

Similar guidance is produced for nurses (Box 23.5) and dentists (Box 23.6) by their registration bodies. Additional guidance is published by the UK Department of Health regarding HIV-infected healthcare workers.[18] This addresses both the infected healthcare worker and the healthcare worker aware of an infected colleague (Box 23.7).

Occupational risks for HIV-infected workers

Potential occupational exposures to opportunistic infection

Healthcare work

Studies early in the 20th century established that healthcare workers were at increased risk of TB. This risk largely disappeared with the advent of effective chemotherapy. However, in the 1990s about a twofold increased risk of TB was found among UK healthcare workers suggesting

Box 23.3 Responsibilities of doctors with HIV infection or at risk of HIV infection

If you know that you have, or think that you might have, a serious condition that you could pass on to patients, or if your judgement or performance could be affected by a condition or its treatment, you must consult a suitably qualified colleague. You must ask for and follow their advice about investigations, treatment and changes to your practice that they consider necessary. You must not rely on your own assessment of the risk you pose to patients.

Extract reproduced from General Medical Council (GMC) guidance, *Good Medical Practice 2006*, paragraph 79, Copyright © General Medical Council.

Box 23.4 Treating patients with HIV infection

Consider and respond to the needs of patients with disabilities and to make reasonable adjustments to your practice to enable them to receive care to meet their needs.

Extract reproduced from 2012 revision of *Good Medical Practice* (subject to consultation) paragraph 61, Copyright © General Medical Council.

Box 23.5 Guidance for nurses

32. You must act without delay if you believe that you, a colleague or anyone else may be putting someone at risk

Extract reproduced from *The code: Standards of conduct, performance and ethics for nurses and midwives*, May 2008, Copyright © Nursing and Midwifery Council.

Box 23.6 Guidance for dentists

If you believe that patients may be at risk because of your health, behaviour or professional performance, or that of a colleague, or because of any aspect of the clinical environment, you should take action. You can get advice from appropriate colleagues, a professional organisation or your defence organisation. If at any time you are not sure how to continue, contact us.

Treat patients fairly and in line with the law. Promote equal opportunities for all patients. Do not discriminate against patients or groups of patients because of their sex, age, race, ethnic origin, nationality, special needs or disability, sexuality, health, lifestyle, beliefs or any other irrelevant consideration.

Extracts reproduced from *Standards for dental professionals*, paragraphs 1.7 and 2.3 May 2005, Copyright © General Dental Council.

Box 23.7 HIV-infected healthcare workers

4.7 A health care worker who has any reason to believe they may have been exposed to infection with HIV, in whatever circumstances, must promptly seek and follow confidential professional advice on whether they should be tested for HIV. Failure to do so may breach the duty of care to patients.

4.16 Health care workers who know or have good reason to believe (having taken steps to confirm the facts as far as practicable) that an HIV infected worker is performing exposure prone procedures or has done so in the past, must inform an appropriate person in the health care worker's employing authority (e.g. an occupational health physician) or, where appropriate, the relevant regulatory body. The DPH should also be informed in confidence. UKAP[a] can be asked to advise when the need for such notification is unclear. Such cases are likely to arise very rarely. Wherever possible, the health care worker should be informed before information is passed to an employer or regulatory body.

[a]UK Advisory Panel for Healthcare Workers Infected with Blood-borne Viruses. (UKAP was set up originally under the aegis of the UK Health Departments' Expert Advisory Group on AIDS in 1991, and in 1993 its remit was extended to cover healthcare workers infected with all blood-borne viruses. UKAP advises physicians of healthcare workers infected with blood-borne viruses, occupational physicians, professional bodies, individual healthcare workers or their advocates; and directors of public health on patient notification exercises.)

Extracts reproduced from *HIV-infected healthcare workers: guidance on management and patient notification*, July 2005, Department of Health, UK © Crown Copyright 2005.

---

continuing occupational risk.[22] For HIV-infected healthcare workers the risk is likely to be even higher and the consequences of infection with TB greater. In view of this, proportionate efforts should be made to protect HIV-infected healthcare workers from exposure to infectious TB patients and material. The British Thoracic Society (BTS) guidelines *Control and prevention of tuberculosis in the UK: code of practice 2000* specifically addressed the case of HIV-infected job applicants and those diagnosed with HIV while in post.[23] The guidance stated that:

> If HIV-infected healthcare workers choose to care for HIV-infected patients, they should understand that they should not care for patients with infectious TB as they put themselves at risk and may then put others at risk should they themselves become infected. . . . Since so many HIV-infected patients are admitted with respiratory symptoms, this will raise practical issues such as implications for staffing and difficulties in maintaining confidentiality.

Decisions about risk should take into account the patient's specific duties in the workplace, the prevalence of TB in the local community and the degree to which precautions designed to prevent the transmission of TB are taken in the workplace. The estimate of risk will affect how and in what capacity the HIV-infected worker should be employed and the frequency with which the worker should be screened for TB. In the UK the employer owes a higher duty of care to any particularly vulnerable employee with a known, pre-existing medical condition (the 'eggshell skull principle') (see Chapter 2). This must be balanced against the wishes and rights of the HIV-infected employee to avoid unfair discrimination.

Regardless of potential risk of exposure to TB-infected patients or material, *all* HIV-infected healthcare workers should be alerted to the symptoms of TB, the need to avoid patients and material suspected or known to be infected with TB, and to seek medical advice immediately if they develop any symptoms suggestive of TB. HIV and occupational health specialists advising HIV-infected healthcare workers should refer to the BTS code of practice[23] for further guidance.

Other occupations

In 2002 the US Public Health Service and Infectious Diseases Society published evidence-based recommendations for preventing opportunistic infections among HIV-infected persons.[24] The guidance referring to different occupations is summarized as follows.

Work in prisons and with the homeless: there is evidence that TB is more common in the prison population than the general population in the USA and several European countries and this is likely to be the case in the UK. Accurate estimates of TB in the UK homeless are difficult to obtain but all available studies point to TB being a particular problem in this group. HIV-infected prison officers and workers in homeless shelters are likely therefore to be at increased risk of TB. As for healthcare workers, similar principles of risk reduction should apply.

Child-care providers: HIV-infected child-care providers are at increased risk for acquiring CMV infection, cryptosporidiosis, and other infections such as hepatitis A and giardiasis from children. The risk for acquiring infection can be diminished by optimal hygiene practices such as hand-washing after faecal contact (e.g. during nappy changing) and after contact with urine or saliva.

Occupations involving contact with animals (e.g. veterinary work and employment in pet shops, farms, or abattoirs): workers in these occupations could be at risk of cryptosporidiosis, toxoplasmosis, salmonellosis, campylobacteriosis, or *Bartonella* infection. However, available data are insufficient to justify a recommendation against HIV-infected persons working in such settings. Optimal hygiene practices should be adhered to.

Working overseas

There are a few particular considerations for the HIV-infected overseas worker. A day trip abroad to an urban office in a developed city should not normally require additional precautions. However, an overseas posting for months or years to a remote area of a developing country needs more thought and planning. Consideration needs to be given to:

- Immigration requirements of the country being visited.
- Risk of exposure to opportunistic pathogens.
- Speed of access to and adequacy of healthcare facilities.
- Repatriation arrangements.

Travel to developing countries might result in substantial risks of exposure for HIV-infected persons to opportunistic pathogens, particularly for patients who are severely immunosuppressed. Consultation with healthcare providers or specialists in travel medicine should help patients plan itineraries.

HIV-infected travellers are at a higher risk for food-borne and water-borne infections than they are in the UK. The usual hygiene precautions recommended for all travellers should be strictly adhered to by those who are infected with HIV. These include steaming hot foods, peeling own fruit, drinking only bottled beverages or boiled water. They should avoid direct contact of the skin with soil or sand (e.g. by wearing shoes and protective clothing and by using towels on beaches) in areas where faecal contamination of soil is likely.

Antimicrobial prophylaxis for traveller's diarrhoea is not recommended routinely for HIV-infected persons travelling to developing countries. Such preventive therapy can have adverse effects and can promote the emergence of drug-resistant organisms. All HIV-infected travellers to developing countries should carry a sufficient supply of an antimicrobial agent, to be taken empirically if diarrhoea occurs. One appropriate regimen is 500 mg of ciprofloxacin twice daily for 3–7 days. Information about vaccination is given later in this chapter.

Countries requiring an entry HIV test

Some countries screen incoming travellers for HIV infection and may deny entry to people with AIDS or evidence of HIV infection. These countries usually only screen people planning extended visits, such as for work or study. Information about policies and requirements can be obtained from the consular officials of individual nations.[25]

Occupational immunizations

Some of the commoner occupational vaccines are described in this section. This advice is based on information from the Department of Health's *Immunization Against Infectious Disease 2006— 'The Green Book'*[26] and the advice should always be checked on their website (<http://www.dh.gov. uk>) for updates. It would also be sensible to check safety with the individual's HIV specialist. Further advice can be obtained from BHIVA.[27]

The majority of occupational vaccines are given to healthcare and laboratory workers and those travelling overseas. As a general rule HIV-infected individuals should avoid live vaccines; however, some are not absolutely contraindicated. Most of the safe vaccines can be given according to the usual schedule in the 'green book'.[26] However an HIV-infected individual may not mount a good immune response. Vaccine efficacy and safety depends on the degree of immunosuppression, which can be quantified by considering CD4 count (Table 23.2).

Varicella zoster vaccine is contraindicated for HIV-infected individuals with severe immunosuppression. This guidance may be relaxed in the near future as evidence is emerging that patients with moderate immunosuppression can be safely vaccinated and will make an adequate response. For HIV-infected individuals with no immunosuppression who are susceptible to varicella, vaccine is indicated to reduce the risk of serious chickenpox or zoster should their condition deteriorate.

Bacillus Calmette-Guérin (BCG) should not be given to those with HIV infection, as there have been reports of BCG dissemination.

Yellow fever vaccine should not be given to HIV-infected individuals. Individuals intending to visit countries requiring a yellow fever certificate for entry, but where there is no risk of exposure, should obtain a letter of exemption from a medical practitioner. Fatal myeloencephalitis following yellow fever vaccination has been reported in an individual with severe HIV-induced

Table 23.2 Measure of immunosuppression by CD4 count

CD4 count/μL (% of total lymphocytes)	
No suppression	≥500 (≥25%)
Moderate suppression	200–499 (15–24%)
Severe suppression	<200 (<15%)

Data from Salisbury D et al. (eds). *Immunisation against infectious disease*, Department of Health, 2006 © Crown Copyright 2006.

immunosuppression. There are limited data, however, suggesting that yellow fever vaccine may be given safely to HIV-infected persons with a CD4 count that is greater than 200 and a suppressed HIV viral load. Therefore if the yellow fever risk is unavoidable, specialist advice should be sought about the vaccination of asymptomatic HIV-infected individuals.

MMR contains live attenuated measles, mumps, and rubella virus but may be given safely provided there are no contraindications, for example, severe immunosuppression with a CD4 count <200 cells/μL. A case of fatal measles-vaccine-associated pneumonitis was reported in a severely immunocompromised HIV-infected man almost a year after measles vaccination.[27] Serious illnesses have not been reported in HIV-infected individuals in association with mumps or rubella vaccination.

Inactivated *poliomyelitis* vaccine (IPV) can be given safely to HIV-infected individuals.

Three *typhoid* vaccines are available:

1 The parenteral ViCPS vaccine, containing purified Vi ('virulence') capsule polysaccharide. Although not required for international travel, the ViCPS vaccine is recommended in all HIV-infected travellers to areas in which there is a recognized risk of exposure to *S. typhi*. One dose of the vaccine should be given at least 2 weeks before expected exposure. Persons who will have intimate exposure (e.g. household contact) to a documented *S. typhi* carrier and laboratory workers exposed to *S. typhi* should also be offered vaccination A booster is recommended every 3 years in those who remain at risk. This interval might be reduced to 2 years if the CD4 count is <200 cells/mL.

2 The oral Ty21a vaccine, containing live attenuated *S. typhi* Ty21a. Although there have been no reports of adverse events associated with Ty21a vaccination in HIV-infected persons, the Ty21a vaccine is contraindicated in immunocompromised persons, including those with HIV infection.

3 A whole-cell inactivated vaccine.

A combined hepatitis A/ViCPS vaccine is also available. Typhoid vaccines are not 100 per cent protective and responses may be further reduced in HIV infection. Travellers should be advised to follow strict food and drink precautions.

Diphtheria containing vaccines should be given according to the usual schedule in the Green Book.[26]

Influenza vaccine contains inactivated virus. It may be given to HIV-infected individuals and is specifically recommended for healthcare workers and for those with immunosuppression including HIV.

Hepatitis B vaccine may be given to HIV-infected patients and should be offered to those at risk, as higher rates of chronic hepatitis B infection have been observed where immunity is suppressed by HIV infection.

Hepatitis A is an inactivated vaccine and should be given to HIV-infected individuals at risk of infection.

Risk of transmitting HIV at work

Transmission from worker to client/patient

Sex workers

The routes of transmission of HIV mean that the only two occupations with potential for transmission of HIV from an infected worker during the normal course of their work are sex work and healthcare. Sex workers in the UK are unregulated. Both they and their client group are difficult to access for routine data collection and research purposes. Therefore little is known about transmission rates from sex workers to their clients.

Healthcare workers

The healthcare industry in developed countries, and in particular in the UK, is regulated. It is possible to investigate healthcare workers and their patients in cases of potential HIV transmission.

Evidence of transmission of HIV from healthcare worker to patient

There have only been four reported incidents world-wide of HIV transmission from an HIV-infected healthcare worker to patient:[28]

+ A dentist in the USA (six patients infected—route of transmission unclear).[29]
+ An orthopaedic surgeon in France (one patient infected).[30]
+ A gynaecologist in Spain (one patient infected).
+ A nurse in France (one patient infected—the route of transmission unclear).

In the first two cases molecular analysis indicated that the viral sequences obtained from the healthcare workers and their HIV-infected patients were closely related. In 1995 the American Centre for Disease Control and Prevention summarized the results of all published and unpublished investigations. Of over 22 000 patients tested who were treated by 51 HIV-positive infected healthcare workers, 113 HIV-positive patients were reported, but epidemiological and laboratory follow-up did not show any healthcare worker to have been a source of HIV for any of the patients tested.[31]

There have been no reported cases in the UK, despite over 30 patient notification exercises between 1988 and 2008 in which nearly 10 000 patients were tested for HIV. There are limitations to this information, for example, only a proportion of patients treated by HIV-infected healthcare workers were tested either because they could not be contacted or because they declined testing. Many look-back exercises undertaken in the UK, USA, and elsewhere since that study have failed to identify further cases.

Occupational restrictions placed on HIV-infected healthcare workers

In the UK, HIV-infected healthcare workers are not allowed to perform exposure-prone procedures or EPPs (see Box 23.2). Department of Health guidance requires 'a healthcare worker who has any reason to believe they may have been exposed to HIV to promptly seek and follow confidential professional advice on whether they should be tested for HIV. Failure to do so may breach the duty of care to patients' (see Box 23.7). This guidance is supported by various regulatory bodies' statements on professional responsibilities (see Boxes 23.3—23.7).[18]

Few other countries (Italy, Ireland, Australia, and Malta) have similar restrictions.[28] In many other countries (Austria, Belgium, Canada, Finland, France, New Zealand, and Sweden), the management of an HIV-infected healthcare worker is decided on a case-by-case basis. The decision about whether to restrict a healthcare worker from performing invasive procedures is undertaken by the employer or the clinician responsible for treating the healthcare worker (independently or in conjunction with an expert committee), or by a local or national expert committee. Germany and Spain do not appear to have national policies in place. Even though there are guidelines published by the US Centers for Disease Control and Prevention and the Society for Healthcare Epidemiology of America, the US has no national policy for managing HIV-infected healthcare workers. French recommendations state that, if a healthcare worker is clinically well and has an undetectable viral load for at least 3 months, they should not be restricted from practice. However, this recommendation has not been adopted by the French Ministry of Health and is not currently national policy.

Proposals to amend the UK guidance is subject to public consultation until March 2012.[28] A tripartite working group including the Expert Advisory Group on AIDS, the Advisory Group on Hepatitis and the UK Advisory Panel for Healthcare Workers Infected with Blood-borne Viruses reviewed national guidance on healthcare workers infected with blood-borne viruses and the available evidence and expert opinion. It concluded that the risk of HIV being transmitted to patients from the most invasive procedures is very low and negligible for less invasive procedures. The proposals include:

- HIV-infected infected healthcare workers should be permitted to perform EPPs if they are on combination antiretroviral drug therapy (cART) and have a plasma viral load suppressed consistently to very low or undetectable levels (i.e. below 200 copies/mL).

- HIV-infected healthcare workers should demonstrate a sustained response to cART before starting or resuming EPPs and should be subject to viral load testing every 3 months while continuing to perform such procedures.

- HIV-infected healthcare workers who wish to perform EPPs whilst on cART should be under the joint supervision of a consultant in occupational medicine and their treating physician.

- Any HIV-infected healthcare worker who fails to comply with monitoring arrangements, or whose plasma viral load rises significantly above 200 copies/mL (i.e. to more than 1000 copies/mL), should be restricted from performing EPPs until their viral load returns to being stably below 200 copies/mL.

HIV testing and healthcare workers

Since March 2007, the UK Department of Health has recommended that all new healthcare workers are offered HIV tests as part of 'standard health clearance' to be completed on appointment.[32] New healthcare workers who will perform EPPs (see Box 23.2) are required to have 'additional health clearance' which includes being non-infectious for HIV (antibody negative). These checks should be completed before confirmation of appointment to an EPP post, as the healthcare worker will be ineligible if found to be infectious. 'New healthcare workers' include those new to the NHS, those moving to a post or training that involves EPPs and those returning to the NHS who may have been exposed to serious communicable diseases. The latter category could include being engaged in research, voluntary service with medical charities, sabbaticals, tours of active duty in the armed forces, locum or agency work and time spent in countries of high prevalence for blood-borne virus infections. The guidance is not intended to prevent HIV-infected healthcare workers from working in the NHS but rather to restrict them from working in those clinical areas where their infection may pose a risk to patients in their care. This guidance is likely to be affected by proposed amendments to the restrictions placed on HIV-infected healthcare workers.[28] It is proposed that new healthcare workers, including students, who will perform procedures, should continue to be tested for HIV when joining the NHS or returning to EPP work in the NHS. If found to be infected, this will no longer automatically restrict them from posts or careers involving EPPs, subject to successful treatment with cART and occupational health clearance. However, the demands of adhering to cART and strict monitoring arrangements would be significant and should be explored in any discussions about career options. It is proposed that existing healthcare workers should continue to remain under a professional duty to promptly seek and follow confidential professional advice on whether they should be tested for HIV in situations where they have reason to believe they may have been exposed to infection, in whatever circumstances. Healthcare workers who are infected with HIV must promptly seek appropriate expert medical and occupational health advice.

A balance between protecting patients and not discriminating against HIV-infected healthcare workers is not easy to achieve and may depend on a number of factors including evidence (or lack of evidence) of scientific risk of transmission, stigma, public opinion, the law and politics.[33]

Patient notification exercise

Newly diagnosed HIV-infected healthcare workers who have been performing EPPs may be subject to a 'look-back' exercise. It is not necessary to notify automatically every patient who has undergone any EPP by an HIV-infected healthcare worker, as the overall risk of transmission is very low. The director of public health has responsibility for deciding on the need for a look-back and which patients to include. They may seek advice from the UK Advisory Panel if there is doubt.[18] Under the new proposals[28] patient notification exercises connected with HIV-infected healthcare workers on cART would only be recommended in circumstances in which their viral load had risen above 200 copies/mL. The need for patient notification would be determined by a risk assessment on a case-by-case basis in line with the principles in existing guidance, and the UK Advisory Panel for Healthcare Workers Infected with Blood-borne Viruses should be consulted for advice.

Care of the HIV-infected healthcare worker

Management of workers with HIV and AIDS should be consistent with the policies and procedures developed for people affected by other serious and potentially progressive medical conditions. Occupational physicians have an important advisory role. This is particularly central in the management of HIV-infected healthcare workers, as emphasized in the UK government guidance on this issue.[18] The new proposals do not include specific reference to the care of HIV-infected healthcare workers, except that those who wish to perform EPPs (see Box 23.2) whilst on cART should be managed by an HIV/genitourinary medicine/infectious diseases physician who liaises closely with the healthcare worker's consultant in occupational medicine.[28] If limitation of practice is necessary, the occupational physician should advise management accordingly but without revealing any clinical information, and with the agreement of the individual concerned. Where possible, redeployment without loss of income should be pursued. This will require a sympathetic approach by management.

The Department of Health guidance also requires all HIV-infected healthcare workers who provide clinical care to patients (even if they have not been involved in performing EPPs) to remain under regular medical and occupational health supervision.[18] It is not clear whether this recommendation will be retained in the proposed amended guidance.[28] HIV-infected healthcare workers are required to follow appropriate occupational health advice, especially if their circumstances change.

No other restrictions are placed on HIV-positive healthcare workers, except at local level where their condition would be managed with the same approach used for other chronic illnesses with potential for immunosuppression.

Confidentiality

Healthcare workers have the same rights of confidentiality as anyone else. Patients can be reassured that the routine precautions taken in their care protect them from the tiny risk of infection from their carers.

For healthcare workers involved in EPPs (see Box 23.2), the possibility of a patient notification exercise is likely to be extremely emotive. Assurances should be given about measures to protect their identity, including seeking an injunction if necessary to prevent publication of their name. Advice on the need to modify their practice can be sought from a specialist occupational physician. The trust's director of human resources and/or the regional postgraduate dean should be approached for advice on retraining and redeployment issues or alternative careers. Other than the special case of HIV-infected healthcare workers performing EPPs, modification of working practices are not necessary to protect others from infection.

Risk of acquiring HIV through work

There are very few occupations and work tasks that have the potential for transmission of HIV to the worker. The two main ones are:

1 Sex work; although there is evidence that in Western Europe the route of transmission is more likely to be through needle sharing in drug addicted sex workers rather than directly through unprotected sex in the course of their work.[34]

2 Healthcare work where the worker is exposed to the blood and other body fluids of HIV-infected patients through percutaneous injury or blood splash on to mucous membranes or non-intact skin.

Unlike sex workers, serosurveys of healthcare workers have not shown a higher prevalence of HIV. However, we know that HIV can be transmitted in the healthcare setting from patient to worker. Large prospective studies have found that the risk of transmission of HIV from an infected patient to a healthcare worker, after a single infected needlestick, is about 0.3 per cent.[35]

Since 1984 five cases of occupationally acquired HIV infections in UK healthcare workers have been documented. In one case the healthcare worker seroconverted despite receiving post-exposure prophylaxis (PEP) with triple therapy. Since 1999, no new cases of occupational transmission of HIV in healthcare workers following percutaneous exposure to HIV have been reported in the scientific literature. However, the lay press reported the death from AIDS in 2007 of a nurse who apparently acquired HIV infection following occupational exposure whilst working in London in 1999.[36] A further 14 healthcare workers with probable occupational acquisition have been diagnosed in the UK. These had no risk factor other than an occupational exposure but they did not have a baseline HIV negative test; 13 of these healthcare workers worked in countries of high HIV prevalence.[37]

Some of the cases in Table 23.3 were reported to voluntary national surveillance schemes. Others were case reports from a variety of other sources. It is likely that the table underestimates

Table 23.3 Occupational transmission of HIV up to end December 2002

	USA	UK	Rest of Europe	Rest of world	Total
Documented seroconversions (specific exposure incident)	57	5	30	14	106
Possible occupational infection (no life-style risks)	139	14	71	14	238

Data from Health Protection Agency. *Occupational Transmission of HIV—summary of published reports*. March 2005 edition (data to the end of December 2002). London: Health Protection Agency, March 2005.

the actual number of occupational infections, particularly in those developing countries with poor infection control practices and reporting systems, but a high prevalence of HIV in the general population.

Despite awareness of the risk among UK healthcare workers, accidental exposure to blood continues to occur. Between 2000 and 2007, 183 centres participating in a national voluntary surveillance scheme reported 889 occupational exposures to HIV.[38] Such exposures can cause great anxiety to employees. Procedures for reporting and managing blood exposure incidents should be set up and publicized widely within the workplace.

Post-exposure prophylaxis

There is evidence from a case-referent study that zidovudine reduces the rate of HIV seroconversion after exposure through needlestick injury.[35] Since 1997 UK guidance, produced by the government's Expert Advisory Group on AIDS (EAGA), has recommended the use of combination antiretroviral drugs as PEP. At the time of writing the recommended regimen is: one truvada tablet (300 mg tenofovir and 200mg emtricitabine) once a day plus two kaletra film-coated tablets (200 mg lopinavir and 50mg ritonavir) twice a day.[39] Other combinations may be appropriate in some circumstances, depending on viral drug resistance in the source patient or relative contraindications in the exposed individual. These should be given as soon as possible, within hours, and certainly within 48–72 hours of exposure. They should be given for 28 days, with follow-up HIV antibody testing at least 12 weeks' post exposure, or if PEP was taken, at least 12 weeks after PEP was stopped. All antiretroviral drugs have side effects, although many of these can be managed symptomatically. Common side effects include nausea, diarrhoea, dizziness, headache, asthenia, and rashes. Those prescribing PEP and/or providing advice should be aware of potential adverse effects and drug interactions, as these can have implications for patient safety and effectiveness of prophylaxis. Further expert advice should be sought where necessary. The Liverpool HIV Pharmacology Group produces interaction charts which are available on their website.[40]

There is no requirement for exposed healthcare workers to stop exposure-prone procedures during the treatment or follow-up period, as the risk of seroconversion is so small (0.3 per cent and lessened by suitable PEP).[39]

The latest EAGA guidance includes advice on healthcare workers seconded overseas and students on electives, managing exposures outside the hospital setting, reporting occupational HIV exposures, and PEP for patients after possible exposure to an HIV-infected healthcare worker.[39]

RIDDOR reporting

In the UK, accidental occupational exposure to HIV is reportable to the Health and Safety Executive under the Reporting of Injuries, Diseases and Dangerous Occurrences regulations 1995 (RIDDOR) as a dangerous occurrence (accidental release of biological agent likely to cause serious human illness) or injury (if three or more days off work). Reporting may be done by telephone, post, or online.

Compensation for HIV infection contracted at work
Industrial injuries disablement benefit

HIV is not a prescribed disease under the Social Security Acts. However, healthcare workers who have acquired HIV because of accidental occupational exposure, e.g. needlestick, may be able to claim.[18]

NHS injury benefits scheme

The NHS injury benefits scheme provides temporary or permanent injury benefits for all NHS employees who lose remuneration because of an injury or disease attributable to their NHS employment. The scheme is also available to general medical and dental practitioners working in the NHS. Under the terms of the scheme it must be established whether, on the balance of probabilities, the injury or disease was acquired during the course of NHS work.[18] These potential benefits support the reporting of *all* accidental blood exposures, as documentation and appropriate blood tests on both the source patient and injured staff member will not only allow access to post-exposure prophylaxis and where necessary HIV treatment, but also eligibility for injury benefit schemes.

Prevention of occupational HIV transmission

Control of Substances Hazardous to Health Regulations

HIV, and the other blood-borne viruses, are covered by the Control of Substances Hazardous to Health (COSHH) Regulations 2002, as 'biological agent(s) . . . which may cause infection'. Therefore the hierarchy of control measures applies. Of particular relevance is the COSHH principle: *Design and operate processes and activities to minimize emission, release and spread of substances hazardous to health*. Applied to HIV in the healthcare setting this can be interpreted as a need to:

◆ Reduce invasive techniques.

◆ Use safe systems for clinical procedures.

◆ Regular and effective training in safe systems of work.

◆ Consider safer needles.

◆ Perform laboratory work at an appropriate containment level (e.g. safety cabinets, eliminate aerosols, eliminate sharps).

Standard precautions

In the healthcare setting prevention relies on safe practice to avoid exposure to blood and body fluids. A 'standard precautions' approach should be adopted. This means that all blood should be considered infectious. Precautions, to avoid needlesticks and skin or mucous membrane exposures to blood, are taken with all patients and with all blood and tissue samples. Local guidelines should be drawn up for safe practice in all situations where contact with blood or body fluids is possible. All employees who may have contact with blood or body fluids should be trained in these practices and adherence to practice guidelines should be regularly reviewed. Protective equipment and clothing, such as gloves, gowns, and eye protection should be provided and usage encouraged. Such an approach will reduce the risk of transmission of HIV (and other blood-borne viruses such as hepatitis B and C) between patients and healthcare workers.

Summary

Despite significant advances in the treatment of HIV infection and dramatic increases in disease-free survival, there has not been a corresponding increase in employment for those infected with HIV. It is likely that drug side effects, psychological barriers, and continuing (but lessening) prejudice among employers contribute.

Occupational physicians working in healthcare require specialist knowledge of guidelines governing the management of HIV-infected healthcare workers. In nearly all other industries HIV-infected individuals can be managed in the same way as any other worker with a chronic, immunosuppressive disease.

If the development of novel drugs outstrips viral resistance, and the disabling side effects of effective treatment reduce, the employment prospects for HIV-infected individuals, at least in developed countries, should continue to improve.

References

1 Health Protection Agency. *HIV in the United Kingdom: 2011. Report*. London: Health Protection Services, 2011.

2 Easterbrook P. The changing epidemiology of HIV infection: new challenges for HIV palliative care. *J R Soc Med* 2001; **94**: 442–8.

3 Fidler S, Spartac Trial Investigators. *The effect of short-course antiretroviral therapy in primary HIV infection: final results from an international randomised controlled trial; SPARTAC* (abstract WELBX06). International AIDS Society, Rome, 17–20 July 2011.

4 Sherr L, Clucas C, Harding R, *et al.* HIV and depression—a systematic review of interventions. *Psychol Health Med* 2011; **16**: 493–527.

5 British HIV Association (BHIVA). *Treatment of HIV-1 infected adults with antiretroviral therapy*, 2012. [Online] (<http://www.bhiva.org>)

6 Panel on Antiretroviral Guidelines for Adults and Adolescents. *Guidelines for the use of antiretroviral agents in HIV-1-infected adults and adolescents*. London: Department of Health and Human Services, 2011. (<http://www.aidsinfo.nih.gov/ContentFiles/AdultandAdolescentGL.pdf>)

7 Terence Higgins Trust website: <http://www.tht.org.uk/>.

8 Waddell G, Burton AK. *Is work good for your health and well-being?* London: The Stationery Office, 2006.

9 Black C. *Working for a Healthier Tomorrow*. London: The Stationery Office, 2008. (<http://www.dwp.gov.uk/docs/hwwb-working-for-a-healthier-tomorrow.pdf >)

10 Rodger A, Brecker, N, Bhagani S, *et al.* Attitudes and barriers to employment in HIV positive patients. *Occup Medi* 2010; **60**(6): 423–9.

11 Office for National Statistics. *Labour Force Survey (LFS)*. London: Office for National Statistics, 2008. (<http://www.ons.gov.uk/ons/dcp171778_250593.pdf>)

12 Wallenius M, Skomsvoll JF, Koldingsnes W, *et al.* Comparison of work disability and health-related quality of life between males and females with rheumatoid arthritis below the age of 45 years. *Scand J Rheumatol* 2009; **38**: 178–83.

13 Khan F, Ng L, Turner-Stokes L. Effectiveness of vocational rehabilitation intervention on the return to work and employment of persons with multiple sclerosis. *Cochrane Database Syst Rev* 2009; **1**:186–92.

14 Directgov work schemes and programmes website: <http://www.direct.gov.uk/en/DisabledPeople/Employmentsupport/WorkSchemesAndProgrammes/>)

15 Direct Gov Jobcentre Plus Programmes and Services Plus website: <http://www.direct.gov.uk/en/Employment/Jobseekers/programmesandservices/index.htm>

16 Equality Act 2010. (<http://www.legislation.gov.uk/ukpga/2010/15/contents>)

17 Kloss D. *Occupational health law*, 5th edn. Chichester: Wiley-Blackwell, 2010.

18 Department of Health. *HIV infected health care workers: guidance on management and patient notification*. London: UK Health Departments, 2005.

19 The Faculty of Occupational Medicine. *Guidance on ethics for occupational physicians*, 6th edn. London: Faculty of Occupational Medicine, 2006.

20 General Medical Council (GMC). *Good Medical Practice*. London: GMC, 2006.

21 General Medical Council. *The review of good medical practice*. [Online] (<http://www.gmc-uk.org/guidance/9879.asp>)

22 Meredith S, Watson JM, Citron KM, *et al*. Are healthcare workers in England and Wales at increased risk of tuberculosis? *BMJ* 1996; **313**: 522–5.

23 Joint Tuberculosis Committee of the British Thoracic Society. Control and prevention of tuberculosis in the United Kingdom: Code of Practice 2000. *Thorax* 2000; **55**: 887–901.

24 Masur H, Kaplan JE, Holmes KK. Guidelines for preventing opportunistic infections among hiv-infected persons—2002: Recommendations of the US Public Health Service and the Infectious Diseases Society of America. *Ann Intern Med* 2002; **137**(5 Pt 2; Suppl.): 435–77.

25 Centers for Disease Control and Prevention. *Yellow book*. (<http://wwwnc.cdc.gov/travel/yellowbook/2012/chapter-3-infectious-diseases-related-to-travel/hiv-and-aids.htm>)

26 Department of Health. *Immunisation against infectious disease 2006—'The green book'*. London: Department of Health, 2006.

27 British HIV Association. *Immunisation of HIV-infected adults*, 2008. [Online] (<http://www.bhiva.org/Immunization2008.aspx>)

28 Department of Health. *Management of HIV-infected healthcare workers—a paper for consultation*. London: Department of Health, 2011. (<http://www.dh.gov.uk/en/Consultations/Liveconsultations/DH_131532>)

29 Hillis DM, Huelsenbeck JP. Support for dental HIV transmission. *Nature* 1994; **369**: 25–5.

30 Lot F, Séguier JC, Fégueux S, *et al*. Probable transmission of HIV from an orthopedic surgeon to a patient in France. *Ann Intern Med* 1999; **130**: 1–6.

31 Laurie M, Chamberland ME, Cleveland JL, *et al*. Investigation of patients of health care workers infected with HIV: the Centers for Disease Control and Prevention database. *Ann Intern Med* 1995; **122**: 653–7.

32 Department of Health. *Health clearance for tuberculosis, hepatitis B, hepatitis C and HIV: new healthcare workers*. London: Department of Health, 2007.

33 Grime P. Blood-borne virus screening in health care workers: is it worthwhile? *Occup Med* 2007; **57**: 544–6.

34 Belza MJ. Prevalence of HIV, HTLV-I and HTLV-II among female sex workers in Spain, 2000–2001. *Eur J Epidemiol* 2004; **19**: 279–82.

35 Cardo DM, Culver DH, Ciesielski CA, *et al*. A case-control study of HIV seroconversion in health care workers after percutaneous exposure. *N Engl J Med* 1997; **337**: 1485–90.

36 Nurse dies from accidental Aids jab. *Metro*, 2007. (<http://www.metro.co.uk/news/98723-nurse-dies-from-accidental-aids-jab>)

37 Health Protection Agency. *Occupational transmission of HIV—summary of published reports*. March 2005 edition (data to the end of December 2002). London: Health Protection Agency, 2005.

38 Health Protection Agency Centre for Infections, National Public Health Service for Wales, CDSC Northern Ireland and Health Protection Scotland. *Eye of the needle. Surveillance of significant occupational exposure to bloodborne viruses in healthcare workers*. London: Health Protection Agency, 2008.

39 Department of health. *HIV Post-exposure prophylaxis: guidance from the UK chief medical officers' expert advisory group on AIDS*. London: Department of Health, 2008.

40 The Liverpool HIV Pharmacology Group website: <http://www.hiv-druginteractions.org/.>

Chapter 24

Drugs and alcohol in the workplace

David Brown and Henrietta Bowden-Jones

Introduction

Drug and alcohol misuse is present at all levels of society and throughout the world although the patterns of use, the substances involved, and the prevailing attitudes vary widely. However it presents, drug and alcohol misuse is a particularly challenging issue for employers, managers, and occupational physicians. These include the effects of drugs and alcohol on health and well-being and the direct and indirect effects on output, performance, and behaviour at work. There are legal implications if employees are under the influence of alcohol or drugs or in possession of illegal drugs where there may be a degree of vicarious liability for the employer. Management may have limited tolerance towards such individuals and there may be significant issues regarding public confidence towards those involved in safety critical industries. Whilst attitudes towards alcohol in society and the workplace appears to be hardening, the distinction between what is acceptable drinking and problem drinking is often blurred.

Prevalence

The largest drug misuse problem in the UK relates to the legal drug alcohol. Over 90 per cent of adults in Britain consume alcohol. Almost one in three men and one in five women consume more than 21 and 14 units a week respectively (the considered upper safe limits). There are an estimated 1.2 million incidents per year of alcohol-related violence and 85 000 cases of drink-driving. Alcohol-related disease accounts for one in 26 National Health Service bed days; up to 40 per cent of all accident and emergency department admissions are alcohol-related and up to 150 000 hospital admissions per year are related to alcohol misuse.[1] In 2009, work-related alcohol misuse was estimated to cost the UK economy up to £6.4 billion per year.[2] In 2007 it was estimated that 43 per cent of employees in managerial and professional occupations exceeded healthy drinking limits as compared to 31 per cent in routine and manual jobs.[3,4] Certain occupations are known to have a high risk of morbidity and mortality from alcohol-related disease, including publicans[5] and recent attention has been focused on the heavy drinking patterns within the armed services, particularly in relation to operational deployment.[6,7]

Information on the pattern of use of drugs other than alcohol in the general and working UK population is poor. The 2010/11 British Crime Survey (BCS) estimated that 8.8 per cent of adults aged 16 to 59 had used illicit drugs (almost 3 million people) and that 3.0 per cent had used a Class A drug in the last year (around a million people). Neither estimates were statistically significantly different from the 2009/10 survey.[8] The majority of those identified were unemployed but of those in regular employment, a significant percentage used drugs recreationally at weekends. Recent research undertaken for the Health and Safety Executive (HSE) found 13 per cent of working respondents reported drug use in the previous year, with an age profile of use similar to that found by the BCS.[9] Cannabis is by far the most commonly used 'illicit' drug and its use in the general population appears to be fivefold higher than any other illicit substance.[10] A 1995 report of psychiatric morbidity suggested a prevalence of drug dependency of 1.5 per cent among workers against a rate in the unemployed of 8.3 per cent.[11]

Impact

The use of drugs and alcohol at work has a negative impact on productivity as well as on the quality of work produced.[12] The UK government estimates that there are up to 17 million working days lost annually in the UK from alcohol abuse. The implications for safety and its cost are more difficult to quantify.

Alcohol

The risk of causing a driving accident increases 3-, 10-, and 40-fold if the blood alcohol exceeds 80, 100, or 150 mg/100 mL respectively. In fact many skills and cognitive processes begin to decline at much lower blood alcohol concentrations (BAC). In the US armed forces a BAC of 50 mg/100 mL or above indicates unfitness for duty and such a level merits disciplinary action. At this level memory transfer from immediate recall to permanent storage may be disturbed, causing impairment of long-term recall. Companies operating oil and gas rigs offshore ban alcohol completely and refuse access to the work site to anyone reporting for duty under the influence of alcohol. Studies of pilots in flight simulators indicate that performance is impaired at a BAC as low as 11 mg/100 mL.[13]

It has been shown that driving at levels below the prescribed BAC introduced in the Road Traffic Act 1967 (80 mg/100 mL) is not free from hazards. Even 'safe' levels of alcohol may be associated with significant impairment of driving ability. Drivers who have consumed moderate doses of alcohol and have BACs of 30–60 mg/100 mL have impaired ability to negotiate a test course with artificial hazards. Furthermore, it has been shown that the combination of alcohol and cannabis (see 'Cannabis'), even at low levels, has a hazardous effect on the driving task. The impairment created by the combination of these two is much greater than that created by either alone.

A strong association has been demonstrated between a raised gamma-glutamyl transferase (GGT) and road traffic accidents in drivers aged over 30, indicating that many of these accidents may be caused by problem drinkers.[14] Of even greater concern is that a high prevalence of raised liver enzyme activity has also been demonstrated in those over the age of 30 who apply for licences as drivers of large goods vehicles (LGVs) and passenger carrying vehicles (PCVs). The findings of a major review of the international literature (the relationship between alcohol and occupational and work related injuries) are shown in Table 24.1.[15]

Drugs

The knowledge base of how drug impairment affects safety in the workplace remains relatively small. Past research in the UK undertaken for the HSE by Cardiff University concluded that there is no association between drug use and workplace accidents. The authors argued, however, that the known effects of illegal drugs on reaction times and cognitive functions such as concentration, and memory are such that they may reduce performance, efficiency, and safety at work.[7] Two major literature reviews have concluded that there is no clear evidence of the deleterious effects of drugs, with the exception of alcohol, on safety and other job performance indicators.[6] In practice, many occupational health practitioners will be able to cite specific cases of the noxious impact of drug use by an employee on both work performance and safety, but this experience is not yet supported by published well designed studies.

Table 24.1 Relationship between alcohol and work-related injuries (from Zwerling14 as summarized by Coomber6)

◆ Acute alcohol impairment is present in about 10% of fatal occupational injuries

◆ Acute alcohol impairment is present in about 5% of non-transport, non-fatal, work-related injuries

◆ A history of alcohol abuse may be weakly associated with occupational injuries (odds ratios ranging from 1.0 to 2.58)

◆ The wide variety of methodological difficulties in the various studies of the association of a history of alcohol abuse and occupational injures should make the reader cautious about drawing conclusions about the data

---

Reprinted from Zwerling C. Current practice and experience in drug and alcohol testing in the workplace, with permission from the United Nations Office on Drugs and Crime, available from <http://www.unodc.org/unodc/en/data-and-analysis/bulletin/bulletin_1993-01-01_2_page006.html>.

Cannabis

There is an extensive literature on human performance under the influence of cannabis and effects on memory, attention span, and perception have been demonstrated. This has implications not only for operating complicated, heavy equipment but also for aircraft pilots, air traffic controllers, train drivers, and signalmen. Cannabis can have an adverse effect on any complex learnt psychomotor task involving memory, judgement, skill, concentration, sense of time, orientation in three-dimensional space, and on the performance of multiple complex tasks. Cannabis can cause temporal disorganization with disruption of the correct sequencing of events in time; therefore work requiring a high level of cognitive integration is adversely affected. A single 'joint' of cannabis can cause measurable impairment of skills for more than 10 hours due to its half-life of 36 hours. This cognitive impairment lasts long after the euphoria has disappeared. Psychophysiological activities impaired by cannabis include: tracking ability, complex reaction time, hand steadiness, complicated signal interpretation, and attention span. Cannabis has a particularly deleterious effect on pilots who have to orientate themselves in three-dimensional space which is particularly crucial for flying a helicopter.[16,17] Amongst the consequences of using cannabis is a dose-related memory impairment effect and even moderate cannabis use is associated with selective short-term memory deficits that persist despite weeks of abstinence. A recent review for the UK Department for Transport concluded that the actual effect of cannabis on real driving performance rather than the effects measured in the laboratory were not as pronounced as predicted.[18] Whilst 4–12 per cent of accident fatalities have levels of cannabis detected, the majority of these cases also have detectable levels of alcohol. There is insufficient knowledge concerning detectable levels of cannabis in non-fatal cases to identify a baseline for comparison. However, the combination of alcohol and cannabis increases impairment, accident rate, and accident responsibility.

Prescribed medication

Sedative psychoactive medication, like alcohol, reduces the overall level of alertness of the central nervous system. Certain antidepressants, anxiolytics, and hypnotics have side effects that reduce skilled performance, concentration, memory, information processing ability, and motor activity as demonstrated in both volunteers and patient populations. All these effects increase the risk of driving accidents. It is for this reason that airline pilots are prohibited from flying while taking prescribed psychotropic medication. It is also known that the use of both prescribed and illicit drugs is associated with an increased liability to road traffic accidents.[19]

The relative contributions of mental illness and psychotropic drug use as causes of accidents have not been analysed in many studies. It is possible that some mentally disturbed patients would pose a greater danger without treatment. On the other hand, after taking their drugs in normal therapeutic doses, these individuals may still present a risk to road safety. Laboratory studies on the effects of psychotropic drugs on driving-related skills of patients on long-term medication are rare. However, it has been demonstrated that patients receiving diazepam perform more poorly, exhibiting impaired visual perception and impaired anticipation of dangerous events when driving.

Laboratory assessments of the effects of psychotropic drugs on sensory and motor skills, steering, brake reaction time, divided attention, and vigilance have shown specific impairment following the administration of benzodiazepines and tricyclic antidepressants. Similar effects have been found to persist the morning after taking benzodiazepine hypnotics. Data from the Netherlands have shown that hypnotics, minor tranquillizers, and tricyclic antidepressants cause driving errors in real-life conditions on the open road, including a tendency to wander across the carriageway. Even fairly low doses of psychoactive drugs have a detrimental effect on the performance of car-driving tests and related measures of psychomotor ability.[20] These detrimental effects have been demonstrated with the hypnotic nitrazepam in a dose as low as 5 mg, and with other psychotropic agents including flurazepam (30 mg), amitriptyline (50 mg), mianserin (10 mg), lorazepam (1 mg), diazepam (5 mg), and chlordiazepoxide (10 mg). The hypnotics were assessed for their residual activity the morning after night-time sedation, whereas the effects of the antidepressants and anxiolytics were measured during the day. The amnesic effect of some benzodiazepines is such that drivers fail to remember routes and cannot read maps competently.

The sleep disturbance caused by jet lag might lead pilots or other people whose work requires vigilance, motor skill, and a high level of decision-making to take a hypnotic. A benzodiazepine with a short half-life might appear to be an attractive option because of the reduction of daytime sedation, but amnesia may persist after the sedation has disappeared. For sedatives or hypnotics, the available data show that their use could more than double the risk of road accidents.

Whereas both amitriptyline and dothiepin impair performance on laboratory analogues of car-driving and related skills, the selective serotonin reuptake inhibitor (SSRI) fluoxetine, in a dose of 40 mg, showed a lack of cognitive and psychomotor effects when administered in an acute dose to volunteers. However, fluoxetine has a long half-life and it is recognized by manufacturers that in the initial stages of a therapeutic period the initial stages may impair driving skills. This is not due to plasma changes as overall once settled on a treatment dose, there is no evidence of significant impairment.

Accidents

In the USA there were several critical accidents involving drugs or alcohol during the 1980s and early 1990s, which are thought to have played a part in the introduction of workplace drug and alcohol testing in safety critical industries. In May 1981, a naval aircraft crashed into an aircraft carrier. Nine of the 14 dead tested positive for cannabinoids at autopsy and the pilot was identified as having taken prescribed antihistamines. In January 1987, there was a rail crash in Maryland that resulted in 16 deaths and 174 people injured. The engineer and brakeman tested positive for marijuana. As a result, testing was brought in for several types of transport workers in the USA. In 1989, the grounding of the Exxon Valdez oil tanker, which caused billions of dollars' worth of property and environmental damage, was linked to alcohol misuse. In 1991, a subway train in New York City derailed, killing five people. The driver had been using alcohol.[15] In the official report of a railway accident in Scotland (March 1974, Glasgow Central Station) it was concluded that the use of diazepam by the train driver was a contributory cause,[21] and Scandinavian researchers have found that serum concentrations of benzodiazepines are significantly greater in drivers involved in road traffic accidents than in control groups. A Dutch case–control study from 2011 analysing all traffic accidents between 2000 and 2007 showed a significant association between road traffic accidents and the use of anxiolytic medication and SSRIs with relative risks of 1.5 and 2 respectively.[22] This study confirms the need for a safety critical workforce to be free of psychotropic medication.

Absenteeism

There is strong evidence that alcohol problems affect absenteeism. Problem drinkers have a rate of absence between two and eight times as high as non-problem drinkers.[23] The UK government estimates that up to 17 million days are lost annually due to alcohol-related absence.[1] The Whitehall II study found that alcohol consumption, even at moderate levels, leads to increased risk for absence due to injury, but with a much weaker relationship to all other absences.[24]

Belief

The research evidence may be limited, but the belief that there are clear-cut deleterious effects of drugs and alcohol on work is very strongly held. Many employers consider that both alcohol and drug use are major causes of absenteeism. Occupational health practitioners will be able to bring cases to mind where drug misuse by an employee had a major effect on their safe working or productivity.

In a survey of drug misuse undertaken in 30 companies by Personnel Today:

- ◆ 27 per cent reported problems of some kind.
- ◆ 31 per cent reported a negative impact on attendance.
- ◆ 27 per cent reported poor employee performance.
- ◆ 3 per cent reported damage to their business.
- ◆ 3 per cent reported accidents at work.

Drug and alcohol at work policies

Major reasons for the introduction of alcohol and drugs policies are to:

- ◆ Mitigate health and safety risks.
- ◆ Promote employee health.
- ◆ Reduce accident levels.
- ◆ Limit employee absence.
- ◆ Respond consistently to alcohol/drug related disciplinary offences.
- ◆ Protect organizational reputation.
- ◆ Enhance employee performance.
- ◆ Protect against the risks from poor decision-making.

Overall, health and safety is the predominant reason for introducing drug and alcohol testing in all employment sectors but particularly safety critical organizations. Non-safety critical organizations are more likely to identify employee health as the reason. A survey of 505 human resources managers in 2007 in the UK showed that about 60 per cent of their companies had policies in place for drug and alcohol problems.[25] This included rules concerning the possession of drugs and alcohol on the premises and alcohol consumption during working time. A quarter of respondents used a capability procedure as part of their approach.

Even if there is no formal policy, certain things will be obvious simply by observing what is acceptable in the workplace. Using alcohol as an example, attitudes range from permitting alcohol to be consumed at work through to a zero tolerance policy that expects employees to have no alcohol in their system during working hours. Some employers may ban alcohol at work but be tolerant of people coming to work regularly with a hangover. The employer may have a differential policy according to the type of work that the employee does. For example, employees in a large company who work closely with the media or who entertain clients may be permitted to drink while involved in this type of work, whereas employees involved in work that has an impact on safe working or product safety may not be permitted to drink at work at all. Where safety is of paramount importance to the organization it is not uncommon for a zero alcohol policy to be in place, at least for those directly involved in activities which may affect safe working or product safety. There may, however, be difficulty in differentiating between groups of workers and the policy must avoid any impression of deliberate targeting of individuals.

Elements of a drug and alcohol at work policy should include:

♦ An explanation of why there is a policy.

♦ The scope of the policy—who it applies to, including whether or not it applies to contractors, consultants, and agencies.

♦ The required code of conduct. This is likely to cover:

- Consumption of alcohol while at work or during meal breaks.

- Consumption, possession, and storage of drugs at work and may also include requirements on the following:

  ▪ Consumption of alcohol while in uniform.

  ▪ Arrival to work when under the influence of drugs/alcohol (zero alcohol, hangovers).

  ▪ An alcohol and drugs testing programme, if used; whether random or routine, and reference to the action that will be taken when an employee has a positive test.

♦ The consequences if the policy is breached.

♦ Any support that the company offers to someone prepared to address an alcohol problem.

♦ The responsibilities of all relevant parties.

♦ A requirement not to bring the company into disrepute by being involved in activities related to drugs at work.

♦ A requirement to find out about the side effects of legal medication and declare the medication to the occupational health practitioner (or manager) if the side effects could affect performance, safety, safety of others or quality of the product.

The policy may also contain reference to the use of alcohol in relation to company cars and the procedure for employees who have been banned from driving due to alcohol. The Faculty of Occupational Medicine has produced guidance on the contents of a drugs and alcohol policy.[26]

Implementation of a new policy

Implementation of a new alcohol and drug policy requires a careful prior assessment of the financial and other implications, and clear agreement on who will be responsible for drawing it up. The workforce should be educated about the content and the implementation of the policy, which should be carefully monitored and reviewed. In setting up company alcohol and drug policies it is essential that wide consultation is held at the draft stages, particularly with staff associations or trade unions. Their acceptance and cooperation is crucial to success and so they should be well-briefed.

Training for managers

As part of the people management training that employees are given, it is useful if training and information on awareness of drug and alcohol related issues is included. This would usually include information about the company's policy, how to recognize potential problems (see Table 24.2), how to arrange testing if this is available, and what support is available. Guidance should also be provided on how to handle those smelling of alcohol at work. Unfortunately surveys have shown that only 33 per cent of managers have received training in handling drug and alcohol misuse at work.[25]

Referral to occupational health

This section assumes that the manager has access to occupational health advice. This is often not the case but this section reviews the process where it does exist. Ideally managers will identify the warning signs described previously, discuss their suspicions with the individual, and refer them for assessment by occupational health. It is common for managers who suspect a problem to find it very difficult to discuss these openly and honestly with the person concerned. Most occupational health practitioners will be familiar with the scenario in which a manager contacts them, describes behaviour that is strongly suggestive of a problem, and then suggests that they refer the person to occupational health

Table 24.2 Possible signs of drug and alcohol misuse

- Short-term sickness absence, especially recurrent Mondays
- Lateness
- Unkempt appearance
- Involvement in accidents and assaults
- Inappropriately aggressive behaviour
- Worsening performance
- Unreliability in someone previously reliable
- Smelling of alcohol
- Shaking/tremor/sweating
- Pinpoint or very large pupils
- Inability to concentrate

Data from Skegg DCG et al. Minor tranquillisers and road accidents. *British Medical Journal*, 1979, 1, pp. 917–19 © BMJ Publishing Group Ltd.

on a pretext 'so that you can just ask about drug use or alcohol use in passing'. This is a recipe for an unsuccessful consultation.

In some companies there is a contractual requirement for employees to attend the occupational health department if their managers refer them. In such companies it is essential for the manager to explain to the individual what they have observed and why they are making a referral, and then confirm this in writing. Even where this occurs in an unequivocal way, the employee may deny it and state that they have no idea why they have been referred. If the manager requests that the employee attend occupational health, and the employee refuses, the manager will need to document this and then take action without the benefit of an occupational health assessment.

Assessment for drug or alcohol misuse and dependency

The assessment is twofold, as is the case for nearly all occupational health assessments. The first part is to identify whether the employee has a significant drug or alcohol problem and if so, the nature and severity of it as well as the individual's willingness to address the issue.

The second part is to advise the employee and their manager on whether they are fit to work and if so, whether adjustments are needed. These assessments are among the most challenging in occupational health practice. Denial is often a prominent feature for those with substance misuse but the employee may have concerns that disclosing the full extent of their dependency might impact negatively on their career prospects. This is a factor observed not just at senior level. One of the aims of the initial session is to get the employee to understand that this is an opportunity to finally sort out an issue that in many cases may be long-standing, often with significant existing negative repercussions on family and personal quality of life.

The assessment by the occupational health adviser usually includes taking a full history of drug or alcohol use and an examination. A variety of questionnaires may be useful—see Table 24.3. For alcohol, blood tests may assist (GGT, alanine transferase (ALT), mean corpuscular volume (MCV), carbohydrate deficient transferring CDT)) but are rarely diagnostic on their own and in some cases, may be normal in employees who subsequently admit to a serious problem.[27] However, a combination of raised test results increases predictive value. Where drug and alcohol testing are available, this can also assist assessment particularly real-time tests such as breathalyser for alcohol.

In one occupational health centre that employs addiction specialists, assessment is undertaken over a period of 3 weeks, using questionnaires, assessment in a series of groups and in one-to-one enquiry, liver function blood tests, and breath or urine testing for alcohol and/or drugs. This is an unusually thorough provision, but gives an idea of the complexity of this area of diagnosis. The degree of alcohol and drug use and misuse lies on a spectrum, from social use not associated with

Table 24.3 Some of the tests available for identification of alcohol or drug misuse[34–37]

- ◆ Substance Abuse Subtle Screening Inventory (SASSI)
- ◆ Michigan Alcoholism Screening Test (MAST)
- ◆ The Alcohol Use Disorders Identification Test (AUDIT)
- ◆ The CAGE Questionnaire
- ◆ Diagnostic interviewing techniques

Box 24.1 Dependence syndrome—seven elements of this biopsychosocial state[33]

1 Narrowing of repertoire of drinking behaviour (so that eventually one day becomes much like another).

2 Salience of drinking behaviour over other priorities in life.

3 Tolerance to alcohol.

4 Repeated withdrawal symptoms.

5 Drinking to relieve withdrawal symptoms.

6 Rapid reinstatement of dependent drinking after a period of abstinence.

7 Subjective experience of 'compulsion' to drink.

Data from Griffith E, Gross MM. Alcohol dependence: provisional description of a clinical syndrome. *British Medical Journal* 1976; 1(6017): 1058–61, © BMJ Publishing Group Ltd.

---

harm through harmful use to dependence. When appropriate treatment is discussed, in some cases of harmful use, an initial brief intervention may be all that is necessary to avoid further misuse of substances, but for most people whose drug and alcohol use is detected at work, the issues may well be far greater, as their use will have escalated from recreational at weekends to daily. An example might be the alcohol-dependent employee who needs a morning drink before leaving for the office (Box 24.1). For cases like these an inpatient alcohol detoxification programme will be recommended.

Features of denial

Alcohol or drug-dependent patients often engage in denial of the nature or extent of their problems, especially when first confronted. Such denial must be dealt with firmly but sensitively. It is rarely productive to engage in directly confrontational arguments about whether or not someone is addicted. However, a carefully considered inquisitorial discussion by an experienced clinician can be helpful. Such confrontation should focus on the evidence available, and on the realities of the workplace. Thus, to say 'the problem is that you have lost 12 hours' work over the last month due to lateness on Monday mornings' is preferable to 'the problem is that you are obviously an alcoholic'. The former can lead to constructive discussion, which may eventually lead to admission of the underlying cause of the problem. The latter is likely to lead to outright denial, anger, and breakdown of trust.

Assessment of fitness to work

It may not be possible for the occupational health adviser to come to a conclusion in their assessment. They may need to refer the individual to an addiction specialist, or to provide pragmatic advice to the manager and individual. Where the person admits a problem and believes that they can address it, a return to full or adjusted duties may be appropriate under regular review. If the person works in a safety critical role, it may be necessary for them to be placed in a non-safety critical role or even to go off sick for the duration of assessment and treatment if it is provided. These decisions involve an assessment of risk, and the involvement of the manager and a health and safety adviser will assist the process. The permission of the individual is, of course, required to reveal the nature of the risk, but will usually be given if it means they are likely to get back to work.

Assessment of immediate fitness to work when the individual is suspected or known to have taken drugs and alcohol is an equally challenging area. It is best addressed by clear guidance in the drug and alcohol policy.

Although the Equality Act 2010 specifically excludes addiction to or dependence on alcohol or any substance (other than the consequences of that substance being legally prescribed), it does cover long-term health effects of alcohol dependency such as liver disease.

Fitness to drive

If a patient has a condition which makes driving unsafe and they refuse to cease driving, General Medical Council guidelines advise breaking confidentiality and informing the Driving and Vehicle Licensing Agency (DVLA). Similarly, if a worker is considered to be under the influence of alcohol or drugs they should be advised not to drive. If they refuse, the company may consider informing the police.

Specific guidance on alcohol misuse and alcohol dependence for Group 1 (car) and Group 2 (LGV/PSV) licence holders is issued by the DVLA. Alcohol misuse normally requires a revocation of a Group 1 licence for 6 months after controlled drinking or abstinence has been achieved, whereas Group 2 drivers require 12 months to elapse. Alcohol dependence requires a year's abstinence for Group 1 and 3 years for Group 2 drivers.[28]

Treatment of dependence

The principles of treatment are initially detoxification, followed by psychological support to enable the individual to admit they have a problem and then develop the skills to address it. Treatment may be residential in the first instance. The '12-Step' philosophy of Alcoholics Anonymous and Narcotics Anonymous is the basis of many treatment programmes. This is based on abstinence and the ongoing support of peers, through mutual help groups. However, this is not the only approach available, and is more prevalent in North America than in the UK. Professional treatment programmes, based upon psychological and medical approaches to treatment, are also available and should be considered as potentially valuable alternative resources. Matching individual patients to particular treatment philosophies is a controversial subject and research evidence provides little information upon which to base such decisions. Patient preference, and availability of treatment programmes with demonstrable results such as outcome data at 3, 6 and 9 months post treatment, should therefore dictate the choice.

Return to work

The detoxification regimen most commonly used for alcohol is the prescribing of chlordiazepoxide in reducing quantities. When the patient is dependent it is not safe to stop drinking suddenly as this may lead to withdrawal seizures and in extreme cases even death. Detoxification in the community is possible for people who are mildly dependent who have significant support and can be reviewed daily. However, the temptation to drink will be harder to resist and the detox may fail.

Drug detoxes vary depending on the substance being abused and the best way of approaching any specific case is to assess each one individually, not forgetting that people using one substance may be using others concurrently, for example, cocaine and heroin. There may be cases where two types of medication are needed to detoxify an individual. Requesting expert advice from an alcohol and drugs specialist has to be a priority if dependence, rather than harmful use, is the problem.

It is often possible to support an employee in their return to work after treatment for addiction. In safety-related jobs this may need ongoing testing, at least for an agreed period of time. A signed 'contract' between the manager and the employee can be helpful, giving written details of expected behaviour. It is very helpful to have the cooperation of the manager, who is usually in a position to identify signs of relapse. There are good success rates from such an approach. A report by the Health and Safety Laboratory (HSL) cites a Civil Aviation Authority estimate that about 85 per cent of professional pilots whose medical certification of fitness has been withdrawn for drug and alcohol problems and have undergone treatment and rehabilitation could be returned to flying.[29]

Drug and alcohol testing at work

Drug and alcohol testing in the workplace is becoming more common in the UK. The 2007 Chartered Institute of Personnel and Development survey showed that 22 per cent of respondent organizations carried out some form of testing (compared to 18 per cent in 2001) with a further 9 per cent who were planning to introduce testing.[25] A comprehensive review of the issues is given in the Independent Inquiry into Drug Testing at Work (IIDTW) published in 2004.[23] Studies in the USA have reported that 40–50 per cent of organizations employ some kind of testing with 85 per cent of major firms doing so.[29] In the USA there is a government body, Substance Abuse and Mental Health Services Administration (SAMHSA), which provides guidance and regulation for the drug testing of federal employees. In Europe there is a European Workplace Drug Testing Society (EWDTS). In the UK there is the UK Workplace Drug Testing Forum, which currently has a membership almost exclusively of laboratories who undertake drug testing.

Drug and alcohol testing should always form a part of a workplace alcohol and drug policy, rather than being in lieu of a policy. It follows that the decision to test, and then how to test, should be made following a risk analysis, looking at the company in question, its activities, and any legislation that may apply.

Organizations must be clear about why they wish to test. The Information Commissioners Employment Practice Code (Data Protection) 2005 (reiterated in recent guidance) states that the collection of information through alcohol or drug testing is unlikely to be justified unless it is for health and safety reasons, and that employers should confine information gathered through testing to those employed in 'safety critical activities'.[30,31] The Human Rights Act 1988 confers a right to privacy and has been cited to support objections to testing; however, case law suggests that justifiable safety grounds will not violate the Act. There may also be a risk of breaching guidelines for good employment practice as recommended in the Data Protection Act 1998. Nevertheless there are obligations on employers and employees with regard to the risk posed by those who might be under the influence of drugs or alcohol whilst at work. These responsibilities are defined within the Health and Safety at Work Act 1974, the Road Traffic Act 1988, the Transport and Works Act 1992, the Compressed Air Regulations 1996, and the Diving at Work Regulations 1997. The following generic criteria are relevant when assessing whether a programme of testing is appropriate:[25]

- ◆ Drug use poses a significant workplace problem.
- ◆ Testing will solve this problem.
- ◆ The benefits of testing will outweigh the costs.
- ◆ The response to a positive test is legally and ethically acceptable.

All testing will require appropriate consent and those people carrying out testing should be appropriately trained in the techniques.

Evidence that testing is effective

The effectiveness of drug testing programmes depends on why they are being implemented. In general the evidence of benefit is inconclusive, but negative studies have often been criticized as being poorly designed. Those studies with very positive findings have been reviewed by Francis et al.[32] and some are described here.

It is argued that testing can have an impact on identifying, controlling, and suppressing corruption within police forces that deal with drug crime.

A review in the US construction industry concluded that companies undertaking testing were able to reduce injury rates by 50 per cent over a 10-year period and that for the average company this reduction was achieved within 2 years of introducing the testing programme.

There is strong evidence of behaviour change in the US military as a result of introducing a drug testing programme. Between 1980 and 1990 the 1-month prevalence of reported drug use fell from 28 per cent to 5 per cent and the proportion of positive drug tests fell from 48 per cent to 3 per cent, although the criteria and techniques varied over this interval.

When to test?

Possible timings for testing are:

+ Pre-employment.

+ Post-accident or incident.

+ Prior to promotion or transfer. This is usual in safety critical industries when employees are first promoted or transferred into jobs with a safety critical element.

+ At random and without announcement. This is commonly used in safety critical industries, but is the most expensive and difficult testing schedule to organize. No prior warning is given to the individuals who are tested. Ideally testing is undertaken at the worksite. It usually requires a visit by a person or team acting as the collecting agent. One option is to test everyone in the workplace but it is more usual to test a sample of the workforce. This requires careful advanced planning, to ensure that the right facilities are available and it is clear who is to be tested. Usually at least one manager needs to be involved. Both staff and managers should be well informed of the procedures. An impartial method of selecting those to be tested is required. This type of testing is often known as 'random' testing, but in fact it may be semi-random, opportunistic, or systematic. Where there is a geographically dispersed workforce or it is too difficult to organize the testing on site, the employee may be advised to attend a centre and may be given a period of notice.

+ For cause or due cause—i.e. where the manager has reason to suspect that drugs or alcohol may be affecting performance or safety, or after an accident or incident at work

+ Voluntary testing can give an employee the opportunity to clear their name or confirm a problem for which help and support could be offered.

+ As part of an employee's rehabilitation programme, in order to monitor their recovery and/or identify otherwise undisclosed relapse to drug use.

Each type of testing has its own practical and ethical issues, which need to be considered in the light of the company's overall alcohol and drugs policy.

Types of test

Tests can either be point of contact (near field/on site) which is used to give an immediate result or via a laboratory or a combination of the two. Sometimes it is important to know immediately whether to suspend a worker from their duties if suspected of abusing substances or alcohol. In these cases the employee will be tested on site but to ensure the reliability of the results on part of the sample should be sent to the reference laboratory for confirmation. Depending on the medium sampled, the test may give a direct reading of the substance present in the body at the time of the test (e.g. blood, breath) or historic from past exposure (urine, hair).

Alcohol screening

This can be conducted in various biological media:

◆ *Breath*. This methodology is similar to that employed for roadside testing of drivers by the police, and uses validated instruments. The breath measurements can be directly related to blood measurements, which themselves can be directly related to the likely degree of impairment of performance.

◆ *Saliva*. Saliva testing involves a real-time read out, based on absorption of saliva on to a pad, with level indications from a change of colour. It relates directly 1:1 to blood alcohol levels and can be regarded as more sensitive than breath testing. It is not widely used in the UK.

◆ *Urine*. Urine testing for alcohol is sometimes used for convenience if drug testing is also undertaken on a urine sample. The disadvantage is that it does not directly reflect the level of alcohol in the blood at the time of testing, but the delayed excretion of alcohol through the renal system.

◆ *Blood*. This represents the definitive measure of alcohol level and can be directly related to likely degree of impairment of performance. It is not usually used in a workplace context though, as it is too invasive.

Drug testing

Urine is the most common form of sample collection in the UK, however, other approaches may be less intrusive and may be indicated depending on the purpose of the test. These include oral fluid, hair, and sweat testing. Table 24.4 summarizes the key types of drug testing and provides details of detection times and reliability. A review of drug testing methods, undertaken for the Railway Safety and Standards Board by HSL, concludes that in addition to urine testing there is a justifiable case for testing oral fluids and hair.[28] The choice of test depends on convenience, cost, and the aim of the testing programme.

What to test for

Testing programmes in the UK usually cover amphetamines, barbiturates, benzodiazepines, cannabis, cocaine, methadone, opiates (including a specific test for heroin), and propoxyphene. The specific profile should be reviewed regularly to reflect drugs in local use. Testing laboratories and toxicologists with an interest in drug misuse can provide useful advice.

LSD (lysergic acid diethylamide) is only found in the urine for 12 hours after use. Heroin is not normally identified more than 24 hours after use. Cocaine and amphetamines can be found in the urine for between 2 and 4 days after use. Cannabis can be found up to 5 days after use in a casual occasional user but can be found up to 30 days after discontinuation of use in a former heavy user. Benzodiazepines are found for 3 days after short-term use, but up to 6 weeks after long-term chronic use.

Table 24.4 Key types of drug testing with detection times and reliability

Type of test	Detection time[a]	Reliability
Urine	2/3 days	Most researched; has been around for 20 years; best test for cannabis use; sample needs to be stored and preserved properly; most open to fraud (substitution of samples); positive result needs laboratory confirmation
Oral fluid	24 hours	Good for recent drug use (cannabis and opiates in particular) but a mouthwash would defeat on-site detection; samples may need refrigeration; dipsticks can be used for on-site results (e.g. can test saliva at the road side); positive tests need to be confirmed
Sweat	24 hours to 2–3 days	Drug patches used mainly for monitoring; when worn, can detect up to a week; drug swipes can detect other use (last 24 hours) but not very reliably
Blood	Up to 31 hours	Vulnerable to fraud; sample needs careful storage and preservation; needs laboratory analysis; on-site results not available
Hair	1 week to 18 months	Cannot detect alcohol; needs laboratory analysis

[a] Length of time test remains positive following drug use.

Adapted with permission from *DrugLink* March/April 2004; 19(2), © DrugScope 2004.

Cut-off levels

The cut-off levels for positivity differ between international authorities. For example, in the USA, SAMHSA has set a much higher cut-off level for opiates in urine (2000 ng/mL) than is set in Europe (300 ng/mL). This is to allow for the possibility of poppy seed in the diet.

Chain of custody

One key aspect of drug testing is to maintain the 'chain of custody'. This is a process that ensures results can indisputably be connected with the person who produced the test sample. It includes the requirement for secure storage of samples. The procedures are based on those used for handling forensic samples.

Refusal of testing

The drug and alcohol policy must include the action to be taken in the event of refusal of a worker to provide a sample. Normally refusal or evidence of adulteration should be regarded as a 'non-negative' or positive sample and appropriate action taken.

Medical Review Officer

The Medical Review Officer (MRO) is a doctor or forensic pathologist who can issue a negative report for a positive analytical result.[29] Where a drug test is classified as positive following laboratory analysis, good practice requires that medical review is arranged. The purpose of this is to tell the individual of the result and confirm that the positive result came from a drug, usually an illicit drug, which was not prescribed by the general practitioner (GP) or other specialist. This advice is based on consultation with the individual, their GP, the laboratory toxicologist, and any information provided at the time the test was undertaken. This stage is an important check. Codeine use, for example, often results in a positive analytical test but a negative report following MRO review.

The experience, skills, and knowledge to undertake the MRO role are covered by US guidelines; as yet these are not well defined in Europe. Training courses on medical review are available in the UK. The company occupational physician is well placed to be the MRO, particularly where individual interviews are concerned, but must avoid giving medical advice when in this role.

Interpretation of results

The interpretation of results for drug tests cannot usually be taken further than confirmation that the drug was taken. Unlike alcohol, it is not usually possible to relate the result to a quantitative estimate of the degree of impairment of performance at the time at which testing was conducted. A positive result may indicate a large dose taken some time ago or a small dose taken recently, and often it is not possible to establish which one of these is the case. One of the underlying objections to the use of drug testing in the workplace is the problem of interpretation. One of the arguments for using oral fluid testing for drugs, rather than urine testing, is that the tests remain positive for a much shorter time and are therefore more likely to be associated with actual impairment in the workplace.

Management of a positive result

The consequences of a positive result, confirmed by the MRO, will depend on the policy of the employer. It can range from no action being taken, through the provision of assistance in addressing an alcohol or drug problem to disciplinary action leading to loss of job. It is important that the employer has decided and communicated to employees the consequences of a positive drug test before drug testing is introduced.

Role of occupational health departments in a drug and alcohol testing programme

There are differences of opinion as to the involvement of occupational health teams in drug and alcohol testing in the workplace, which is a balance between avoiding a perception of acting in a policing capacity and maintaining the trust of the workforce. However, they may be better placed than an external contractor to ensure the process is carried out in a fair way and to acceptable professional standards. There is a requirement for medical involvement in drug screening programmes and there are benefits in maintaining an in-house MRO. If the OH team is involved, they must not assist in determining who is tested or have any part in the disciplinary process as this will compromise their professional relationship with employees

In pre-employment screening, which can be done at the same time as the standard new entrant medical assessment, the drug screening process should be regarded as a management responsibility, delegated to the occupational health department. Separation of function can be achieved by separately reporting results so that the drug screening test is not perceived as part of the clinical procedure. It is possible to delegate collection of samples for 'random' and 'for cause' testing to an external company which might avoid any concerns over separation of policing and rehabilitation roles. If this is the case, the occupational physician should be involved in selection of the company and agreeing the necessary procedures.

Testing for impairment

As discussed earlier, breathalyser testing for alcohol can be related to impaired performance, but the same is not true of the results of most other types of testing for drugs in the workplace.

Direct tests of impairment would be more acceptable, and could be followed up with a drug test if impairment were demonstrated. Although there is potential for this in the future and various tests have been trialled in the USA, within the UK it is only possible to say whether drugs are present rather than what their effect is.

Conclusions

The management of work-related drug and alcohol problems and misuse requires careful consideration, a high level of people management skills, and up-to-date knowledge of what is good practice. It is an area where even the most experienced managers, occupational health specialists, and addiction specialists sometimes struggle. It is important that processes are carefully developed and then regularly reviewed with full involvement of all stakeholders.

Useful websites

<http://www.alcoholconcern.org.uk> Alcohol Concern website.

<http://www.drugsmeter.com> Self-help resource.

<http://www.drugscope.org.uk> UK independent centre of expertise on drugs.

<http://www.ewdts.org> European Workplace Drug Testing Forum.

<http://www.hse.gov.uk> Information and resources on drugs and alcohol at work.

<http://www.ilo.org> An international perspective.

<http://www.talktofrank.com> Resources on recognizing effects and risks of drugs and alcohol.

References

1 UK Government Strategy Unit. *National harm reduction strategy. Interim analysis. Executive summary*, 2003. [Online] (<http://www.number-10.gov.uk/output/Page77.asp>)
2 Alcohol Concern. *Factsheet: alcohol in the workplace*. Cardiff: Alcohol Concern, 2009.
3 Cabinet Office Strategy Unit. *Interim analytical report*. London: Cabinet Office, 2003.
4 Office of National Statistics. *Public service output, inputs and productivity: healthcare triangulation*. London: Office of National Statistics, 2010. (<http://statistics.gov.uk/pdfdir/ghs0109.pdf>)
5 Romeri E, Baker A, Griffiths C. Alcohol-related deaths by occupation, England and Wales, 2001–05. *Health Stat Quart* 2007; **35**: 6–12.
6 Henderson A, Langston V, Greenberg N. Alcohol misuse in the Royal Navy. *Occup Med* 2009; **59**(2): 5–32.
7 Jones E, Fear NT. Alcohol use and misuse in the military – a review. *Int Rev Psych* 2011; **23**: 166–72.
8 Smith K, Flatley J (eds). *Findings from the 2010/11 British Crime Survey England and Wales*. London: Home Office Statistical Bulletin, 2011. (<http://www.homeoffice.gov.uk/publications/science-research-statistics/research-statistics/crime-research/hosb1211/hosb1211?view = Binary>)
9 Coomber R. *A literature review for the independent inquiry into drug testing at work*. Available from Drugscope, 2003. (<http://www.drugscope.org.uk/>).
10 Smith A, Wadsworth E, Moss S, *et al*. *The scale and impact of illegal drug use by workers*. Norwich: HSE Books, 2004.
11 Melzer H, Gill B, Pettigrew M, Hinds K. *OPCS surveys of psychiatric morbidity in Great Britain. Report 1 the prevalence of psychiatric morbidity among adults living in private households*. London: HMSO, 1995.
12 HM Government. *Drug Strategy 2010*. London: Home Office, 2010.
13 Davenport M, Harris D. The effect of low blood alcohol levels on pilot performance in a series of simulated approach and landing trials. *Int J Aviat Psychol* 1992; **2**: 271–80.

14 Whitfield, JB. Gamma glutamyl transferase. critical reviews in clinical laboratory sciences 2001; **38**(4): 263–355.

15 Zwerling C. *Current practice and experience on drug and alcohol testing in the workplace*. Geneva: International Labor Office, 1993.

16 Calder IM, Ramsey J. A survey of cannabis use in offshore rig workers. *Br J Addict* 1987; **82**: 159–61.

17 Yesavage JA, Leirer VO, Denari M, *et al*. Carry-over effects of marijuana intoxication on aircraft pilot performance: a preliminary report. *Am J Psychiatry* 1985; **142**: 1325–9.

18 Department for Transport. *Cannabis and driving: a review of the literature and commentary (12)*. London: Department for Transport Report, 2003. (<http://www.dft.gov.uk>)

19 Skegg DCG, Richards SM, Doll R. Minor tranquillisers and road accidents. *BMJ* 1979; **1**: 917–19.

20 Hindmarch I.The effects of psychoactive drugs on car handling and related psychomotor ability. In: O'Hanlon JF, de Gier JJ (eds), *Drugs and driving*, pp. 71–9. London: Taylor and Francis, 1986.

21 Department of Environment. *Railway accident report on collision at Glasgow Central Station on 29 March 1974*. London: Department of Environment, 1975.

22 Ravera S, van Rein N, de Gier JJ, *et al*. Road traffic accidents and psychotropic medication use in the Netherlands: a case-control study. *Br J Clin Pharmacol* 2011; **72**(3); 505–13.

23 Joseph Rowntree Foundation Drug and alcohol research programme. *Drug testing at work. Report of independent inquiry into drug testing at work*. York: York Publishing Services Ltd, 2004. (<http://www.jrf.org.uk>)

24 Head J, Martikainen P, Kumari M, *et al*. *Work environment, alcohol consumption and ill-health. The Whitehall II study*. Norwich: HSE Books, 2002.

25 Chartered Institute of Personnel and Development. *Managing drug and alcohol misuse at work*. London: Chartered Institute of Personnel and Development, 2007.

26 Faculty of Occupational Medicine. *Guidance on drug and alcohol misuse in the workplace*. London: Faculty of Occupational Medicine, 2006.

27 Wolff K, Walsham N, Gross S, *et al*. *Road safety research report no. 103. The role of carbohydrate deficient transferrin as an alternative to gamma glutamyl transferase as a biomarker of continuous drinking: a literature review*. London: Department for Transport, 2010.

28 Driving and Vehicle Licensing Agency. *At a glance guide to the current medical standards of fitness to drive*. Swansea: DVLA, 2011

29 Akrill P, Mason H. *Review of drug testing methodologies, prepared for Railway Safety and Standards Board*. London: Health and Safety Laboratory, 2005.

30 Information Commissioner. *The employment practices data protection code: part 4 information about workers' health*. Wilmslow: Information Commissioner, 2004.

31 Information Commissioner. *Quick guide to employment practice codes*. Wilmslow: Information Commissioner, 2011.

32 Francis P, Hanley N, Wray D. *A literature review on the international state of knowledge of drug testing at work, with particular reference to the US*. Newcastle: University of Northumbria, 2003. (<http://www.drugscope.org.uk/>)

33 Edwards G, Gross MM. Alcohol dependence: provisional description of a clinical syndrome. *BMJ* 1976; **i**: 1058–61.

34 Fact Sheet. *DrugLink* 2004; **19**(2). Reproduced in IIDTW (Ref 23).

35 Miller FG. SASSI: application and assessment for substance-related problems. *J Substance Misuse* 1997; **2**: 163–6.

36 Poorny AD, Miller BA, Kaplan HB. The brief MAST: a shortened version of the Michigan Alcoholism Screening Test. *Am J Psychiatry* 1972; **129**: 342–5.

37 Babor TF, de la Fuente JR, Saunders J, *et al*. *AUDIT The Alcohol Use Disorders Identification Test. Guidelines for use in primary health care*. Geneva: World Health Organization, 1992.

Chapter 25

Medication and health in the workplace

Caroline L. Swales and Jeffrey K. Aronson

Medication allows many to pursue productive employment when they would otherwise be unable to work safely and effectively, particularly older workers who represent an increasing part of the workforce. Others require short courses of medicines which can occasionally cause harm. Although occupational health clinicians are generally not regular prescribers, they have a vital role in ensuring safe use of medications at work. Here we review the positive and negative effects of medication in the workplace and consider how occupational health can support employees taking medications.

Epidemiology of medication use

The use of medications continues to rise in developed countries. The number of prescription items dispensed by community pharmacies in England in contract with Primary Care Trusts (PCTs) to dispense National Health Service (NHS) prescriptions was 510 million in 2000–2001 and 813 million in 2009–2010, a 59 per cent increase.[1] The total cost of UK NHS prescriptions at 2010 prices rose from £9.4 billion in 2000 to £12.4 billion (about £200 per head) in 2010.[2] In 1995, the working population in England received six prescriptions per head while elderly people received 22 prescriptions per head.[3] This figure will increase further as the working population ages. Increased use of medications will probably cause more adverse reactions. Prescribing patterns have also changed, and the use of prescription-only medicines (PoMs) increases with age, whereas over-the-counter (OTC) purchases reduce.

Medication prevalence in the workplace

In a 1972 study,[4] 55 per cent of a sample population had taken or used some medication during the 24 hours before the interview; in a later study,[5] 20 per cent of a factory population were taking medications, and in 1999, 22 per cent of employees at a chemical plant had taken a PoM and 27 per cent an OTC medicine in the preceding fortnight.[6]

Classification of medications

There are three legitimate ways of obtaining licensed medicines in the UK, defined in the 1968 Medicines Act (Box 25.1). Medications are most commonly taken orally; other routes include inhaled, topical, transdermal, intravenous, subcutaneous, and intramuscular routes, and administration by pessary or suppository.

Box 25.1 Ways of obtaining licensed medicines in the UK

1 PoM: prescription-only medicines from qualified prescribers (doctors, dentists, nurse or pharmacist independent prescribers, or supplementary prescribers).

2 P: pharmacy-only medicines, obtained without a prescription from, or under the supervision of a qualified pharmacist.

3 GSL: general sales list medicines, obtained without a prescription from, for example, a pharmacy or a supermarket.

P and GSL (over-the-counter) medicines can also be prescribed in the usual way.

Reclassification

Reclassification of many PoMs to pharmacy use in the 1980s led to easier accessibility to some drugs, with potentially hazardous effects.[7] Pharmacists had to provide increasing amounts of customer advice, leading to greater emphasis on communication and counselling skills in pharmacy courses,[8] and also a requirement from the Royal Pharmaceutical Society for counter staff to undertake accredited training programmes.[9] Medications are also available now for purchase via the Internet, requiring electronic advice in public information resources. No data from a central source are as yet available for access to Internet resources, but in 1999, 30 per cent of employees taking OTC medications had not read the information provided, of whom 57 per cent were taking OTCs that could have caused adverse reactions.[6]

Harms from medications

Workers need to fulfil their duties safely, effectively, and responsibly. Harms from medications that are trivial for non-workers can affect employees' safety. Common reasons for adverse events are listed in Box 25.2.

Classification of adverse drug reactions

Harms from medications can be categorized as adverse effects (the physiological or pathological effects that drugs have at the molecular, cellular, or tissue levels) and adverse reactions (the signs and symptoms that occur as a result). The modern classifications of adverse outcomes called EIDOS and DoTS involve descriptions of the mechanisms by which they occur, their clinical features, their uses in pharmacovigilance planning, risk management, and prevention of adverse reactions.[10]

Box 25.2 Common reasons for adverse events

♦ Medications taken at an incorrect time or inappropriately.

♦ Incorrect dosage regimen.

♦ Changes to dosages.

♦ Introduction of a new medication.

♦ Self-prescribing.

Unwanted reactions may also result from interactions with other drugs, herbal medicines, foods, alcohol, specific chemicals at work, and some medical devices. The effects of such reactions on performance are of particular concern in safety critical jobs, (for example, drivers and machine operators).

Frequencies of adverse drug reactions in the workplace

In 1999, 11 per cent of a study population had adverse reactions that they felt could have affected their safety. Of those who reported such reactions, 30 per cent were working in high-risk occupations and 25 per cent moderate risk. For men, the most frequent adverse reactions were drowsiness (29 per cent), poor concentration (18 per cent), and dizziness (12 per cent). Among women, visual deterioration was the most common adverse reaction. Of those with adverse reactions, only 40 per cent informed any medical personnel, and only 23 per cent informed occupational health. Such reactions may be minimized by better understanding of their mechanisms, better reporting of reactions by employees, and much improved guidance on using OTC medicines.

Patient information

European Commission (EC) Directive 92/97 requires information, including a description of possible adverse reactions, to be provided for the consumer, either in a leaflet or on the packaging, for all medicines licensed by the Medicines and Healthcare products Regulatory Agency (MHRA) including PoM, P, and GSL medicines. The MHRA is an executive agency of the Department of Health, responsible for ensuring that medicines and medical devices work and are acceptably safe (<http://www.mhra.gov.uk>).

In a study of PoMs used by employees in a chemical plant,[6] 74 per cent reported having read and understood advisory information, 17 per cent had not understood, and 6.5 per cent had not consulted the information; 75 per cent reported that their general practitioner (GP) had not warned them about possible adverse reactions that could affect safety at work; of these, 43 per cent were taking medications with potentially disabling adverse effects.

Clinical pharmacology relevant to harms

Drug elimination

Drugs are eliminated by the kidneys and liver and in the lungs, saliva, sweat, and breast milk. Many drugs are inactivated by hepatic detoxification and the metabolites are primarily excreted via the bile and kidneys. Hepatic and renal impairment can reduce the elimination of drugs and doses should be altered accordingly.

Drug interactions

Drug interactions occur when one drug (the precipitant or perpetrator drug) alters the disposition or actions of another (the object or victim drug). Certain foods can also be precipitants.

Drugs that commonly interact with other medications include:

◆ Drugs that act as hepatic enzyme inhibitors, such as erythromycin, fluconazole, and ritonavir, which increase the effects of other medications, such as warfarin.

◆ Diuretics, such as hydrochlorothiazide and furosemide, which can cause hyponatraemia and hypokalaemia and potentiate the actions of lithium and digoxin respectively.

Dietary effects include:

♦ Inhibition of gut and liver enzymes by grapefruit, reducing the metabolism of many medications, including ciclosporin, felodipine, nifedipine, and carbamazepine.

♦ Hypertension due to monoamines in foods, such as red wine and hung meats, when taken with monoamine oxidase inhibitors.

♦ Reduced absorption of antibiotics, such as tetracycline and ciprofloxacin, when taken with milk or antacids.

♦ Additive effects of alcohol with other central nervous system (CNS) depressants, such as antipsychotic drugs and antihistamines.

Abuse of medications

Problems can arise from abuse of prescribed or unprescribed drugs, often associated with impaired mental health. Alcohol abuse in the UK is more common than abuse of other drugs, of which cannabis is the commonest. In a 2004 HSE study, 13 per cent of working respondents reported drug abuse in the previous year.[11]

Influence of legislation/guidance

The Health and Safety at Work etc. Act 1974[12] and the Management of Health and Safety at Work Regulations, 1999 require employees to take reasonable care of their own health and safety and that of any other person who may be affected by their actions or omissions at work. These provisions encompass medications and their effects. Furthermore, employers risk prosecution if they knowingly allow employees who misuse drugs, and whose behaviour places them or others at risk, to continue working.

The Equality Act 2010 (see also Chapter 3)

The Equality Act prohibits discrimination and requires employers to make reasonable adjustments to enable qualifying employees to remain at work.[13] Such adjustments may relate to the actions of medications. The successful control of a disability by medications does not invalidate the protection afforded to the employee by the Equality Act, if there is evidence that the employee would be significantly affected if their treatment was discontinued. In addition, whereas drug addiction is normally excluded from the Act, any addiction that was originally the result of medically prescribed drugs or other medical treatment is covered. While the Equality Act prohibits employers from asking applicants about their health before offering positions, those who apply for safety critical roles should still have pre-placement assessments, with opportunities to discuss prescription medications. There is also standardized/national guidance or specific screening for some employment, reducing the likelihood that the effects of medications will remain unrecognized.

SEQOHS standards

National accreditation standards are being introduced to support the achievement of Safe Effective Quality Occupational Health Services (SEQOHS), including standards for management of medications relating to storage and dispensing. Section D4 describes the minimum advisory standards.[14]

Effects of medications on performance

Performance testing

Testing the effects of a specific drug on performance can be complex and time consuming. Tests fall into two categories: those that measure the effects of drugs on individual components of psychomotor function and those that measure their effects on activities of everyday life, such as driving. It is difficult to simulate most working conditions, other than flying and driving, and laboratory testing is relied on. There is much evidence that laboratory tests of psychomotor function can reliably detect the effects of drugs that may affect activities such as driving. Laboratory tests of psychomotor function include cognitive information processing, short-term memory and learning, motor functions, and activities involving sensory, central, and motor abilities. In theory, similar approaches could be used to screen workers taking essential long-term medications, such as anticonvulsants, in safety critical professions. However, marked variability in responses between individuals reduces the precision of such tests.

Comparatively little is known about the effects of antidepressants on cognition and performance, particularly in depressed patients, as most studies have been performed in healthy volunteers. In such studies, the effects on performance largely correlate with the sedative properties of the antidepressants, but this produces such blanket impairment that more detailed testing of the finer points of cognition is often precluded.

The Institute of Aviation has developed a list of safe medicines for pilots, and the Department of Transport Research Laboratories have designed a battery of sensitive tests for measuring driving impairment by drugs and alcohol.

Circadian rhythms

Circadian variation affects performance. Scores for most simple tasks peak at 12.00–21.00 hours and fall to a minimum at 03.00–06.00 hours,[15] correlating with body temperature. There is diurnal variation in pulmonary function, and circadian rhythms may affect administration of asthma medications and the timing of medical procedures, particularly since patients with asthma have nocturnal worsening of pulmonary function and an early morning dip in peak expiratory flow rate.

Performance can be affected by shift working and travel across time zones, causing fatigue, disorientation, and insomnia. Whilst adaptation occurs within a few days employees are often required to work shortly after arrival. Additional health effects can occur through poorer control of a health condition, because of altered timing of medication. There is evidence that melatonin, properly administered, and other measures can mitigate the effects of jet lag.[16]

Circadian rhythms can influence the effects of some medications;[17] for example, serum amitriptyline concentrations are higher after a morning dose than an evening dose;[18] however, the most significant effects are associated with the effects of medications on circadian variation, for example, responses to corticosteroids.

Occupational exposures and medications

Exposure to harmful substances at work should be controlled by protective measures, but workplace exposure limits have generally been derived from animal experiments and experiments on humans not taking medications. Work environments that can influence medications include extremes of temperature, when adverse reactions can occur, particularly to cardiovascular medications; when there has been an unexpected or unknown exposure to CNS depressants, such as solvents; and when unknown exposure has occurred to gases or fumes. Interaction with a CNS depressant may increase the risk. Many environmental chemicals are also enzyme inducers, including polycyclic aromatic hydrocarbons, organochlorines, and organophosphorus compounds. Workers engaged in pesticide manufacture may have enzyme induction.[19] Organophosphorus compounds inhibit the enzyme cholinesterase, leading to accumulation of acetylcholine in nerve tissues and other organs, with effects on many systems. Employees working in the manufacture of pharmaceuticals and staff handing cytotoxic drugs in the workplace require appropriate safety measures to reduce exposure and avoid adverse reactions that can result in further harm when other medications are used.

Effects of medications on specific occupations

Medications may affect cognition, mobility, and dexterity, and therefore actions such as walking, driving, sitting, and the operation of computerized equipment. There should be a focus on maintaining such functions despite the effects of medications. Not all occupations have regulated and standardized guidance in relation to medication and fitness to work, and there is a requirement to establish standards for employees in some safety critical roles. An outline is provided here, and the reader is referred to specific chapters for comprehensive guidance.

Drivers

With over 21 million private driving licences in the UK, doctors should assume that most of their adult patients drive, some of whom will drive for work. Drowsiness is a major cause of road traffic accidents (RTAs) and may be aggravated or caused by medications. A driver may not only fall asleep but also suffer loss of attention or slowing of reactions during critical driving manoeuvres. Sedation caused by benzodiazepines results in compromised steering, road positioning and reaction times in both laboratory and road tests.[20] A study in Dundee [21] showed a significant increase in the risk of RTAs among those taking anxiolytic benzodiazepines and the short-acting hypnotic zopiclone; users of hypnotic benzodiazepines were not at increased risk. The authors suggested that anyone taking long half-life anxiolytic benzodiazepines or zopiclone should be advised not to drive. Zopiclone, a cyclopyrrolone that acts on the same receptors as benzodiazepines, had residual effects that impaired driving, despite a relatively short half-life (5 hours). There was no increase in rates of RTAs among users of tricyclic antidepressants or selective serotonin re-uptake inhibitors.

Section 4 of the Road Traffic Act 1988 does not differentiate between illicit and prescribed drugs; hence, anyone in an unfit condition is liable to prosecution. The Poisons Rule (1972) requires a number of substances containing antihistamines to be labelled with the words 'Caution, may cause drowsiness; if affected do not drive or operate machinery'. A Driver and Vehicle Licensing Agency (DVLA) publication provides guidance on the fitness to drive for Group 1 or Group 2 licences.[22] Advice from the Drivers Medical Unit of the DVLA for medical practitioners on medication, states that:

♦ Driving while unfit through drugs, provided or illicit, is an offence and may lead to prosecution.

♦ Doctors have a duty of care to advise their patients of the potential dangers of adverse effects from medications and interactions with other substances, especially alcohol.

♦ All CNS-active drugs can impair alertness, concentration, and driving performance, particularly within the first month of starting or increasing the dose. It is important to stop driving during this time if adversely affected.

- Benzodiazepines are the most likely psychotropic drugs to impair driving performance, particularly the long-acting compounds. Alcohol potentiates their effects.
- Drivers with psychiatric illnesses are often safer when well and taking regular psychotropic medications than when they are ill.
- Antipsychotic drugs, including depot formulations, can cause motor or extrapyramidal effects, as well as sedation or poor concentration, which may, either alone or in combination, be sufficient to impair driving.
- The older tricyclic antidepressants can have pronounced anticholinergic and antihistaminic effects, which may impair driving. The more modern antidepressants may have fewer effects.
- The epileptogenic potential of psychotropic medications should be considered, particularly when patients are professional drivers.

DVLA Group 2 drivers

Stricter criteria apply to certain drivers (Group 2), including those who drive large goods vehicles and taxis, since they drive for longer hours and are at greater risks of the effects of adverse drug reactions or interactions. In the case of short-term medications, if it seems likely that the treatment might impair driving, it is safest to certify the driver as unfit for an initial period. If treatment has to continue, a decision about returning to driving is then taken, with awareness of any adverse reactions that may have occurred during the initial stage of treatment. If long-term medication is required, both the medical condition and the prescribed treatment should be considered in respect of Group 2 driving.

Shift workers

Sixteen per cent of all UK employees are shift workers. Shift working itself can cause sleepiness, and additive effects can occur from medications because of adverse reactions or hangover effects. Shift patterns and changes to them should be discussed with the prescribing physician and occupational health. The Working Time Regulations 1998 require employers to carry out periodic health assessments for night workers, which should take account of medications and their effects.

Physicians

Physicians have professional responsibilities, as determined by the General Medical Council, to safeguard their own health. They should also be registered with a GP. Nevertheless, inappropriate self-treatment by physicians is widespread and is a serious threat to professionalism.[23,24] In a survey of the attitudes of trainee GPs to self-care, 30 per cent had not consulted a GP within the previous 5 years, 65 per cent felt unable to take time off when ill, and 92 per cent self-prescribed medications on at least one occasion. Almost half felt that they neglected their own health. While many clinicians do seek appropriate advice, interventions to raise awareness and to manage the problem of self-treatment are required, such as access to occupational health.

Occupational travellers

Fatigue, changes in time zones and climate, and altered dietary and fluid intake can all affect control of medical conditions and the effects of medications. Careful preparation is essential in relation to health and provision of medical care overseas. It is advisable not to start new prescription medications shortly before travel, in case of adverse reactions, and to ensure that medical conditions are under good control. When necessary, advice should be sought from a travel medicine clinic, GP, or occupational health.

Aircrew (see also Appendix 1)

Any medications that reduce performance are considered hazardous to aircrew, including OTC medications. The Air Navigation Order states that individuals are not entitled to act as flight crew members or as air traffic control officers if they know or suspect that they may be unfit to do so. The Civil Aviation Authority's circular *Modern Medical Practice and Flight*,[25] states that 'any regular use of medication' requires the advice of a CAA authorized medical examiner (AME) before duty resumes. Changes in medications or dosages may temporarily affect fitness to fly. Environmental factors, such as changes of pressure, gravity, and temperature, can all affect performance and add to the effects of medications.

Restrictions to flying are required for the following medications:

◆ *Potent analgesics.*

◆ *Tranquillizers, antidepressants, and sedatives*: owing to their effects on performance, although the pilot's underlying mental state may also be incompatible with flying. Temazepam is the only hypnotic approved by the RAF for pilot use, although it can only be taken occasionally and should not be taken less than 12 hours before flying. It is short acting (4–6 hours) and reportedly has no residual effects on performance.[26,27]

◆ *Stimulants (for example, caffeine and amphetamine)*: the use of such 'pep' pills while flying is not permitted.

◆ *Anaesthetics*: at least 24 hours should elapse before return to flying after a local anaesthetic and 48 hours after a general anaesthetic.

Advice from an AME is also required for:

◆ *Antihypertensive drugs*: unexpected hypertension is a restriction to flying; advice about treatment is required from the AME before returning to flying.

◆ *Antihistamines*: the less sedative medications are required.

Similar advice is given by the CAA regarding medications and air traffic controllers.[26] This guidance also advises against the use of pseudoephedrine for nasal congestion, because of adverse reactions, such as anxiety, tremor, and tachycardia.

The position regarding cabin crew is different; such staff are unlicensed, and each company sets its own health standards. However, Air Navigation (No. 2) Order 1995: article 57(2) states:

> A person shall not, when acting as a member of the crew of any aircraft or being carried in any aircraft for the purpose of so acting, be under the influence of drink or a drug to such an extent as to impair his capacity so to act.

The CAA publication Safety Sense Leaflet 24 *Pilot Health* provides further advice on medications and flying.[28]

Merchant navy employees (see also Appendix 2)

The fitness of merchant seafarers is subject to regular approved doctor medicals. Having sufficient supplies of treatment while at sea is important. When medications are acceptable for use, reserve stocks may be held with the agreement of the ship's master.

Malaria prophylaxis

Recommended malaria prophylaxis varies according to the destination and the local sensitivity of the parasite. Specialist travel advice must be sought. Drug prophylaxis should ideally begin a week before travel, although a fortnight is advised for mefloquine. Medication should be continued for at least 4 weeks after returning. See Appendix 5 for advice regarding medical care of overseas employees.

Offshore workers (see also Appendix 3)

The UK Offshore Operators Association provides *Guidance for medical aspects of fitness for offshore work*. Referring to medications, it states the following:

♦ Individuals taking anticoagulants, cytotoxic agents, insulin, anticonvulsants, immunosuppressants, and oral steroids are unacceptable for offshore work.

♦ Individuals on psychotropic medications, for example, tranquillizers, antidepressants, narcotics, and hypnotics, are also unacceptable and a previous history of such treatment will require further consideration.

♦ Individuals taking medications must ensure they have an adequate supply and must report any adverse drug reactions to the offshore medic.

Divers (see also Appendix 4)

Any medication that reduces performance is a potential hazard to divers. Environmental hazards of temperature, pressure, and the use of gas combinations, for example, oxygen/helium, may cause further problems. Form MA1 from the Employment Medical Advisory Service (EMAS) on the medical examination of divers, provides further guidance: 'The diver should be asked specifically for details of any current medication'. The effects and use of drugs can cause practical problems when treating sick divers under hyperbaric conditions. Cox[29] lists drugs that have been used by divers, the depths to which they have been used, and the extent of any untoward effects. Those who work in the Norwegian and Dutch sectors of the North Sea come within similar legislation in those countries.

Management of clinical conditions

There can be a fine balance between the need to manage a condition by medication and the risk of adverse reactions. Patients who have an unfavourable response to a particular medication may be impaired by both the medication and the disease, and the most hazardous effects involve impaired function in safety critical roles. Particular attention should be paid to the benefit to harm balance with psychological medications, strong analgesics, and cardiovascular medications. The following is an overview of specific effects of medications for some of the more common disorders.

Central nervous system

For mental health conditions, the ability to maintain employment depends on the effectiveness of the treatment in reducing any performance and behavioural aspects of the condition while trying to limit adverse drug reactions. This is particularly the case for bipolar disorder.

Antidepressants

The major classes of antidepressants are the tricyclics, the selective serotonin re-uptake inhibitors (SSRIs), and the serotonin-noradrenaline reuptake inhibitors (SNRIs). Many produce sedation, especially at the start of treatment, which is markedly potentiated by alcohol. Amitriptyline and doxepin are the most sedative tricyclics and imipramine and nortriptyline the least. The

SSRIs, such as fluoxetine and paroxetine, and the SNRIs, such as venlafaxine, do not usually produce sedation and appear to have little effect on performance. Monoamine oxidase inhibitors, although now rarely used, have a stimulant effect, although phenelzine can sometimes be sedative. Tolerance to these sedative effects usually develops. Consider appropriate restrictions in employees who could be affected by sedation during the first few treatment days. Tricyclic antidepressants with anticholinergic effects produce blurring of near vision, and can cause a tremor, potentially affecting work performance. Hyponatraemia due to inappropriate secretion of antidiuretic hormone has been associated with all antidepressants, but is more common with SSRIs. Severe hypertension can occur if monoamine oxidase inhibitors interact with certain foods or drugs, such as mature cheese or pethidine.

Hypnotics and sedatives

Hypnotics and sedatives are CNS depressants and most can inhibit psychomotor function, retard responsiveness, and impair motor skills, coordination, and responses concerned with self-preservation. As a result, they may affect ability for safety critical roles. The duration of effect depends on the half-life of the drug, but most hypnotics produce residual effects the following morning, which may impair tasks such as driving. Effects persist during long-term administration and tolerance or habituation can occur; it is more marked in elderly patients and is potentiated by alcohol.

Barbiturates, rarely used today, have a larger effect on performance than benzodiazepines. Individual benzodiazepines differ in their effects on psychomotor performance; as hypnotics, short-acting drugs, such as temazepam, are less likely than nitrazepam to have hangover effects; as anxiolytics, clobazam appears to have less effect on performance, particularly memory, than lorazepam and diazepam. Benzodiazepines and newer hypnotics and anxiolytics, such as zaleplon, zolpidem, and zopiclone (the 'Z drugs') can also cause dizziness, light-headedness, confusion, and visual disturbances. Benzodiazepine withdrawal can produce a characteristic syndrome, including anxiety, sleeplessness, perceptual disturbances, and depersonalization; withdrawal should be controlled.

Antipsychotic drugs

Antipsychotic drugs include the phenothiazines (such as chlorpromazine), the butyrophenones (such as haloperidol), and similar drugs (such as pimozide and fluspirilene); so-called 'atypical drugs' include clozapine, olanzapine, risperidone, and quetiapine. Many impair psychomotor performance, depending on the degree of sedation produced. Flupentixol has a predominantly alerting effect and hence less effect on performance than the more sedative phenothiazines. Such effects should be considered when advising about the risks of employment tasks during antipsychotic drug therapy, maintenance of performance being a balance between benefit and adverse reactions.

Extrapyramidal symptoms, such as Parkinsonian symptoms and tardive dyskinesia, are common effects of fluphenazine and haloperidol and can interfere significantly with performance. Interference with hypothalamic temperature regulation and cholinergic control of sweating can occur in locations with extreme environmental temperatures, leading to hypo or hyperthermia. Visual disturbances can occur with chlorpromazine and thioridazine; chlorpromazine causes blurred vision, and corneal and lens opacities are possible with chronic high-dose therapy. Thioridazine can cause a pigmentary retinopathy and reduced visual acuity.

Lithium

Specialist prescription and careful monitoring is required for treatment of bipolar disorder with lithium, owing to its narrow therapeutic/toxic ratio. Toxicity is aggravated by hyponatraemia; diuretics should be avoided and adequate fluid intake maintained, with avoidance of dietary changes that might alter sodium intake. Postural hypotension can cause problems, particularly in hot environments. Lithium can also cause polyuria and polydipsia, resulting in further toxicity, and also confusion with symptoms of diabetes and renal or prostatic disease. Lithium is associated with only mild cognitive and memory impairment during long-term use, but reduced performance, increased morbidity, and sickness absence can result because of adverse reactions.

Antiepileptic drugs

Antiepileptic drugs allow normal careers for most epilepsy sufferers, although some employees' occupations will be affected. The most hazardous time is during dosage adjustment, when safety critical roles should be restricted. Employees require appropriate monitoring to ensure that plasma concentrations remain within the target ranges. Employees on well-controlled, long-term monotherapy usually have few adverse reactions. Studies of cognitive function in healthy volunteers and patients taking chronic anticonvulsant therapy have shown some impairment of cognition and concentration but impairment is greater in patients taking polytherapy, with increased effects with phenytoin than carbamazepine. Excessive doses of phenytoin, carbamazepine, and newer drugs such as lamotrigine or gabapentin can produce drowsiness, tremor, ataxia, and double vision. Lamotrigine is also now licensed for use as a mood stabilizer.

Antihistamines

Antihistamines are used in the treatment of allergic rhinitis, pruritus, insect stings and bites, and the prevention of urticaria. They are available in a variety of formulations and OTC. Most older compounds are short-acting and associated with sedation and antimuscarinic effects, such as dry mouth and blurred vision; they also potentiate the actions of alcohol. The newer, non-sedating antihistamines, such as cetirizine, fexofenadine, and desloratadine, cause less sedation and psychomotor impairment. Antihistamines that produce less blurred vision and sedation are recommended when driving cannot be avoided; otherwise, employees should be warned that their ability to drive or operate machinery is likely to be impaired.

Antimigraine drugs

The $5HT_1$ agonists (such as naratriptan, sumatriptan, and zolmitriptan), used to treat acute migraine, can cause drowsiness and should be used with care in patients with cardiac disease. Other drugs, such as isometheptene and pizotifen are associated with dizziness and postural hypotension.

Drugs for Parkinson's disease

Parkinson's disease is the second commonest neurodegenerative disorder after Alzheimer's disease; 40 per cent of those affected are under 65 years and 5–10 per cent under 45 years. 60 per cent can have depression, and cognitive problems can be the first effect noticed at work. Levodopa, the mainstay of treatment, improves motor function; occasionally it may cause confusion or hallucinations. Younger patients are more likely to be taking a dopamine receptor agonist, and

10 per cent can be affected by dopamine dysregulation syndrome, which includes pathological gambling and overspending without insight, for which the risk is highest at the start of treatment and times of dosage change. It can take time to achieve the optimum treatment regimen. Hypotensive reactions can occur during the initial days of treatment with dopamine receptor agonists and sometimes with levodopa and selegiline; hence, particular care should be taken when driving or operating machinery at such times. Blurred vision can complicate the use of most anti-Parkinsonism drugs, including amantadine and antimuscarinic drugs, such as benzhexol. It is rare to see advanced Parkinson's disease or the Parkinson's plus syndromes in the workplace, owing to their marked effects on function.

Medications for multiple sclerosis

Multiple sclerosis is the commonest neurological condition in young adults (see Chapter 6). Treatment currently focuses on reducing relapse rate; none is available to prevent long-term disability or reverse existing impairment. Natalizumab, an intravenous monoclonal antibody, reduces the relapse rate by 80 per cent, allowing increased function and return to work; it is associated with a 1:1000 risk of progressive multifocal encephalopathy (PML), a fatal viral infection of the brain. Fingolimod, a sphingosine-1-phosphate receptor modulator, is claimed to reduce relapse rates by 60 per cent, can be taken orally, and has not been associated with PML. Employers may need to consider adjustments to allow attendance for injection-administered treatment and absences secondary to side effects from treatment, for instance, the flu-like symptoms associated with interferon.

Stimulants and appetite suppressants

Amphetamines and other stimulants increase risk-taking behaviour, diminishing work performance and safety, especially if combined with alcohol. Their use should be discouraged, as dependence and psychosis may result.

Autonomic nervous system

Antimuscarinic medications (such as oxybutynin and flavoxate for urinary incontinence and pilocarpine for dry mouth) can cause blurred vision, which can affect night driving. Mydriatic eye-drops, such as homatropine and cyclopentolate, paralyse accommodation and produce blurred vision.

Anaesthetics

The effect of anaesthesia on fitness for work relates to recovery time from general anaesthesia. For inpatient anaesthesia, the symptoms of the condition usually necessitate sickness absence until after the anaesthetic effects have abated. Following day surgery, patients should not drive or operate machinery for 24 hours after general anaesthesia; they should be given written instructions at discharge.

Cardiovascular medications

Disabling adverse reactions from cardiovascular medications are relatively uncommon, but dizziness and hypotension can occur, especially when first prescribed. It is advisable to start such medications or to have dose increments at weekends or during breaks in shifts. Visual disturbances may occur with disopyramide, flecainide, propafenone, and the lipid-regulating agent, gemfibrozil, and most patients taking amiodarone develop corneal microdeposits, sometimes with night glare. Fibrates, statins, and dipyridamole can cause myalgia or myositis, which can affect physical performance.

Antihypertensive drugs

Antihypertensive treatment is common in those of working age. Most antihypertensive drugs can cause hypotension, such as alpha-blockers and beta-blockers with vasodilatory properties, such as carvedilol and labetalol. Some beta-blockers also increase the adverse effects of cold exposure. Diuretics increase the risk of dehydration at high temperatures and are not the antihypertensive drugs of choice for employees working in hot environments. Most modern antihypertensive drugs (low-dose thiazides, calcium channel blockers, angiotensin-converting enzyme inhibitors) do not have important central effects and do not appear to affect performance, whereas older drugs, such as methyldopa and clonidine, produce sedation; methyldopa can impair driving performance.

Beta-blockers, especially the more lipophilic agents, such as propranolol, can affect psychomotor functions, which return to normal after about 3 weeks. Aircrew are permitted by the CAA to take specified beta-blockers, but only after careful specialist evaluation and simulation testing. A period of ground duties is necessary after starting treatment, to allow stabilization. In a small proportion of patients, beta-blockers cause adverse reactions that can impair work capacity, such as fatigue (reported in about 5 per cent). Reduced exercise tolerance has been reported with all beta-blockers, without significant differences between cardioselective drugs and non-selective drugs. Both types significantly increase the sense of fatigue during exercise, and a given workload appears subjectively more difficult to achieve. Beta-blockers can produce bronchospasm in susceptible people; this should be considered when prescribing for patients working in irritant atmospheres.

Anticoagulants

Employees taking anticoagulants who perform occupations that involve physical hazards, such as labouring have an increased risk of injury and bleeding. Anticoagulant therapy usually requires only short-term adjustments to an employee's role or alternative duties. Foreign travel requires restriction until dosage stabilization is achieved, and provision of sufficient medications while abroad. The medical problem and the available medical facilities at the destination can determine whether travel is advisable. Specific jobs, because of safety or isolation issues, require particular consideration. Flight crew taking anticoagulants require assessments by an AME; similarly, offshore workers may be restricted because of the risks associated with both the underlying medical condition and the unsupervised taking of anticoagulants for long periods in an isolated environment. Employees are advised to carry anticoagulant treatment cards and to have informed their employer. The British Society for Haematology's guidelines on significant haemorrhage are reproduced in the *British National Formulary*.

Analgesics and non-steroidal anti-inflammatory drugs

Analgesics and non-steroidal anti-inflammatory drugs (NSAIDs) allow many employees to remain productive, by reducing pain and increasing range of movements. The most safety critical adverse reactions are marked sedation and reduced clarity of thought associated with opioid analgesics such as morphine. Employees taking such medications should not undertake safety critical roles. Codeine and dihydrocodeine can affect driving-related skills. The effects vary between employees and between the different strengths of codeine formulations. Alcohol potentiates the effects of all opioid analgesics. NSAIDs, including OTC formulations, such as ibuprofen, can cause dizziness and vertigo. Indometacin impairs laboratory tests of driving-related skills. NSAIDs, even the COX-2 inhibitors, can cause gastrointestinal irritation and sometimes gastric bleeding. High doses of salicylates can be ototoxic and increase the harmful effects of noise exposure. Other drugs used to treat arthropathies can affect morbidity, attendance, and performance. For example, methotrexate allows patients to continue in work, but adverse effects, such as macrocytosis and impaired liver function, can require dosage reduction or withdrawal, with resultant adverse effects on function.

Hypoglycaemic drugs (see also Chapter 28)

Hypoglycaemia and the loss of associated warning signs are the most incapacitating effects of treatment for diabetes mellitus, especially in those taking insulin but it may also occur in those taking the sulphonylureas such as gliclazide. Many RTAs caused by hypoglycaemia occur because drivers continue to drive despite warning symptoms of hypoglycaemia. Assessment of an employee's degree of control is essential, especially for safety critical roles, and particular care is needed to ensure that employees recognize the warning signs and act accordingly. Where hypoglycaemic awareness has been lost and there are no warning signs driving may be restricted. Beta-blockers can also blunt the peripheral effects of hypoglycaemia, apart from sweating. Further guidance on driving and diabetes is provided in Chapters 15 and 28.

Anticancer medications

Many employees continue working while undergoing chemotherapy. Oral rather than parenteral treatment, when possible, reduces the need for hospital attendance, but increasing numbers of employees want to continue working while receiving medications by continuous ambulatory infusion or via a central line. Those in safety critical work may require restrictions until successful treatment and resumption of an appropriate level of function is possible. Employees whose work involves overseas travel are often unable to work during treatment, since continuity of therapy is essential. The oestrogen receptor antagonist tamoxifen is associated with light-headedness and visual disturbances (corneal opacities, cataracts, and retinopathy) and an increased risk of thromboembolism.

Anti-infective agents

Gastrointestinal symptoms are common adverse reactions, although they rarely cause significant problems. The fluoroquinolones, such as ciprofloxacin, can affect performance of skilled tasks, such as driving, and also enhance the effects of alcohol. The risk of convulsions is increased, particularly if they are used with NSAIDs. Many antimicrobials (for example, the cephalosporins and metronidazole) can cause dizziness, which can affect performance. The antituberculosis drug ethambutol can cause reduced visual acuity and colour blindness; immediate discontinuation of therapy is required in such circumstances. Ototoxic drugs, such as gentamicin, can cause vestibular damage, increasing the harmful effects of noise exposure.

Travel medications

Chloroquine used for malarial prophylaxis can be associated with visual disturbances. Mefloquine often causes mild symptoms such as dizziness or disturbed balance but can also be associated with more severe transient neuropsychiatric reactions with an estimated frequency of one in 13 000 during prophylactic use and one in 215 with therapeutic use. Symptoms include disorientation, mental confusion, hallucinations, agitation, and reduced consciousness. A single dose can initiate such reactions. Unpredictable reactions can be provoked by concomitant use of CNS-active drugs and alcohol, and medical assessment is advised. Starting mefloquine a fortnight before travel can detect adverse reactions early, allowing replacement with an alternative medication before departure.

Good occupational health practice

It is important to consider the benefits of medication and the value of supporting employees to encourage correct use of medications in order to reduce the risk of harm (see Box 25.3). Most employees take their responsibilities seriously, but some fail to report problems that may affect their fitness for work, whether poorly controlled illnesses or adverse drug reactions. The occupational physician's main information source of medication details is usually the employee, and those with repeat prescriptions can be encouraged to bring printouts to assessments. Use of medications by the self-employed and employees without occupational health provision requires particular consideration, as such employees can be in safety critical roles.

Workplace solutions and adjustments

Occupational health strategies to assist employees to manage medication are listed in Box 25.4.

Box 25.3 Measures to encourage safer use of medications

- Specific enquiry about employees' medications, including OTC medicines.
- Education of employees as to possible adverse reactions to medications.
- Support for employees when reporting reactions.
- Ensuring a clear and easy method to report medication concerns.
- Encouragement to employees taking new or long-term treatment to report changes to medications or dosages.
- Enquiry at opportune moments about medication problems; for example, employees attending for annual surveillance; medication as a topic of health and well-being assessment days.
- Development of improved links with prescribers.
- Encouragement to employers to maintain a self-referral option.
- Inclusion of a question in requests for reports from treating physicians relating to use of medications.
- Provision of advice on alternative OTC medications with fewer adverse reactions.

Box 25.4 Occupational health strategies to assist manage medication

- Highlighting medication times with written or electronic instructions on the person, at the workstation, or with use of a personal alarm system.
- Use of a pill-dispensing container.
- Advising the employer/supervisor, with the employee's consent, if there is a risk of serious adverse drug reactions.
- Ensuring the employee is aware to avoid operating machinery or vehicles if drowsiness is a possible adverse reaction with new medications or changes to doses.
- Adjustment of employee's work routine to accommodate medication needs.
- Encouraging the employer to provide safe, secure storage for medications, including fridges and private space for administration of medications or continuous infusions.

Prescribing in occupational health

Common types of prescriptions in occupational health are listed in Box 25.5. Occupational physicians prescribe less frequently than other specialists, but they still have responsibilities to:

- Prescribe treatment only when they have adequate knowledge of the patient's health and are satisfied that the treatment serves the patient's needs.
- Provide effective treatments based on the best available evidence and a proper assessment of the benefit to harm balance.
- Keep clear, accurate and legible records, including details of any drugs prescribed.
- Inform the primary care physician what has been prescribed.

Many medications in the workplace are prescribed using patient group directions; some, such as post-exposure prophylaxis, require patient specific directions. Good communication with pharmacists and specialist teams, such as respiratory medicine and immunology, ensures good compliance with prescribing policies. A robust policy for sourcing post-exposure prophylaxis is essential, especially out of hours, as early treatment is essential. Good links with travel medicine resources, such as the Medical Advisory Service for Travellers Abroad,[30] ensures that up-to-date information is available.

Box 25.5 Common prescriptions in occupational health

- Vaccinations for healthcare workers, for example MMR, hepatitis B.
- Vaccinations for travel overseas.
- Mantoux test/BCG inoculation.
- Antimalarial drugs.
- Post-exposure prophylaxis (PEP) for high-risk, needle-stick injuries.

> ## Box 25.6 *British National Formulary* (<http://www.bnf.org>)
>
> The BNF is a joint publication of the British Medical Association and the Royal Pharmaceutical Society, published biannually under the authority of a Joint Formulary Committee. Online access to full publication with regular newsletters is available with free registration; there is also access via software applications. The BNF includes key information on the selection, prescribing, dispensing, and administration of medicines in the UK. Information is drawn from manufacturers' product literature, medical and pharmaceutical literature, UK health departments, regulatory authorities, and professional bodies. The BNF also takes account of authoritative national guidance and guidelines and emerging safety concerns.

It is good practice to keep abreast of the more commonly used prescription medications and to have reference resources, such as the *British National Formulary*, readily available (see Box 25.6).

Summary

Medications are essential to maintain health and thus employability, productivity, safety, and effectiveness in the workplace. Occupational health can significantly influence the safe management of medications. The future lies in developing processes into standard assessment practices, so that enquiry about medications becomes routine and to encourage employees to discuss medication concerns. Recent approaches to improve service quality, such as SEQOHS, will provide effective platforms to support improved management of medications. Further development of links between occupational health and prescribers is under way, together with improvement of the relationship between occupational health and primary care. Focus is also required on improving clinician well-being with proper adherence to standard treatment practices. Technology is an increasingly important resource, for both communication and education and software applications, such as for the BNF, are enhancing mobile communications, which are of particular value for peripatetic clinicians. Future research should continue to investigate the influence of medication in the workplace.

References

1 The NHS Information Centre, Prescribing Support Unit, Lloyd D. *General pharmaceutical services in England 2000–01 to 2009–10*. Version 1.0. London: NHS Information Centre, 2010.

2 Office of Health Economics. *Health services data*. (<http://www.ohe.org/page/health-statistics/access-the-data/health-service/data.cfm>)

3 Department of Health. *Statistics of prescriptions dispensed in the Family Health Services Authorities: England 1985 to 1995*. London: Department of Health Statistical Bulletin, 1996.

4 Dunnell K, Cartwright A. *Medicine takers, prescribers and hoarders*. London: Routledge and Kegan Paul, 1972.

5 Rennie IG. *Accidents at work—risks from medication*. Royal College of Physicians, Faculty of Occupational Medicine, MFOM Dissertation, 1985.

6 Swales CL. *A study to determine the prevalence of adverse side effects arising from the use of prescription and non-prescription medication on a chemical manufacturing site*. Royal College of Physicians, Faculty of Occupational Medicine, MFOM Dissertation, 1999.

7 Aronson JK. From prescription-only to over-the-counter medicines ('PoM to P'): time for an intermediate category. *Br Med Bull* 2009; **90**: 63–9.

8 Hargie ODW, Morrow NC. Introducing interpersonal skill training into the pharmaceutical curriculum. *Int Pharm J* 1987; **1**: 175–8.

9 Moclair A, Evans D. Vocational qualifications for pharmacy support staff. *Pharm J* 1994; **252**: 631.

10 Aronson JK. Adverse drug reactions: history, terminology, classification, causality, frequency, preventability. In: Talbot J, Aronson JK (eds), *Stephens' detection and evaluation of adverse drug reactions: principles and practice*, 6th edn, pp. 1–119. Oxford: Wiley-Blackwell, 2011.

11 Smith A, Wadsworth E, Moss S, *et al*. The scale and impact of illegal drug use by workers. Sudbury: Health and Safety Executive, 2004. (<http://www.hse.gov.uk/research/rrpdf/rr193sum.pdf>)

12 *The Health and Safety at Work etc. Act 1974*. London: The Stationery Office. (<http://www.legislation.gov.uk/ukpga/1974/37/>)

13 *The Equality Act 2010. London*: The Stationery Office. (<http://www.legislation.gov.uk/ukpga/2010/15/contents>)

14 Faculty of Occupational Medicine. *Occupational Health Service, Standards for Accreditation*, January 2010. [Online] (<http://www.facoccmed.ac.uk/library/docs/standardsjan2010.pdf>)

15 Nicholson AN, Stone BM. Disturbance of circadian rhythms and sleep. *Proc R Soc Edin Sect B Biol Sci* 1985; **82B**: 135–9.

16 Herxheimer A, Waterhouse J. The prevention and treatment of jet lag. *BMJ* 2003; **326**(7384): 296–7.

17 Aronson JK. Chronopharmacology: reflections on time and a new text. *Lancet* 1990; **335**(8704): 1515–6.

18 Nakano S. Time of day effect on psychotherapeutic drug response and kinetics in man. In: Takahashi R, Holberg F, Walker CA (eds), *Towards chronopharmacology*, pp. 51–9. Oxford: Pergamon Press, 1982.

19 Hunter J, Maxwell JD, Stewart DA, *et al*. Increased hepatic microsomal enzyme activity from occupational exposure to certain organochlorine pesticides. *Nature* 1972; **237**(5355): 399–401.

20 Hindmarch I. Psychomotor function and psychoactive drugs. *Br J Clin Pharmacol* 1980; **10**(3): 189–209.

21 Barbone F, McMahon AD, Davey PG, *et al*. Association of road-traffic accidents with benzodiazepine use. *Lancet* 1998; **352**(9137): 1331–6.

22 Driver and Vehicle Licensing Agency. *At a glance guide to the current medical standards of fitness to drive*. Swansea: DVLA, 2011. (<http://www.dft.gov.uk/dvla/medical/ataglance.aspx>)

23 Oxtoby K. Doctors' self prescribing. *BMJ Careers* 2012; 10 January. (<http://careers.bmj.com/careers/advice/view-article.html?id = 20006142>)

24 Montgomery AJ, Bradley C, Rochfort A, *et al*. A review of self-medication in physicians and medical students. *Occup Med* 2011; **61**(7): 490–7.

25 Civil Aviation Authority. *Modern medical practice and flight: aeronautical information circular United Kingdom*, AIC 96/2004. [Online] (<http://www.alantyson.com/aics/4P069.PDF>)

26 Vermeeren A. Residual effects of hypnotics: epidemiology and clinical implications. *CNS Drugs* 2004; **18**(5): 297–328.

27 Donaldson E, Kennaway DJ. Effects of temazepam on sleep, performance, and rhythmic 6-sulphatoxymelatonin and cortisol excretion after transmeridian travel. *Aviat Space Environ Med* 1991; **62**(7): 654–60.

28 Civil Aviation Authority. *Safety sense leaflet 24: Pilot health*. [Online] (<http://www.caa.co.uk/application.aspx?catid = 33&pagetype = 65&appid = 11&mode = detail&id = 1178>)

29 Cox RAF (ed). *Offshore medicine: medical care of employees in the offshore oil industry*, 2nd edn. Berlin: Springer-Verlag, 1987.

30 Medical Advisory Service for Travellers Abroad website: <http://masta-travel-health.com>

Chapter 26

The older worker

Henry N. Goodall and John Grimley Evans

Age will not be defied.
Francis Bacon (1561–1626) English Philosopher
Essays, 'Of Regiment of Health'[*]

Introduction

Throughout the world, populations are ageing, as birth rates fall and people live longer. This 'demographic transition' brings about a permanent change in population structure and an increase in the ratio of people traditionally regarded as being of 'retirement age' to those traditionally regarded as being of 'working age'. Both for the productivity of a population and for the funding of pensions and other social benefits, the whole trajectory of working life and the social structures that underpin it have to change to match labour resources to needs. In particular, people in the developed world must expect to continue working to later ages than in the past, a change that has implications both for the employed and for employers. Occupational physicians have an important role to play in making longer working lifetimes possible, productive, and pleasant.

The demographic background

It is estimated that by 2050, the numbers of people aged over 60 in Europe will have doubled to 40 per cent of the population. As shown in Figure 26.1, populations that have not yet undergone full economic development show a broad-based rapidly tapering structure characteristic of high birth and infant mortality rates. Figure 26.1 also shows the very different pattern established in the developed world and, assuming no major global disasters, the future of populations responding to the effects of economic advance in reducing birth rates and prolonging life.

Against the background of this general trend, European nations are undergoing shorter-term changes due to the large numbers of children who were born between the late 1940s and the mid-1960s. They have produced fewer children than their parents and so as they age, there will be a relative decline in the proportions of people of working age following on behind them (Figure 26.2). The 'age dependency ratio', that is the number of people past retirement age compared with the number of people of working age, will virtually double from about 1:3 to about 2:3. This forms the basis of the so-called 'pensions crisis'. The mass immigration of younger workers since 2000 is not

[*] Reproduced with permission from Kiernan M (ed). *The Oxford Francis Bacon XV. The Essayes or counsels, Civill and Morall.* Oxford: Oxford University Press, 2000.

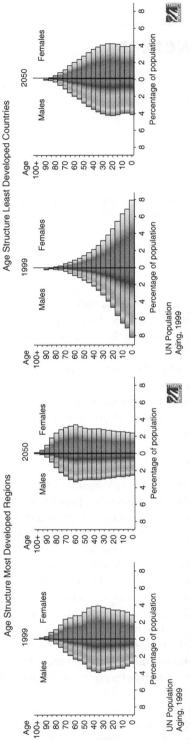

Figure 26.1 The changing age structure of developed and developing countries. Reproduced with permission from Professor David Wegman, from the keynote speech, Society of Occupational Medicine, Annual Scientific Meeting, 2003. Data from UN Population Aging, 1999.

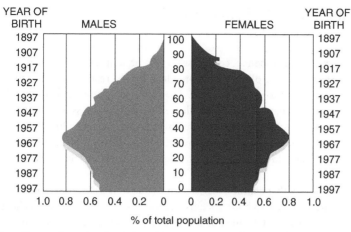

Figure 26.2 How Europe is ageing (based on 11 European member states). Reproduced from <http://europa.eu.int/comm/eurostat/> Copyright © European Union, 1995–2012.

a sensible response to this challenge, especially for the UK, with its already high population density. Young workers grow old, so the problem is merely postponed, not solved. Hence the primary need is for all workers to increase their lifetime contribution to the funding of social substructure including pensions. This means working more productively—not necessarily harder—and longer, but not necessarily full-time. It also means increasing opportunities for citizens under-represented in the current workforce, such as women and people with disabilities, to be productively employed.

The United Kingdom

In a position paper on age and employment, the Faculty of Occupational Medicine has drawn attention to particular issues in the UK:[1]

> The majority of non-working men [in the UK] aged between 50 and 65 are economically inactive (i.e. retired, sick or caring for others and unavailable for work) rather than unemployed (one in ten of this non-working age group). The number of people over 50 and on Incapacity Benefit has trebled in the last 20 years. Of those not seeking work, approximately half are on sickness or disability benefit (over 1 million people) and nearly half a million, mainly women, are full time carers. Individuals in this age group are more likely to experience low self-esteem, ill health and poverty. Thirty-seven per cent of 55–64 year olds say they have a limiting long-standing illness. Depression, social exclusion, and marital problems are also more common in this age group. Most of those not working have been out of employment for long periods, many having previously been in long standing jobs. Involvement in other activities (such as charitable work) is also declining in this age group.

This probably presents too gloomy a picture. Disability benefit is more generous than unemployment benefit and it is well documented that in places where traditional industries, such as steel making, have closed down, redundant workers rationally seek status as disabled rather than unemployed. However, the resulting statistics can mislead policy-makers, challenged by the need for socio-economic change to meet increases in longevity.

In this chapter we review some of the implications of the employment of older workers for occupational medicine. The first section outlines age-associated changes in health and function, the second deals with the adaptations in occupational health services, and the third raises some broader issues relating to the organization of industries and companies.

General age-associated changes

Ageing

Ageing, in the sense of senescence, comprises a loss of adaptability of an individual organism over time. As we become older we become less able to respond adaptively to challenges from our external or internal environments. The homoeostatic responses on which survival depends become on average less sensitive, slower, weaker, and less well sustained. For most human beings, loss of adaptability may not be obvious until very late in life, as we live in non-challenging environments that rarely bring individuals to the limit of their functional capacity. Nonetheless, as we grow older, most of us go about our work and daily life with diminishing functional reserves.

The loss of adaptability that characterizes ageing is due to the accumulation of un-repaired or only partially repaired damage to body systems, organs, tissues, cells, and intracellular organelles. The longevity of a species is determined by the efficiency of its damage control systems—damage control comprising prevention, detection, and repair or replacement. Resources used for damage control and longevity cannot be used for reproduction, so long-lived species breed more slowly than short-lived ones. Slower reproduction provides for opportunities to improve the survival of progeny to their own sexual maturity, for example, by timing reproduction to seasonal availability of food or providing parental care. As it is successful reproduction that leads to evolutionary success, natural selection will favour longevity in species that live in safe environments.[2]

In the human species, senescence first becomes apparent about the age of 12, where mortality rates turn upwards, and is a continuous process thereafter. It is indeed a lifelong process, not something that starts mysteriously around the age of retirement; determinants of disease and disability in middle age can be identified in childhood and even foetal life.

Differences between younger and older people

A starting point for the scientific appraisal of human ageing is to compare young people with older people and the general view of ageing is derived, explicitly or implicitly, from such comparisons.[3] However, the result can be deceptive because differences between young and old people can arise through processes other than ageing (Table 26.1).

Differences not attributable to ageing

Some differences have come about, not because old people have changed due to ageing, but because they have always been different from younger people with whom they are being compared.

Table 26.1 Differences between young and old

Non-ageing	True ageing
Selective survival	**Primary:**
Cohort effects	Intrinsic
Differential challenge	Extrinsic
	Secondary:
	Individual adaptation
	Specific adaptation

♦ *Selective survival* is the result of people with advantageous genes or social environment, or healthy lifestyles, surviving longer than the less fortunate people born at the same time.

♦ *Cohort effects* are the differences between generations of people born at different times and therefore exposed, especially in developing societies, to different influences and experiences, particularly early in life. Such cohort differences can be considerable. A study in the 1960s demonstrated that a major part of what appears in cross-sectional studies to be age-associated change in some types of psychological functioning was due to cultural, especially educational, differences between generations.[4] Although prominent in the sphere of psychological function, which reflects educational standards and practices during childhood, cohort effects will contribute to cross-sectional estimates of age-associated variation in physical variables such as height, serum lipids, and obesity, as well as to risk of diseases such as lung cancer. Cohort comparisons reflect differences between generations in their lifestyle and behaviour as well as in changes in the physical environment.

♦ *Differential challenge.* If ageing is to be defined in terms of reduced adaptability, it can only be assessed by offering equal challenges to people at different ages. Social policy often leads to our offering more severe challenges to older people than to younger ones and then attributing differences in outcome to the effects of ageing. Ageism, in its various guises, is so deeply engrained in British society that discrimination against older people is universal.

Differences attributable to ageing (true ageing)

There has long been debate about distinguishing 'diseases' from 'normal ageing', but the distinction is meaningless in scientific terms.[5] True ageing comprises all the ways in which individuals change as time passes. Some of the responsible processes, for reasons that range from the medical to the political, may come to be called 'diseases'.

Primary ageing is loss of adaptability due to the effects of many different processes in the tissues and organs of the body. These ageing processes are the product of interactions between *extrinsic* (environmental and lifestyle) influences and *intrinsic* (genetic) factors. Some of these interactions may be specific: for example, it is likely that excess dietary salt raises blood pressure only in people with particular genes. Other interactions are more general: habits of physical exercise, for example, affect a wide range of body systems, presumably through genetically determined pathways. Diet is important in healthy ageing, notably through deficiencies and imbalance. Dietary factors are also probably involved in ageing effects, due to the generation and insufficiently rapid destruction of free radicals (highly active oxygen molecules) generated in mitochondria that damage cell components including DNA.

Secondary ageing is a term usefully reserved to designate those adaptations made by individuals—or by a species through natural selection—that counter the effects of ageing. At the individual level, secondary ageing is most obvious in the realm of psychological and behavioural functioning. Mildly obsessional behaviour making an ordered environment substitute for memory is a common and successful adaptation. (If we always put our car keys on the hall table, we do not have to waste brain-power remembering where we have left them today.) Older workers may develop apparently idiosyncratic ways of carrying out familiar tasks that are efficient—for them—in conserving effort and circumventing specific problems, such as a stiff joint.

Social factors are important extrinsic determinants of ageing. One of the most significant and much studied correlates of healthy ageing is higher educational level. This will partly reflect the health benefits of relative affluence and occupations that are less damaging physically. Education will also be relevant to the ability of the individual to know of medical advances and to understand their implications for prevention or therapy, and to profit from them. Social class effects on health and disability are highly complex and there may be subtle psychosocial and work-related determinants of health in middle and later life. People in lower grade jobs have less sense of control over their patterns and pace of working, and this leads to chronic 'stress' arousal, associated with changes in endocrine and immune function, that may have pervasive effects on susceptibility to age-associated illness and disability, especially cardiovascular disease.[6]

Obviously, the effects of ageing processes on body functions depend in part on how good those functions were initially. Both men and women lose muscle tissue at the same rate with ageing but, because women start with less muscle (on average) than men, they are more likely (on average) to become immobile and dependent in later life. A similar model applies to bone tissue, and to the high rates of fractures in older women, although women also experience a higher rate of bone loss with ageing. Two determinants of how soon brain damage, produced by Alzheimer's disease, for example, shows itself in the clinical syndrome of dementia, are the original intelligence and the education level of affected individuals.[7] The better the brain, perhaps, the longer it can compensate for progressive damage.

Because we start from different baselines, carry different genes and live different lives, we age at different rates and in different ways. Although, on average, we deteriorate with age, some people in their 80s will be functioning better than would be regarded as normal for people in their 30s. It is therefore unscientific, as well as unjust, to make judgments about individuals' capabilities simply on the basis of their age—as unjust in fact as to make such judgments from their sex, skin colour, or social class. In all the discussion of age-associated changes in health and function in this chapter, we describe what happens *on average* in the population; it must not be assumed that such changes affect every ageing individual.

Is the pattern of ageing changing?

Data from the USA indicate that, over the last two decades, people there have been living longer on average but that the prevalence of disability in later life has been falling.[8] This is presumably partly due to the adoption of healthier lifestyles by significant sections of the population—notwithstanding a general increase in obesity—and partly due to better medical care, and the development of less demanding environments, but there are probably other factors that have caused a decline in disabling diseases, especially of the cardiovascular system since the 1960s. It is not clear whether similar improvements in general health and function in middle and later life are occurring in the UK, although reductions in cigarette smoking among men and control of urban and industrial smoke pollution have reduced the prevalence of limiting pulmonary disease in the last three decades. Less reassuringly, British data suggest that social class differences in mortality and morbidity have been widening. The reasons for this are complex, and include changes over time in the composition of the various classes, but will also include failure of some members of the population to benefit as much as others from social and medical advances.

There are encouraging signs that the epidemic of cardiovascular disease has peaked, although the incidence may still be rising in some population groups, notably immigrants from the Indian subcontinent. If the improvements in the patterns of disability in older people seen in the USA could be made to happen here, there would be good prospects for people being fit enough to work longer for their pensions, while yet living to enjoy a sufficient and active period of retirement.

How old is an 'older worker'?

The World Health Organization has recommended that 'older people' should replace the depersonalizing term 'the elderly'. In the population at large the age at which one becomes 'older' has, quite properly, moved on with the growth in the expectation of life. Anxieties (largely ill-founded or tendentious) about the medical implications of ageing populations are usually expressed in terms of the numbers of people aged over 80. Certainly, in the developed world, the traditional male retirement age of 65 would now be regarded as a continuation of middle age rather than the onset of senility.

The retirement age of 65 for men was originally computed in 19th-century Germany, on the assumption that pensions would be paid by a levy on the wages of men still working—a 'pay-as-you-go' system. Conceptually, the developed world is moving toward the assumption that future pensions will be based on an insurance model (private or social), in which individuals will in effect pay in advance for their own pensions. Logically this would lead to a system in which the average (not necessarily compulsory) retirement age would be adjusted to take account of the expectation of life in later years, so that a levy of 'x' per cent of one's earnings over an average of 'y' years would be seen as 'purchasing' an average of 'z' years of adequate income after retiring. Even more challenging than the actuarial intricacies of such a scheme would be equity issues raised by social class and occupation differences in life expectancy. Whatever happens, however, it is reasonable to expect that for the immediate future the 'older worker', of practical concern to occupational health services, will be aged 55–70, rather than over 75 years of age.

Age-associated changes in function

Any attempt at a comprehensive catalogue of age-associated changes and illnesses would easily fill a large textbook. This chapter is necessarily restricted to major topics related to work capacity and to illustrative examples of how illnesses may present in a work-related context.

Physical activity

Muscle mass declines in both sexes from the third decade onwards. As already noted, because women start life with less muscle than men, they are more likely to suffer from limitation in muscle strength and power in later life.[9] In addition to muscular strength and power, endurance and joint flexibility also decline with age. The last can be partly compensated for by deliberately putting joints through a full range of movement before working.[10] The collective warm-up exercises required of workers in some Far Eastern factories have a physiological as well as ideological function.

Endurance, the ability to maintain high levels of physical activity over prolonged periods, is limited by muscular power and exercise tolerance, and also by pulmonary and cardiac function, all of which decline on average with age. Although breathlessness is usually the dominant symptom in strenuous activity, the limits on exercise capacity are usually muscular or cardiac rather than pulmonary, except in smokers or individuals with lung damage due to other causes.

Older workers in physically strenuous jobs may be working closer to their physical limits than younger colleagues keeping to the same pace, and they may become more readily fatigued. Older workers can cope with heavy muscular exertion,[11] so long as the work is interspersed with recovery periods sufficient in frequency and duration, but they find the demands of continuous fast paced lighter work more difficult to sustain. Older workers may prefer to move away from externally paced or 'piecework' jobs into hourly paid jobs, if the choice is available. Part of the age-associated loss of muscular function observed in the population is due to lower levels of exercise in older age groups. Training can recover some of the loss by increasing muscle bulk and blood supply, as well as improving muscle metabolism.[12]

Hearing

Some age-associated loss of sensitivity to high frequencies is virtually universal in western societies, and is probably partly due to chronic exposure to noise rather than intrinsic ageing processes.[13] Those who have worked in noisy industries for many years, with inadequate hearing protection, are almost certain to have significant hearing loss, by the time they reach their mid-fifties. High frequencies are important in the comprehension of speech but, before the process becomes severe enough to produce overt deafness, it can result in slower 'decoding' of speech. This in turn can produce functional cognitive impairment due to slowing of processing and the missing of some information.[14] (Detection and correction of 'minor' hearing loss is a necessary first step in the assessment of someone suspected of early dementia.) In the workplace, this effect may be compounded by high ambient noise levels.[15]

Sufferers lose the ability accurately to distinguish particular consonants, notably 'b', 'd', 't', and 's' sounds. They may misidentify words or fail to make sense of what they are hearing. An additional problem is difficulty in reliably following one speaker when other voices are also audible, as in many social and work situations. The natural reaction when talking to someone perceived as deaf is to speak more loudly, but this may not help. The sufferer's cochlea may show a disproportionate response to increase in volume known as 'recruitment', and loud sounds can become both painful and distorted. In some working environments, loss of accurate comprehension of verbal instructions will have implications for safety and production costs, if process or other errors result. Some individuals can compensate for hearing loss by lip-reading, and colleagues can be helpful by making use of gesture and facial expression. In some working environments, more use of visual material in the communication of crucial information can improve safety. This becomes easier and more accurate with electronic communication systems. A wide range of adaptive technologies now exist to support the hard of hearing at work (see Chapter 10).

Up to a third of older people suffer from tinnitus, of which the commonest cause is sensorineural deafness due to previous noise exposure. Most people manage to ignore the problem but for others it can become distressing, at least intermittently. The clinician also needs to be alert to recognize depression when it presents as preoccupation with previously ignored tinnitus.

Vision

There are age-associated changes in visual perception, due to both peripheral and central factors. With increasing age, the lens becomes less elastic and the intrinsic muscles weaker, so that accommodation for near vision becomes limited. This effect can begin as young as the mid-forties in otherwise healthy workers and is sometimes a missed cause of what the older worker puts down to 'eyestrain'. The lens and vitreous of the eye become less transparent and acquire a yellowish tinge that can interfere with colour perception. Owing to the loss of transparency, and also because of changes in the retina, the older eye requires higher light intensities and greater contrast in print for accurate reading. This has important implications for the design of work environments for older employees. Cataracts become common, reducing acuity and also scattering incoming light, causing dazzle. This last factor is especially significant for night driving.

Also relevant to driving safety is a tendency for the functional visual field to contract, so that stimuli in the periphery of vision may not be noticed, even though formal static testing of the visual field shows no defect.[16] This is thought to be one factor in the increase with age in low-speed lateral car collisions at road intersections.[17] Some studies have found it possible to reverse this phenomenon by specific training, and it presumably represents some form of central inattention. Although less clear than in the case of hearing, minor degrees of visual impairment can manifest as slower or less accurate understanding of written material or misinterpretation of environmental cues that can present as apparent cognitive impairment.

Macular degeneration is a further affliction that an older worker may suffer. Treatment is at present of limited benefit and access to advice and suitable visual aids less than perfect. Modifications to computer keyboards and visual display units, and scanning cameras to assist in reading are, however, available and may be of help in prolonging a sufferer's working life.

Touch and proprioception

Dexterity and fineness of touch may deteriorate over time, especially if chronic exposure to trauma leads to thickening of the skin and subcutaneous tissues of the hands. The risk of falls increases in both sexes after the age of 65. The risk is higher, at all ages, in women, who also show a bimodal risk with an earlier transitory peak around the age of 50.[18] Although the risk of falls is related to muscle strength and joint stiffness, as well as any neurological disease, there seems to be a general age-associated impairment of global proprioception.

Proprioception, as tested by standard clinical examination (joint position sense or Romberg test, for example), is unlikely to be manifestly impaired in the absence of specifically diagnosable conditions, such as vitamin B12 deficiency or cervical myelopathy. Global proprioception, in the sense of accurate awareness of the body's position, orientation, and movement in space, is the product of continuous integration of input from eyes, inner ear, and a range of peripheral proprioceptors, especially in cervical joints, the feet, and the Achilles tendons. As a consequence of degeneration in cervical joints and peripheral nerves, the information from these various sources may be attenuated or may not arrive simultaneously in the central nervous system. In later life, this probably underlies the common symptom of non-rotatory dizziness that is epidemiologically associated with a risk of falls.[19]

Mental function

Dementia is rare at ages under 70, except in people with a family history of an early-onset form. There are, however, some differences in mental functioning between middle-aged people and young adults that may need to be considered in matching older workers to occupational tasks (by choosing the workers or designing the tasks) and in developing training programmes. As noted already, some of the differences observed between younger and older workers may be due to cohort effects rather than ageing and so will change with time. One of the first things we learn at school is how to learn, so cohort effects must be expected to be significant in designing training programmes for older workers.

The various processes and aptitudes that comprise human intelligence have been polarized between the 'crystalline' and the 'fluid'. Crystalline intelligence solves problems by applying learned strategies or paradigms. Fluid intelligence solves problems by innovation and analysis from first principles. As we grow older, we tend to rely more on crystalline than on fluid processes. As long as the paradigm chosen, often by recognition of analogies between present and past situations, is appropriate, crystalline intelligence is efficient. It may, however, fail, and indeed be a positive hindrance, in rising to a totally new challenge that requires original thinking. An older individual in a problem-solving situation may need to be made explicitly aware of the need for a new approach, not a ready-made solution from past experience.

Subjectively, the dominant problem in mental ageing is difficulty with memory. It is a clinically useful oversimplification to visualize human memory as comprising an immediate working memory, possibly subserved by active inter-neuronal transmission, linked to a long-term memory based on some permanent neuronal change such as modification of synapses. Some material from the first passes into the second, from whence if adequately filed and labelled, suitable cueing can bring it forth. Both types can show deterioration with age and difficulties with shorter-term memory are obvious enough. In age-associated memory impairment and in the early stages of Alzheimer's disease, a dominant feature is an apparent problem in the link between shorter-term and longer-term memory, so that material is not written into longer-term store or cannot be recalled from there. This difficulty is commonly, albeit somewhat misleadingly, labelled as a defect in short-term memory—even though the subject's ability to remember telephone numbers long enough to dial them ('digit span') may still be normal.

Increasing attention paid to Alzheimer's disease in the media has led to middle-aged people with subjective difficulties with memory becoming worried or even depressed, by a fear of incipient dementia, especially those with a family history of dementia, even though the risk for relatives of someone with late-onset dementia is very little higher than average. A middle-aged person manifesting or complaining of memory problems therefore needs skilled and empathetic evaluation. Employers of older workers should encourage the appropriate use of memory supporting strategies—note-taking, notice boards, and electronic prompters, for example. This will help to prevent problems, both directly and also indirectly, so that individuals, fearful of memory loss, do not feel stigmatized by making use of such supportive devices. The value of checklists, for workers of all ages, is formally recognized for airline pilots and surgeons.

Ageing is also associated with a slowing of mental processing and a reduction in channel capacity—essentially the capacity to process several different sequences of data simultaneously and rapidly. Decisions may take longer and mistakes may be made in complex situations. These processes contribute to the rise in accident rates among older car drivers, for example. Compounding the channel capacity problem with ageing is a failure to identify and suppress irrelevant factors when analysing a situation or performing a complex task.

Specific age-associated problems

Cardiovascular function

Age-associated changes are prominent in the structure and function of the cardiovascular system. Cardiovascular diseases increase in incidence and fatality with age and are leading causes of death and of premature retirement.

The heart With ageing, heart muscle becomes stiffer, so that diastolic filling may be impaired.[20] In response to exercise, cardiac output rises less through increasing heart rate and more by increased stroke volume, in comparison with a younger heart. Cardiac reserve falls with age, even in the absence of demonstrable ischaemic disease.

Ischaemic heart disease is common in middle age and beyond, especially so in men. Risk factors include hypertension, smoking, high low-density lipoprotein cholesterol, diabetes, obesity, and lack of exercise, all of which interact. Risk of ischaemic heart disease can be reduced by modification of risk factors at any age and there is no justification for excluding older people from preventive programmes. For reasons that are not yet clear, when ischaemic heart disease is present, pain may be a less prominent symptom in older people than at younger ages. In later life limited cardiac output, due to ischaemic disease or other causes, may present as a sensation of muscular fatigue on exertion rather than as dyspnoea.

Blood pressure In Western populations, systolic blood pressure tends to rise with age although this is associated with an increase in variance because some individuals show no rise. Blood pressure is positively associated with increase in risk of cardiovascular disease, especially stroke. The age-associated rise is due to both increased stiffness of the arterial walls, affecting chiefly systolic pressure, and arteriolar tension influencing diastolic pressure. The old notion that only diastolic pressure is relevant as a risk factor for cardiovascular disease is now discredited and high systolic pressure needs treatment even if the diastolic is 'normal'.

Epidemiological evidence suggests that the rise with age is largely due to extrinsic factors. A high intake of dietary salt contributes, at least in genetically susceptible individuals, and obesity is another remediable factor. As a risk factor for vascular disease, hypertension interacts powerfully with other risk factors such as smoking, and the combination of hypertension and diabetes is particularly problematic. The benefits of treatment are at least as great for older people as for younger. For older people, drug treatment is essentially along conventional lines but beta blockers are sometimes less effective and less well tolerated than with younger patients.

Cerebrovascular disease

Epidemiological data suggest that cerebrovascular disease has been diminishing in incidence for many decades in Western populations, but some specific forms have only been identified comparatively recently. Stroke with temporary or permanent neurological deficit, as a presenting feature of cerebrovascular disease, is well-recognized by both medical and lay members of the public. Diagnostic errors more often involve failure to identify non-cerebrovascular causes of an apparent stroke. Hypoglycaemia in a treated diabetic is an example requiring urgent exclusion; cardiac arrhythmia or hypotension, possibly iatrogenic, are others. An unwitnessed epileptic attack followed by Todd's paresis can have serious consequences, especially in a work situation, if mistaken for a transient ischaemic attack (TIA). A cerebral tumour presenting as a stroke syndrome will usually come to light in the course of subsequent assessment, as will emboli from atrial fibrillation or valvular disease of the heart.

Cerebrovascular disease is a cause of dementia either through the accumulation of small strokes, or by the less well understood 'small vessel disease' thought to underlie the periventricular white matter damage (leucoaraiosis) seen on magnetic resonance imaging of the brain. TIAs are often recurrent and need investigation and, usually, preventive treatment. They are characterized by focal neurological defects lasting less than 24 hours. It is unwise to assume that some kind of syncopal or confusional episode, without focal neurological signs, is a TIA; other conditions, especially cardiovascular syncope, and the increasingly recognized syndrome of transient global amnesia[21] need to be excluded.

Peripheral vascular disease shares risk factors with other forms of vascular disease but smoking and diabetes are especially important. The typical presentation is intermittent claudication—pain in the lower legs induced by walking and passing off within 10 minutes of rest. The chief differential diagnosis is neurogenic intermittent claudication due to spinal stenosis (see 'Skeletal changes'). If the lower aorta is involved in severe atherosclerotic disease some variant of the Leriche syndrome may occur, including buttock claudication and erectile dysfunction.

Neoplasms

Recognition of cancer as a cause of health problems presenting in the workplace is a matter of normal clinical vigilance. Virtually all cancers increase in incidence with age, a fact well-known to older patients for whom fear of cancer may be an unspoken element in any medical consultation. Lung, large bowel, prostate in men, and breast in women, are currently the commonest sites of cancers in the UK.

Work-related cancer remains a concern and an ageing workforce risks longer periods of exposure. The occupational physician therefore still needs to be ready to respond appropriately and with due discretion to unusual types or frequencies of neoplasms in his or her workforce.

Discretion is necessary as the statistical distinction between a true 'cluster' and the simple play of chance is strictly a matter for experts.

Skeletal changes

Osteoarthritis is a common problem in later middle age and beyond. One factor is damage due to overuse, an issue in occupational and legal medicine. The knee, shoulder, and hands are susceptible to occupational damage, as is the hip; also, non-occupational factors (e.g. obesity, preexisting minor congenital or developmental abnormalities) contribute to many cases of large joint arthritis.[22]

Apart from pain arising from damaged joints, cervical disc prolapse can produce acute and extremely painful entrapment neuropathies. Chronic disability due to other brachial neuropathies is also common, but the most damaging consequence of cervical spondylosis is cervical myelopathy, affecting the long tracts of the spinal cord. Among subtler effects of cervical spondylosis, as already mentioned, is the loss of proprioceptive feedback from cervical joint receptors that contributes to control of body stability and movement.

Pain in the lumbar spine is a leading cause of disability in the general population and of lost productivity in industry. Acute syndromes involving spinal nerves may merit neurosurgical opinion, but for the great majority of chronic or recurrent lumbar pain not radiating down the legs, treatment remains initial analgesia with as little rest as is necessary to control pain before active exercise is gradually resumed. With the older male worker, the possibility of metastatic prostatic disease needs to be borne in mind but until more specific tests for metastasizing prostatic cancer become available investigation has to be undertaken with care. Lumbar spine stenosis, especially in association with a midline disc protrusion may produce a syndrome of neurogenic intermittent claudication that can closely mimic vascular disease of the legs. An infrequent but suggestive feature is the association of paraesthesiae with the pain. The pain is produced because the vasa nervorum of the cauda equina nerves cannot dilate in response to increased neural activity associated with walking. Decompressive surgery can be effective for this condition.[23]

Osteoarthritis of the spine is more common in the cervical and lumbar regions than in the less mobile thoracic division. However, in occupations that involve much twisting of the upper body, pain radiating from thoracic spondylosis can mimic cardiac pain. Other diseases of thoracic vertebrae, including metastases and osteoporotic collapse can cause a similar diagnostic problem.

Osteoporosis is largely but not exclusively a problem for older women, rather than men. Both sexes lose bone tissue on average throughout adult life but women start with less and experience accelerated loss following the menopause. The older female worker is more likely to suffer a forearm fracture in a fall, or to experience the effects of spinal osteoporosis. Thoracic and lumbar vertebrae are vulnerable, the most commonly affected vertebrae being those near the thoracolumbar junction. Spinal osteoporosis may follow a painless and insidious course of kyphosis and loss of height. At the other extreme, acutely painful vertebral collapse may occur in a fall or follow apparently minor activity such as pushing a vacuum cleaner. As already noted, the pain of a thoracic vertebral collapse may occasionally mimic an acute cardiac syndrome. Although most spinal fractures in middle-aged women will reflect osteoporosis, the clinician has always to consider the possibility of metastatic disease, especially from the breast.

Genitourinary problems

Older men and women may experience various urinary difficulties. Urgency, frequency, and incontinence—or the fear of incontinence—can interfere with work as well as with sleep and social life.[24] Affected individuals may be loath to discuss their symptoms, even with their general practitioner (GP), and urinary difficulties are typically worsened by anxiety. Older workers with such problems will appreciate frequent rest periods from externally paced work. Surveys have indicated that people with incontinence in the general population have often not received expert advice on managing their problem. Incontinence advisors are now appointed in many districts.

Depression

Opinions differ over whether the ageing brain is more or less susceptible to depression. Late middle age is, however, a time of life when particularly depressing experiences are liable to happen. Bereavements, awareness of lost opportunities and fading sexual attractiveness, anxiety about future (or present) income and vicarious involvement in the misfortunes of children are all common. Although behaviour may change with the maturing of more recent age cohorts, older people are less willing than younger adults to countenance the idea of being mentally ill and tend to somatize their feelings of depression. Persistent pain, tinnitus, or paraesthesiae may become the focus of depressive rumination. The occupational physician responsible for a multiethnic workforce needs to be aware that there are also important cultural differences in the physical and behavioural manifestations of depressive illness.

Suicide as a consequence of depression increases in risk with age. Middle-aged and older men, living alone, are particularly vulnerable to successful suicide when severely depressed. The presence of chronic symptomatic illness and higher social class are also recognized risk factors, as is accessibility of means of self-harm, such as prescribed tricyclic antidepressants.

Iatrogenic factors

Geriatricians have long recognized the high frequency of iatrogenic disorders among older people. The taking of a careful drug history is important for older workers. Most problems arise from lack of fine-tuning in prescribing and interactions between multiple medications. Special enquiry should be made about the use of over-the-counter or alternative medicines, especially by people from ethnic minorities. With regard to pharmacokinetic issues, drugs excreted by mainly renal mechanisms can cause problems, but in the absence of unusual renal impairment this is unlikely to create problems at working ages. More relevant are some pharmacodynamic problems, especially an age-associated increased sensitivity to the effects of sedatives, such as benzodiazepines. Benzodiazepine prescription has been linked to road traffic accidents and to falls, and must be suspected as a probable cause of industrial accidents and errors. The drugs are addictive, and withdrawal effects can be unpleasant and sufficient often to interfere with work. Their duration varies with the actual benzodiazepine responsible. The so-called 'Z-drugs', e.g. zopiclone, are shorter acting than currently licensed benzodiazepines. Although chemically distinct from benzodiazepines and marketed as an alternative, they act on the same receptors in the brain and must be expected to have a similar profile of adverse effects and potential for dependency.

The *British National Formulary*, now accessible online, is an indispensable resource of information on drugs.[25] Among older patients, adverse effects from medications prescribed to control high blood pressure are common, and include hypotension, impotence and depression. Impairment of exercise capacity by beta-blockers may be significant for older workers in physically demanding occupations, especially in externally paced work.

Alcohol presents a range of challenges to the occupational physician. Alcohol-related health and behaviour problems can affect all age groups. At a physiological level, tolerance of alcohol diminishes with age, owing in part to reduction in the size and blood supply of the liver, and many heavy social drinkers adjust their intake accordingly. Lowered tolerance can also result in habitual intakes starting to cause sleep disturbance in middle age, and drinkers may recognize this effect and reduce their intake. Not all heavy drinkers are dependent, and it has often been noted how workers in heavy industry may give up drinking abruptly and without difficulty, when they retire and can no longer afford the habit. There is a particular risk of alcoholism being overlooked in older female workers, partly as a result of cultural expectations, but also because the volume of alcohol consumed need not be as great as for a male colleague. In general, however, the problems associated with alcohol and the means of dealing with them are the same for workers of all ages and are dealt with in Chapter 24.

Drug problems

Iatrogenic problems have already been discussed. Misuse of illegal 'recreational' drugs is still rare among older workers, and does not seem to have increased with the maturing of the generation that was young in the 1960s. This may be partly because use of illegal drugs is largely associated with the social ambience of late adolescence, and partly because individuals with a serious drug habit leave the workforce, one way or another. But culturally determined patterns of drug use must be expected to vary. Anecdotal evidence suggests that the present-day occupational physician is more likely to encounter a problem with cocaine among the managers than with heroin among the workers.

Health maintenance and service issues

Nutrition, diet, and exercise

Conventional wisdom has it that, as we age, we need less food and more exercise, less sleep and more rest. Few of today's older workers received any advice about diet and nutrition during their early lives. Nonetheless, research suggests that older workers are likely to have a greater understanding of nutrition than younger workers.[26] Evidence from the USA suggests that the most successful education interventions are aimed at families, neighbourhoods, and communities, especially when supported by legislation, the media, and marketing efforts. Within the ageing population, those with greatest health needs include members of minority groups and recent immigrants. These groups are often overlooked when designing and implementing health promotion programs.[27,28]

During the 1960s and 1970s, government health education encouraged the UK population to reduce salt, sugar, and fat in their diets. Quality protein, salads, and fruit were then more expensive than foods containing high concentrations of saturated fats. Ready-to-eat meals, containing large quantities of salt, sugar, and saturated fats, became popular with the spread of home microwave ovens. The widening food and lifestyle habits of the different socio-economic groups in the population resulted in wealthier groups eating a healthier diet. This divergence is seen in today's poorer older workers, in higher rates of heart, lung, and liver disease, diabetes and bowel disorders and in reduced life expectancy. Only those with particular eating habits (e.g. vegetarians and vegans) have bucked the trend of a widening gap between the life expectancy of rich and poor.

In the past 30 years, year-round salads, fruit, and frozen food became available to almost all of the population. However, habits (and atheroma) developed in the 1960s and 1970s have been hard to change, with those in the poorer socio-economic groups changing least. Smoking has continued longer in these same (poorer) groups, reducing average life expectancy still further. Toxins, such as the breakdown products of tobacco and alcohol, weaken the body's defences and addiction to them worsens the user's chances of a long and healthy life.

There is evidence that workers over 50 have more positive health behaviours, stronger beliefs about the value of healthy behaviour and better self-assessed health. In addition, they are more likely to hold attitudes associated with participation in worksite health promotion activities. Physical activity should continue in older workers, even though strength may diminish. Regular exercise is key, at least three times a week, to raise the heart rate according to age, taking due account of concurrent medical conditions. There is evidence that those with a body mass index of 30 or more die earlier and that all age groups benefit from regular exercise. The BMI should ideally be kept under 25, even though there is a natural tendency for body weight to move centrally, with age. Accumulation of omental fat inside the abdomen is especially prominent in men.

Daily fruit and vegetables, adequate supplies of protein and a good intake of water (said to be ideally 1.5 L per day, although there is no empirical evidence to support this recommendation) are essential for good health. For the older worker, keeping the immune system healthy, active, and effective against viruses, bacteria, and early cancers, may well be a matter of life and death, and the advice of a qualified nutritionist or dietician should be considered.[29]

Health surveillance

Studies in Scotland in the 1960s demonstrated that much disease and disability among older people was unknown to their GPs. General practice was then response based; if patients did not complain they were assumed to be well. In addition, older people did not appreciate that some afflictions of later life were not simply due to ageing but were the consequence of potentially remediable disease. Often, some older people dreaded the undignified and unpleasant processes of medical investigation and treatment more than the illness and the prospect of premature death. One response to this problem was to institute various kinds of surveillance.

The issue of surveillance may arise in occupational medicine, with the increase in numbers of older workers, many of whom will not wish to seek medical attention if they thereby risk both investigation and possible loss of employment. While it might seem logical to consider special surveillance for older workers, both to safeguard their health and also to prevent accidents or loss of production due to unrecognized impairments, there are ethical questions, and a blanket policy which is not risk-based and easily defensible cannot be endorsed. It is prudent to be vigilant for problems that an older worker is more likely than a younger colleague to encounter, but if certain groups of workers are subject to regular review, to ensure that they meet minimum physical and health standards for their particular assigned tasks and are not adversely affected by their work, then review procedures should cover members of that group equally and not discriminate by age.

Links with primary care

Evidence following the introduction of the new 'fit note' suggests that, to date, employers are no better informed than before about their employees' fitness for work, and that few notes are issued with practical additional advice which is of use to the employer.[30] Larger employers commonly obtain the advice of a specialist occupational physician, working in the private healthcare sector.

There is often an understanding between GP and hospital consultant and an acceptance as to who is managing a patient's treatment at any one time. This may not be the case between a GP and an occupational physician. Healthy alliances (as described in the government documents *Health of the* Nation[31] and *Our Healthier Nation*[32]) will be especially necessary for effective and efficient patient care of older workers, who are more likely to be taking regular long-term medication for chronic conditions.

More occupational health services and GPs (providing part-time occupational health services) will be needed in the future. The quality of these services will need to be monitored, through revalidation and SEQOHS,[33] to ensure that appropriate standards are maintained with faster, more accurate communication and wider dissemination of relevant medical information and knowledge via e-mail, health information systems and continuing medical education. However, ethical and legal concerns arising from GPs passing health information about their patients to occupational physicians, without obtaining patients' specific consent, will remain.

Workability and employability

Degenerative disease and the chronic illnesses of middle age, even if manageable and treatable, often impair working capacity and lead to restricted activity and reduced productivity at work. In the past, medical restrictions on the work of individuals have been advised by occupational physicians, aimed at preventing exacerbation of existing conditions and avoiding injury, but employers find these onerous. Many large employers have responded to the challenge responsibly, by investing heavily in lifting and handling aids and ergonomically improved workstations over the past decade. However, the future numbers of older workers may prove overwhelming to smaller employers with resources too meagre to effect change. The concept of 'workability', rather than 'disability', as advocated in the Faculty of Occupational Medicine position paper on 'Age and Employment', is the way forward and will require a change of mind set on the part of employers, away from the concept of medical restrictions.[1]

Job analysis, skill assessment, job coaching (and retraining), and job matching are all components of an effective management system. There are now several job content and employee capability assessment computer programs under trial in Europe, e.g. the IMBA scheme, developed by the German government.[34,35] These construct a worker capability profile, and match this with a list of job requirement profiles. A list of jobs results, that the worker should be able to carry out, with minimal risk of exacerbating existing medical conditions. The benefits include transparency, flexibility of labour, retaining older workers in suitable jobs and producing an audit trail. Substantial initial investment is required, as is frequent re-assessment of workers recovering from recent incapacity, but early signs are that the investment will prove worthwhile.

Ageing and recovery from illness or injury

Age-associated loss of adaptability not only increases the risk of disease and injury, but increases the risk of secondary complications and lengthens the time needed for healing and recovery. This can be compensated for by the deployment of enhanced rehabilitation programmes to speed an older employee's return to work. While rest may initially be necessary to assist pain control after injury, for example, inactivity is detrimental to older people, as any loss of fitness brings them closer to their functional limits on return to work. Active rehabilitation and physiotherapy is a sound investment in restoring older individuals to the workforce. Psychological, as well as physical, needs may require attention. Specifically, older workers may suffer a loss of confidence following an accident or illness. Active *and repeated* encouragement and reassurance may prevent unnecessary invalidism combined with a phased return to work.

Although, owing to comorbidity, older people may recover more slowly than young people from illness, injury, or surgery, wide variations occur, dependent upon previous health, availability of suitable treatment, motivation, status and enjoyment of work, support of colleagues and family, managers' attitudes, and the opportunity for a graded or phased return to work, monitored by trained medical staff.[36] The myth that workers should be pain-free before returning to (suitably restricted) work, should be actively debunked. Functional assessments in the work environment are key to early and successful reintegration into work, following sickness absence, especially for acute musculoskeletal conditions.

Few employers today can afford the cost of delayed treatment and even fewer employees can afford the loss of income or job. Early access to assessment, active rehabilitation, and treatment services, preferably on-site or close by the place of work and managed by an occupational health practitioner, will expedite a successful return. Proactive intervention (e.g. instruction by physiotherapists in individually tailored exercise programmes, reinforced by other medical and nursing staff) may also prevent significant injury in those at risk and those displaying early symptoms.

It is the authors' experience that, if managers and supervisors are educated in the benefits of maintaining older workers' fitness and have free physiotherapy assessment and treatment services available and see their impact on sickness absence reduction, they will refer workers directly and proactively. Workers welcome early access to assessment and treatment, enabling them to stay in work and avoid sickness absence (and the consequent loss of income), giving improved control over their working lives and the business reaps the benefit.

There is evidence that older workers have longer absences from work due to illness than younger workers, as major medical problems increase with age, but they have fewer short-term spells of absence, which prove more disruptive to employers. Overall, older workers do not have more absence from the workplace than workers of other ages[1] and are careful to conserve sick leave as a 'cushion' for serious illness.[37] They are also less prone to accidents. However, if absence is prolonged, colleagues, supervisors, working patterns, and the workplace may have changed, posing a greater challenge to the older worker, returning to what is effectively a different job. Older workers are less confident and require more support when adapting to change.

An integrated approach comprising: (1) early completion of outpatient investigation and specialist assessment of the illness (ideally, within 6 weeks); (2) a supportive treatment and work hardening plan (involving an individual physical or psychological training plan, to return the worker to their own work, or to suitable alternative work); and (3) a graded or phased return to work on reduced hours, agreed with management, is the most cost-effective and efficient way of returning people safely to work. A reduction in long-term sickness absence usually results. Ideally, close cooperation and dialogue between the GP and the occupational physician will support the objective of reaching a decision point, regarding a return to work or if appropriate a medical ill health retirement, as soon as practicable.

There is a considerable cost-benefit, taking into account all employment costs, in proactively expediting early outpatient investigation and specialist assessment, ahead of normal NHS waiting times.

Retraining and redeployment

Older workers, once trained, are often more reliable and make fewer mistakes than younger workers. Initially, older workers may need help to avoid making mistakes, as these may have to be unlearned before the correct track is established. Time invested in training and re-training older workers is well spent. Lower staff turnover in older age groups has financial benefits in reduced recruitment costs and yields better returns from training initiatives. Content and delivery of older workers' training needs to be structured differently from that for younger workers. Trainers need to understand and utilize the differing learning strengths and weaknesses of both groups and tailor their programmes accordingly.[38]

In this adaptive society, multiple career changes and continuous retraining are now the norm in a longer working life to age 70 and beyond. Today's cutting edge new technologies will become routine tomorrow and will be handed on to workers with specific skills. The latter will still require core skills, enabling them to adapt to new changes as they appear; otherwise their skill base will become obsolete, rendering them at a disadvantage. Ring-fenced retraining funds will enable older workers to continue working, especially if they can no longer remain in their full-time job because of chronic illness or disability. These necessary costs will rise over the next 20 years.

Many semi-retired workers seek part-time employment to supplement their pensions. Part-time and flexible work in the UK service industry sector now provides many jobs (but often low rates of pay). However, personal safety for older people, where direct contact with the public is an integral part of the work, is a growing concern. When handling cash is involved, the older worker may be physically more vulnerable to injury or threats than the younger worker; assaulting and robbing older people may be seen as relatively risk-free by young assailants.

Older workers tend to work closer to their homes and not commute as far as younger workers. If these habits are to change, to satisfy demand for labour as the population ages, improved public transport will be required, designed to accommodate older workers with disabilities and special needs.

Ethical issues and retirement: duties to employers, responsibilities to employees

Expectations and norms will need to change for the manager, the worker, the GP, the occupational physician, the worker's family and dependents, and for all age groups in society. Most importantly, politicians who have ordered things so that people have to work longer to earn their pensions have an ethical duty to ensure that there are sufficient employment opportunities for older people. Employment options for older workers may well become more varied and flexible as the retirement age rises.

Ethical dilemmas will also become more frequent and challenging for occupational physicians. The continuing desire of many larger employers for manpower reductions, to meet cost requirements (downsizing, voluntary redundancy programmes, etc.), can result in both active and passive discrimination against the older worker.[39] Age discrimination is often based upon inaccurate and outdated assumptions and stereotypes about older workers or job applicants, which all work against the interests of both workers and their employers.[40,41]

The Faculty of Occupational Medicine position paper on Age and Employment (2004)[1] states:

> Older workers often have accumulated experience or learned strategies that may be valuable in contributing to business success. The published literature does not support the popular misconception that work performance declines with age. Older workers are noted to perform generally more consistently and to deliver higher quality, matching the performance of younger colleagues. In practice, despite an age related decline in physical strength, stamina, memory and information processing, this rarely impairs work performance. Older workers may use knowledge, skills, experience, anticipation, motivation and other strategies to maintain their performance. Older workers also bring the benefits of often being more conscientious, loyal, reliable and hard working and having well developed interpersonal skills. On balance, older workers do not have more absence from the workplace than workers of other ages. Older workers are also less prone to accidents. Lower staff turnover in the older age groups has financial benefits in reduced recruitment costs, and also in terms of better returns from training initiatives.

In a 2003 survey by 'Maturity Works', it was reported that 80 per cent of staff between the ages of 34 and 67 years say they have been victims of age discrimination. Conversely, one major UK national retail store chain has made a virtue out of positive age discrimination, recruiting older workers, for their greater experience of customers' needs. UK legislation has now removed the traditional default retirement age, thereby outlawing active age discrimination. However, whether employers will conform or seek ways around the legislation remains to be seen.

Some managers assume and promote the myth that all workers with cancers or those undergoing radiotherapy or chemotherapy will either die soon or will never return to productive work. Younger managers often have little or no personal experience of serious illness. Many older workers expect and want to stay in work, in spite of serious illness.[42-44] They appreciate that work may take more time and that recovery may take longer. They are often surprised and shocked when this is deemed unacceptable by managers.

The issue of ill health retirement is covered in detail in Chapter 27. There are many differing definitions and criteria for 'ill health or medical' retirement, in different occupations and work environments. Under pressure from managers, criteria for eligibility can become 'flexible', if organizational accommodations (reasonable adjustments) are believed to be too difficult to achieve. Older workers may then be judged to be failing in their jobs and can feel threatened if they are considered for dismissal on the grounds of capability.

The occupational physician must retain an independent and consistent position in such cases, always willing to consider and modify advice if and when relevant new evidence comes to hand, but resolute in the face of management pressure to remove an individual from the organization if he or she is simply perceived as being unlikely to return to productive work. All relevant information should be gathered to build up a complete picture of the patient's health and long-term prognosis. Although a recommendation for ill health retirement may be the outcome, this should always remain the last resort. In difficult circumstances it is often useful to discuss the case with a more experienced specialist occupational physician colleague.

If people expect to work longer, then the attitudes society holds on career trajectories will need to change. The question of whether large employers, whose core business requires much heavy or repetitive externally paced work, should be required by government to make lighter work available is as yet unanswered. Recent outsourcing by large organizations of non-core staff (e.g. caterers, janitors, and security staff) could be reversed, providing a possible method of retaining older workers in employment. Pre-retirement courses, run by many large employers, should always include a session on staying healthy in retirement, delivered by a competent and experienced healthcare worker. Such courses provide a valuable opportunity to guide prospective retirees in lifestyle choices and to encourage them to remain active and healthy.

Organizational issues

Management and social aspects

There is a perception among UK managers that older workers are more expensive than younger workers. This may change, particularly with the growth of fixed-term contracts in which overhead costs are unaffected by the age of the employee. There is an understandable ambivalence in the attitude of trades unions (TUs) to older workers, or to any development that may increase the availability of manpower, such as older workers remaining economically active into their later years. Governments, too, are happy to have a 'sink' of retirement in which to hide excessive unemployment. Society will need to address this issue and one option is for positive discrimination in favour of the older worker. However, if it is perceived that older workers are receiving preferential treatment within the group or company at the expense of younger workers, TUs will experience a difficult conflict of interest.

Increasingly, retirement is anticipated as a time for new interests and the pursuit of new goals. Part-time working, job-sharing, and other innovative semi-retirement packages can all help the older worker to achieve what is for them a preferred work pattern that suits their capability and personal circumstances as they move from full-time work into full-time retirement. These enable retiring workers to retain the social contact and support network of the working environment without the pressure and commitment to full-time work. However, in a mass production environment, such flexibility may be difficult to achieve as employers find job-sharing expensive (due to taxation, employment and training costs) and time consuming, especially if illness or family responsibilities disrupt the agreed work pattern and employees require additional support.

Shift work

Many workers find shift work more difficult as they age, especially if night work is involved, and may seek medical approval to withdraw from work at night.[45] People aged over 40 starting shift work for the first time experience difficulty adapting to different sleep and eating times, while those who have worked shifts for decades may suddenly notice fatigue at night and feel lethargic and less well. The performance on night shifts of older workers may be less than that in younger workers.[46] There is evidence that the time to exhaustion is reduced by a significant amount (20 per cent) for older shift workers during the recovery period from night shift.[47] In addition, evidence exists that a fast forward rotating shift schedule is more suitable for older workers than a slower backward rotating system.[48]

Sleep disorders are more common in older workers.[49] In extreme cases the older worker may be at risk of losing his or her job if regular day shift work cannot be provided. In addition, older workers, who travel regularly back and forth across several time zones by air either as aircrew or passengers, take longer to recover their circadian rhythm with increasing age. However, older individuals who have wider natural circadian rhythm swings and the apparent ability to reset their body clocks more quickly appear to cope better than others with this work and lifestyle. If performance is affected adversely to an unacceptable degree, redeployment within the employing organization may prove difficult, e.g. for pilots. Employers should be sympathetic to making reasonable adjustments to accommodate such requests.

Temporary reorganization of shift patterns may be necessary for individual workers after depressive illness or while still recovering on medication. This is especially necessary during the winter months at higher latitudes when 'Zeitgeber' (time-of-day) cues are reduced or absent and when the risk of relapse, after stopping medication at this time of year, may be increased. Diabetics and sufferers from seasonal affective disorder (SAD syndrome) will have their own additional difficulties with alterations in diurnal rhythm associated with shift changes. These can usually be overcome by good planning and a disciplined approach, both of which are more commonly observed in older workers. Bright desk lamps can be used by office workers with SAD syndrome to assist alertness and productivity.

Hours of work

The EU Working Time Directive (implemented in the UK by the Working Time Regulations 1998[50]) requires written consent from workers required to work an average of more than 48 hours per week over a (normally 3-month) reference period. In addition, other requirements include a minimum daily rest period of 11 consecutive hours a day and that night working must not exceed 8 hours a night on average.

A culture of long working hours is more prevalent in the UK than in other European countries. Additional hours of work (e.g. 12-hour shifts, weekend overtime, and additional shifts) are often welcomed by the younger worker for the earnings they bring. Older workers are often less enthusiastic, especially those in poor health. The incentives for the self-employed to work longer hours and to take less time off for illness remain. Access to occupational health services for the self-employed has always been inferior to that for employed workers and this may need to be rectified. The Turner Report[51] urged the UK Government to consider incentives to keep older workers in work for longer. Such incentives will need to be flexible, regarding part-time working, and accompanied by suitable alterations in taxation and employment legislation to ensure that they achieve the desired result. In addition, the older self-employed and teleworkers will need to be included in these arrangements.

Upstream ergonomics: input into the design of processes

Mass production and service industry job design requires early occupational health involvement and effective monitoring of process developments and changes. Feedback of information, learned from current processes, incorporating ergonomic improvements into new manufacturing and service delivery processes is in the interests of all workers, regardless of age.

Occupational physicians should make strong representation to be consulted regularly during the job design phase of new components and products as this has been inconsistent in the past. In particular, the occupational physician *must* be involved at the earliest possible design stage of repetitive work. Late changes and alterations in the product should not be made without the occupational physician being consulted. Failure to involve the occupational physician, can lead to costly subsequent work reorganization and/or legal claims from workers, affected by repetitive overuse injuries or psychological illness. The older worker who develops such conditions is likely to take longer to recover than the younger worker, and is more likely to develop a chronic state, requiring permanent redeployment, always assuming that such alternative work is available.[52]

Ergonomic improvements should ideally be innovative, individual and inexpensive. Adaptation of the majority of workplaces is needed to accommodate physically restricted older workers. Ideally, job rotation needs to be 2–4-hourly, rather than daily or weekly, to accommodate all temporarily or permanently restricted and disabled workers. A worker who is recovering from a laparotomy, a myocardial infarction, or a prolapsed intervertebral disc may be restricted with regard to manual handling for several weeks or months whatever their age. The introduction of robots or other mechanical equipment (preferably under the worker's control) and improved workplace and component design, and 'lazy seats' allowing the worker to move more easily around a production line while sitting, thereby avoiding standing and repeated bending, are examples of improvements that will preferentially protect older workers and improve their overall flexibility and status in the workforce.

While much mechanical back pain is now avoided by ergonomic workplace improvements, ergonomic design aimed at preventing neck, shoulder, and upper limb pain and fatigue is only now in the ascendant. Additional training is needed for ergonomists to enable them to understand the abilities and limitations of older people in respect of capabilities, muscular strength, static loads, the risk of injury, and the effect of shift patterns and rest periods in relation to fatigue. Expert ergonomic input into process and risk assessments will ensure that both are relevant and appropriate for workers of all ages.

Older workers and younger managers

This is the first generation in which a majority of younger managers and supervisors, in their 30s and early 40s, are commonly managing groups of people, of whom half or more are from their parents' generation. Commonly, the younger manager has no concept of what it feels like to live with chronic pain and the effect that this has on performance and on a worker's enjoyment of work.

Research has shown that managers rate older job applicants as less economically beneficial to the organization than younger applicants.[41] The older worker is sometimes seen by the younger manager as being slow, work-shy, uncooperative, and resistant to change. The younger manager, in turn, is sometimes seen as unpredictable, overbearing, inconsistent, and arrogant. Inflexible handling of misunderstandings by the younger manager can lead to resentment, mistrust, and, ultimately, demotivation. Older workers may fear for their job security, especially if already coping with discomfort and disability associated with long-standing degenerative illness, either in themselves or in a spouse or partner.

This can lead to emotional crisis or depression and, commonly, to sickness absence. Aggressive or blame cultures can exacerbate such situations. Individual productivity inevitably suffers. In an ageing population, such situations may occur more frequently in the future. All parties can benefit from improved training in communication, conflict resolution, and in improved knowledge and understanding of the strengths, capabilities, and reasonable expectations of different age groups. The occupational health practitioner will often require patience and great sensitivity in such situations (assisted by human resources staff and expert counselling services, as necessary), to re-establish the older worker's self-esteem, if prolonged sickness absence is to be avoided.

Possible actions and solutions

In 2004, The National Statistical Office estimated that the UK population would rise by about 5 million people over 20 years, with immigrants accounting for two-thirds of this growth. Net migration into the UK during this period was projected to be about 135000 a year. Labour market gaps and government spending on public services to support this increase will create a need for more nurses, teachers, doctors, and other skilled workers.

Importing young people indiscriminately from abroad may be thought at first sight to represent a solution. However, this can produce a net drain on resources if they do not have skills that enable them immediately to contribute to the economy. In addition, once migrants are settled, they tend to adopt the habits and lifestyle of the host country and grow older. More new immigrants are then needed to support them and the cycle is repeated.

For two decades, societal attitudes, consumer pressures and tastes and legislation have all been driving business organizations towards becoming 'lean, mean, and young'. The skills and experience of older workers have been largely sidelined by the movement of information away from books and older people into information technology systems. This has been driven by computerization, the (global) standardization of processes across businesses, and by the need to reduce manufacturing process variability, all driven by consumer pressures for higher quality and reliability of goods and services at reduced cost.

As the population ages further, social institutions now need to be re-based; expectations and norms will need to change. John Stuart Mill[53] recognized a tolerant society, which was fundamentally individualist but in which individual members accepted obligations towards other people. In an increasingly competitive world, all age groups will need to provide for themselves and for one another, and for their own potential periods of low productivity and earnings (e.g. pregnancy, sickness, retirement), throughout their lives. A social model of older and retired workers being provided for by the relatively diminishing cohorts of younger workers is no longer realistic.

Concepts of 'rights' and 'entitlements' will undergo necessary evolution, as Britain's earning capacity in the world alters, relative to the developing economies, primarily in China, and the Far East. However, the global picture is complex; for example, China also has a large older segment of its population.[54] Economic competitiveness of the EU with the 'BRIC' economies (Brazil, Russia, India, and China), which have significantly younger age profiles, will require the UK workforce to 'work smarter', as 'working harder' may not be practicable as the working population ages.

This change *can* be accommodated within a culture of inclusion for the older worker, at the same time as meeting and maintaining manufacturing and service industry requirements, but the change will not be swift or easy. Older workers with scarce skills will remain in demand and will be economically self-sufficient; those who cannot embrace the computer age or who suffer from chronic illness and/or live in areas of higher unemployment will fare less well. There is good evidence of a link between unemployment and ill health, with older economically inactive people between 50 and 65 years of age being less fit than their working counterparts. In the future, people will have to work longer but not necessarily harder, up to the age of 70 and, if they wish beyond, in order to provide for their old age. This concept is now promoted by the UK government and a retirement age of 70 is likely to be in place before 2030.

A recent survey of UK employers showed that 86 per cent believe that care issues (for older relatives) will be a key concern in the future. As a result, the career expectations, earnings, savings, and work trajectories of older workers will all need to alter, as will training, legislation, age discrimination, taxation, the provision for pensions, and arrangements for the care of older workers' elderly relatives living into their nineties. (See web-listed references in Boxes 26.1 and 26.2, after G. Glover, Society of Occupational Medicine Annual Scientific Meeting, 2003, personal communication.) Business, government, and TUs must jointly and severally acknowledge their responsibilities for integrating older people into the working community.

Box 26.1 What businesses require of government as the population ages

Businesses need the Government to:

- Develop a strategic position on the demographic issue.
- Develop health services aimed specifically at supporting older workers remaining in work.
- Consider funding/subsidizing individuals who cannot cope with full-time (first-tier) employment as they become older.
- Provide tax incentives and other means of support for employing organizations to safeguard training budgets, especially for older workers.
- Ensure that pension arrangements support worker mobility.
- Be aware of the pressures on organizations for 'ill health retirement' as the retirement age rises.
- Provide flexible labour policies enabling employers to release employees, often at short notice and for extended periods, for elder care (parents and relatives).

Box 26.2 What businesses need to do to accommodate an ageing workforce

Businesses need to:

+ Consider their most effective strategic plan and direction—as well as employment legislation.

+ Examine and change individual and institutional attitudes towards older employees.

+ Review all policies, procedures, practices, and then customise them to meet the needs of the older employee.

+ Consider how best to support the rising number of staff caring for elderly parents and relatives.

+ Regard flexibility as key for employees seeking changes, to maintain an acceptable work-life balance.

+ Review methods needed to sustain employee motivation over longer careers and to transform organization cultures away from a 'youth culture'.

+ Increase the emphasis on improving health, safety, and well-being, as part of a drive towards greater productivity and efficiency, especially for the older worker.

+ Refine and embed strategies in their organization to deal with foreseeable absence and periods of prolonged illness in older workers.

+ Challenge organizational norms about what workers can do, as they age.

+ Challenge established national norms about when employees leave (and return to) organizations.

+ Harness new technologies, innovative work practices and job design to support and keep older workers at work.

+ Promote an environment and culture of continuous personal improvement and lifelong learning.

+ Establish a position as an employer of choice, not just for the young but for all age groups.

References

1 Faculty of Occupational Medicine. *Position paper on Age and Employment*, 2004. London, Faculty of Occupational Medicine.

2 Kirkwood TBL, Rose MR. Evolution of senescence: late survival sacrificed for reproduction. *Phil Trans R Soc Lond B* 1991; **332**: 15–24.

3 Grimley Evans J. How are the elderly different? In: Kane RL, Grimley Evans J, Macfadyen D (eds), *Improving the health of older people: a world view* pp. 50–68. Oxford: Oxford University Press, 1990.

4 Schaie KW, Strother CR. A cross-sequential study of age changes in cognitive behavior. *Psychol Bull* 1968; **70**: 671–80.

5 Grimley Evans J. Ageing and disease. In: Evered D, Whelan J (eds) *Research and the ageing population* pp. 38–57. Chichester: John Wiley and Sons Ltd, 1988.

6 Steptoe A, Marmot M. The role of psychobiological pathways in socio-economic inequalities in cardiovascular disease risk. *Eur Heart J* 2002; **23**: 13–25.

7 Ott A, Breteler MB, van Harskamp F, *et al.* Prevalence of Alzheimer's disease and vascular dementia: association with education. The Rotterdam study. *BMJ* 1995; **310**: 970–3.

8 Manton K, Gu X. Changes in the prevalence of chronic disability in the United States black and non-black population above age 65 from 1982 to 1999. *Proc Nat Acad Sci USA* 2001; **98**: 6354–9.

9 Aittomaki A, Lahelma E, Roos E, *et al.* Gender differences in the association of age with physical work-load and functioning. *Occup Environ Med* 2005; **62**: 95–100.

10 Raab DM, Agre JC, McAdam M, *et al.* Light resistance and stretching exercise in elderly women: effect upon flexibility. *Arch Phys Med Rehabil* 1988; **69**: 268–72.

11 Snook SH. The effects of age and physique on continuous-work capacity. *Hum Factors* 1971; **13**: 467–9.

12 Orlander J, Aniansson A. Effects of physical training on skeletal muscle metabolism, morphology and function in 70–5 year old men. *Acta Physiol Scand* 1980; **109**: 149–54.

13 Goycoolea MV, Goycoolea HG, Rodriguez LG, *et al.* Effect of life in industrialized societies on hearing in natives of Easter Island. *Laryngoscope* 1986; **96**: 1391–6.

14 Pichora-Fuller MK. Cognitive aging and auditory information processing. *Int J Audiol* 2003; **42**(Suppl. 2): S26–32.

15 Pichora-Fuller MK, Schneider BA, Daneman M. How young and old adults listen to and remember speech in noise. *J Acoust Soc Am* 1995; **97**: 593–608.

16 Ball K, Owsley C, Beard B. Clinical visual perimetry underestimates peripheral field problems in older adults. *Clin Vis Sci* 1990; **5**: 113–25.

17 Owsley C, Ball K, McGwin G, *et al.* Visual processing impairment and risk of motor vehicle crash among older adults. *JAMA* 1998; **279**: 1083–8.

18 Winner SJ, Morgan CA, Grimley Evans J. Perimenopausal risk of falling and incidence of distal forearm fracture. *BMJ* 1989; **298**: 1486–8.

19 Grimley Evans J. Transient neurological dysfunction and risk of stroke in an elderly English population: the different significance of vertigo and non-rotatory dizziness. *Age Ageing* 1990; **19**: 43–9.

20 Lakatta EG. Cardiovascular aging without a clinical diagnosis. *Dialogues Cardiovasc Med* 2001; **6**: 67–91.

21 Sander K, Sander D. New insights into transient global amnesia: recent imaging and clinical findings. *Lancet Neurol* 2005; **4**: 437–44.

22 Felson DT. Epidemiology of hip and knee osteoarthritis. *Epidemiol Rev* 1988; **10**: 1–28.

23 Zucherman JF, Hsu KY, Hartjen CA, *et al.* A multicenter, prospective, randomized trial evaluating the X STOP interspinous process decompression system for the treatment of neurogenic intermittent claudication: two-year follow-up results. *Spine* 2005; **30**: 1351–8.

24 Wu EQ, Birnbaum H, Marynchenko M, *et al.* Employees with overactive bladder: work loss burden. *J Occup Environ Med* 2005; **47**: 439–46.

25 British National Formulary, 2005. (<http://www.bnf.org/bnf/bnf/current>).

26 Meck Higgins M, Barkley MC. Barriers to nutrition education for older adults, and nutrition and aging training opportunities for educators, healthcare providers, volunteers and caregivers. *J Nutr Elder* 2004; **23**: 99–121.

27 Bagwell MM, Bush HA. Improving health promotion for blue-collar workers. *J Nurs Care Qual* 2000; **14**: 65–71.

28 Infeld DL, Whitelaw N. Policy initiatives to promote healthy aging. *Clin Geriatr Med* 2002; **18**: 627–42.

29 Bozzetti F. Nutritional issues in the care of the elderly patient. *Crit Rev Oncol Hematol* 2003; **48**: 113–21.

30 Fit note gets lost in translation, says research. *Occup Health* 2011; **63**(9): 5.

31 Secretary of State for Health. *The Health of the Nation. A Strategy for Health in England.* Cm1986. London: HMSO, 1992.

32 Secretary of State for Health. *Our Healthier Nation. A Contract for Health.* CM 3852. London: The Stationery Office, 1998.

33 Faculty of Occupational Medicine. *SEQOHS—Occupational Health Service Standards for Accreditation.* London. January 2010. ISBN 978-1-86016-374-6.

34 de Zwart BHC, Frings-Dresen MHW, van Duivenbooden JC. Test-retest reliability of the Work Ability Index questionnaire. *Occup Med* 2002; **52**: 177–81.

35 Greve J, Jochheim KA, Schian HM. Assessment methods for vocational integration of disabled persons– from ERTOMIS methods to the IMBA information system [in German]. *Rehabilitation* 1997; **36**: 34–8.

36 Bongers PM, de Winter CR, Kompier MAJ, *et al.* Psychosocial factors at work and musculoskeletal disease. *Scand J Work Environ Health* 1993; **19**: 297–312.

37 Cant R, O'Loughlin K, Legge V. Sick leave—cushion or entitlement? A study of age cohorts' attitudes and practices in two Australian workplaces. *Work* 2001; **17**: 39–48.

38 Wetherick NE. Changing an established concept: a comparison of the ability of young, middle-aged and old subjects. *Gerontologia* 1965; **11**: 82–95.

39 Vahtera J, Kivimäki M, Pennti J. Effect of organisational downsizing on health of employees. *Lancet* 1997; **350**: 1124–8.

40 McMullin JA, Marshall VW. Ageism, age relations, and garment industry work in Montreal. *Gerontologist* 2001; **41**: 111–22.

41 Finkelstein LM, Burke MJ. Age stereotyping at work: the role of rater and contextual factors on evaluations of job applicants. *J Gen Psychol* 1998; **125**: 317–45.

42 Kinne S, Probart C, Gritz ER. Cancer-risk-related health behaviors and attitudes of older workers. Working Well Research Group. *J Cancer Educ* 1996; **11**: 89–95.

43 Verbeek J, Spelten E, Kammeijer M, *et al.* Return to work of cancer survivors: a prospective cohort study into the quality of rehabilitation by occupational physicians. *Occup Environ Med* 2003; **60**: 352–7.

44 Spelten ER, Sprangers MA, Verbeek JH. Factors reported to influence the return to work of cancer survivors: a literature review. *Psychooncology* 2002; **11**: 124–31.

45 Harma MI, Ilmarinen JE. Towards the 24-hour society-new approaches for aging shift workers? *Scand J Work Environ Health* 1999; **25**: 610–5.

46 de Zwart BC, Bras VM, van Dormolen M, *et al.* After-effects of night work on physical performance capacity and sleep quality in relation to age. *Int Arch Occup Environ Health* 1993; **65**: 259–62.

47 Tepas DI, Duchon JC, Gersten AH. Shiftwork and the older worker. *Exp Aging Res* 1993; **19**: 295–320.

48 Hakola T, Harma M. Evaluation of a fast forward rotating shift schedule in the steel industry with a special focus on ageing and sleep. *J Hum Ergol (Tokyo)* 2001; **30**: 315–19.

49 Reid K, Dawson D. Comparing performance on a simulated 12 hour shift rotation in young and older subjects. *Occup Environ Med* 2001; **58**: 58–62.

50 Working Time Regulations 1998 (Statutory Instrument 1998/1833).

51 The Pensions Commission. *Pensions: challenges and choices.* The first and second reports of the Pensions Commission. (<http://www.pensionscommission.org.uk/publications/2004/annrep/index.asp> and <http://www.dwp.gov.uk/publications/dwp/2005/pensionscommreport/annrep-index.asp>)

52 Salvendy G, Pilitsis J. Psychophysiological aspects of paced and unpaced performance as influenced by age. *Ergonomics* 1971; **14**: 703–11.

53 Mill JS. *On liberty.* London: John W Parker and Son, West Strand, 1859.

54 Zhai Z. Urbanization and the aging of urban population in China: trend and countermeasures. *Chin J Popul Sci* 1997; **9**: 35–44.

Further reading

Bromley DB. *The psychology of human ageing*, 2nd edn. Harmondsworth: Penguin, 1996.

Buchan J. The 'greying' of the United Kingdom nursing workforce: implications for employment policy and practice. *J Adv Nurs* 1999; **30**: 818–26.

Healy ML. Management strategies for an aging work force. *AAOHN J* 2001; **11**: 523–9.

Hearnshaw LS. The psychological and occupational aspects of ageing. Liverpool researches (1953–70). London: Medical Research Council, 1971.

Heron A. Ageing and employment. In: Schilling RSF (ed), *Modern trends in occupational health*, 209–29. London: Butterworth, 1960.

Jamieson GH. Inspection in the telecommunications industry: a field study of age and other performance variables. *Ergonomics* 1966; **9**: 297–303.

McGee JP, Wegman DH. *Health and safety needs of older workers: Committee on the Health and Safety Needs of Older Workers*. Washington, DC: National Academies Press, 2004.

Macheath JA. *Activity, health and fitness in old age*. London: Groom-Helm, 1984.

Wegman DH. Older workers. *Occup Med* 1999; **14**: 537–57.

Welford AT. *Ageing and human skill*. Oxford: Oxford University Press, 1958.

Woollams C. *Everything you need to know to help you beat cancer*, 2nd edn. Gawcott, Buckingham: Health Issues Ltd, 2003. (<http://allyouneedtoknowaboutcancer.com>)

Chapter 27

Ill health retirement

Jon Poole

Demographics

In the UK the number of people of pensionable age has been rising as life expectancy has increased and fecundity has fallen. The number of workers to the number of retirees, which is known as the support ratio, is falling in most developed counties. In the UK, the crude ratio was 4.3 in the 1970s, but fell to 3.6 in 2010 and is expected to fall to 3.0 in 2025. If the number of unemployed people is removed from the numerator then the ratio falls even further.[1] Governments and pension scheme managers are addressing the problem of a falling support ratio by increasing the retirement age, increasing contribution rates, and moving from 'defined benefit' to 'defined contribution' schemes. Figure 27.1 provides an example of a low support ratio for a large national occupational pension scheme with many more pensioners than active members.

During the 1980s early retirement due to ill health rapidly increased, with rates of 10–20/1000 contributing members in most public sector schemes.[2,3] The reasons for these increases are unknown, but were probably influenced by changes to working practices and some employers' desire to use the pension scheme for workforce management. Currently, only a small proportion of people work after the age of 65, but this is likely to increase with the removal of default retirement ages, changes to the normal pensionable age, relaxation of tax rules on the receipt of pension benefits while continuing to work, and lifting of the maximum number of pensionable years of service.

Wide variations in rates of early retirement have been reported between employers and even within different parts of the same organization.[3] While some variation is to be expected, such as a higher rate in jobs that require high levels of physical fitness, or in an older workforce, most variation is inexplicable on medical grounds alone. For example, a concurrence of modes of ill health retirement (IHR) age with dates of enhancement in benefit can only be explained by the influence of non-medical factors on decisions to retire. There is no medical reason why increases of ill health (mainly in the form of minor psychiatric and musculoskeletal disorders) should occur at these times. It is reasonable to assume therefore that other reasons, such as lack of motivation to remain at work and an exaggerated declaration of incapability, have been contributory factors.

In general, rates of retirement due to ill health, rather like sickness absence, are higher in the public sector than the private sector. The reasons are likely to be multifactorial, but probably include a sharper focus by the latter on performance and attendance, with greater readiness to dismiss on incapability grounds. However, in response to the Treasury's review of IHR in the public sector,[4] pension schemes have tightened up their processes and eligibility criteria for granting early pensions. Occupational physicians are now more likely to be involved and conflicts of interest for other doctors reduced. In most schemes permanent incapacity has been defined as up to normal pensionable age and most schemes have more than one tier of benefits, with maximum

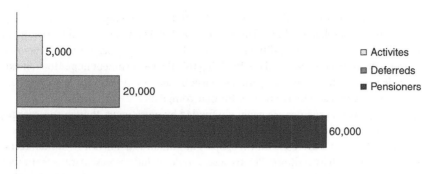

Figure 27.1 A UK pension scheme membership profile with a very low support ratio. Data from the Office of National Statistics.

benefits being awarded to those incapable of undertaking any work whatsoever, not just their current job. Consequently, the rate of IHR in, for example, the National Health Service (NHS) has fallen from 3.8/1000 employed members in 2001–2002 to 1.4/1000 in 2010–2011 (personal communication) and the Home Office has estimated that it saved £42m in pension payments to firefighters between 2005 and 2010 (personal communication).

Is retirement good for your health? Early studies suggested that retirement led to a doubling of the risk of myocardial infarction,[5] but mental health was likely to improve, particularly for those with high socio-economic status.[6] More recent longitudinal studies, that have controlled better for health selection effects prior to retirement, have shown that mortality after retirement depends on the health of the retiree and not on early retirement per se.[7,8] So for most people retirement makes no difference to their health, although some will feel better.

State pensions

The state scheme in the UK is two tiered, consisting of a basic pension and an additional state pension known as the State Second Pension (previously SERPS). Individuals may opt out of this additional scheme in favour of an occupational, stakeholder, or personal pension. It is funded directly from National Insurance contributions from both the employer and the employee. Currently the state pension is payable from age 65 for men and from age 60 for women, but will increase gradually for women born after 1949 from 2010 until it has been equalized to age 65 in 2018. The pensionable age for both sexes will then move to 66 in 2020 and to 68 in 2046. An online calculator to determine an individual's state pension age is available.[9] The state pension cannot be taken early (other than for bereaved spouses), but can be deferred until age 70, with a percentage increase for each week of deferment. The value of the basic pension has been declining since the link to earnings was replaced with inflation linkage two decades ago. Concerns about growing poverty in old age and the affordability of current benefit levels has resulted in a re-examination of the fundamental principles underpinning the current arrangements.[10]

Occupational and personal pensions

Occupational pension schemes in the UK have traditionally been offered by the larger and longer-established employers. Since October 2001 it has been mandatory for employers with five or more employees to offer a 'stakeholder pension' if a suitable occupational or personal scheme does not exist (see the Welfare Reform and Pensions Act 1999). However, employers were not required to contribute to such a scheme. Under The Pensions Act 2008 employers will be required from 2012 to enrol their workers into 'qualifying pension schemes' into which both the employee and the employer will contribute 8% of salary. By doing this the Government hopes that an extra 10 million people will be enrolled in occupational pension schemes. A Pensions Regulator has been appointed to oversee this and there are fines for non-compliance.[11]

Occupational pension schemes are generally funded by investment, though some large public sector schemes are funded from taxation. They are generally run by representatives of the employer in the form of trustees, with the help of administrators, investment managers, and external consultants such as auditors. The trustees should include representatives from staff and pensioners. Occupational and personal pension schemes tend to be more flexible than the state scheme, with the possibility of taking benefits early, such as age 35 for sportsmen, or later, up to age 75. Trustees have discretionary powers over eligibility to an early pension and in the case of ill health they will base their decision on information submitted by the member and from independent doctors. Pension schemes must have a formal internal dispute resolution procedure (IDRP) for complaints and appeals. These are usually divided into two stages, firstly at the level of the employer and secondly at the level of the pension scheme's administrators.

The Pensions Advisory Service

Advice about pensions can be obtained in the UK from the Pensions Advisory Service, an independent organization that is grant-aided by the Department for Work and Pensions. Complaints, disputes, or appeals which cannot be resolved by an IDRP can be referred to this service, which may in turn refer the case to the Pensions Ombudsman. He will determine whether trustees or administrators have: (1) incorrectly interpreted the scheme rules or regulations; (2) misdirected themselves in law; (3) taken into account all the relevant factors but no irrelevant ones; or (4) come to a perverse decision, i.e. one that no reasonable body would make. The Pensions Ombudsman receives 30–40 complaints per year about early retirement due to ill health, mostly disputing the non-permanence of their incapacity. These represent about 12% of complaints referred to this office.[12]

Defined benefit and defined contribution schemes

The model for most occupational pension schemes through the 20th century was that of defined benefits (DB). Individuals and employers pay a proportion of salary into a general fund from which pensions are then paid out. Characteristically each year of service with the organization would qualify the individual for a proportion (e.g. 1/80 or 1/60) of their final salary at retirement as a pension—such schemes may also be referred to as final salary schemes. These arrangements favour individuals who accrue long service with a single organization and whose earnings peak at the end of their career. They also provide the individual scheme member with substantial certainty about the value of the pension they are likely to receive at retirement, so risk falls on the employer or their pension scheme provider to pay a contractual sum at retirement.

The main alternative model is the defined contribution (DC) scheme. Here individuals and employers pay a proportion of salary into a fund of which each member has a share dependent upon their contribution. Upon retirement the individual is free to use the sum accumulated to purchase an annuity that will provide an income—such schemes may be described as money purchase schemes. These arrangements are more favourable to individuals whose earnings do not vary substantially, or whose peak income occurs some time before their retirement age. The value of the annuity is dependent upon market conditions at the time of purchase, so the employer or their pension scheme provider has a much greater certainty regarding their potential liability and risk falls mainly on the employee. UK employers in the private sector are moving towards DC pension schemes and such a move, with a common framework of provisions, has been recommended for the public sector as well.[10]

Most schemes include a provision for compensating members who have to give up work early because of ill health or injury. They typically pay a pension immediately, rather than at the normal retirement age, without actuarial reduction of benefits and often with an enhancement to the pensionable years of service.

Criteria

Eligibility for an early and enhanced pension is dependent on the member meeting criteria set out by the trustees or regulators of the pension scheme. Criteria vary between schemes, but most require the applicant to be permanently incapable of undertaking their job, or any work as a consequence of ill health, illness, or injury. It is essential for the doctor to understand the precise criteria for the scheme on which they are advising and the interpretation that is applied to the wording (Box 27.1). Reference should always be made to the scheme regulations, and any statutory guidance or other guidance that has been written by the trustees or the scheme's administrators.

Permanence is usually defined as until the scheme's normal pensionable age, which can vary by scheme, date of joining, length of service, and job (Table 27.1). Most pension schemes allow for flexible retirement whereby members can draw an occupational pension while continuing to work for the same employer. The removal of the default retirement age does not affect a pension scheme's normal pensionable age, which is likely to be the same for both men and women and some patients may need to have this explained to them.

Most schemes require that the applicant has undergone reasonable treatment before ill health or injury is said to be permanent. If the applicant has not engaged in such treatment then the doctor should either defer judgement about permanency, or say whether treatment would normally be expected to be effective. Reasonable adaptations, aids in the workplace, or adjustments to the job should have been tried and found to have been unsuccessful for medical rather than non-medical reasons before permanency of incapacity is confirmed. That is, the doctor may have to make a judgment about engagement with treatment and motivation when a patient fails to respond to treatment or adjustments, that normally would be expected to be effective, when there is an incentive to remain incapacitated.

Box 27.1 Impact of scheme rules on eligibility for ill health retirement

Scheme A states that to qualify for ill health retirement an individual must be *incapable by virtue of permanent ill health* while Scheme B states that one must be *permanently incapable by virtue of ill health*. Someone experiencing an acute exacerbation of a chronic condition, such as diabetes or epilepsy, which renders them unfit for work now but which is expected to improve over time might arguably qualify for ill health retirement under the rules of Scheme A but not under those of Scheme B.

Table 27.1 Ill health retirement in public sector pension schemes 2009–2011

Pension scheme	NPA	Tiers	Number of IHRs in 1 year	Number of contributing members in same year	Rate of IHR/1000 members
NHS	55, 60, 65	2	1845	1 368 215	1.4
Local Government	65	3	2952	1 684 000	1.8
Teachers	60, 65	2	651	658 351	1.0
Civil Service	55, 60, 65	1 or 2	652	528 160	1.2
Fire	50–60	1 or 2	44	39 754	1.1
Police	50–60	1 or 2	306	141 486	2.2

NPA, normal pensionable age, but subject to change. IHR, ill-health retirement.

A number of pension schemes in both the private and public sectors have more than one tier of eligibility criteria for IHR. Characteristically the lower tier (lower benefits) requires evidence of incapacity to undertake the job for which the member is employed and the upper tier (higher benefits) requires evidence of incapacity to undertake any gainful employment. A common arrangement is that, while a pension is paid immediately for both tiers, only benefits of the upper tier are enhanced. The job may be defined in various ways, for example, for NHS staff as their contracted duties for that employing Trust; for teachers as teaching in any school (including part-time) and for police officers as the ordinary duties of an officer in any force (not just the one for which they are employed).

In general, incapacity for all work is more clear-cut than incapacity for their job. Furthermore, in most schemes capability to undertake a job other than the contacted one need not be restricted to one of similar earning capacity, e.g. a patient may not be capable of working as a director, but if they are capable of working as an administrator or driver this would make them ineligible for a higher-tier pension. Determining incapacity from an individual's own job requires the advising doctor to have a good knowledge of the functional requirements of the job, working practices, and the sort of adjustments that can reasonably be accommodated by the employer. This should be made explicit by the doctor in their report.

Terms such as ill health or infirmity of body or mind are rarely defined in regulations themselves so doctors are advised to become familiar with the explanatory guidance of the scheme. Conditions that are not contained within the current International Classification of Diseases,[13] such as stress or burnout, should not be accepted as medical illnesses for the purpose of IHR. Care should also be taken to ensure that there is a direct causal link between any incapacity and ill health. Some applicants will declare incapability for carrying out tasks for which they are employed and a long-standing coexisting illness may be convenient for terminating employment on favourable terms funded by the pension scheme.

An area of particular difficulty is that of secondary ill health. Employees with performance, attendance, or disciplinary problems may absent themselves from work citing 'stress', anxiety, or depression and choose to pursue IHR as the solution to their employment problems. Some schemes insist that the ill health qualifying for a pension must be primary (i.e. unrelated to any effects of a reasonable employment process), rather than secondary and require that issues related to employment be resolved before eligibility to a pension is considered. In any case, reactive ill health is unlikely to be permanently incapacitating unless it occurs shortly before the normal pension age. So, although it may be in the employee's best interest to retire, the eligibility criteria for a medical pension must be met.

Evidence

The optimum means of determining whether an individual is likely to meet the criteria for IHR will vary by case. However, it will be usual for evidence to include an assessment of capability, matched to the requirements of the job, as well as medical evidence about the illness or injury that allows the formulation of a diagnosis and prognosis. In most cases, sufficient medical evidence can be gleaned by examining the patient and from the patient's medical records, general practitioner, or specialist but, where this is deficient, an independent examination or additional investigations may be needed to provide the necessary quality of evidence. When requesting a report it should be made clear that it is information on diagnosis, treatment, and prognosis which is being sought, and not a view on employment issues or entitlement to a pension, the terms of which may not be known to the treating doctor.

Where the illness is terminal, prognosis should be ascertained as pension benefits may be commuted when life expectancy is less than 12 months. Most pension schemes require a certificate of eligibility to be completed by the independent doctor but it is good practice to include a report as well, so that at any subsequent appeal the evidence on which the doctor's inferences were made and the reasons for subsequent recommendations about IHR can be seen.

In a few cases, providing a professional opinion when a patient wishes to avoid work or to gain a pension or injury award may be problematic for the doctor. This is because the relationship between doctor and patient is not a normal therapeutic one, but is for the purposes of providing specific advice to a third party. Guidance on the ethical issues for doctors with such a dual responsibility has been published by the General Medical Council and the Faculty of Occupational Medicine (see also Chapter 5). Whilst it is the duty of all doctors to put the care of the patient first, this should be for medical and not economic purposes. In the process of the examination the doctor may identify inconsistencies in the history or examination, abnormal illness behaviour, entrenched beliefs or views about prognosis, undiagnosed psychological (rather than medical or psychiatric) ill health, or illness deception. Such findings should be documented and taken into account when formulating a professional opinion. The patient should be given an opportunity to comment on a draft medical report before it is submitted to the pension scheme trustees or administrators and given an explanation of the grounds for the decision not to award a pension. Recommendations should be made on the basis of a balance of probabilities rather than beyond reasonable doubt, i.e. what is likely, rather than what is possible or almost certain.

Conflicts of interest

Those charged with advising a pension scheme about eligibility to IHR must remember that they have a contractual duty to the trustees of the scheme or the taxpayer, but not to the individual scheme member or to the employer. Advice must be objective and evidence based. Factors such as expediency or social circumstances should be disregarded. Doctors who may be involved in the treatment of the patient, or are the patient's general practitioner, should not advise the pension scheme about eligibility because of the inherent potential for a conflict of interests. Such a doctor may provide factual information about the patient's health, treatment and prognosis, but should not be asked whether eligibility criteria have been met and should avoid offering an unsolicited opinion. Pension scheme medical advisers or trustees may reasonably disregard such opinions, as opposed to factual information.

In larger pension schemes it is usual to separate occupational health advice to the employer from advice to the pension scheme. Smaller schemes may have to rely on the employer's medical adviser as the only source of competent advice on health related to employment, so those undertaking such a role must be assiduous in acting impartially. For this reason it is good practice for two or more doctors to be involved in the process of IHR and for those doctors not to be colleagues.

Competence

Advice on eligibility for IHR must be given only by doctors who have sufficient knowledge of the job and working environment. Many pension schemes require their medical advisers, rather than doctors solely providing information about the patient's health, to have a qualification in occupational medicine. The minimum qualification varies between schemes but should not be less than the Diploma in Occupational Medicine (DOccMed), supplemented by training in the application of the scheme criteria. Such doctors should be overseen by an accredited specialist (i.e. MFOM or FFOM in the UK, or equivalent qualification issued by a competent authority in an EEA State). An appeal against an initial decision should be considered by an accredited specialist in occupational medicine.

Appeals and complaints

All IHR assessment processes should have an appeal mechanism. The scheme member should be advised of the grounds for the original decision and have an opportunity to appeal, with or without further medical evidence. The appeal may be considered by a doctor or panel of doctors who should include an accredited specialist in occupational medicine with sufficient knowledge and experience to judge the issues. Some schemes require appellants to present for medical examination, but most appeals are conducted on a 'papers only' basis, partly for logistical reasons, but also because further examination may not provide new objective evidence. Appeal reports should demonstrate that all relevant evidence and no irrelevant evidence has been considered, the regulations or rules of the scheme have been correctly understood, and the rationale applied in the decision explained in lay language.

Assessment of eligibility for IHR can result in a complaint by the patient against the doctor. This is most likely to occur if the application has been unsuccessful. It is essential not only to have a robust complaints procedure running alongside the appeal procedure but also one which identifies potentially vexatious or vindictive complaints. Requests to remove factually relevant material that is not supportive of the patient's case should be resisted, as should requests to assess a case without medical reports unfavourable to the case, or without sight of the previous doctor's rationale for their opinion. A request not to send a report because it does not support an appellant's case should be resisted, and if asked to remove relevant clinical information, the doctor should make it clear in the report where such information has been deleted.

Guidelines

No controlled trials have been undertaken on retirees, so existing written guidance is based on consensus opinions of senior occupational physicians.[2,14] Some large, public sector pension schemes (e.g. run by the Civil Service, Home Office, Communities and Local Government, and the Department of Education), have produced guidance, which should be read before undertaking work for their pension scheme. The occupational physician should obtain all the relevant information about the patient's illness, including diagnosis, treatment (current and proposed), and prognosis. A checklist for doctors undertaking this work is shown in Table 27.2 (with contributions from Dr A.D. Archer).

The *true* functional ability of the patient should be ascertained, as well as details of their job or workplace. If the doctor believes that the true functional ability of the patient has not been ascer-

Table 27.2 Permanent incapacity checklist

Name_____	Date of birth_____
Scheme_____	Job title_____

		Comments
1	Do you know which pension regulations or rules apply to this application? This may vary according to the age, job & membership (deferred) status of the applicant.	
2	Have you read the relevant statutory or medical guidance for the pension regulations or rules? Do you have the correct certificate?	
3	Do you know the eligibility criteria for ill health retirement in this scheme and how it varies by tier?	
4	Is the applicant working and if not, how long have they been off sick? Some applicants have more than one job.	
5	Do you have a job description that includes reference to functional capacity requirements?	
6	Do you have sufficient information about diagnosis, treatment and prognosis?	
7	Have all investigations been completed?	
8	Have all reasonable treatments been tried and given for a therapeutic period of time and has there been adequate time for recovery and rehabilitation?	
9	Is there a credible explanation for failure to respond to treatment or rehabilitation? Failure to respond may be for non-medical reasons.	
10	Has a medical assessment of functional capabilities, impairment and disability in relation to the job and alternative jobs been undertaken?	
11	Would you recommend rejection of the applicant, even with adjustments, for another job? If yes, then applicant likely to be unfit for any work.	
12	If applicant is still employed, is there evidence that the employer has explored reasonable adjustments and redeployment?	
13	If alternative work was offered, is there an explanation as to why it was not accepted or successful?	
14	Is there an unresolved employment issue such as misconduct, a grievance or an investigation? If yes, decision about IHR should wait until employment issue resolved.	
15	Has the applicant included a statement of his or her own medical condition and functional impairments? (optional)	
16	Have you explained the grounds for supporting or rejecting the application?	

tained, despite reasonable efforts, or the degree of disability declared by the patient is more than would be normally expected for that illness or injury, it is recommended that the doctor bases their advice on what would normally be expected by way of function or prognosis in a patient with the same diagnosis but who is not seeking early retirement.

Reasonable adjustments, aids, or workplace adaptations should have been tried to accommodate the patient's disability or illness, as well as opportunities for redeployment before a decision is made about IHR. Adjustments might include adaptive technology, involvement of the Access to Work team and 'permitted' or 'supported' employment. IHR is also a dismissal in law, so failure to make reasonable adjustments may constitute grounds for a claim of unfair dismissal. Workplaces and the people who work in them are in constant flux, so refusal by an employee to return to a particular workplace should not merit IHR unless there is a demonstrable inability to do so because of permanent incapacity for medical reasons.

Advice should, whenever possible, be based on objective medical evidence and non-medical factors contributing to the patient's ill health (e.g. anger, embitterment, or disaffection with the employer, or a lack of motivation to return to work) should generally be disregarded. Illnesses that are the most difficult to assess objectively are those that rely entirely on subjective complaints (e.g. chronic fatigue syndrome, fibromyalgia, post-traumatic stress disorder, and some mental health disorders). Advice on these illnesses in relation to IHR is given elsewhere.[14]

Audit

The additional cost to the pension scheme of IHR has been estimated at about £50000/case.[4] Great variability in outcome has been shown, which is disconcerting for scheme trustees, administrators, and patients,[3] and indicates the need for audit. This can be done in two ways. Firstly, by comparing a doctor's rate of recommended IHR to the national rate of IHR for that scheme, or, if this information is unavailable, to that in other schemes with similar criteria. Where there are tiered benefits, the distribution of the doctor's cases by tier is also auditable. Figure 27.2 shows the

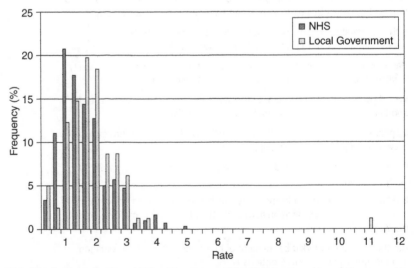

Figure 27.2 Distribution of rates of ill health retirement by NHS trust and Local Government administering authority 2009–2010.

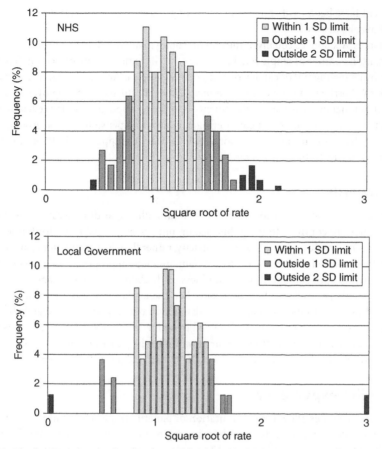

Figure 27.3 Distribution of normalized rates of ill health retirement with standard deviations (SDs) by NHS trusts and Local Government administering authorities 2009–2010.

distribution of IHR by trust in the NHS (but excluding ambulance trusts) and by administering authority in Local Government (LG). The median and interquartile range for the NHS is 1.28 (0.84–1.86) and that for LG 1.56 (1.13–2.14). These rates are significantly different ($p = 0.02$) and lower ($p < 0.001$) with less spread than when last measured by the author in 2003.[14] Doctors can also compare their rate of IHR with the normalized (square rooted) data in Figure 27.3. Where a doctor's rate of IHR lies more than one standard deviation outside the mean, they (or ideally someone else) can audit their practice for a sample of their cases against published diagnostically-specific guidance on IHR.[14]

Medico-legal aspects

Employees and managers often view ill health retirement as an alternative to resignation, redundancy, or dismissal. In fact it is not an employment issue but rather a process for paying pension benefits once a decision to terminate an employee's contract has been made. Even if the individual applies for the benefit, the employer must be satisfied that all decisions relating to employment have been made fairly and according to due process, otherwise a case for unfair dismissal may be justified.

The Equality Act applies equally at the end of employment as it does at recruitment and during employment. Examples of employers being found to have unlawfully discriminated against an employee by giving them IHR can be found in case law such as *Kerrigan* v. *Rover Group Ltd* (1997) and *Meikle* v. *Nottinghamshire County Council* (2004). Dismissing an employee with illness or injury without making reasonable adjustments or offering opportunities for redeployment, with or without an IHR pension, or not considering eligibility to a pension, may be grounds for unfair dismissal. In these circumstances a doctor should be wary of supporting IHR, or of not making a comment about eligibility to a pension.

Injury awards

These are benefits paid by pension schemes for injury, illness, or disease caused by the employee's work. They are confined to the public sector and privatized public sector bodies. They are designed to compensate for loss of earning capacity, rather than loss of function, pain, or suffering for which Industrial Injury Benefit and a civil claim might be appropriate. Judgements about injury awards involve apportionment between illness or disability due to work and any pre-existing illness or disability, as well as calculations based on the applicant's pre-injury salary and current or projected earnings in the job market. The distinction between an injury aggravating or accelerating a pre-existing condition may also need to be made, and the Home Office has published guidance on this and the calculation of injury awards for the police and fire services. Access to the patient's medical records and experience in making these judgements is recommended.

Limited life expectancy

Most pension schemes allow for commutation of benefits (replacement of monthly payments with an augmented lump sum) for members in employment, but not usually for deferred members, with a life expectancy of less than 12 months. Trustees or administrators may apply this discretion if it is within the scope of their scheme, but it is also governed by tax rules. The Inland Revenue has stated that such commutation is intended for the benefit of the scheme member rather than their dependants or estate. Consequently, well-intentioned efforts to secure commutation for individuals who are terminally ill are potentially unlawful and, if repeated across several cases, could result in the withdrawal of the concession by the Inland Revenue for that scheme. Unfortunately, the patient or a relative has the task of requesting commutation, which creates difficulty if they are unaware of or are sensitive about the prognosis. A doctor will need to confirm the prognosis in writing. Most schemes offer some form of death benefit for the dependants of members employed at the time of death. Doctors should avoid acting as financial advisers, even though they may be trying to act in the patient's best interests.

Conclusions

Doctors who give advice to pension scheme trustees or administrators should be aware of the eligibility criteria for that scheme and the meaning of terms used in the regulations, the statutory guidance, or explanatory notes published by the scheme. Most schemes require that the doctors who act as their medical advisors have a qualification in occupational medicine. The evaluation of evidence in support of an application for IHR should be robust but fair and care should be taken to avoid conflicts of interest for doctors involved in the treatment of the patient. The medical standards to which doctors work in making these judgements should be explicit and they should audit their rate of IHR against national data, if equitable decisions are to be made and confidence in the process is to be maintained.

References

1 Office for National Statistics: <http://www.ons.gov.uk>.

2 Poole CJM, Baron CE, Gunnyeon WJ, *et al.* Ill health retirement-guidelines for occupational physicians. *Occup Med* 1996; **46**: 402–6.

3 Poole, CJM. Retirement on grounds of ill health: cross sectional survey in six organisations in United Kingdom. *BMJ* 1997; **314**: 929–32.

4 HM Treasury. *Review of ill health retirement in the public sector.* London: HM Treasury, 2000.

5 Casscells W, Hennekens CH, Evans D, *et al.* Retirement and coronary mortality. *Lancet* 1980; i, 1288–9.

6 Mein G, Martikainen P, Hemingway H, *et al.* Is retirement good or bad for mental and physical health functioning? Whitehall II longitudinal study of civil servants. *J Epidemiol Community Health* 2003; **57**: 46–9.

7 Brockmann H, Muller R, Helmert U. Time to retire—time to die? A prospective study of the effects of early retirement on long-term survival. *Soc Sci Med* 2009; **69**: 160–4.

8 Hult C, Stattin M, Janlert U, *et al.* Time of retirement and mortality—a cohort study of Swedish construction workers. *Soc Sci Med* 2010; **70**: 1480–6.

9 The Pension Service: <http://www.thepensionservice.gov.uk>

10 *Independent Public Service Pensions Commission: Final Report* (J. Hutton, Chair). London: Independent Public Service Pensions Commission, 2011.

11 The Pensions Regulator: <http://www.thepensionsregulator.gov.uk>

12 The Pensions Advisory Service: <http://www.pensionsadvisoryservice.org.uk>

13 World Health Organization. *International Statistical Classification of Diseases and Related Health Problems*, 10th revision. Geneva: WHO, 1992.

14 Poole CJM, Bass CM, Sorrell JE, *et al.* Ill health retirement: national rates and updated guidance for occupational physicians. *Occup Med* 2005; **55**: 345–8.

Chapter 28

Health and transport safety: fitness to drive

Tim Carter, Heather G. Major, Sally A. Evans, and Andrew P. Colvin

Introduction

Fitness to work in all modes of transport, where this may put members of the public or other workers at risk, has long been an area of public concern. Because inadequate performance may endanger fellow workers or the public and put expensive assets at risk, frameworks for statutory regulation have been developed. This chapter uses fitness to drive, the area of widest interest, as an example, but each mode of transport has its own pattern of performance requirements and hence fitness standards, although they have much in common. Separate appendices cover fitness to work in the rail industry, as a seafarer, and in aviation.

The risks to the safety of others posed by performance deficits or incapacitation has meant that decisions on fitness are frequently taken not for the benefit of the person examined but to safeguard those at risk as a consequence of their actions. Hence hard decisions often have to be taken and for this reason standards for medical aspects of fitness are usually formal and often published. They are usually applied by physicians acting on behalf of regulatory authorities and have associated review or appeal mechanisms available to those who have been failed or restricted. Standards are necessarily based on the balance between public risk and potential loss of employment, with the former predominating.

The evidence base for current standards is of variable quality and this is often a cause of contention. Patient groups and equal opportunities organizations may find it difficult to accept the concept of standards based on epidemiological evidence of risk. They may cite equality legislation to encourage applicants to demand individual assessment of risk and job adaptations to allow employment, often in situations where this is impossible.

In addition to long-term health problems that are handled by reference to such formal standards, transport workers may also have short-term decrements in performance from injury, minor illness, or medication. In some areas, e.g. aviation, even short-term decreases in medical fitness are subject to national or international regulation.

Safety critical tasks

The term 'safety critical task' can generally be taken to mean one where certain forms of personal impairment can put other people at risk. It is a useful general concept, but one open to slightly differing interpretations in different situations and so the rationale for its use should always be explored before assumptions are made. Driving provides a good example of a 'safety critical' transport task:

♦ Information about the vehicle, other road users, and the road are perceived, mainly using vision.

♦ This is cognitively processed against a learned background of skills and intentions for the journey.

♦ Based on this the speed, direction, and signalling of the vehicle are determined by hand and foot controls.

♦ The results of these actions are, in turn, processed to determine subsequent control requirements.

Lack of experience, inattention, behavioural traits such as risk taking, and impairment, including that from a medical condition, may interfere with this loop. Interference will increase the risk of error and accident.

A similar perceptual, cognitive, and motor loop is relevant to rail drivers, aircraft pilots, and seafarers when navigating. However, the nature of the visual and auditory environment, the sensory inputs, and the response to control actions all vary greatly. In addition there are differing safety support systems, either in human terms, as with the presence of a co-pilot in passenger aircraft, or engineered, such as protective signalling and automatic braking systems on the railways.

Health-related impairment does not appear to be a major direct contributor to transport accidents, although there is no recent definitive study on this. Other forms of impairment such as fatigue and alcohol are much more significant, as is being an inexperienced driver, and risk-taking behaviour, particularly of young male drivers. All forms of impairment and driver behaviour taken together are, however, much more important as causes of crashes than the condition of either the vehicle or the road.[1,2]

Impairing disabilities and medical conditions

Performance decrement may be permanent, for instance, the static disability of an amputated limb or reduced visual acuity. It may also be episodic as in a seizure, cardiac event, or episode of hypoglycaemia. Many conditions also present with a mix of characteristics, for example, the fluctuating impairments of multiple sclerosis or the progression of a malignancy or of motor neurone disease. Treatments frequently reduce risk, but some such as insulin, psychoactive medications, or warfarin can create new risks of their own.

The approaches to static and to episodic conditions are different. In a static condition, given sufficient evidence linking the level of impairment to risk, it should be possible to make an assessment of the individual that includes any appliances used to reduce the impairment, such as corrective lenses or modified car controls. This can then be used to determine task-specific capabilities. In practice, the level of impairment often cannot be precisely linked to the excess risk of accident, as is the case with impaired visual acuity.[3] An assessment of driving performance may be the most practically useful arbiter of road safety and it has good face value for the participant, although its predictive value has not been formally evaluated.

When a condition is episodic it will not be possible to make an individual assessment of performance and the best that can be achieved is a valid estimate of the future risk of recurrence derived from epidemiological data on the relevant condition. There is good information on recurrence rates for seizures and for cardiac events, which can be used for stratification. Assessment may be more difficult where there are variables in disease management that are under individual control, as with the risk of hypoglycaemia from insulin treatment.

One of the key features with an episodic condition is the time taken to become incapacitated, the level of awareness, and the ability to take action during this time. Thus, while a seizure may be instantly incapacitating with no warning, cardiac events usually only incapacitate once blood flow to the brain has been severely reduced, and so there is frequently a warning period. For drivers on roads this is often sufficient to pull over to one side of the road and stop. Where an incapacitating episode is not perceived, either through lack of awareness of the prodromal symptoms or because cognition is clouded by the early stages of the episode, as with hypoglycaemia, then driving may continue as incapacitation increases.

The period over which the incapacity arises can also determine the scope for action by others. Incapacity in aircraft pilots in a multicrew operation or watchkeepers on dual-manned ships' bridges should result in the command being taken over, while on the railways safeguards in the signalling system will come into play. A particular problem arises for seafarers because illness, even when developing over several hours, cannot be referred for medical attention. Hence standards include restrictions on those at excess risk of a recurrence or complication, for instance, from renal stones, strangulation of a hernia, or dental abscess. While primarily aimed at reducing risk to the individual such restrictions also reduce risk to others since helicopter evacuation, diversion of a vessel and the operational consequences of having to nurse a seriously ill person on a modern ship with the minimum required crew can increase both risk and costs.

Occupational driving: public highways

Space on the roads, in the air, or on the water is shared between those at work and those using the medium for leisure activities. The latter are sometimes required to meet less stringent fitness standards or, in some cases, none at all.

There is great diversity in the risks and performance requirements for driving tasks at work. In the UK, work-related driving is estimated to result in 25–33% of all fatal and serious accidents on public roads. This amounts to around 500–600 road fatalities per annum and thus is the major cause of work-related fatal accidents.

The implications of employment on responsibilities for meeting standards are a complex one in transport. This is addressed in several ways. For road transport in Great Britain, the Driver and Vehicle Licensing Agency (DVLA) makes no statutory distinction between drivers at work and other road users. Vehicle size, structure, and use form the basis for differential standards. Vehicle definitions and associated medical fitness requirements for drivers are standardized across the European Union (EU).[4] More stringent fitness levels apply to drivers of Group 2 vehicles: those weighing over 3.5 tonnes or with more than eight passenger seats. The rationale for this is that there is good evidence of higher consequential damage from such vehicles. In addition, the worst-case accident, involving large numbers of passengers, will likely lead to more fatalities. These statutory minimum standards are supplemented by a local licensing system for taxis, for which the more stringent Group 2 standards are recommended as best practice, despite use of smaller (Group 1) vehicles. In addition, some employers have their own enhanced standards, in particular the emergency services where high-speed driving may be anticipated.

For all other drivers the less stringent, Group 1, medical licensing standards apply. The basis for control in all cases is by the issue, revocation, or restriction of the person's driving licence. This is only applicable to longer-term health conditions and it is up to the individual driver to avoid driving if they have a short-term impairment. This is something that some drivers find difficult to handle responsibly, especially when their livelihood depends on driving. It is one of the reasons why some employers have established corporate driving risk-reduction programmes that include provision for declaration of short-term incapacity and temporary cessation of driving without penalty.[5]

Occupational driving: off-road

Many workers drive vehicles off the public roads as part of their job. These include farmers, dockworkers, and forklift truck drivers in many sectors. There are also highly specialized vehicles used, for instance, in mines, quarries, airports, and at container ports. Where vehicles are operated occupationally, and the activities are not carried out on the public highway, there is often confusion about the application of medical fitness standards. Examples include lift trucks, cranes, construction site vehicles.

The legal requirement of the Health and Safety at Work etc. Act 1974 is that the employer has a safe system of work. This applies to all those who drive at work, whether on highways or off-road. Although there is no specific legal requirement for medical assessment, there is a clear implication that medical fitness may be a prerequisite of ensuring such a safe system. Health and safety law is applicable to all workplaces. The employer will normally require the advice and assistance of a competent person, in this case an occupational physician, for both the setting of medical fitness standards and their implementation.

In setting occupational standards, there is merit in using an existing set of fitness criteria rather than setting new standards from scratch and a logical choice would be either the Group 1 or 2 medical standards. It should be remembered, however, that these standards are developed for users of the public highway, and the DVLA has no jurisdiction over driving on private property. If part or all of the driving activity takes place on the public highway, then the DVLA standards generally apply, but with some limited exemptions for agricultural vehicles.

In setting standards for occupational drivers who are not using the public highway, it is possible to use the DVLA Group 1 and 2 standards as benchmarks, and to deviate from them based on a task-specific risk assessment.[6] A risk assessment that uses DVLA standards just for benchmarking is advised, as direct application of DVLA medical standards may not be suitable, resulting in challenges under the Equality Act 2010.

Medical aspects of licensing

Within the UK, each mode of transport has its own licensing arrangements. All are linked to EU or international agreements. For aviation and seafaring, a central authority is responsible for the oversight of fitness assessments and there is a network of doctors approved by the authority who undertake medicals on all but the lowest risk groups (see Appendices 1 and 2). For road drivers, licensing is formally a responsibility of the Secretary of State for Transport. In practice, in Britain it is delegated to the DVLA, where the medical aspects are the responsibility of the Drivers' Medical Group. There is a comparable agency in Northern Ireland. The legal basis for the standards and for their enforcement lies in the Road Traffic Act 1988.[7] This specifies certain disabilities, known as 'relevant disabilities', which bar a person from driving, and 'prospective disabilities', which may then require regular medical licensing review. In both instances, the fact of the disability places an obligation on the driver to notify the DVLA of the medical condition, its nature, and extent. The standards are aligned with the EC driver licensing directives but, across Europe, there are national variations in the ways in which they are applied and in which compliance is checked. The

UK, unlike most other member states has a single driver licensing centre, with its own medical staff who make decisions based on clinical information obtained from drivers, their clinicians, and sometimes from commissioned investigations and examinations. Records of about 43 million drivers are held, of whom approaching 4 million have had contact with the medical group over the last decade. Around 130,000 new enquiries are received each year, with year on year growth above 10%. Nearly 20% of cases now arise from licence renewal in those aged 70 or over, highlighting the consequences of an ageing population of drivers. About 90% of cases are handled by administrative staff, while the more complex cases, often involving Group 2 applicants or those with multiple medical conditions are assessed by one of the medical advisers. The advisers are also available to health professionals by telephone and letter to discuss individual cases.[8]

The medical standards used are published in the *At a Glance Guide to the Current Medical Standards of Fitness to Drive* which is revised every 6 months.[9] The DVLA is advised by six expert honorary medical panels covering the most common problem areas: vision, heart disease, diabetes, neurology, psychiatric illness, and the effects of drug and alcohol misuse. The members are appointed by the Secretary of State and they both advise on the medical standards and review any particularly difficult cases or ones where the standards are not working effectively.[10] Standard setting is also supported by review and research programmes undertaken within the Department[11] and by reports from elsewhere in the world literature.

A new applicant for a Group 1 licence has a legal obligation to declare whether or not they suffer from an impairing illness. Basic visual performance is assessed at the practical driving test based on reading a car number plate at a distance of 20 metres. The terms of the licence issued require drivers to inform the DVLA of any significant illness arising while they hold their licence. This remains their personal responsibility but the General Medical Council recommends a process for a doctor to follow if one of their patients does not notify when they have been advised to do so.[12] The Group 1 licence expires at the age of 70 (although the photo must be updated every 10 years) and then has to be renewed every 3 years with the submission of a new medical declaration.

From January 2013, Group 2 licences will carry a maximum 5-year administrative validity. Group 2 drivers (vehicles over 3.5 tonnes for a new licence but over 7.5 tonnes for those holding a Group 1 licence issued prior to 1997) are currently required to supply a medical examination form (D4), which may be completed by any doctor, but usually comes from their general practitioner or occupational physician. This is needed on first application, then on 5-yearly licence renewals from age 45 to 65 and annually thereafter. From 2013, self-declarations of health will also be required on 5-yearly licence renewals below age 45. None of these interactions absolves the drivers from the requirement to self-declare a new condition in the interim. From this date there will also be some changes in the criteria for licensing those with visual impairment, diabetes, and seizures—the details have yet to be finalized.

Any declaration of a relevant illness on application, during the currency of a licence or found at the time of a Group 2 medical assessment will be followed up with a medical enquiry. For Group 1 this normally involves the driver completing a factual questionnaire with similar questionnaire enquiry to the doctor(s) involved in their treatment. Specialist referral may be required, particularly so for Group 2 licences. The information received is assessed by the staff of the DVLA Drivers Medical Group, who will then reach a licensing decision. Options include issuing or continuing a full licence, issuing one for a shorter period with review, restricting a licence to the use of certain vehicles or use of vehicle adaptations, refusing a licence application, or revoking the existing licence. Appeals against any licensing decision are heard in the local Magistrates Court in England and Wales or the Sheriffs Court in Scotland. Such appeals are rare and only about 25 cases proceeded to full hearing in 2010.

Specific medical conditions

Details of the standards may be found in the *DVLA 'At a Glance' guide.*[9] The evidence on which they are based is widely scattered in the literature but the evidence linking medical conditions to accidents has been reviewed in detail and summarized in a guide for health professionals.[13,14] Other chapters of this book discuss most of the conditions of concern. The following are standards where there are important features specific to driving, and to a varying extent, to other modes of transport.

Cardiac events and strokes

Arterial disease poses a risk of both progressive impairment and relatively sudden incapacity. Standards are based on current capabilities and especially on likelihood of recurrence. For Group 1 drivers, little more than a period without driving after satisfactory recovery from an event is required but for Group 2 drivers, the additional probability of recurrence must be stratified, based on the Bruce protocol exercise electrocardiogram or other equivalent functional test. Driving may resume if this is satisfactorily completed, though then subject to periodic review.

A cautious approach has been adopted to implanted defibrillators in any driver because they may discharge without warning. Their internal memories can be used to determine frequency of discharge and if this is very low it may allow Group 1 driving. The need for an implanted defibrillator is at present a bar to Group 2 entitlement.

Seizures

There is good evidence about the probability of a repeat seizure at various times after the last one, both with and without medication. This has enabled standards to be set based on a quantitative risk of recurrence. The level used is a probability of less than 20% in the next year for Group 1 and less than 2% for Group 2. The difference reflects the time likely to be spent at the wheel and the consequential damage likely if an accident occurs. More generally, the scope for applying quantitative approaches to assessing the accident risk from medical conditions has been investigated but because of the inherent limitations of the data it will never be a precise tool.[15] (Also see Chapter 8.)

Diabetes

The major risk is from insulin-induced hypoglycaemia, although sulphonylureas and glinides may also cause 'hypos'. Risk data on diabetes is complex. The medical causes of road accidents are not readily identifiable and, while there is no clear evidence that hypoglycaemia is a cause of overall excess risk, each year the DVLA receives around 300 police notifications of presumed impairment from this cause while driving, some leading to serious accidents. This is an area of considerable concern as many otherwise fit people are affected and any threat of a restriction on driving may lead to less than optimal treatment of the disease to avoid the risk of 'hypos'.

Vision

Vision and the use of visual information is a multistage process. The tests currently used are limited to the assessment of acuity and visual fields, for which there are few clear correlations between degree of impairment and accident risk. For on-road driving there is good evidence that colour vision is not a requirement; conversely impairments of twilight vision, contrast sensitivity, and glare may have greater relevance but, as yet, cannot easily be assessed nor standards defined.

One of the most contentious areas is visual field loss, associated with stroke, glaucoma, and certain retinopathies. Here decisions have to be taken on a wide variety of defects, each of which can be mapped in detail but for which the consequences in terms of current risk and progression are not predictable.

Sleep disorders

The majority of sleep-related road accidents are in those with sleep deficits that do not have a medical cause. However, two medical conditions, obstructive sleep apnoea and narcolepsy, are important. Sleep apnoea is particularly prevalent in the overweight, middle-aged male and is reliably associated with an excess risk of road crashes. The detection of undiagnosed sleep apnoea in professional drivers is important and can be improved by driver education and its recognition by company managers and medical advisers. Treatment with continuous positive pressure ventilators (CPAP) during sleep is acceptable and has been shown to reduce the risk of accidents.[16] The severity of narcolepsy may be reduced by medication; where satisfactory control can be objectively demonstrated, e.g. by the Osler wakefulness test, driving may be permitted.

Psychiatric illness, drugs, and alcohol

Severe psychoses are normally a bar to driving but for less severe illness there may be other potentially debarring issues, which relate to the side effects of the medication used as much as to the risks from the disease. There are no good correlations between non-psychotic mental illness and road accidents. Substance abuse as a short-term impairment is normally handled by police sanctions. The assessment of longer-term dependency and misuse arises as a medical issue and there are provisions for certain classes of driving offences in 'high-risk offenders' to require medical clearance before returning to driving.[17]

Fixed disabilities

People with fixed disabilities such as paralysis, cerebral palsy, spina bifida, and amputations can often drive safely once they have been trained to use a modified vehicle. Assessments and advice on vehicle adaptations are provided by a network of Mobility Centres.[18] Any clinician can arrange a referral.

The role of the occupational health professional

Medical factors, as currently controlled, appear to be only very small contributors to road accident risk. Any organization that has staff with driving duties needs to consider the introduction of policies on driving at work. Health risk management is only one part of such policies but one where occupational health (OH) advice is needed both to set policies and to handle decisions on fitness.

Checks on return to work after illness and surveillance to detect new health problems, to check vision, and to ensure that existing medical conditions are controlled are commonly used. Compliance with therapy and self-management are important aspects of risk reduction for conditions such as diabetes and sleep apnoea. It is now possible to record objective information about the quality of self-management from data logging devices such as blood glucose monitors and CPAP machines. This can improve the quality of risk assessment in occupational drivers.

It is important to ensure that health risk management does not just relate to long-term conditions that may put the driving licence at risk. Short-term impairment from acute illness, injury, or the use of impairing medications must also be included. This requires rapid access to OH advice to ensure that appropriate decisions are taken.

In furthering the well-being and return to work of their patient, clinicians often see a conflict between their patient's interests and giving advice on fitness to drive that may limit work and mobility. Those advising on fitness to return to work need to be aware of this conflict as well as of clinicians' limited knowledge of fitness standards, despite their ready access to information from the DVLA and elsewhere. OH advisers often need to communicate with clinicians to obtain a full and up-to-date view on a person's condition in order to support both employees and managers by giving valid advice and ensuring relevant job adaptations are made if there is a temporary limitation on fitness to drive.

References

1 Taylor JF (ed). *Medical aspects of fitness to drive*, p. 7. London: Medical Commission on Accident Prevention, 1995.

2 Department for Transport. *The casualty report: contributory factors. Statistics*. Department for Transport, 2009. [Online] (<http://webarchive.nationalarchives.gov.uk/+/http://www.dft.gov.uk/excel/173025/221412/221549/227755/503336/RCGB2009Article4.xls>)

3 Charman WN. Vision and driving—a literature review and commentary. *Ophthal Physiol* 1997; **17**: 371–91.

4 European Union Directive on driving licences 91/439/EC and amendments 97/26/EC and 2009/112/EC (which came into force 15 September 2010), to be replaced by: European Union Directive on driving licences 2006/126/EC, from 19 January 2013. (<http://ec.europa.eu/transport/road_safety/behavior/driving_licence_en.htm>)

5 Department for Transport, Health and Safety Executive. *Driving at work: managing work-related road safety*, 2004. [Online] (<http://www.hse.gov.uk/pubns/indg382.pdf>)

6 An example of how this can be applied is provided in the Health and Safety Executive publication *Safety in working with lift trucks* (HSG6). London: Health and Safety Executive, 2000. [Appendix 2 deals with medical standards and explains the benchmarking process in relation to lift truck operators.]

7 Road Traffic Act 1988 (Section 92). [More detailed provisions are in the Motor Vehicles (Driving Licence) Regulations 1999.]

8 Contact for use by medical professionals only. DVLA 01792 782337 or email via medadviser@dvla.gsi.gov.uk. Driver and Vehicle Licensing Northern Ireland 028 703 41369.

9 Drivers Medical Unit. *At a glance guide to the current medical standards of fitness to drive*. Swansea: DVLA, May 2012. Updated 6-monthly at: <http://www.dft.gov.uk/dvla/medical/ataglance.aspx>

10 Agendas, minutes, and annual reports of the medical panels can be accessed at: <http://www.dft.gov.uk/dvla/medical/medical_advisory_information/medicaladvisory_meetings/>

11 Research reports can be found at: <http://www.dft.gov.uk> under science and research, road safety.

12 General Medical Council. *Confidentiality*, 2009. [Online] (<http://www.gmc-uk.org/guidance/ethical_guidance/confidentiality.asp>) [Reporting concerns about patients to the DVLA or the DVA.]

13 Charlton J, Koppel SN, O'Hare MA, *et al. Influence of chronic illness on crash involvement of motor vehicle drivers*. Monash University Accident Research Centre Report 213. Clayton: Monash University Accident Research Centre, 2004. (<http://www.general.monash.edu.au/muarc>)

14 Carter T. *Fitness to drive: a guide for health professionals*. London, RSM Press, 2006.

15 Spencer MB, Carter T, Nicholson AN. Limitations of risk analysis in the determination of medical factors in road vehicle accidents. *Clin Med* 2004; **4**: 50–3.

16 Carter T, Major H, Wetherall G, *et al.* Excessive daytime sleepiness and driving: regulations for road safety. *Clin Med (London, England)*, 2004; **4**(5): 454–6.

17 The Motor Vehicles (Driving Licences) Regulations 1999 s74.

18 Forum of Mobility Centres: <http://www.mobility-centres.org.uk>. [Details of services and locations.]

Chapter 29

Health screening

Tar-Ching Aw and David S. Q. Koh

Introduction

Screening refers to 'a test or a series of tests to which an individual submits to determine whether enough evidence of a disease exists to warrant further diagnostic examination by a physician'.[1] Health screening has been defined by the US Commission on Chronic Illness as 'the presumptive identification of unrecognized disease or defect by the application of tests, examinations or other procedures which can be applied rapidly'. The Commission describes screening tests as tests that 'sort out apparently well persons who probably have a disease from those who probably do not' although cautioning that 'A screening test is not intended to be diagnostic. Persons with positive or suspicious findings must be referred to their physicians for diagnosis and necessary treatment'.

There are several types of health screening, including:

◆ Mass screening of the whole population.

◆ Multiple or multiphasic screening, employing several tests on the same occasion.

◆ Prescriptive screening for the early detection of specific diseases that have better prognosis if detected and treated early.

In occupational health practice, health screening programs can be aimed at:

◆ Detecting effects resulting from workplace exposure to hazards; or

◆ Using the workplace to provide general health screening for health effects that may not be directly related to specific occupational exposures; or

◆ Detecting pre-existing unrecognized ill health that may pose a risk to the individual or to third parties (co-workers, members of the public).

Wilson and Jungner[2] suggested several criteria which screening should meet. These relate to the condition to be screened, and the test to be used for screening (Table 29.1). The principles are applicable to screening for occupational as well as non-occupational diseases. With the advent of new screening tools, these criteria have been reviewed.[3] However, they remain applicable, especially for occupational health where there are limited advances in procedures for effective screening.

Characteristics of a screening test

Sensitivity, specificity, and predictive value

The *sensitivity* of a test is its ability to detect those with the condition being tested. A test with 100% sensitivity will produce a positive test result for everyone affected by the condition. Thus, it will not produce any false negative results.

Table 29.1 Characteristics of diseases and tests that are appropriate for screening

The disease	The screening test
• Clinically important	• Acceptable
– significant morbidity/mortality	• Safe
– prevalent	• Sensitive
• Has recognizable latent stage	• Specific
	• Easily done
• Amenable to treatment	• Relatively cheap

The *specificity* of a test is its ability to detect those who do not have the condition for which testing is being done. A test with 100% specificity will produce a negative result for everyone not affected by the condition. Thus, it will not produce any false positive results.

No test is 100% sensitive and 100% specific. The likelihood of anyone with a positive test result actually having the disease, the *positive predictive value* (PPV) of the test, depends on the prevalence of the disease in the population being tested. While sensitivity and specificity are often described as constant characteristics of any screening test, the PPV of a test will vary with the population in which the test is being applied. If the disease prevalence is low in the population tested, there will be a greater likelihood of false positive results, so that a given positive test has a low PPV.

The *negative predictive value* (NPV) of a test is the probability that a person is disease free in the presence of a negative screening test result. This value will also be affected by the disease prevalence in the population that is tested. For a rare disease, the NPV is expected to be high, as virtually all who are screened will be disease free. Besides the disease prevalence, the sensitivity and specificity of the test will also affect the predictive values. In summary (see Table 29.2):

♦ *Sensitivity* = $a/(a + c) \times 100\%$

   is the probability of a positive test in people with the disease.

♦ *Specificity* = $d/(b + d) \times 100\%$

   is the probability of a negative test in people without the disease.

♦ *PPV* = $a/(a + b) \times 100\%$

   is the probability of having the disease when the test is positive.

♦ *NPV* = $d/(c + d) \times 100\%$

   is the probability of not having the disease when the test is negative.

Table 29.2 Sensitivity, specificity, and predictive value of a screening test

Test result	Disease or condition	
	Present (+)	Absent (–)
Positive (+)	a	b
Negative (–)	c	d

a = true positive, b = false positive, c = false negative, d = true negative.

Table 29.3 How disease prevalence, sensitivity, and specificity of a screening test affect its positive predictive value. Consider screening tests for two diseases in a population of 1000 people: let a = true positive, b = false positive and PPV = a/(a + b)

	True + ve *(a)*	False + ve *(b)*	PPV [*a*/(*a* + *b*)]
Rare disease (20 cases in 1000)			
Sensitivity low (20%)	4		
Specificity low (20%)		196	2.0%
Specificity 50%		490	0.8%
Specificity high (80%)		784	0.5%
Sensitivity and specificity 50%	10	490	2.0%
Sensitivity high (80%)	16		
Specificity low (20%)		196	7.5%
Specificity 50%		490	3.2%
Specificity high (80%)		784	2.0%
Specificity low (20%)		196	
Sensitivity low (20%)	4		2.0%
Sensitivity 50%	10		4.9%
Sensitivity high (80%)	16		7.5%
Specificity high (80%)		784	
Sensitivity low (20%)	4		0.5%
Sensitivity 50%	10		1.3%
Sensitivity high (80%)	16		2.0%
Common disease (400 cases in 1000)			
Sensitivity low (20%)	80		
Specificity low (20%)		480	14.3%
Specificity 50%		300	21.1%
Specificity high (80%)		120	40.0%
Sensitivity and specificity 50%	200	300	40.0%
Sensitivity high (80%)	320		
Specificity low (20%)		480	40.0%
Specificity 50%		300	51.6%
Specificity high (80%)		120	72.7%
Specificity low (20%)		480	
Sensitivity low (20%)	80		14.3%
Sensitivity 50%	200		29.4%
Sensitivity high (80%)	320		40.0%
Specificity high (80%)		120	
Sensitivity low (20%)	80		40.0%
Sensitivity 50%	200		62.5%
Sensitivity high (80%)	320		72.7%

The relationship between disease prevalence, sensitivity, specificity, and predictive value is shown in the worked example in Table 29.3, where:

♦ PPV increases with increasing disease prevalence.

♦ PPV increases with increasing sensitivity of the screening test.

♦ PPV decreases for a rare disease, but increases for a common disease with increasing specificity of the screening test.

A similar example can also be worked out for NPV.

Likelihood ratios

Likelihood ratios (LRs) of tests indicate how many times more likely patients with a disease are to have that particular result, compared to those without the disease. It is the ratio of the probabilities of specific test results among the diseased to those who are disease free.

A test with a LR above 1 indicates that it is associated with presence of the disease. Conversely, a test with a LR below 1 is associated with absence of the disease. As a rule of thumb, a test with a LR of 10 or more provides good evidence to indicate the presence of disease, while a test with a LR of less than 0.1 gives a good indication to rule out the disease.

Receiver operating characteristic curves

There are often practical difficulties in the definition of a positive or negative screening result. If the screening test result is a variable measured on a continuous scale, the cut-off point for a positive result can be varied to produce a test with either high sensitivity and low specificity, or high specificity and low sensitivity. An important question is, 'How does one determine an appropriate cut-off point for the screening test?'

One method is to express these values of the test in a visual form as a receiver operating characteristic (ROC) curve. In a ROC curve, the vertical axis of such a plot is the sensitivity of the test,

Table 29.4 Blood concentration of chemical X, presence of clinically significant toxicity, and sensitivity and false positive rate of a screening test at different cut-off points

Blood concentration of chemical X	Sensitivity	1 – specificity (false positive)
21.5	0.941	0.550
24.0	0.882	0.500
27.5	0.882	0.300
32.5	0.765	0.200
37.5	0.765	0.150
41.0	0.647	0.150
43.5	0.588	0.150
46.5	0.412	0.100
49.0	0.412	0.050
52.5	0.294	0.050
55.5	0.235	0.050
57.0	0.176	0.050
59.0	0.059	0.050
61.0	0.000	0.000

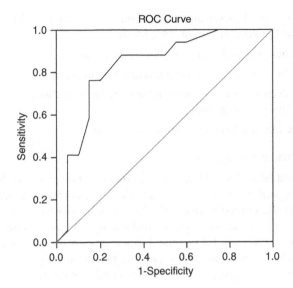

Figure 29.1 ROC curve for blood concentration of X as a screening test.

while the horizontal axis is (1 – specificity). The individual points represent the sensitivity and specificity obtained using different cut-off values, and the optimal cut-off value for the screening test is the point that is furthest from the 45° diagonal.

As an example:

An occupational physician needs to determine an effective cut-off point for the blood level of chemical X to screen workers with significant exposure and a high likelihood of developing toxic effects. They conduct a study and measure the blood concentration in workers who either have or do not exhibit clinically significant toxicity to chemical X. From these data (Table 29.4), a ROC curve can be plotted (Figure 29.1). Based on the curve and the table:

◆ If a blood concentration of 41 is adopted as a cut-off point, the test would have a sensitivity of 65%, and a 15% false positive rate.

◆ If a blood concentration of 37.5 is adopted as a cut-off point, the sensitivity is increased to 76%, while the false positive rate remains at 15%.

This method to determine the most appropriate cut-off point is not applicable for a test with a dichotomous outcome. The method also assumes an equal weight (or value, or importance) for sensitivity and specificity. An equal weight given to sensitivity and specificity may not necessarily be desirable, depending on the nature and natural history of the disease, and also the consequences of false positive and false negative results.

Practical and ethical aspects of screening

Scope of the screening examination

Screening procedures could include symptom review, clinical assessment, medical examination, and special investigations. The physical examination is unlikely to reveal significant abnormalities in an apparently healthy person. However, the consultation presents an opportunity to review lifestyle practices that impact on health, such as smoking habit, alcohol consumption, diet, and exercise behaviour. Unfortunately, this aspect of the clinical encounter is often not used fully and obviously it should not be at the expense of controlling exposure to workplace hazards.

A wide range of ancillary tests and laboratory investigations are available to screen for health disorders such as vascular, neoplastic, metabolic, haematological, ophthalmological, otological, mental disorders (and substance abuse), and infectious diseases. Useful website addresses for guidance include that of the US Preventive Services Task Force (The guide to clinical preventive services 2010-201: <http://www.uspreventiveservicestaskforce.org/recommendations.htm>) and the website of the Canadian Task Force on Preventive Health Care (<http://www.canadiantask-force.ca/>)

Frequency of examination

The frequency of screening and whether the tests are performed on specific occasions will depend on the conditions to be detected, the resources available, and on presenting opportunities. For situations where screening can be effective, the recommended frequency of examination varies with age and the natural history of the disease. Commonly, frequency of examination varies from annually to once in 3–5 years.

In occupational asthma, if sensitization to an inhaled agent in the workplace occurs, it is more likely in the early stages of employment and exposure. Hence the UK Health and Safety Executive (HSE) advice on lung function testing for workers exposed to asthmagens puts emphasis on greater frequency of screening during initial employment. For diseases with a long latent period between first exposure and subsequent health effects, there are no clinical reasons for advocating screening in the earlier years following initial exposure.

Advantages and disadvantages of health screening

Health screening may detect sentinel cases of disease in populations exposed to hazardous materials. The detection of these cases will signal the need for preventive measures. The principle behind instituting health screening is therefore appealing: detect disease early, and take preventive action. In practice, there are good examples where this is effective, e.g. screening for cardiovascular risk factors followed by measures to reduce risk. There are also examples where the benefits of screening are limited. Periodic chest x-rays for exposure to fibrogenic dusts such as silica particles or asbestos fibres may enable earlier detection of pulmonary fibrosis, but there may be little that can be done to halt the progression of the disease. Early detection of disease may produce an apparent gain in the duration of life between detection and death, although the mean age at death of those screened is not altered. All that screening does in these cases is to alert the screened individuals to the occurrence of disease, without necessarily affecting disease outcome. This has been suggested previously in a study of periodic chest x-rays in chromate-exposed workers.[4] Earlier diagnosis as a result of screening can cause an improvement in survival time (interval from diagnosis to death), but this can be due to lead time and length time bias, instead of actual prolongation of life.[5] In any case, early detection is part of secondary prevention. Prevention of occupational disease through reduction of exposure (primary prevention) is preferable.

Adverse effects of screening can arise with the indiscriminate use of screening tests. A false positive test result causes unnecessary anxiety and worry in the subject. A false positive test often leads to further investigations, with their associated risk of morbidity and further expense.

False negative results can provide false reassurance and cause complacency. They may be viewed as an 'all-clear' until the next round of screening and can even lead to the person ignoring future early warning symptoms.

For example, the exercise electrocardiogram (stress ECG), when used for screening coronary heart disease in an apparently healthy general population, has a PPV of <30%.[6] Hence, seven of ten persons who are stress ECG positive are subjected to unnecessary and potentially harmful further investigations. In addition to causing anxiety, a false positive stress ECG may also have negative consequences for occupational and insurance eligibility, or other leisure opportunities. Even in cases of suspected coronary artery disease, the PPV for stress ECG is only 51%.[7]

There is an evolving range of opinions on screening of asymptomatic workers in occupational groups. Various organizations and expert groups have recommended exercise electrocardiography for job categories including airline pilots, firemen, police officers, bus and truck drivers, and railroad engineers. For athletes, there is a suggestion that stress ECG could be considered for younger (aged <45 years) asymptomatic individuals if they have multiple cardiovascular risk factors.[8] The American College of Cardiology and the American Heart Association[9] indicate that exercise testing in healthy asymptomatic persons is not recommended, but may be considered in occupations where public safety may be affected. In the UK, exercise tolerance testing may be indicated for applicants for a Group 2/Category C (large goods or public service vehicles) driving licence, if there is possible underlying cardiovascular disease.[10] The US Preventive Services Task Force also recommend against routine screening with exercise ECG for asymptomatic adults. However, they also suggest that for people in certain occupations involving public safety, considerations other than benefit to the individual may influence the decision to perform screening.[11] A review for this task force of the published evidence on ECG screening of asymptomatic adults concluded that ECG abnormalities are associated with a risk of cardiovascular events, but 'the clinical implications of these findings are unclear'.[12]

Ethical considerations

There is a key difference between clinical consultation and health screening. In the clinical consultation, the patient approaches the doctor for advice or treatment for a health complaint and has to give consent to certain diagnostic procedures and therapy having been advised of some limitations or even possible adverse effects. In health screening, however, the doctor reviews an apparently healthy person for the possible presence of asymptomatic disease. In so doing, there must be a good understanding of the efficacy and safety of the screening tests, and patients should similarly be informed of the possible consequences of false positive and false negative results following screening.

A test procedure that is ethically justifiable on diagnostic grounds may not necessarily be applicable when used for screening asymptomatic people. Holland points out that there is lack of evidence that some health screening procedures are beneficial.[13] Indeed, there is positive evidence that they may lead to increased anxiety, illness behaviour, and also inappropriately utilize and deplete healthcare resources.

From a preventive perspective, the energy and expense of general health screening could perhaps be better diverted to promote measures to encourage proper diet, weight control, regular exercise, smoking cessation, moderation in alcohol consumption, and stress management, or control of workplace hazards. Modifications in lifestyle behaviour require motivation and effort on the part of the individual, whereas health screening is essentially a passive process, where an individual is seemingly reassured that all is well after a negative examination. This is perhaps the reason why general health screening has popular appeal.

Screening in occupational health practice

In occupational health settings, screening examinations are performed at different times and for various purposes.

Pre-placement examination

Pre-employment and pre-placement examinations are often required of persons embarking on a new job. The distinction between the terms is that pre-employment examination is usually performed before an individual is offered a job, and confirmation in the post is contingent upon passing the 'medical examination'. In pre-placement examination, the clinical assessment is conducted after a person is offered a job based on qualifications, experience, recommendations, etc. rather than health considerations. The purpose is to determine whether there may be health reasons why an individual should not be placed in a particular workplace, and/or make any necessary workplace adjustments. The reason that is often stated for excluding an individual from a specific job is that the safety of the individual or third parties may be compromised because of the health status of the prospective employee, e.g. an infectious hepatitis B carrier proposing to perform surgical procedures.

For a proper evaluation of fitness, the examining doctor should be aware of the requirements of the job and the working environment, in addition to assessing the health status of the person. In some countries, pre-employment examinations are prohibited under disability discrimination laws. However, there may also be national regulations that stipulate pre-employment and periodic medical examination for specific occupational groups, or persons exposed to specific hazards at work, e.g. workers exposed to inorganic lead. In the UK, the Equality Act 2010 stipulates that, with few exceptions, employers should now not ask about the health of prospective employees before a job offer.

Another often stated reason for the pre-employment examination is to establish baseline health information for subsequent health surveillance. It could also be used to assess health status for medical insurance purposes, and to defend or support a subsequent compensation claim for occupational illness. It is uncertain how much use is made of such baseline information, or whether the records are readily retrievable should there be a need to refer to baseline findings from pre-employment assessments.

Many occupations do not require high standards of physical fitness. The probability of discovering disease that might significantly impair job performance in apparently healthy job applicants, especially among young adults, is low. Thus, the rejection rate for fitness to work based on medical grounds is generally low. In a national audit of pre-employment assessments for healthcare workers, the rejection rate for applicants was less than 1%.[14]

The components of any pre-employment assessment should be justified on the basis of necessity and risk, and based on sound evidence that the specific questions asked or examinations performed are warranted for the proposed job.

If warranted, instead of subjecting every job applicant to the same general pre-employment screening, the examination should be tailored to the specific demands of the job. A self-administered health declaration or questionnaire that is processed by an occupational health adviser may be adequate for most clerical or administrative jobs. However, it has been advocated (albeit, with controversy) that more comprehensive screening be conducted for selected 'high flier' candidates, where substantial investment in training and resources is required. A recent evidence-based review on pre-employment examinations indicated that there was conflicting evidence on whether these procedures prevent injury, ill health or reduce sickness absence. It reaffirmed the view that, if indicated, pre-employment examinations should be job specific.[15]

Health screening prior to job transfers

Health screening is often performed for employees prior to job transfers or job reassignment, especially in large multinational organizations. In cases of posting overseas for a prolonged period, the employee may be accompanied by their family, and therefore the examination can also be offered to accompanying family members (often for health insurance purposes or where the employer has responsibility for healthcare costs of the individual and the family) (see Appendix 5).

Health screening for return to work after illness

Health screening can be conducted prior to return to work, especially after prolonged or serious illness. Knowledge of the natural history and prognosis of the illness is essential. It may be necessary to recommend an interim period of modified work, to allow time for the employee to readjust to the 'normal' work schedule and workload. For example, a person working in a hot environment who has been away from work for health reasons for a prolonged period would benefit from health screening, relevant advice, and provision of time for re-acclimatization.

Specific screening tests

A variety of laboratory and clinical investigations are used for screening of individuals exposed to specific hazards. Examples include:

◆ *Exposure to noise*: audiometric screening is required under noise regulations in many countries. (See Chapter 10.) Noise surveys to determine and reduce sources of excessive noise should have precedence over audiometry as a means for effective prevention.

◆ *Exposure to hand-transmitted vibration*: UK legislation and guidance on screening for hand–arm vibration syndrome requires an initial screening questionnaire for all workers before they start work involving exposure to vibration, and an annual screening questionnaire for surveillance of exposed workers. Different tiers of screening are required for those reporting symptoms. (See Appendix 6.)

◆ *Lung function tests*: spirometry, serial peak flow readings, and other tests of lung function are considered in workers exposed to the risk of obstructive or restrictive lung disease. Some of these tests are also used for diagnostic purposes, e.g. serial peak flow rates for occupational asthma, or for following up the efficacy of treatment or prevention. (See Chapter 18.)

◆ *Vision screening*: in the UK, workers who regularly use computers and other display screen equipment in the course of their work are entitled to vision testing. (See Chapter 9.)

◆ *Tests of liver or renal function*: attempts have been made to explore the use of bile acid clearance to indicate acute and chronic liver damage from chemicals but this remains experimental. Serum transaminases and transferases are elevated in liver disease but they are not specific enough for use as a screening tool. Similarly there is no good indication for the use of indices of renal function, such as blood urea and electrolytes, for occupational health screening. (See Chapters 14 and 19.)

◆ *Other specific screening procedures*: such as periodic chest x-rays for exposure to fibrogenic dusts, urinary screening for microscopic haematuria and detection of malignant cells in those exposed to bladder carcinogens, and examination of the skin in workers exposed to mineral oils are covered in greater detail elsewhere.[16]

Executive health screening

The periodic medical examination for managerial and senior posts in an organization is sometimes termed 'executive health screening'. The screening may involve determination of biochemical profiles, exercise ECGs, scans, and endoscopies. These periodic multiphasic medical examinations may be advocated by some patients and their physicians with the rationale that early detection of disease in highly paid executives has economic benefit to the company; but there is only anecdotal evidence to support this.[17,18]

As executive medicals are usually offered on a voluntary basis, the tendency would be for the highly motivated and health conscious to participate in the examination. In contrast to these 'worried well', those who are less concerned with their personal health (and who may have a greater need for counselling and lifestyle interventions), seldom participate in screening. Hence, any illness that may be present in this latter group remains undetected. This paradoxical phenomenon has been called the 'inverse care law'.[19] In time, executive health screening may well have a benefit in regards to the individual or to the organization as a return on investment,[20] but for the moment they are viewed as a 'perk' for selected groups within an organization. If there is any benefit in these screening procedures at all, then they should be made available for all.

Genetic screening

Several markers have been developed that attempt to detect those at higher risk of disease following specific exposure. Examples are alpha-1-antitrypsin deficiency as an indicator of increased risk of emphysema in those exposed to cadmium, and human leucocyte antigen (HLA) gene markers, specifically HLA-DBP1, as a factor associated with the development of chronic beryllium disease.[21] There is no indication that these methods are sufficiently well developed to warrant their routine use in occupational health practice. There are also ethical constraints over the use of such tests.

In regard to other screening for susceptibility, the determination of atopic status for workers who may be exposed to asthmagens, for example, is of limited use for screening in occupational health. Since atopy in the general population is common, this would result in exclusion of a significant proportion of job applicants.

Screening for drugs and alcohol

In occupational health practice, this is best considered in the context of a clear organizational policy on the consequences of a positive result, on whether testing is voluntary or mandatory, and whether it should apply to all levels of staff regardless of seniority (see also Chapter 24.).

Biological monitoring and biological effect monitoring

Biological monitoring and biological effect monitoring are procedures used as part of screening in occupational health practice:[22] biological monitoring screens for exposure, and biological effects monitoring attempts to detect early effects. As in other forms of screening, the principle is to detect adverse exposure or early alterations in biochemical parameters following workplace exposures, and then to take appropriate preventive measures to prevent the onset of overt health effects or clinical disease.

Biological monitoring involves the analysis of biological samples (urine, blood, or breath) for the presence of the chemical to which the individual worker is exposed, or for a metabolite. Examples amenable to monitoring are lead and mercury, and organic solvents such as trichloroethylene and xylene. Metabolites of organic solvents that can be detected in urine samples are trichloroacetic acid for trichloroethylene and 1,1,1,-trichloroethane, and mandelic acid for styrene. Some metabolites are non-specific and can result from several different exposures, both occupational and non-occupational, e.g. hippuric acid in the urine can occur from benzoate in foods or from occupational exposure to toluene. Other metabolites are more specific, e.g. methyl-hippuric acid in urine following exposure to xylene.

Biological effect monitoring attempts to detect changes in one or more biochemical parameters as an early effect of occupational exposure. Examples are the detection of elevated free erythrocyte protoporphyrin level in blood among those exposed to inorganic lead, and depression of serum cholinesterase in workers exposed to organophosphates. Tests such as the detection of DNA adducts in biological samples for exposure to carcinogens[23] and markers of oxidative stress in workers exposed to pesticides[24] are available, but are not indicated for routine biological effect monitoring.

Health surveillance

The periodic clinical and physiological assessment of workers for exposure to workplace hazards[25] or for monitoring general health status forms an integral part of occupational medicine practice. For the prevention of work-related illness, emphasis should be on the former. Some of the components of health surveillance for specific purposes have been covered in the preceding sections.

Evaluation of screening programmes

A common error in evaluating the potential of a screening test is to adopt the sensitivity and specificity of the test when it is first evaluated in people with the disease. As the population considered for screening by occupational health practitioners consists mainly of asymptomatic persons who may or may not have disease, the application of findings of the screening test in a diseased population to the general population is not appropriate and could lead to erroneous conclusions about the usefulness of the test.

In evaluating screening programmes the potential for bias should be considered. Different categories of possible bias are summarized in Table 29.5. Screening programmes should also be reviewed and audited periodically to ensure that the basis and procedures for such screening remain valid.

Table 29.5 Possible biases in the evaluation of screening programmes

Selection bias	Occurs when those who participate in screening programmes are volunteers. Such volunteers are generally more health conscious than those who do not participate in screening programmes. As such, even without screening, these persons who volunteer for the screening test are more likely to have better health outcomes from their disease as compared with the general population or those who do not participate in the screening
Lead-time bias	The evaluation of the usefulness of screening examinations may sometimes be influenced by the apparent long survival of a patient (e.g. a patient with cancer) who is diagnosed early by screening. This long survival in fact may only be a manifestation of *lead-time bias*, where screening brings forward the time of diagnosis and thus lengthens the disease knowledge time without actually prolonging life
Length bias	There is a tendency for screening to detect the less serious conditions. More rapidly advancing illnesses, by their nature, will only be present in the population for a relatively short time, and so miss being detected. As more slowly progressing illnesses than aggressive conditions are found on screening, this also gives the erroneous impression that detecting these conditions early has improved survival

Conclusions

Health screening is a useful tool in occupational health practice, but theoretical and practical issues bear consideration before beginning such screening for any group of workers. Legal requirements will vary from country to country and will influence what is provided. Proper communication with the workforce, employer, and occupational health and safety professionals is essential for implementing successful health screening programmes.

References

1 Blumberg MS. Evaluating health screening procedures. *Operations Res* 1957; **5**: 351–60.

2 Wilson JMG, Jungner G. *Principles and practice of screening for disease.* Geneva: World Health Organization, 1968.

3 Andermann A, Blancquaert I, Beauchamp S, *et al.* Revisiting Wilson and Jungner in the genomic age: a review of screening criteria over the past 40 years. *Bull World Health Organ* 2008; **86**: s317–19.

4 Schilling CJ, Schilling JM. Chest X ray screening for lung cancer at three British chromate plants from 1955 to 1989. *Br J Ind Med* 1991; **48**: 476–9.

5 George PJM. Delays in the management of lung cancer. *Thorax* 1997; **52**: 107–8.

6 Petch MC. Misleading exercise electrocardiograms. *Br Med J* 1987; **295**: 620–1.

7 Maffei E, Palumbo A, Martini C, *et al.* Stress-ECG vs. CT coronary angiography for the diagnosis of coronary artery disease: a "real-world" experience. *Radiol Med* 2010; **11**: 354–67.

8 Freeman J, Froelicher V, Ashley E. The ageing athlete: screening prior to vigorous exertion in asymptomatic adults without known cardiovascular disease. *Br J Sports Med* 2009; **43**: 696–701.

9 American College of Cardiology/American Heart Association Task Force on Practice Guidelines. ACC/AHA guidelines for exercise testing: executive summary. *Circulation* 1997; **96**: 345–54.

10 Drivers Medical Group. *At a glance guide to the current medical standards of fitness to drive.* Swansea: DVLA, 2011. (<http://www.dft.gov.uk/dvla/medical/ataglance.aspx>)

11 The US Preventive Services Task Force. *The guide to clinical preventive services 2010–2011.* [Online] (<http://www.uspreventiveservicestaskforce.org/recommendations.htm>)

12 Chou R, Arora B, Dana T, *et al.* Screening asymptomatic adults with resting or exercise electrocardiography: a review of the evidence for the U.S. Preventive Services Task Force. *Ann Intern Med* 2011; **155**: 375–85.

13 Holland WW. Screening: reasons to be cautious. *BMJ* 1993; **306**: 1221–2.

14 Whitaker S, Aw TC. Audit of pre-employment assessments by occupational health departments in the National Health Service. *Occup Med* 1995; **45**: 75–80.

15 Mahmud N, Schonstein E, Schaafsma F, *et al.* Cochrane review—pre-employment examinations for preventing injury and disease. *Cochrane Database Syst Rev* 2010; **8**: CD008881.

16 Aw TC. Health surveillance. In: Sadhra SS, Rampal KG (eds), *Occupational health: risk assessment and management*, pp. 288–314. Oxford: Blackwell Science, 1999.

17 O'Malley PG, Greenland P. The annual physical: are physicians and patients telling us something? *Arch Intern Med* 2005; **165**: 1333–4.

18 Oboler SK, Prochazka AV, Gonzalez R, *et al.* Public expectations and attitudes to annual physical examinations and testing. *Ann Intern Med* 2002; **136**: 652–9.

19 Hart JT. The inverse care law. *Lancet* 1971; **i**: 405–12.

20 Komaroff AL. Executive physicals: what's the ROI? *Harv Bus Rev* 2009; **87**: 28.

21 McCanlies EC, Ensey JS, LefantJr JS, *et al.* The association between HLA-DBP1^{Glu69} and chronic beryllium disease and beryllium sensitization. *Am J Ind Med* 2004; **46**: 95–103.

22 Aw TC. Biological monitoring In: Gardiner KG, Harrington JM (eds), *Occupational hygiene*, pp. 160–9. Oxford: Blackwell Publishing Ltd, 2005.

23 Al Zabadi H, Ferrari L, Laurent A-M, *et al*. Biomonitoring of complex occupational exposure to carcinogens: the case of sewage workers in Paris. *BMC Cancer* 2008; **8**: 67. (< http://www.biomedcentral.com/1471-2407/8/67>)

24 Astiz M, Arnal N, de Alaniz MJ, *et al*. New markers for screening for pesticide exposure—oxidative stress biomarkers? *Env Toxicol Pharmacol* 2011; **32**: 249–58.

25 Koh DSQ, Aw TC. Surveillance in occupational health. *Occup Environ Med* 2003; **60**: 705–10.

Chapter 30

Managing and avoiding sickness absence

Richard Preece and Dean Royles

Sickness absence is an important issue for workers, managers, and occupational health services. Most employees suffer health problems at some time during their career and face decisions on fitness in relation to their work. All employers will occasionally be concerned about the fitness to work of absent employees and what actions they might take to address this. Advising on sickness absence management and the fitness to work of absentees, individually and collectively, is a major activity for occupational health specialists.

Epidemiology of sickness absence

An estimated 175 million working days are lost each year in the UK due to sickness absence.[1]

Data on sickness absence are not gathered systematically and the quality of summary statistics reflects this weakness. The most recent surveys by the Chartered Institute of Professional Development (CIPD) and Confederation of British Industry (CBI) found rates of 7.7 days and 6.5 day per employee per year respectively.[2,3] Rates vary markedly across different organizations. International comparisons of sickness absence rates are uncommon. The data, although of limited validity, imply marked variations. For example, rates of absence of at least 1 day in the past year range across Europe from 6.7 per cent to 24.0 per cent, the UK rate being 11.7 per cent.[4] Two groups of factors have been found to explain between-country differences: objective factors, such as the health status and employment rates, and the generosity of sickness absence compensation systems.[5]

Sickness absence rates vary by sex, age, occupation, sector, region, pay grade[6] (see Figure 30.1) and the size of the workplace[2,3,7] and a large number of other psychosocial factors relating to employees' attitudes and behaviour—e.g. motivation[8] and the degree of control they have over their work.[9]

The principal causes of long-term sickness absence among manual workers (across all sectors in the UK) are acute medical conditions, followed by back pain, musculoskeletal injuries, stress, and mental health problems. Among non-manual workers (across all sectors), the leading causes are stress, acute medical conditions, mental health problems (such as depression and anxiety), musculoskeletal injuries, and back pain.[2]

Whilst many different factors influence sickness absence, illness is usually accepted as the reason for an episode of sickness absence. A recent CBI survey reported 'illness is still the major cause of absence'.[3] However, very little of the variance in absence rates amongst individual employees is explained by illness. In a recent large study in Wales, only 4 per cent of the variance in sickness absence rates was explained by illness.[10,11] This observation is important as it emphasizes the importance of addressing the non-biological elements of the biopsychosocial model.

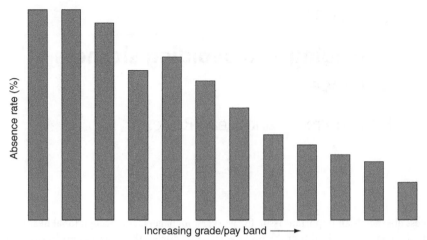

Figure 30.1 Absence rate relationship with grade/pay. Data from Managing Sickness Absence in the NHS Health Briefing February 2011 Copyright © Audit Commission 2011.

Theoretical models of sickness absence management

Three models of sickness absence are popular: the expected utility model of absenteeism, the stress model, and the organization model.[12]

The *expected utility model* assumes that workers have some choice whether or not they will report sick and that they consider the costs and rewards in making a decision to attend or not. Approaches based on this model should aim to set a high threshold for being absent and a low threshold for resuming work when absent.

The occupational *stress model* focuses on the negative effects of the work environment and the coping abilities of workers. Some people are more resilient and have better coping strategies than others. Approaches based on this model focus on reducing stressors, improving social support, and building resilience.

The *organization model* focuses on rewarding work, including job content, fairness, status, and social relationships, to improve satisfaction and motivation. Approaches based on this model focus on promoting well-being.

These three models all have merit. In practice they are often combined to form an *integrated model* which aims to alter the balance of costs and rewards, reduce stress, and promote resilience and well-being.

Promoting attendance

Engagement

[Engagement is] a workplace approach designed to ensure that employees are committed to their organisation's goals and values, motivated to contribute to organisational success and are able at the same time to enhance their own sense of wellbeing.[13]

In recent years, measures of staff engagement have been increasingly recognized as important indicators of performance across the private and public sectors. Macleod et al.[13] found that engaged employees have lower sickness absence rates than those who are disengaged with beneficial effects

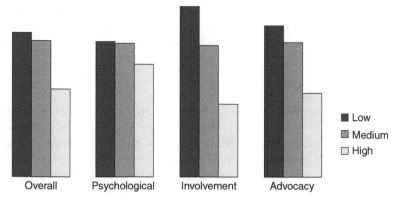

Figure 30.2 Relationship between absence rate (%) and high, medium and low levels of staff engagement (n = 154726) Adapted from West M et al, NHS Staff Management and Health Service Quality, Department of Health, London © Crown Copyright 2011.

on competitiveness and performance. Staff with high levels of engagement displayed a number of positive behavioural traits:

♦ Increased commitment.

♦ A belief in their organization.

♦ A desire to work to make things better.

♦ Suggesting improvements.

♦ Working well in a team.

♦ Helping colleagues.

♦ A likelihood to 'go the extra mile'.

Four broad enablers are critical to employee engagement: leadership (strategic narrative), enabling managers, employee voice, and, integrity.[13]

A positive working environment is good for health and well-being with evidence from the largest staff survey in the UK that higher levels of staff engagement are associated with lower levels of sickness absence (Figure 30.2).[14]

Manager attitudes and behaviour

Line managers are important to promoting attendance. They are responsible for:

♦ Setting objectives.

♦ Designing work arrangements.

♦ Supporting employees (whether they face health issues or not).

♦ Making adjustments to work.

The behaviour of line managers is a major influence on whether employees remain in work and resume work successfully following a period of sickness absence.[15] The most important attributes of managers are good people management skills, including effective communication, sensitivity to, and understanding of, the individual and the context.

Managers who do not believe that sickness absence can be reduced tend to underestimate its impact and are less likely to proactively tackle the problem. This may be a particular issue for managers who have only ever worked in a sector with a relatively high sickness absence rates and have not experienced anything different. In these circumstances, managers' attitudes will undermine the effectiveness, and bring into doubt, the value of interventions. It becomes critical to understand and change managers' beliefs about improving attendance if improvement is to be achieved.[16]

What is good work?

In his review of the most effective evidence-based strategies for reducing health inequalities, Marmot reported that being in 'good' employment is protective of health and getting people into work is therefore of critical importance. The longer sickness absence continues, the more likely that job loss will ensue.[17] Returning employees promptly to work after illness should prevent this.

Marmot described ten core components of work that protect good health and promote health[18] (Box 30.1).

Box 30.1 Characteristics of good work

'Good' work (is):

- Free of the core features of precariousness, such as lack of stability and high risk of job loss, lack of safety measures (exposure to toxic substances, elevated risks of accidents) and the absence of minimal standards of employment protection.

- Enables the worker to exert some control through participatory decision-making on matters such as the place and the timing of work and the tasks to be accomplished.

- Places appropriately high demands on the worker, both in terms of quantity and quality, without overtaxing their resources and capabilities and without doing harm to their physical and mental health.

- Provides fair employment in terms of earnings reflecting productivity and in terms of employers' commitment towards guaranteeing job security.

- Offers opportunities for skill training, learning and promotion prospects within a life course perspective, sustaining health and work ability and stimulating the growth of an individual's capabilities.

- Prevents social isolation, discrimination, and violence.

- Enables workers to share relevant information within the organisation, to participate in organisational decision-making and collective bargaining and to guarantee procedural justice in case of conflicts.

- Aims at reconciling work and extra-work/family demands in ways that reduce the cumulative burden of multiple social roles.

- Attempts to reintegrate sick and disabled people into full employment wherever possible by mobilising available means.

- Contributes to workers' well-being by meeting the basic psychological needs of experiencing self-efficacy, self-esteem, sense of belonging and meaningfulness.

Reprinted with permission from *Fair Society, Healthy Lives: The Marmot Review*, February 2010, pp. 112, Copyright © The Marmot Review.

Although good work is desirable there is a danger that its importance is both overstated and idealistic leading everyone to conclude that their own work and the work of those they manage is not good. Although it is difficult to show the health benefits of work there is very little evidence that work is bad for health as in most circumstances occupational risks are low or well controlled.[17] In encouraging and supporting attendance the focus should emphasize work is usually good for health and that with some effort it can often be even better.

Measuring and monitoring absence

The starting point in managing sickness absence is to measure and report it. The system of measurement should reflect the size and complexity of the organization. In smaller businesses the impact of absence is often immediate and stark—there is simply nobody else to do the work.

For larger organizations managers will need to measure and respond to the impact on their teams' activities. The immediate and short-term impact may seem small as work carries on. Senior managers in larger organizations will need to measure and respond to the wider organizational impact on performance and productivity.

The act of measuring and reporting absence accurately can serve to prompt intervention and to identify trends. Typically organizations will measure sickness absence rates in terms either of days of absence or percentage of lost working time. However, this seemingly simple measure may not be straightforward, for example, in counting:

- The number of working days (e.g. public holidays and weekends).
- Absence for only part of a working day.
- Absences of part-time workers.
- Absences of those working variable length shifts.

$$\text{Sickness absence rate}\,(\%) = \frac{\text{Total absence}\,(\text{hours or days})\,\text{in the period}}{\text{Possible total}\,(\text{hours or days})\,\text{in the period}} \times 100$$

Many organizations prefer instead to emphasize and report the positive measure of attendance rate.

The second typical measure is one that provides an indication of the frequency of periods of sickness absence.

$$\text{Frequency rate} = \frac{\text{No. of spells of absence in the period}}{\text{No. of employees}} \times 100$$

These two measures give some indication of the impact of sickness absence on the organization. However, they offer little insight into the nature of the underlying absence in terms of causes, patterns, and the impact arising from absent subgroups within the workforce.

The cause of absence can be monitored by recording the reasons cited by employees and their doctors on certificates, but data gathered in these ways can be difficult to interpret. The actual reason or reasons for sickness absence may not be the one(s) declared. Moreover, the impact of work and potential for intervention at work may not be clear.

A summary sickness absence rate gives no indication of the underlying pattern of absence. Other measures are needed to demonstrate the contribution from distinct episodes of short and long duration. Long periods of absence usually contribute most to the overall lost time but may not have such a dramatic effect on business continuity as managers have time to make plans in response and maintain output. In contrast, short frequent episodes may contribute less to overall lost time but may be highly disruptive with a disproportionate impact on productivity.

Inception rates indicate the number of new episodes starting in the measurement period—expressed as a proportion (%) of the average number of staff employed in that period. This may be useful as a measure of longer periods of absence. (Termination rates, the number of episodes ending in the measurement period, are a related alternative and have a potential advantage as the reason for absence may be known.)

$$\text{Inception rate} = \frac{\text{No. of spells of absence which start in the period}}{\text{No. of employees}} \times 100$$

Many workers will not be absent at all during a monitoring period and some will be absent on several occasions. The overall rates do not give any indication of absence behaviour. Frequent absences may be an indication of a long-term underlying health problem but more often it is because the worker has a lower threshold for not attending (for example, due to carer responsibilities or illness behaviour). Measuring the organizational impact of workers taking frequent episodes of sickness absence can prompt management intervention.

$$\text{Frequent episodes rate} = \frac{\text{No. of employees absent on more than x occasions in the period}}{\text{No. of employees}} \times 100$$

Whilst some workers will be absent frequently the majority will not. Many workers rarely take any sickness absence. Some illness is inevitable and it is not possible for all employees to attend all the time. In some cases attending when ill can have a detrimental impact on productivity (presenteeism) or on colleagues and customers (e.g. due to infectious diseases). Full attendance during a time period does, however, provide some indication of engagement and commitment.

$$\text{Full attendance rate} = \frac{\text{No. of employees who take no sickness absence at all in the period}}{\text{No. of employees}} \times 100$$

Recording sickness absence in 'real time' enables managers to intervene swiftly to provide support and to take action to encourage attendance.

Trigger points

Typically, management protocols will define 'trigger points' at which managers should consider formal action to require improved attendance. Trigger points can provide a consistent approach to attendance management but there is a risk that they institutionalize absenteeism by establishing an acceptable level of absence. In setting trigger points it is important to emphasize that the objective is full attendance of all employees and to emphasize the importance of management discretion in considering the period(s) of absence within the whole picture for an individual employee.

Trigger points may be based upon any or all of:

◆ The cumulative number of days absence in a time period.
◆ The number of episodes of absence in a time period.
◆ The pattern of episodes (e.g. on a public holiday or immediately before or after a holiday/weekend).

Organizations may adopt a trigger point based on a combination of days and episodes. The best known example of this is the Bradford score (also known as factor, formula, and index) which is designed to provide an indication of the disruption caused by persistent periods of short-duration sickness absence. The Bradford score combines measures of both frequency and duration of absence, with a greater emphasis placed on frequency. The formula S2D or $S \times S \times D$, is used to calculate a score or index for a given period (usually a rolling year), where S is the number of spells of absence, and D is the aggregate number of days absent.

The Bradford score appears to have been derived from Bradford's law (of scatter). Samuel Clements Bradford (1878–1948) was a practising librarian and one of the pioneers of bibliometrics. He found that most of the papers on a certain subject were published in a few journals and some articles were scattered in many borderline journals and proposed a mathematical formula to describe the large contribution from a small number.[19]

The utility of the Bradford score is even less certain than its provenance. Its effectiveness has not been demonstrated. There is a danger that use of the Bradford score, or another scoring system, leads to undue focus on employees with long-term health conditions who are prone to short-term exacerbations but whose overall attendance is above average and employees with significant carer responsibilities.

For example, an employee taking five individual days of sickness absence in a year would have a higher Bradford score ($5 \times 5 \times 5 = 125$) than an employee having two episodes each totalling 4 weeks ($2 \times 2 \times 20 = 80$). The first employee's absence may be significantly below average and the second employee's well above average, but if the organization has set a trigger point of 100 then only the first employee would face formal management action. However, many employers are comfortable with this as they place greater weight on disruptive periodic absences.

Policy and procedure

Employers should establish a policy that explains the responsibilities of managers and employees when an employee is absent due to sickness. This should describe the expectations, actions, and terms and conditions of employment (Box 30.2 provides a model policy statement designed by ACAS). Organizations pay employees to attend work, so attendance is accepted as the norm. Whilst employers recognize that some limited absence is inevitable their aim is to facilitate a return to work at the earliest opportunity when provided with appropriate support and assistance.[20]

Box 30.2 ACAS sample policies

Policy statement

We are committed to improving the health, wellbeing and attendance of all employees. We value the contribution our employees make to our success. So, when any employee is unable to be at work for any reason, we miss that contribution. This absence policy explains:

- what we expect from managers and employees when handling absence
- how we will work to reduce levels of absence to no more than xx days per employee per year.

Box 30.2 ACAS sample policies *(continued)*

This policy has been written after consultation with employee representatives. We welcome the continued involvement of employees in implementing this policy.

Key principles

The organisation's absence policy is based on the following principles:

1　As a responsible employer we undertake to provide payments to employees who are unable to attend work due to sickness. (See the Company Sick Pay scheme.)

2　Regular, punctual attendance is an implied term of every employee's contract of employment—we ask each employee to take responsibility for achieving and maintaining good attendance.

3　We will support employees who have genuine grounds for absence for whatever reason. This support includes:

　a　'special leave' for necessary absences not caused by sickness

　b　a flexible approach to the taking of annual leave

　c　access to counsellors where necessary

　d　rehabilitation programmes in cases of long-term sickness absence.

4　We will consider any advice given by the employee's GP on the 'Statement of Fitness for Work'. If the GP advises that an employee 'may be fit for work' we will discuss with the employee how we can help them get back to work—for example, on flexible hours, or altered duties.

5　We will use an occupational health adviser, where appropriate, to:

　a　help identify the nature of an employee's illness

　b　advise the employee and their manager on the best way to improve the employee's health and wellbeing.

6　The company's disciplinary procedures will be used if an explanation for absence is not forthcoming or is not thought to be satisfactory.

7　We respect the confidentiality of all information relating to an employee's sickness. This policy will be implemented in line with all data protection legislation and the Access to Medical Records Act 1988.

Notification of absence

If an employee is going to be absent from work they should speak to their manager or deputy within an hour of their normal start time. They should also:

◆ give a clear indication of the nature of the illness and

◆ a likely return date.

The manager will check with employees if there is any information they need about their current work. If the employee does not contact their manager by the required time the manager will attempt to contact the employee at home.

An employee may not always feel able to discuss their medical problems with their line manager. Managers will be sensitive to individual concerns and make alternative arrangements,

Box 30.2 ACAS sample policies *(continued)*

where appropriate. For example, an employee may prefer to discuss health problems with a person of the same sex.

Evidence of incapacity

Employees can use the company self-certification arrangements for the first seven days absence. Thereafter a 'Statement of Fitness for Work' is required to cover every subsequent day.

If absence is likely to be protracted, ie more than four weeks continuously, there is a shared responsibility for the Company and the employee to maintain contact at agreed intervals.

'May be fit for some work'

If the GP advises on the Statement of Fitness for Work that an employee 'may be fit for work' we will discuss with the employee ways of helping them get back to work. This might mean talking about a phased return to work or amended duties.

If it is not possible to provide the support an employee needs to return to work—for example, by making the necessary workplace adjustments—or an employee feels unable to return then the Statement will be used in the same way as if the GP advised that the employee was 'not fit for work'.

Return to work discussions

Managers will discuss absences with employees when they return to work to establish:

- the reason for, and cause of absence
- anything the manager or the company can do to help
- that the employee is fit to return to work.

If an employee's GP has advised that they 'may be fit for work' the return to work discussion can also be used to agree in detail how their return to work might work best in practice.

Formal review

A more formal review will be triggered by:

- frequent short-term absences
- long-term absence.

This review will look at any further action required to improve the employee's attendance and wellbeing. These trigger points are set by line managers and are available from Personnel.

Absence due to disability/maternity

Absences relating to the disability of an employee or to pregnancy will be kept separate from sickness absence records. We refer employees to our Equality Policy—covering family policies and disability discrimination policies.

Reproduced from Managing attendance and employee turnover booklet, Department of Work and Pensions and ACAS, September 2010 Copyright © ACAS, Euston Tower, 286 Euston Road, London NW1 3JJ under the Open Government Licence v1.0. Available from <http: //www.acas.org.uk/CHttpHandler.ashx?id=241&p=0>

Prerequisites to interventions

The National Institute for Health and Clinical Excellence (NICE) described a number of prerequisites for effective action:

* Appropriate health support for absentees should be available from their general practitioner (GP) and other relevant clinicians.
* Absentees should provide consent to share some confidential information with specified parties.
* Absentees and employers should be in regular contact to plan and execute any agreed activities.
* The person planning, coordinating, or delivering support should have the relevant experience, expertise, and credibility.
* Account should be taken of the employee's age illness, and the nature of their work.
* Activities need to be tailored to the individual's condition and perceived (or actual) barriers to returning to work.
* Organizational sickness absence policies and health and safety practices should be implemented.

NICE suggests that there is evidence that actively helping to implement something (e.g. physiotherapy) can be more effective than encouraging the absentee to do something for themselves (e.g. advising regular physical activity or to make contact with another organization).

Managing short- and medium-term absence

Short-term absences can be highly disruptive. In some organizations these absences may be common. They have the potential to significantly influence attendance culture, potentially legitimizing absence amongst peers and setting a benchmark that encourages workers to expect even longer periods of absence in the event of more serious illness.

There is no commonly agreed definition of short-term absence. It is useful to distinguish between a short-term absence (e.g. up to 7 days) and a medium-term absence (8 days up to 4 weeks), as the reasons for the shortest absences that are self-certificated are likely to differ from those that are slightly longer and certificated by the employee's GP.

In the past two decades two interventions have been popularized for preventing short-term sickness absence—the use of triggers and return-to-work interviews. However, their popularity is founded on reputation rather than persuasive evidence.

The CIPD annual survey has been influential in developing management practice. Respondents to the survey have repeatedly shared their opinions that triggers and return-to-work interviews are effective but this has not been substantiated by empirical research. Practice experience has strengthened a belief in the effectiveness of these two interventions and they are widely used (Table 30.1).[21,22] However, the value of return-to-work interviews is not certain.

Irrespective of the evidence on effectiveness there is an expectation that managers both talk to an employee who has been absent on his/her return (a return-to-work interview) and use some sort of threshold to initiate a discussion about improved attendance (trigger point). The focus of these activities is to identify the support that might enable an employee to attend work more consistently. In some cases the discussion between the employee and the manager will identify a health need that may result in referral for occupational health advice. Referrals should not be

Table 30.1 Employers' experience of managing short-term absence

	Proportion of respondents using this approach (%)		Proportion believing it to be amongst the most effective interventions (%)	
	2003	2010	2003	2010
Triggers	68	83	28	56
RTW interviews	77	88	60	68

Data from Employee absence 2003: A survey of management policy and practice, the Chartered Institute of Personnel and Development, London, Copyright © 2003 and Annual survey report 2010: absence management, the Chartered Institute of Personnel and Development, London, Copyright © 2010.

automatic as unnecessary consultations are not likely to be valued by the employee, the manager, and the occupational health specialist.

The use of return-to-work interviews and triggers is not without difficulty. Return-to-work interviews can be time consuming especially if formally recorded. Many such interviews take place without the evidence that they improve future attendance. A large amount of management time is invested for each employee ultimately dismissed for poor attendance and, even if effective, there should still be doubt about their cost-effectiveness and the effort to conduct them as efficiently as possible. These concerns should be balanced against the importance of taking action and the need to reinforce the responsibility of managers in promoting a healthy workplace and attendance culture.

A trigger point approach to management action can be useful but can also over-simplify attendance management. Setting the threshold too low generates a considerable volume of work of doubtful value for managers, while setting it too high defeats its purpose.

The role of occupational health services in the management of short-term absence is usually limited. In many cases there will only be a pattern of unrelated and relatively minor ailments. Occupational health advice is likely to be limited to confirmation that the patient is fit for work and could potentially provide regular and effective attendance and performance in the future. In some cases it will be possible to confirm that a cause of recent absences has been addressed and so should not give rise to further episodes.

Where short-term absences arise from an underlying long-term health condition the occupational health team will provide advice to both the manager and the patient on actions that might promote well-being and attendance. The advice may include an opinion as to whether, taking account of health factors, the patient is likely to provide regular and effective attendance and performance in the future.

In all cases the report should only be issued with the consent of the patient and managers and human resources advisers should understand that consent is a prerequisite.

Short- and medium-term absence is common. The lack of evidence of effectiveness for interventions in short-term absence is an important and costly gap in knowledge that should addressed by new research.

Predicting future absence

A large number of factors associated with sickness absence have been reported in epidemiological studies. Some are related to working conditions and may be modified by the employer, such as the flexibility and support provided at work. Most of the factors related to the individual employee cannot be modified, including age, gender, location, and type of occupation (skilled vs. unskilled).

The individual factors that can be modified include the treatment for any underlying conditions and the behaviours associated with health.

An important role for occupational health practitioners in managing sickness absence is to identify whether an employee has any underlying medical conditions and make sure that the appropriate treatment and advice is being provided. However, improving treatment of underlying medical conditions is unlikely to significantly improve attendance most of the time (as differences in health explain very little of the variation in individual sickness absence). Interventions that change individual behaviour, in response to health and well-being issues, may have a more enduring impact on attendance in many situations.

Employees' beliefs about when they might be justified in taking sickness absence directly influences future absence. Those whose perception of their own health means they believe they would have been justified in taking time off work at least five times the past year are likely to be absent more often in the future.[23]

Past sickness absence is an important and possibly the most important indicator of future absence. In a study of low back pain the strongest prognostic indicator was found to be the history of sickness absence during the preceding 10 years.[24] A similar result has been reported for cumulative sickness absence from all causes in the preceding year.[25]

The risk of future sickness absence increases with the number of prior episodes.[26] Sixty per cent of workers, who had four or more episodes in a baseline period of 1 year, repeated this number of episodes per year at least once during a follow-up period of 4 years.[27] Frequency of sickness absence is better predicted by the history of sickness absence than the duration in terms of days of sickness absence.[28]

A recent systematic review concluded that sickness absence data from the past 2 years helps to identify employees who are likely to have above average sickness absence and it is not necessary to go further back than 2 years in an employee's history to predict this.[29] The review found that:

♦ Days of sickness absence in the past year predict future days of sickness absence.

♦ Episodes of sickness absence in the past 2 years predict future episodes of sickness absence.

Identification of employees who are frequently absent enables attempts to influence health behaviour. Changing health behaviours is possible in theory, but difficult in practice. This is a major reason why there is limited evidence of effectiveness for interventions for frequent episodes of absence.[30] However, the potential for success will be greater with approaches that focus on the psychosocial context rather than underlying health.

Long-term absence

NICE has defined long-term sickness absence as absences from work lasting 4 or more weeks.

Long-term absence explains a significant proportion of total sickness absence. The proportion varies according to the type of work, the business sector, and the size of organization (Table 30.2).[2] The proportion of total absence is likely to be closely related to the amount of (paid and unpaid) time a worker's terms and conditions of employment allow before an absentee's contract is terminated. The proportion of absence due to long-term sickness absence is biggest in large and public sector organizations. For example, more than half of the total days of sickness absence incurred by the UK's largest employer, the National Health Service (NHS), are due to periods of long-term sickness absence.[31]

There is a richer evidence base to indicate the appropriate actions to manage long-term sickness absence. Two important reviews of attendance management have been published. The first

Table 30.2 The proportion of total days of absence due to short-, medium-, and long-term periods for different employees and employers

	1–7 days (%)	8–28 days (%)	>28 days (%)
All employees	64	16	19
Manual employees	62	17	22
Non-manual employees	73	12	15
Industry sector			
Manufacturing and production	71	16	14
Private sector services	72	14	14
Public services	52	18	29
Non-profit organizations	57	20	22
Number of UK employees			
1–49	78	12	9
50–249	70	16	14
250–999	61	16	23
1000–4999	56	20	25
5000+	46	20	34

Reproduced from the Chartered Institute of Personnel and Development (2011) Annual survey report 2011: absence management, CIPD, Lond on with the permission of the publisher, the Chartered Institute of Personnel and Development, London (<http: //www.cipd.co.uk>).

in 2002 by BOHRF considered reports dating from the 1970s onwards although some of the evidence may be somewhat out of date.[32] More recently, NICE conducted a review and published guidance on interventions in the workplace and community to help people return to work after sickness absence and/or incapacity.[30,33] The evidence reviews that NICE commissioned to inform the guidance aimed to identify any relevant interventions, policies, strategies, or programmes that help people return to work after sickness absence and/or incapacity.[30,33]

The NICE recommendations were informed by the most appropriate available evidence of effectiveness and cost-effectiveness provided by research using any study design that evaluated the status before and after the intervention has been effected.[34] The literature review considered thousands of reports. More than 50 met well-defined criteria for inclusion, quality, appropriateness to the scope, and applicability to specific populations and settings in England. The evidence was considered by a multidisciplinary committee comprising professional, lay, and academic experts.

This review is the most comprehensive to date and provides a robust foundation for managing sickness absence. It suggests a three-step approach:[34] initial enquiries, detailed assessment, coordinating and delivering interventions and services.

Initial enquiries

1 Identify someone who is suitably trained and impartial to undertake initial enquiries with the relevant employees.

2 Make sure that initial enquiries are undertaken in conjunction with the employee, ideally between 2 and 6 weeks of a person starting the period of sickness absence:

- To determine the reason for the sickness and their prognosis for returning to work (that is, how likely it is that they will return to work) and if they have any perceived (or actual) barriers to returning to work (including the need for workplace adjustments)
- To decide on the options for returning to work and jointly agree what, if any, action is required to prepare for this.

3 If action is required consider identifying:

- Whether or not a detailed assessment is needed to determine what interventions and services are required and to develop a return-to-work plan.
- Whether or not a case worker should be appointed to coordinate a detailed assessment, deliver any proposed interventions, or produce a return-to-work plan.

Detailed assessment

1 Arrange for a relevant specialist/s to undertake an assessment (or different components of it) in conjunction with the employee (and in communication with the line manager) which include referral to an occupational health adviser or another appropriate health specialist.

2 Conduct a combined health and work assessment that evaluates the following:

- The employee's health, social, and employment situation: this includes anything that is putting them off returning to work, for example, organizational structure and culture (such as work relationships) and how confident they feel about overcoming these problems.
- The employee's current or previous experience of rehabilitation.
- The tasks the employee carries out at work and their physical ability to perform them (dealing with issues such as mobility, strength and fitness).
- Any workplace or work equipment modifications needed in line with the disability provisions of the Equality Act 2010 (including ergonomic modifications).

3 Prepare a return-to-work plan that identifies the type and level of interventions and services needed (including any psychological support from someone trained in psychological assessment techniques) and how frequently they should be offered. The report could also specify whether or not any of the following is required:

- A gradual return to the original job by increasing the hours and days worked over a period of time.
- A return to some of the duties of the original job.
- A move to another job within the organization (on a temporary or permanent basis).

The detailed assessment should be coordinated by a suitably trained case worker (Box 30.3).

Coordinating and delivering interventions and services

NICE further recommends that the delivery of planned health, occupational, or rehabilitation interventions or services and any return-to-work plan developed following initial enquiries or the detailed assessment is coordinated. People who have a 'poor' prognosis for returning to work are likely to benefit most from more 'intensive' interventions and services; those with a 'good' prognosis are likely to benefit from 'light' or less intense interventions and services.

Box 30.3 Case worker

A case worker has been defined as a person responsible for managing an assessment and coordinating delivery of interventions and services to help a person return to work (NICE).[34] The purpose of the role is to make sure that support and intervention is coordinated so that it is provided in a timely way to help employees to resume their usual or adjusted work as soon as they can. Whilst there is no commonly agreed description of case working there is some emerging consensus on the importance of:

- Monitoring absence data in real time.
- Coordinating any required assessments.
- Timetabled actions to eliminate delays between milestones.
- Initiation of formal interventions.
- Prompt and tracked actions.
- Providing periodic reports to stakeholders.

Liaison of all parties (e.g. line managers and occupational health staff) should occur. NICE advises:

1 Where necessary, arrange for a referral to relevant specialists or services. This may include referral via an occupational health adviser (or encouragement to self-refer) to a GP, a specialist physician, nurse, or another professional specializing in occupational health, health and safety, rehabilitation, or ergonomics. It could also include referral to a physiotherapist.

2 Where necessary, employers should appoint a case worker to coordinate referral for any required interventions and services. This includes delivery of the return-to-work plan including modifications to the workplace or work equipment if required. The case worker does not necessarily need a clinical or occupational health background. However, they should have the skills and training to act as an impartial intermediary and to ensure appropriate referrals are made to specialist services.

3 Ensure employees are consulted and jointly agree all planned health, occupational, or rehabilitation interventions or services, and the return-to-work plan (including workplace or work equipment modifications).

4 Encourage employees to contact their GP or occupational health service for further advice and support as needed.

5 Consider offering people who have a poor prognosis for returning to work an 'intensive' programme of interventions (e.g. counselling about a return to work, workplace modifications, and vocational rehabilitation including training).

6 Consider offering specific interventions for common psychological and musculoskeletal problems where the evidence supports the success of such intervention.

The annual CIPD[2,21,22,35,36] survey has indicated that some of the recommendations made by NICE are becoming more commonplace (Table 30.3), especially the availability of work adjustments (changes), rehabilitation, and psychological support (e.g. counselling). However, despite the evidence of benefit, active case management is still relatively uncommon.

Table 30.3 Options adopted by managers in cases of long-term absence

	% of surveyed organizations using this approach				
	2003	**2008**	**2009**	**2010**	**2011**
Referral to Occupational Health	66	64	60	77	74
Stress counselling	36	37	36	45	43
Employee Assistance Programme	24	34	35	46	47
Rehabilitation	28	38	36	46	40
Changes to work	41	48	51	63	61
Nominated case manager	17	15	17	22	26
Return-to-work interviews	74	75	74	85	86

Data from *Annual survey report 2011: absence management*, the Chartered Institute of Personnel and Development, London, Copyright © 2011; *Employee absence 2003: A survey of management policy and practice*, the Chartered Institute of Personnel and Development, London, Copyright © 2003; *Annual survey report 2010: absence management*, the Chartered Institute of Personnel and Development, London, Copyright © 2010; National Institute for Health and Clinical Excellence, *Management of long-term sickness and incapacity for work (PH19)* NICE, London, Copyright © 2009; and *Annual survey report 2008: absence management*, the Chartered Institute of Personnel and Development, London, Copyright © 2008.

The CIPD surveys indicate that almost all interventions are more commonly used in the public sector where sickness absence rates are measured and long-term absence is more common. A notable exception is the provision of private medical insurance which is provided by up to 43 per cent of private sector employers but by only 4 per cent in the public sector.[2]

Timeliness

A consistent theme in guidance on managing attendance is the need for early intervention. Studies have not yet been conducted that provide evidence for the best timing for intervention. However, it is assumed that in many cases there is not likely to be benefit from delaying the provision of effective advice and treatment and in some cases this will be detrimental. For example, back pain is a common cause of sickness absence and patients benefit greatly from receiving authoritative advice on back care.[37] The longer someone is not working, the less likely they are to return to work; consequently, most benefit claimants absent for 6 months or more have an 80 per cent chance of being off work for 5 years.[17]

NICE suggested the time to intervene was within the first 2–6 weeks.[34] Others have concluded there is sufficient evidence to recommend intervention within the first 1 or 2 weeks (Figure 30.3).[38]

Dame Carol Black, in her report, *Working for a Healthier Tomorrow*, highlighted the importance of early intervention[1] and identified three key principles:

- A biopsychosocial approach that simultaneously considers the medical condition, the psychological impact and the wider social determinants including work, home, or family situation.
- Multidisciplinary teams able to deliver a range of services tailored to the needs of the individual patient.
- Case workers who can help the individual navigate the system and facilitate communication.

Effective early intervention combines action by managers with early support from occupational health services. It is helpful to measure the timeliness of actions by managers and occupational

---

Scope: Any new episode of any musculoskeletal pain that interferes with work and lasts more than a day or two if severe, or up to a week if not severe.

Note: Over-reaction to mild or resolving episodes should be avoided

<u>**Stage 1**</u>: **Within one week from onset**

      Initial discussion, assessment and planned action with employer or their services

↓

Any modifications considered

↓

Involvement of health professional (if concerned)

↓

<u>**Stage 2**</u>: **Within two weeks from onset**

↓

Reassessment and revised action plan for recovery

↓

Monitoring and amendment of staged recovery plan – together with employer and with particular attention to activity and function (as distinct from pain alone) – until recovery achieved.

Figure 30.3 Recommended care pathway for early management of musculoskeletal disorders. Reproduced from Breen et al, Improved early pain management for musculoskeletal disorders, Health and Safety Executive Research Report 399 under the Open Government Licence v1.0.

health services. The timeliness of referrals to occupational health services has been best described by audit in the NHS. Even in this setting, where all employees had access to occupational health support, one third were not assessed until they have been absent for more than 3 months.[39] Only one-quarter of NHS organizations routinely measured the time from start of absence to referral to occupational health (Figure 30.4).[40]

The timeliness of intervention is an important component to monitor in judging the effective case management and quality of service provision in occupational health.

Occupational health reports

Effective attendance management relies on collaboration between line managers, human resources managers, occupational health advisers, and others. The main output from occupational health is usually a report providing advice to the manager.

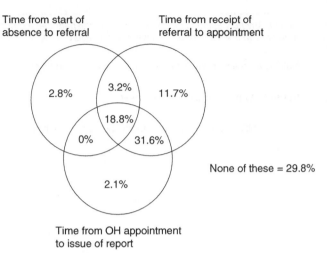

Figure 30.4 Proportion of English NHS organizations measuring the timeliness of intervention. Reproduced from Royal College of Physicians and Faculty of Occupational Medicine. *Implementing NICE public health guidance for the workplace: a national organisational audit of NHS trusts in England*. London: RCP, 2011. Copyright © 2011 Royal College of Physicians. Reproduced by permission.

There is no commonly agreed standard for occupational health reports although guidance has been published (Box 30.4).[41] There is a clear expectation that the report is issued with the informed consent of the patient and that medical information is omitted unless there is a good reason it must be brought to the attention of the recipient.

Communication with other specialists

The benefit of good advice from experts on health and work must not be underestimated. Studies in the UK and elsewhere have shown the importance of occupational health specialists influencing colleagues in secondary care to change the work-related illness behaviour of patients (and potentially the sickness certification behaviour of primary care clinicians).[42,43]

It should not be assumed that patients receive good health and work advice from their specialists. A substantial proportion of professional advice is out of line with the research literature.[44] Professional advice is more likely to be correct when it refers to up-to-date research literature. Occupational health advisers who ask for professional advice should always ask for the evidence supporting the advice and should provide information to colleagues that might improve their practice.

There is a growing body of resources providing evidence-based and consensus based guidance on when patients can return to work (e.g. from the Royal College of Surgeons and Royal College of Obstetricians and Gynaecologists—see Chapters 20 and 21).

Occupational rehabilitation

Employees do not always need to be 100 per cent fit to continue to work or return to work. Work can contribute to recovery.[45]

Occupational rehabilitation is whatever helps someone with a health problem stay at, return to, or remain in work.[46] It is an approach more than an intervention or a service and considers all of a person's needs for getting or keeping work. Early intervention is important because the challenge of returning an employee to work only increases as a period of sickness absence continues.

Box 30.4 Ingredients of a suitable occupational health report

a Must use language that can be easily understood by a non-medical audience and be of practical value to managers and the employee.

b Should be focused and deal with matters of employment and fitness for work.

c Should, with the employee's consent, contain relevant and appropriate medical information, including any interventions being planned to allow management to achieve a full understanding of the employee's situation.

d Should include details of any functional limitations or relevant disabilities that may temporarily or permanently affect the employee's ability to carry out their job.

e Should include guidance in relation to the timescale for a return to full or restricted duties, expected duration of any limitations and whether a review is necessary.

f Should indicate if further information needs to be obtained from the employee's GP or hospital doctor to enable a better understanding of the underlying medical condition.

g Should advise whether the condition is likely to be covered by the disability provisions of the Equality Act, if adjustments to the job would be appropriate, and if these are likely to be temporary or permanent.

h Should indicate if it appears that the employee's medical condition is related to their work, including any allegations of internal disputes that may require management assessment.

i Should provide an opinion on the impact of the employee's health condition on future attendance or performance and whether retirement on health grounds may be appropriate.

j Should indicate if a meeting between the occupational health adviser and management would be helpful, or if a workplace visit would provide further information that would assist in providing advice.

Reproduced with permission from Addley K et al. Occupational health reports: Top 10 tips, *Occupational Health* 2009; 61: 28, Copyright © Reed Business Information.

In their review of occupational rehabilitation[46] Waddell, Burton, and Kendall suggested there is strong evidence that:

◆ 'Occupational outcomes for most people with most musculoskeletal disorders are improved by increasing activity, including early return to some form of work.

◆ Return to work process and vocational rehabilitation interventions are more effective if they are closely linked to, or located in, the workplace.

◆ Vocational rehabilitation is more effective if all players recognize their roles in the return to work process, take responsibility and play their parts when appropriate.

◆ Commitment and coordinated action from all the players is crucial for successful vocational rehabilitation.

◆ Communication between all players leads to faster return to work and less sickness absence overall, and is cost-effective.

- Temporary provision of modified work reduces duration of sickness absence and increases return to work rates.
- Early intervention through delivery of appropriate treatment, positive advice/reassurance about activity and work, and/or workplace accommodation is sufficient for many people with musculoskeletal disorders.
- Structured multidisciplinary rehabilitation programmes, including cognitive behavioural principles to tackle psychosocial issues, are effective for helping people with persistent musculoskeletal disorders return to work.'

They suggested that effective occupational rehabilitation is dependent on coordinating work-focused healthcare with accommodating workplaces.

Occupational health specialists should provide advice on rehabilitation that combines guidance for both the patient and the employer.

The rehabilitation plan should describe the capabilities of the patient on resuming work and the adjustments that might need to be accommodated by the employer to enable this. Research by the Health and Safety Executive suggests the rehabilitation plan should describe the complete patient journey—including intermediate milestones—from resuming adjusted work to resuming all the usual work activities (or to resuming all the work activities with any permanent adjustments that might be needed)[47,48] (Box 30.5). The expectations of employee and employer should be clearly defined. In short, an effective rehabilitation plan should have a start, middle, and crucially an end.

The types of adjustments that employers might consider include:

- Altering the employee's working hours.
- Making physical adjustments to the workplace.
- Allocating some of the employee's activities to another person.
- Allocating different work activities to the employee.
- Providing support or equipment.
- Providing training.

Presenteeism and productivity

Presenteeism is defined in terms of the lost productivity that occurs when employees come to work ill and perform below par because of that illness.[48] The cost of presenteeism may exceed the cost of absenteeism. Reduced productivity due to reduced health at work is important but its

---

Box 30.5 Key features of a Return to Work plan

- Details of any temporarily adjusted work arrangements with a timeframe.
- Clearly specified goals which are achievable and can be measured as milestones.
- A timeframe which provides a start and end point, with appropriate steps.
- Defined review points.

Data from Hanson et al. The costs and benefits of active case management and rehabilitation for musculoskeletal disorders, RR493 Health and Safety Executive, London, © Crown Copyright 2006.

impact has not been fully established.[49] There is limited evidence from the UK on the costs of presenteeism.[48]

It has been suggested that rigorous management of sickness absence may increase presenteeism and could, in theory, be counterproductive.[50] However, there is very little evidence to suggest this happens in practice.[51]

The risk of presenteeism should not be used as a justification for neglecting management of attendance. The risk of presenteeism is a justification only for providing the appropriate support for employees with health needs at work and for trying to change beliefs about capability of those workers. Most employees with health needs if appropriately supported will remain productive and the impact of presenteeism will be minimized.

Most workers face health concerns at certain times during their career. It is important that employers invest in the health of their workforce to enhance performance and productivity. The foremost solution to presenteeism should be to encourage action that enables employees to continue their activities when health problems arise, by making adjustments and providing effective occupational health support.

References

1 Black C. *Working for a healthier tomorrow*. London: The Stationery Office, 2008.

2 Chartered Institute of Personnel and Development. *Annual survey report 2011: absence management*. London: CIPD, 2011.

3 Confederation of British Industry. *Healthy returns? Absence and workplace health survey*. London: Confederation of British Industry, 2011.

4 Gimeno G, Benavides FG, Benach J, *et al*. Distribution of sickness absence in the European union countries. *Occup Environ Med* 2004; **61**: 867–9.

5 Osterkamp R, Röhn O. Being on sick leave: possible explanations for differences of sick-leave days across countries. *CESifo Econ Stud* 2007; **53**: 97–114.

6 Audit Commission. *Managing sickness absence in the NHS, health briefing*. London: Audit Commission, 2011.

7 Barham C, Begum N. *Sickness absence from work in the UK. Labour market trends*. London: Office for National Statistics, 2005.

8 Styron JF, Barsoum WK, Smyth KA, *et al*. Preoperative predictors of returning to work following primary total knee arthroplasty. *J Bone Joint Surg Am* 2011; **93**: 2–10.

9 Johansson G, Lundberg I. Adjustment latitude and attendance requirements as determinants of sickness absence or attendance. Empirical tests of the illness flexibility model. *Soc Sci Med* 2004; **58**: 1857–68.

10 Wynne-Jones G, Buck R, Varnava A, *et al*. Impacts on work absence and performance: what really matters? *Occup Med* 2009; **59**: 556–62.

11 Preece R. (Lack of) Impacts on work absence and performance. *Occup Med* 2010; **60**: 81.

12 Steensma H. Sickness absence, office types, and advances in absenteeism research. *Scand J Work Environ Health* 2011; **37**: 359–62.

13 MacLeod D, Clarke N. *Engaging for success: enhancing performance through employee engagement*. London: Department for Business, Innovation and Skills, 2008.

14 West M, Dawson J, Admasachew L, *et al. NHS staff management and health service quality*. London: Department of Health, 2011.

15 Yarker J, Hicks B, Munir F, *et al. Managing rehabilitation: a competency framework for managers to support return to work*. London: BOHRF, 2010.

16 Walker V, Bamford D. An empirical investigation into health sector absenteeism. *Health Serv Manage Res* 2011; **24**: 142–50.

17 Waddell G, Burton A. *Is work good for your health and wellbeing?* London: The Stationery Office, 2006.

18 Marmot M. *Fair society, healthy lives: the Marmot review.* London: UCL: 2010.

19 Bradford SC. Sources of information on specific subjects. *Engineering* 1934; **137**: 85–6.

20 Chartered Institute of Personnel and Development. *Absence measurement and management: fact sheet.* London: CIPD, 2011.

21 Chartered Institute of Personnel and Development. *Employee absence 2003: a survey of management policy and practice.* London: CIPD, 2003.

22 Chartered Institute of Personnel and Development. *Annual survey report 2010: absence management.* London: CIPD, 2010.

23 Bergström G, Bodin L, Hagberg J, *et al.* Sickness presenteeism today, sickness absenteeism tomorrow? A prospective study on sickness presenteeism and future sickness absenteeism. *J Occup Environ Med* 2009; **51**: 629–38.

24 Müller CF, Monrad T, Biering-Sørensen F, *et al.* The influence of previous low back trouble, general health, and working conditions on future sick-listing because of low back trouble. A 15-year follow-up study of risk indicators for self-reported sick-listing caused by low back trouble. *Spine* 1999; **24**: 1562–70.

25 Bergström G, Bodin L, Bertilsson H, *et al.* Risk factors for new episodes of sick leave due to neck or back pain in a working population. A prospective study with an 18-month and a three-year follow-up. *Occup Environ Med* 2007; **64**: 279–87.

26 Navarro A, Reis RJ, Martín M. Some alternatives in the statistical analysis of sickness absence. *Am J Ind Med* 2009; **52**: 811–6.

27 Koopmans PC, Roelen CAM, Groothoff JW. Risk of future sickness absence in frequent and long-term absentees. *Occup Med* 2008; **58**: 268–74.

28 Dekkers-Sánchez PM, Hoving JL, Sluiter JK, *et al.* Factors associated with long-term sick-leave in sick-listed employees: a systematic review. *Occup Environ Med* 2008; **65**: 152–7.

29 Roelen CA, Koopmans PC, Schreuder JA, *et al.* The history of registered sickness absence predicts future sickness absence. *Occup Med* 2011; **61**: 96–101.

30 Rick J, Carroll C, Hillage J, *et al. Review of the effectiveness and cost effectiveness of interventions, strategies, programmes and policies to reduce the number of employees who take long term sickness absence on a recurring basis.* Brighton: IES, 2008.

31 National Audit Office. *Managing sickness absence in the NHS Health briefing.* London: NAO, 2011.

32 Spurgeon A. *Managing attendance at work: an evidence-based review.* London: BOHRF, 2002.

33 Hillage J, Rick J, Pilgrim H, *et al. Review of the effectiveness and cost effectiveness of interventions, strategies, programmes and policies to reduce the number of employees who move from short-term to long term sickness absence and to help employees on long-term sickness absence return to work.* Brighton: IES, 2008.

34 National Institute for Health and Clinical Excellence. *Management of long-term sickness and incapacity for work (PH19).* London: NICE, 2009. (<http://www.nice.org.uk/PH19>)

35 Chartered Institute of Personnel and Development. *Annual survey report 2008: absence management.* London: CIPD, 2008.

36 Chartered Institute of Personnel and Development. *Annual survey report 2009: absence management.* London: CIPD, 2009.

37 Burton AK, Waddell G, Tillotson KM, *et al.* Information and advice to patients with back pain can have a positive effect. A randomized controlled trial of a novel educational booklet in primary care. *Spine* 1999; **24**: 2484–91.

38 Breen A, Langworthy J, Bagust J. *Improved early pain management for musculoskeletal disorders. HSE Research report 399.* London: Health and Safety Executive, 2005.

39 Health and Work Development Unit. *Depression detection and management of staff on long-term sickness absence—Occupational health practice in the NHS in England: A national clinical audit—round 2.* London: RCP, 2010.

40 Health and Work Development Unit. *Implementing NICE public health guidance for the workplace: a national organisational audit of NHS trusts in England.* London: RCP, 2011.

41 Addley K, Hannah I, McQuillan P. Occupational health reports: top 10 tips. *Occup Health* 2009; **61**: 28.

42 Clayton M, Verow P. A retrospective study of return to work following surgery. *Occup Med* 2007; **57**: 525–31.

43 Jensen LD, Maribo T, Schiøttz-Christensen B, *et al.* Counselling low-back-pain patients in secondary healthcare: a randomised trial addressing experienced workplace barriers and physical activity. *Occup Environ Med* 2011; 2012; **69**: 21–8.

44 Schaafsma F, Verbeek J, Hulshof C, *et al.* Caution required when relying on a colleague's advice; a comparison between professional advice and evidence from the literature. *BMC Health Serv Res* 2005; **5**: 59.

45 Bevan S, Passmore E, Mahdon M. *Fit for work?* London: The Work Foundation, 2007.

46 Waddell G, Burton AK, Kendall NAS. *Vocational Rehabilitation: What works, for whom, and when?* London: The Stationery Office, 2008.

47 Hanson MA, Burton K, Kendall NAS, *et al. The costs and benefits of active case management and rehabilitation for musculoskeletal disorders RR493.* London: Health and Safety Executive, 2006.

48 Cooper C, Dewe P. Well-being—absenteeism, presenteeism, costs and challenges. *Occup Med* 2008; **58**: 522–4.

49 Preece R. Is health and productivity an issue for all employers? *J Occup Environ Med* 2009; **51**: 989.

50 Roelen CAM, Groothoff JW. Rigorous management of sickness absence provokes sickness presenteeism. *Occup Med* 2010; **60**: 244–6.

51 Preece R. Effective absence management *Occup Med* 2010; **60**: 575.

Chapter 31

Health promotion in the workplace

Steve Boorman and Ian Banks

Introduction

Whilst there are a number of subtly different definitions for health promotion, at its simplest, health promotion aims to give people the awareness, capability, and skills to control and thereby improve their own health.

Health is a complex concept and in recent years has become inextricably linked with the equally complex concept of well-being. Both concepts have a continuum between positive (good health and well-being) and negative (ill health or poor well-being) and both are subjective in terms of having an individual focus and potential for variation.

Defining health promotion

The World Health Organization (WHO) defined health in 1946 as a 'state of complete, physical, mental and social well-being and not merely the absence of disease or infirmity'.[1] This was developed further in 1986, with the Ottawa Charter for Health Promotion, in which WHO proposes that, rather than being a static state, health should be regarded as 'a resource for everyday life, not the objective of living. Health is a positive concept emphasizing social and personal resources, as well as physical capacities'.[2]

Successive conferences and statements from WHO global assemblies since Adelaide in 1988 to Bangkok in 2005[3] have refined and built upon the Ottawa Charter—emphasizing health as a basic human right and establishing health promotion as a process of enabling people to increase control over their health and its determinants. This is inextricably linked with public health improvement and recognizes that reducing health inequalities and improving public health is vital to economic success and sustainability. Political, economic, and cultural influences play significant roles creating a supportive environment to help people make positive health choices which will underpin successful healthy public policy.

Being aware that there have been many attempts to clearly define 'well-being', it is perhaps simpler to consider well-being as subjective contentment with similar physical, mental, and social components.

Whatever the definitions used it is clear that both concepts are more than just about presence or absence of disease or injury, and authors have repeatedly reinforced the importance of the 'health triangle'—physical, mental, and social well-being components, interacting to influence health and well-being status.

Whilst some influences on health may be predetermined, such as sex and genetic predisposition to disease, others are clearly features of individual behaviours or lifestyles, such as alcohol use, drug consumption, smoking, and exercise. Others may be features of the broader environment the individual is within, both past and present, such as social status and income, education, and employment conditions. A further component may be access to healthcare or support, which may be influenced by economic, political, and cultural considerations.

It follows therefore that some determinants of health may be difficult to modify or change, although in the case of genetic or sex-determined components, awareness may enable choices to modify or reduce risk of impact. For example, if an individual knows they have a genetic predisposition to cardiovascular disease, they can choose to modify other risk factors that may act to express the disease.

Other health determinants may be modified by personal decision or behavioural change, such as increasing exercise to reduce risk of disease related to being overweight. These factors, often described as 'lifestyle risk factors', are popularly targeted in traditional workplace health promotion campaigns. The simple underlying principle is that increased awareness of risk behaviour can enable and encourage an individual to modify that behaviour.

Environmental risk factors may be modified by personal intervention (individual awareness and control), or may be beyond individual control with varying ability to influence directly. For instance, working conditions may be influenced by negotiation and political decisions will depend on systems of administration, both of which offer opportunities to change, but macro environmental factors, such as temperature, rainfall, or availability of local resources, may be less easy to influence.

Health promotion and public health

Health promotion is often interpreted as simply offering advice to individuals, but increasingly broader opportunities to influence public health have seen the concept extended to encompass societal, environmental, and organizational interventions. This is exemplified by the concept of 'health promoting workplaces'.

The detailed Marmot review, *Fair Society, Healthy Lives: A Strategic Review of Health Inequalities in England Post-2010*, explored the underlying basis of health inequalities across the UK.[4] The review highlighted that productivity losses due to health inequalities cost the UK £31–33 billion a year with a further £20–32 billion of cost to the economy from lost taxes and increased welfare payments and direct cost to the National Health Service (NHS) of £5.5 billion. The Marmot review also concluded that without measures to address risk factors for ill health this situation may worsen—increasing obesity, for example, was associated with £2 billion of illness costs in 2010, but this could rise to £5 billion by 2025.

Marmot identified six policy areas where improvement was needed to reduce health inequalities. These were: giving every child the best start in life, enabling people of all ages to maximize capabilities and control their lives, creating fair employment and good work, ensuring a healthy standard of living, creating and developing healthy and sustainable places and communities, and improving ill health prevention. Giving every child the best start in life was the highest priority recommendation, focusing on reducing inequalities in early development, better maternity and childcare services, and building resilience in young children.

Marmot clearly identified components of work which contribute to reducing ill health, effectively defining 'good work'. Subsequent work by Waddell and Burton, *Is Work Good for Your Health & Well-being?*, provides evidence for the ill health created by 'worklessness' and concluded that good work was beneficial to health.[5] Marmot's work identified the components of good work, concluding that ten features ranging from job security, individual control, and workload through to issues around work/life balance are important (see Chapter 30, Box 30.1 'Characteristics of good work').

Two key areas, relevant to this chapter, included the workplace as a health and well-being promoting environment, and the opportunity for work to reintegrate those with sickness or disability. It is possible therefore to think of health promotion as addressing needs at different levels—individual, organizational, and societal.

At a societal level, governments are responsible for establishing conditions to create environments in which the populations they serve can lead healthy lives. Social justice is a key part of this, and the case has been made that healthy public policies in the short term will drive the conditions to improve health, creating increased productivity and economic success. Technology, changes in population demographics, globalization, and political, economic, and ecological change all represent significant challenges to which public health policy will need to adapt.

Throughout the emergence of the modern health promotion agenda a number of key themes have remained:

+ The creation of supportive environments, where people can live and work with reduced exposure to hazardous agents.

+ The need to improve food and nutrition and access to safe water, reducing hunger and malnutrition and enabling healthy food choices.

+ The reduction of dependence on harmful substances such as alcohol, tobacco, and other drugs hazardous to health.

+ The improved capacity of communities to support enhanced personal skills to improve health.

+ The development of health services orientated to support health-promoting communities.

Health promotion in the workplace

Work is a major component within this agenda. Not only does work create the economic success needed to fund improvements, it creates social cohesion and forms the place where many in a community spend a significant proportion of their waking time, providing the opportunity for effective health promotion awareness.

Many workplaces still consist of workforces with a high proportion of one sex; for instance, men predominate in heavier manufacturing, labouring, and the armed forces whereas women predominate in some service industries such as the NHS. In addition to gender diversity, some types of work may also involve workers in lower social classes, for instance construction. Work of this nature may also have geographical and ethnic variation.

Research confirms that different groups in society access health information in different ways and to a variable extent. Throughout global societies women are consistently more receptive and interested in health messages. Public health policy has sought to exploit this, targeting women's networks to carry health messages to communities and using women as health-promoting 'champions'.

In the UK there is a clear differential in the use and access to health services—women either in themselves or in their role as the main carer for dependents are more likely to attend clinics, pharmacies, or other health services. Literature targeted at a female audience contains more health content than that targeted at men. There is a wealth of evidence that suggests that men's health behaviours are different, with a tendency to minimize symptoms and present later for health advice. This differential results in a number of common health conditions having generally higher morbidity and mortality among men, whilst being no more frequent in incidence.

At a societal level the health promotion agenda relies on political decisions to influence the allocation of resources to create the environment to support positive change. To some extent this is also true of the approach needed to health promotion at an organizational level. Developing health-promoting workplaces has featured in successive government public health policies recognizing that quality employment is important in maintaining a healthy population. This recognition is not new! Historically a number of forward thinking employers have recognized this and also understood that a healthy workforce is good for business—with better overall productivity.

Workplace health promotion examples

Royal Mail appointed a workplace doctor in 1855, with objectives which included 'improving and maintaining the health of the Royal Mail workforce'. Another well-known example lies in the Cadbury business; after nearly 70 years of trading in the 19th century, George Cadbury, the son of John Cadbury who started the business in 1824, recognized that the developing rail network enabled his business to develop away from the poor conditions workers experienced in many parts of London. As he built the business in south Birmingham he recognized an opportunity 'to alleviate the evils of modern more cramped living conditions' and purchased 120 acres of land around their factory to create a village to house their workers—Bournville. Aside from the improved living conditions for workers afforded by the 313 cottages built across the estate, the Cadbury Quaker beliefs also banned alcohol. This example of a health-promoting workplace is a good one as it clearly recognizes the social dimension of good health as well as seeking to raise awareness of lifestyle risk factors that may adversely impact on physical or mental health.

Whilst Royal Mail's approach was initially a traditional 'medical model', with a company doctor examining and advising sick employees, this business also recognized the impact that social distress had on its workforce and importantly the potential for this to reduce business success. In the mid 20th century Royal Mail created a welfare service, training workplace 'welfare officers' to support workers. This support deliberately extended beyond the walls of the workplace, helping staff to find cost-effective housing, supporting those with debt or relationship problems, providing advice in crisis, and helping with bereavement or legal problems. In some organizations trades unions provided similar functions, in others, philanthropic employers recognized that looking after their workers enabled them to retain a committed and loyal workforce.

Aside from the health benefits, caring for workers' health is associated with psychological benefits—reinforcing the 'psychological contract'. This concept recognizes that as well as any formal contractual relationship between employer and employee, workers' commitment to an employer or a business has psychological elements. In circumstances where employees feel they share common perceptions and beliefs with their employer, enhanced loyalty is generated and this may be associated with enhanced productivity, quality, and reduced losses associated with grievance or absence. This is increasingly referred to as 'engagement'.

MacLeod and Clarke formally examined this association in their 2008 review, '*Engaging for Success: enhancing performance through employee engagement*'.[6] The review provided multiple business case studies to support its findings and the authors concluded that 'the correlation between engagement, well-being and performance is repeated too often for it to be a coincidence'. The MacLeod review encouraged employers to consider the value of developing better bonds with workers and reinforced evidence that employers who support the health of their workers have higher engagement and better business performance. The recommendations of this review were accepted in full by the UK government.

The association between worker well-being and productivity and performance was also illustrated by the 2009 Department of Health commissioned review of the health and well-being of the NHS workforce.[7] The review was part of the government's response to the Black report, *Working for a Healthier Tomorrow*, which highlighted the economic losses associated with ill health amongst the working age population.[8] With over 1.3 million workers, the NHS is one of Europe's largest employers and research was undertaken exploring the association between NHS workers' health and organizational performance. The review highlighted that those NHS trusts which had better staff health and well-being also had improved financial performance including lower sickness absence costs, reduced turnover, and less need for investment in agency staff cover. Importantly they also had improved patient outcomes including satisfaction and less illness from hospital acquired infection and better performance against regulatory targets for quality of service and use of resources. The review drew on research from Aston University which has also shown that patient outcomes are better in NHS organizations that have better staff feedback relating to their own health.

National campaigns

Business in the Community (BiTC), a third-sector organization, has studied this association in many national and international major businesses.[9] Its Workwell campaign, supported by numerous business case studies from large employers, promotes the role of health promotion in securing successful business.

The Workwell model has been developed with support and involvement of leading businesses and has four dimensions supporting better workplace health—'better work, better relationships, better specialist support and better physical and psychological health'. Supported by a metric system encouraging self-assessment of performance across these areas, the model affirms an integrated strategic approach to health promotion at an organizational as well as an individual level. The Workwell model cites research from the Work Foundation suggesting that increased investment in employee engagement would significantly improve UK business profitability.

These themes are echoed in a number of national initiatives. Under the auspices of public health improvement The Responsibility Deal seeks to engage business, government, and specialist stakeholders by signing up to health improvement-related pledges.[10] Its targets include producers, retailers, employers, and communities and its aims include to encourage healthy eating, responsible alcohol use, increased exercise, and healthy workplaces. Organizations participating in the workplace health strand are encouraged to make pledges to actively support their workforces to lead healthier lives. This includes pledges to measure and report employee health, target smoking cessation, provide healthier workplace nutritional programmes, provide good quality advice on common health issues, and use good quality (accredited) occupational health services.

A number of schemes actively promote and reward workplace health promotion. The Investors in People scheme now incorporates health management and health promotion within its measurement framework of good management practice. In England, the Workplace Wellness Charter seeks to encourage organizations to measure and recognize good support for workplace health.[11] There are equivalent health workplace awards schemes in Scotland and Wales. The Scottish Health at Work Scheme encourages organizations to support individual employees, seek measures to improve the working environment, and to intervene to improve organizational structures and working practices.[12] Participation in schemes such as these help employers to access simple toolkits with good quality health awareness advice and by their nature these schemes seek to involve workers in getting actively involved in health-improving activities.

Communication techniques

Health promotion seeks to firstly raise awareness amongst its target audiences, be they individuals, employers, politicians, or leadership role models. This is an exercise in good communication and the most effective communication is planned in the knowledge of how best to attract the attention of the recipient. Unless health promotional materials are targeted to their audience they risk being ignored or discarded. For instance, male-dominated blue-collar workforces may respond better to material that includes humour and simple cartoons.

As well as raising awareness, the factual content of health promotion messages needs to convince of the need to modify behaviours, supporting change. Factors influencing behaviour may be complex—stark messages such as 'smoking may kill' are not always persuasive and individual risk perception may vary based on past experiences, cultural beliefs, or other influences, such as the attitude of peers.

Effective planning has a key role to play in increasing the impact and efficacy of health promotion messages. Simple considerations may make a big difference to the priority and retention of information materials. For example, delivering a health promotion event to manual workers at the end of a working shift, or on the same evening as a key sports event may generate significantly fewer attendees than an event scheduled during working time or whilst workers are less tired.

The approach to delivery may also clearly influence uptake—visually attractive material with an obvious presence in a prominent part of the workplace is more likely to attract attention than a low key presence in a remote location. However, for some health promotion or health surveillance programmes the latter may be preferable—for example, in a large, male-dominated manual workforce a mobile cervical screening programme achieved significantly better uptake from female workers when the screening vehicle was parked 'discreetly' (allowing access without male workers overlooking).

Creativity is needed to attract attention. This may involve a 'tagline'—a catchy phrase or branding that encourages recognition. The Health and Safety Executive (HSE) campaign 'Good health equals good business' is a good example.[13] 'The mindful employer' is another simple phrase carrying a clear message informing of a campaign's aims.[14] The language and style of campaigns also needs consideration—jargon or slang can in some cases improve accessibility, but if its use confuses the message the converse may be true. Associating a health message with a product or service, particularly one linked to the workplace concerned, may strengthen the message.

The Men's Health Forum is a charitable organization promoting men's health in the UK.[15] It worked with the Royal Mail to raise awareness of a forthcoming health promotion week. Millions of stamps were cancelled with the words 'Delivering male health'—a pun on the function of the mail service provider whilst deliberately raising awareness of the series of events.

Knowing the target audience can also influence the best mode of communication to use for effective health promotion. Some groups respond best to face-to-face communication, whilst other groups may favour provision of online electronic information that can be accessed with privacy, particularly where a health topic may be seen as embarrassing or 'sensitive'.

Gimmicks, giveaways, and gadgets can also be used to promote retention of material and messages. These include items directly contributing to the issue being promoted, for example, a pedometer being used to promote exercise. Alternatively, the health message may be attached to a commonly used item that is likely to be retained, such as notepads, pens, or memory sticks.

There is much commonality here between the skills of the advertising/marketing professions, and those designing health promotion campaigns. In both cases the aim is to generate sufficient attention and interest from the recipient that a key message is understood and then retained, with the aim of influencing future behaviour.

As with other disciplines, health promotion must embrace the benefits of technology, which allows a wider range of audiences to be reached. Digital information can be amended and updated more easily and with lower cost, may be replicated and widely dispersed, and can be designed to be interactive. Interactivity has benefit in allowing health promotion messages to be further tailored or targeted to individual need (e.g. generating specific nutrition or lifestyle information), and can also engage other techniques to improve retention and interest. Computer technology-based programmes can, for example, generate an element of competition or challenge to encourage participation. By introducing fun to repetitive tasks such as exercise they can help to reduce attrition associated with lost interest. Increasingly such programmes may also include follow-up or prompts—emails or other contact to remind participants of tasks and encourage compliance.

The advent of social media, and increasingly sophisticated portable technology such as 'smartphones' and tablet PC technology further increases the flexibility of communications media to deliver health promotion messages. Whilst some working populations (lower income groups, for example) may traditionally have been excluded from access to such modes of communication, increasingly the ubiquitous nature of games, access to music, and video media, mean that such technology now reaches substantial proportions of the population and cannot be ignored as a mode of health promotion delivery.

Although it may be more difficult to measure the positive impact this has on families of workers, many businesses interested in workplace health promotion will extend programmes to include families. This may originate from knowledge that health issues in dependents may impact on the productivity of the worker. This can be from the perspective of sickness absence, leave requested to support an ill family member, or from the direct impact on worker health from worrying about issues arising. The family unit may also be a more receptive target for health promotion messages. Delivering health promotion materials to the home may enable other family members or contacts to use their awareness to influence the worker's behaviour more effectively.

Examples of health promotion in the workplace

An example of this is a large UK organization that successfully ran smoking cessation programmes involving the individual worker's spouse. Providing smoking cessation materials to the home enabled the spouse and other family members to help motivate change. This approach has recently been echoed in effective television advertising campaigns—children in the household being used to promote a positive message regarding smoking cessation.

Targeting is now generally considered essential rather than just a good idea. This can be based on a number of criteria such as occupation, age, geographical location, culture, and gender. Male specific targeting of health information and services is a relatively new concept. The Men's Health Forum has pioneered UK approaches, working in recent years to articulate the business case for targeting male health promotion in the workplace (see Box 31.1). There are sound social and economic reasons for an effective programme of health promotion in the workplace.[16]

Recent work would suggest that the delivery of services, including health promotion, is in fact 'hard to reach' for many men and is a contributory factor for the significant differences in morbidity and mortality between the sexes. Although men are more than one and a half times as likely to develop bowel cancer, they remain less likely to participate in the NHS Bowel Cancer Screening Programme (57 per cent female uptake compared with 51 per cent male uptake).[17] A recently published European Commission report into the health of men in Europe had similar conclusions.[18] Many of the key issues concerning gender differences in access to health services are set out in a 2008 Department of Health commissioned report, *The Gender and Access to Health Services Study.*[19]

Box 31.1 Men's Health Forum: National Men's Health Week policy paper 2008

Health improvement initiatives delivered in the workplace are of particular importance for men because:

♦ Men are less likely than women to make use of almost all other forms of primary health provision. For example, men see their GP an average of only three times annually compared to five times for women; men are less likely than women to have regular dental check-ups (just over half of men compared with two-thirds of women); and are less likely to seek health advice at a pharmacy. Men are also acknowledged to be less likely to participate in public health improvement programmes of all kinds.

♦ Men spend far more of their lives in the workplace. Overall there are more men than women in paid employment (15.9 million men compared with 13.5 million women) and men are twice as likely to work full-time (14.1 million men, 7.8 million women). Men also work much more overtime (30 per cent of men work more than 45 hours per week compared with 10 per cent of women) and because of the traditional differential in the retirement age, men still tend to work to a greater age.

♦ Men develop many serious illnesses earlier than women—10–15 years earlier in the case of heart disease, for example (there are nearly five times as many male deaths as female deaths from coronary heart disease in the 50–54 age group). Sixteen per cent of men compared to 6 per cent of women die while still of working age.

♦ There is an increasing and convincing body of evidence that health improvement initiatives in the workplace are not only effective at engaging men but are also welcomed and valued by men. In this sense, workplace interventions have gained an endorsement from men that may have been lacking in previous population-level initiatives.

Reproduced with permission from Men's Health Forum, Copyright © 2012. <http://www.menshealthforum.org.uk/>

The importance of actions tailored to meet the needs of different groups within the workforce, including men, has been recognized more widely. Dame Carol Black's review of the health of the working age population, *Working for a Healthier Tomorrow*, observed that successful health programmes are those that are specifically designed to meet employee needs—'there is no *one size fits all*'.[8]

The Black report also acknowledged the potential importance of gender-sensitive approaches in enhancing the effectiveness of workplace health improvement initiatives, a point also made in a report from the World Economic Forum (WEF), *Working Towards Wellness: Practical Steps for CEOs*[20,21] This report highlighted the successful health improvement initiatives undertaken by a UK-based telecommunications company in support of its global workforce and acknowledged both that 'different strategies and messaging are required for men and women' and that 'men are a much more resistant audience and require special attention'.

The workplace is considered to be an ideal setting for health promotion initiatives; approximately one-third of waking hours are spent at work and it provides regular access to a relatively stable population, many of whom are men.[6] Importantly, workplace health promotion is associated with a reduction in health risks, and with improvements in economic and productivity factors including reduced medical costs, compensation benefits, employee absenteeism, and increased job satisfaction. The value of workplace health promotion was identified in the Health Promotion Strategy[7] and 'Developing a Health Promoting Workplace'[6] provides a framework and guidelines for the development of workplace health promotion policies.

A prostate health awareness programme run for postal workers in the West Midlands not only produced a significant increase in awareness levels, it also gathered a range of qualitative data that demonstrated men's willingness to engage with this sort of initiative. An academic analysis of the project concluded that 'it has shown that the workplace can provide an ideal setting in which to deliver health promotion to men'.[22]

A study of men and indigestion, conducted by Bournemouth University found that, overall, nearly 70 per cent of the men sampled felt that health issues should be discussed at work and concluded that 'going to where men are' with health campaigns and services would be useful in terms of improving their health and offering screening.[23]

The 'Work Fit' project is another example of a 'male-friendly' approach to health improvement. A UK-based telecommunications company (BT) worked with a specialist provider to help the company target public health issues linked to obesity, an ageing workforce, sedentary lifestyles, and the associated health implications.

The overall aim of Work Fit was to contribute to the development of a healthy workplace culture within BT by encouraging staff to make sustainable improvements to their lifestyle. Key objectives included encouraging and enabling BT staff to maintain a healthy weight, to seek advice from their general practitioner (GP) if needed, and to develop a model for health improvement interventions, usable within BT and other workplace settings.

Liaison with the two main trade unions, Connect and the Communication Workers Union (CWU), was identified as crucial to the project's ability to succeed and they were both involved from the outset. Focus groups were also undertaken to involve employees in the development process, to test proposed resources, and to gain feedback on how best to market health improvement messages to the workforce.

Work Fit was designed as a lifestyle-management programme focusing on nutrition and physical activity. It was delivered entirely through the BT company intranet and open to all 90 000 male and female employees as individuals or as part of a team. The 16-week programme incorporated weekly challenges, email prompts, and online help from independent health advisors. Information supplied allowed participants to monitor their own progress online and gave the project team the ability to review progress and trends against critical success factors. On registration, participants were sent a tool kit including a pedometer, tape measure, and a health advice booklet designed to look like a Haynes' car manual.[24]

It was also recognized that to be effective all employees needed to be aware of the programme and any fears concerning confidentiality should be allayed. Over 20 half-day road-shows were organized, in conjunction with the CWU and with active support from Connect, as a form of community outreach and incorporated an information stall providing background information, general advice, and health 'MOTs' to employees. Internal and external marketing channels were also used to get the message across, including the in-house newspaper, workplace posters, and the national press.

Work Fit was extremely successful. Its target of 5000 participants was achieved within 24 hours of going live. Over 16 000 participants were eventually registered, 75 per cent of whom were male, accurately reflecting the ratio of male/female workers at BT; 4377 of these lost a combined weight of over 10 000 kg representing an average of 2.3 kg per person. Most significant is that up to two-thirds of participants reported sustained changes to their lifestyle as a direct result of the Work Fit programme.

Other workplace-based diet and physical activity initiatives aimed at men have also achieved positive results. The 'Keeping It Up' campaign in Dorset aimed at middle-aged men resulted in almost three-quarters of participants reducing their BMI, 58 per cent increased their physical fitness (as measured by a step test), and almost half reduced their percentage of body fat.[25] The Bradford Health of Men project has also successfully engaged with men at workplaces.[26]

Business benefits of health promotion can be hard to calculate but a study by PricewaterhouseCoopers commissioned by the Health Work Wellbeing Executive in 2008 suggested that improving employee health is good for business.[27] The study identified a number of benefits of staff wellness programmes including reduced levels of sickness absence, lower staff turnover and greater employee satisfaction. Where these benefits were costed against staff performance, they demonstrated a measurable return against the financial investment. The study concluded that 'workplace wellness makes commercial sense' and suggested that the workplace offers considerable untapped potential as a setting for the improvement of population health.

These are not just theoretical assertions. The potential of action to improve health at work is clearly shown by work to reduce absenteeism undertaken by the Royal Mail. The Royal Mail employs 180 000 people. A report by the London School of Economics (LSE) found that the company achieved significant reductions in absence—from 7 per cent to 5 per cent—between January 2004 and May 2007, equivalent to an extra 3600 employees in work.[28] Raising the health awareness of staff formed an important element of the Royal Mail's approach. The LSE calculated that if the 13 sectors in the economy with the highest absence rates followed Royal Mail's example, the resultant reduction in absenteeism would be worth £1.45 billion to the UK economy.

The arguments for cost benefits associated with health promotion have been better developed in the USA, where the financial differences in healthcare organization place greater emphasis on the potential benefits of prevention. US literature contains many references to cost benefit analysis of health promotion programmes. Burton et al. document the increased likelihood of lost working days and productivity losses linked to identified health risks.[29] Loeppke et al. have published data showing the benefits of health promotion in modifying health risks,[30] and further work from Burton cites the productivity improvements gained by modifying health risks.[31] Edington's research cites an annual saving of $143 per annum per person (from 2001) for each health risk reduced.[32]

An occupational health scheme pilot commissioned by the HSE and carried out in Leicestershire between 2004 and 2006 demonstrated that it is possible to achieve a high take-up of voluntary health checks in another industry with workers that may be hard to access with healthcare messages.[33] More than 1700 construction workers had health checks during the programme. One-third of those checked suffered from general health issues such as high blood pressure and respiratory illness. Problems arising from occupational health risks, such as vibration or excess sound levels, were also common. Overall, one-third of those checked needed to be referred to their own general practitioners. Significantly, the pilot found that the main barrier to delivering occupational health to construction workers was at the managerial level, and not a lack of interest from workers.

Another project with construction workers—addressing skin cancer prevention—also achieved positive results. One hundred per cent of the workers considered the workplace an appropriate setting in which to address health issues with men, 68 per cent of the men attending awareness-raising workshops said they were now more aware of the dangers of sun exposure and 69 per cent said they would now protect themselves in sunlight.[34]

A 2003 study found that delivering self-testing kits for chlamydia screening via workplaces is potentially an effective way of increasing take-up among men.[35] Of those people submitting urine samples for analysis in the study, 78 per cent were male, compared with only 13 per cent of those screening for chlamydia in the National Chlamydia Screening Programme at the time. The proportion of men being screened in the National Chlamydia Screening Programme has increased significantly since this work due to better targeting. The programme's men's strategy, *Men Too*, published in 2007, identifies workplaces as one of several accessible venues for men.[36]

A study commissioned by the Food Standards Agency found that a workplace intervention can produce positive change in awareness of the impact of salt on health and can contribute to positive changes in workers' health behaviours.[37] For example, there were significant increases between baseline and follow-up in the proportion of workers who believed salt intake to be associated with heart disease (51 per cent to 62 per cent), heart attack (46 per cent to 61 per cent) and stroke (32 per cent to 43 per cent). There were also significant increases in the proportion of workers who were able to correctly identify the advised maximum daily intake of salt between baseline and follow-up (29 per cent to 64 per cent). The evaluation showed that men are likely to value different methods of delivery from women and concluded that gender sensitivity is therefore important in both the design and implementation of a workplace intervention.

A health initiative run by Lambeth Primary Care Trust (PCT) at two ARRIVA bus garages also produced positive results.[38] The interventions used in this project included nurse-led 'MOT' health checks, advice, support, signposting to relevant services, on-site interventions such as stop smoking support, and a weight-loss competition. The MOT consisted of a cardiovascular check (body mass index, blood glucose, blood pressure, smoking status, nutrition, alcohol, and physical activity), counselling, advice, support, service referral and a 3-month post contact follow-up. The checks also provided an opportunity for sexual and mental health issues to be addressed through health education and signposting. The PCT confirmed that engaging with men in the workplace about their health was effective: 162 men had MOT checks at both garages, 20–30 per cent of whom were referred for lifestyle support because of their cardiovascular risk.

Summary

This chapter has sought to provide a summary of the development of modern approaches to health promotion in the workplace, illustrated by a number of case studies from UK businesses active in this area. The workplace is an effective forum for health promoting activities and the examples highlight that careful planning and targeting may increase the likelihood of success. Many employers expect such programmes to have high cost, or be difficult to organize, but the increasing resources available from third-sector and public health programmes may be accessed by partnership approaches to deliver high-quality programmes, with minimal cost.

Comprehensive occupational health should encompass prevention and health promotion, within the continuum ranging from pro-active health support to more reactive intervention to address injury or illness.

Acknowledgement

The authors would like to thank David Wilkins from The Men's Health Forum for support and research contributing to this chapter.

References

1 Preamble to the Constitution of The World Health Organization as adopted by the International Health Conference, New York, 19 June–22 July 1946; signed on 22 July 1946 by the representatives of 61 States (Official Records of the World Health Organization, no. 2, p. 100) and entered into force on 7 April 1948.

2 World Health Organization. *Ottawa charter for health promotion.* First International Conference for Health Promotion, Ottawa, 1986.

3 World Health Organization. *Milestones in health promotion: statements from global conferences.* Geneva: World Health Organization, 2009.

4 Marmot M(chair). *Fair society, healthy lives. A strategic review of health inequalities in England post-2010* (The Marmot Review). London: The Marmot Review, 2010. (http://www.instituteofhealthequity.org/Institute-work)

5 Waddell G, Burton AK. *Is work good for your health & well-being?* London: TSO, 2006.

6 MacLeod D, Clarke N. *Engaging for success: enhancing performance through employee engagement. A report to government.* London: Department for Business, Innovation & Skills, 2009.

7 Boorman S (lead reviewer). *NHS health & well-being, final report.* London: Department of Health, 2009.

8 Black C. *Working for a healthier tomorrow.* London: Department of Work & Pensions, 2008.

9 Business in The Community. *Public reporting guidelines: employee wellness and engagement.* London: BiTC, 2011.

10 Public Health Responsibility Deal, Department of Health, 2011: <http://responsibilitydeal.dh.gov.uk/>

11 Liverpool NHS Primary Care Trust. *The workplace wellbeing charter.* Liverpool: Liverpool NHS Primary Care Trust, 2011.

12 Healthy Working Lives, Scotland: <http://www.healthyworkinglives.com>

13 Entec UK Ltd. *Evaluation of the good health is good business campaign.* London: Entec UK Contract Research report for HSE No 272/2000, 2000.

14 Mindful Employer®. *Line managers' resource. A practical guide for supporting staff with a mental health condition.* Exeter: Devon Partnership NHS Trust, 2011.

15 Men's Health Forum: <http://www.menshealthforum.org.uk>

16 Men's Health Forum. *Improving male health by taking action in the workplace: a policy briefing paper.* Men's Health Week Policy Paper. London: Men's Health Forum, 2008.

17 Wilkins D. *Slow on the uptake? Encouraging male participation in the NHS Bowel Cancer Screening Programme.*London: Men's Health Forum, 2011.

18 White A. *The state of men's health in Europe: extended report.* Brussels: European Commission, 2011.

19 Men's Health Forum/Bristol University report for Department of Health. *The gender and access to health services study: final report.* London: Department of Health, 2008.

20 World Economic Forum. *Annual Report 2007/2008.* Geneva: World Economic Forum, 2008.

21 Litchfield P. *Working towards wellness: practical steps for CEOs.* Geneva: World Economic Forum, 2003.

22 Dolan A, Staples V, Summer S, *et al.* 'You ain't going to say . . . I've got a problem down there': workplace-based prostate health promotion with men. *Health Educ Res* 2005; **20**(6): 730–8.

23 Hemingway A, Taylor G, Young N. *Quit bellyaching: the men and indigestion pilot study.* London: Men's Health Forum, 2004.

24 http://www.menshealthforum.org.uk/mini-manuals/19009-mens-health-forum-mini-manuals> [One of a series in this format].

25 Wilkins D. Promoting weight loss in men aged 40–45: the 'keeping it up' campaign. In: Davidson N, Lloyd T (eds), *Promoting men's health.* London: Bailliere Tindall, 2001.

26 White, AK, Cash, K. Conrad, P. Branney, P. *The Bradford & Airedale Health of Men Initiative: a study of its effectiveness in engaging with men.* Leeds: Leeds Metropolitan University, 2008.

27 Price Waterhouse Coopers LLP for Department of Work and Pensions. *Building the case for wellness.* London: Price Waterhouse Coopers LLP, 2008.

28 Marsden D, Manconi S. *The value of rude health; a report for the Royal Mail Group.* London: London School of Economics, 2008.

29 Burton W, Chen CY, Conti DJ, *et al.* The association of health risks with on-the-job productivity. *J Occup Environ Med* 2005; **47**(8): 769–77.

30 Loeppke R, Edington D, Beg S. Impact of the prevention plan on employee health risk reduction. *Popul Health Manag* 2010; **13**(5); 275–84.

31 Burton W, Chen CY, Conti DJ, *et al.* The association of health risk change and presenteeism change. *J Occup Environ Med* 2006; **48**(3): 252–63.

32 Edington R. Emerging research: a view from one research center. *Am J Health Prom* 2001; **15**(5): 341–9.

33 Institute of Employment Studies. *Constructing better health: final evaluation report.* London: Health and Safety Executive, 2007.

34 Twardzicki M, Roche T. Addressing skin cancer prevention with outdoor workers. In: Davidson N, Lloyd T (eds), *Promoting men's health: a guide for practitioners.* London: Bailliere Tindall, 2001.

35 Men's Health Forum. *The men and chlamydia project 2002–2004.* London: Men's Health Forum, 2005.

36 National Chlamydia Screening Programme. *Men too: strategy to support equitable access to chlamydia screening for men within the national chlamydia screening programme.* London: Health Protection Agency, 2007.

37 Men's Health Forum. *With a pinch of salt: men and salt—a workplace intervention.* London: Food Standards Agency, 2008.

38 *All Aboard for Better Health* at Local Government Improvement and Development website: <http://www.idea.gov.uk>

Chapter 32

Cancer survivorship and work

Philip Wynn and Shirley D'Sa

Introduction

About 5 per cent of the overall UK cancer burden can be attributed to occupational exposures.[1] However, occupational physicians in clinical practice are most likely to be called upon to support and advise employed patients with non-occupational cancers. Each year in the UK, 109 000 people aged between 15 and 64 are diagnosed with cancer.[2] More than 60 per cent of adults and 78 per cent of children live for at least 5 years after diagnosis.[3] There are currently 2 million people living with cancer in the UK and this number is set to grow by over 3 per cent every year, reflecting an increase in the incidence of cancer and an improvement in survival rates (Table 32.1).[4] Support services in the UK are being reconfigured to help this growing population of cancer survivors to live full and active lives for extended periods. Returning to the workplace is a part of this goal, and occupational physicians are likely to see increasing numbers of adults seeking work after treatment for conditions that in the past would have led to ill health-related retirement.

Set against these improvements in clinical outcome, and the increasing emphasis on support for patients who achieve long-term survival, is evidence that many working-age adults treated for the common cancers subsequently encounter financial and occupational difficulties. People with cancer often experience a loss in income as a result of their condition. In one meta-analysis, 34 per cent of adult cancer survivors in employment at the time of diagnosis were unemployed at follow-up, being 1.4 times more likely to be unemployed than healthy controls.[5] Thus, although most working adults diagnosed with primary cancer return to work, a significant minority do not.

Cancer is increasingly seen as an illness that can be effectively treated, but functional outcomes vary considerably. The model of potential outcomes in Box 32.1 has been termed the 'survivorship framework'. Cancer survivorship is considered to encompass people who are undergoing primary treatment, in remission following treatment, show no symptoms of the disease following treatment, or are living with active or advanced cancer (Figure 32.1). Within this framework occupational physicians may be requested to assess work capability and provide advice on workplace support for cancer survivors in any of the survivorship states, including:

- Pre-employment health assessment of job applicants who have survived cancer in adult or childhood.
- Advice on the vocational rehabilitation of employees newly diagnosed with cancer.
- Advice on long-term adjustments for employees returning to work after diagnosis and treatment, but affected by one of the long-term sequelae of the condition or its treatment.
- Advise on health and safety implications of cancer diagnosis and treatment.
- The likely duration of cancer-related sickness absence.
- Advice on whether the ill health retirement provisions of occupational pensions are met.

Table 32.1 Numbers of people living in the UK who have had a cancer diagnosis[2]

	UK	% of total
Total	2 000 000	100
Male	800 000	40
Female	1 200 000	60
Age 0–17	16 000	0.8
18–64	774 000	38.7
65+	1 210 000	60.5
Breast	550 000	28
Colorectal	250 000	12
Prostate	215 000	11
Lung	65 000	3
Other	920 000	46

Data from Maddams J et al. Cancer prevalence in the United Kingdom: estimates for 2008. *British Journal of Cancer*, 2009: 101: 541–7, Nature Publishing Group © 2012 Cancer Research UK.

Box 32.1 Outcomes after primary cancer diagnosis

◆ All evidence of cancer eliminated following primary treatment, have a period of remission, and are not affected by the illness for the rest of their lives. (For example, the majority of people diagnosed with breast cancer, colorectal cancer, and many other cancers show no evidence of the disease following treatment.)

◆ Treated successfully but giving rise to long-term side effects that a person has to cope with for many years or the rest of their life.

  • Problems with urination, bowel control, and sexuality in survivors who have had cancers of the uterus, bladder, or prostate.

  • Problems with insufficient hormone production in patients who have had cancers of the lymph glands or the brain.

  • An increase in incidence of heart disease in patients who have had breast or prostate cancer.

◆ Live with active cancer following treatment—for example, patients with lung and pancreatic cancer. Others will develop active and advanced cancer after a period of remission. Some of these people will enter further periods of remission after secondary or subsequent treatment.

◆ Diagnosed with active or advanced cancer—may die from their illness within a matter of weeks or months.

◆ Live with cancer for many years without developing significant symptoms—they might die 'with' cancer but 'from' another cause.

◆ Patients whose cancer relapses after a period of months or years may respond to a secondary or subsequent treatment. Typically, however, cancers become less responsive to treatment over time, partly because the most effective treatments are used first.

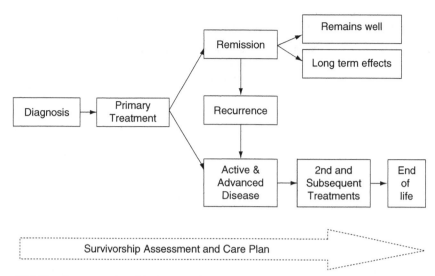

Figure 32.1 The Cancer survivorship framework.

In the UK, 98 per cent of public sector and 30 per cent of private sector employers have access to occupational health services. Employers will normally seek guidance from these services on how to manage employees who have developed a serious illness such as cancer. This means that occupational physicians can be in a key position to coordinate the vocational rehabilitation of cancer survivors.[6] This chapter offers an overview of the evidence on work capability, rehabilitation, and occupational risk assessment that may apply to adults diagnosed with a range of cancers. (Specific cancers are addressed under the relevant systems chapters within this book.)

Cancer, cancer treatment, and work capability

The impact of cancer may not end after treatment. On average, long-term survivors of cancer report poorer health and well-being than the general population, sometimes substantially.[7] The long-term effects of cancer or cancer treatment can be defined as symptoms or changes to physical, psychological, or social function. This definition embraces a broad range of problems, the natures of which depend upon the primary site of the cancer and treatments administered. Approximately 25 per cent of people treated for cancer experience a late effect that reduces their quality of life.[8] Of childhood cancer survivors, 67 per cent go on to develop one or more late morbidities.[9] Survey data suggest that awareness of these late effects is low in patients surviving initial treatment and in their treating doctors.[10]

Estimates of the proportion of cancer survivors who return to work after diagnosis vary widely. However, the likelihood of return to work after cancer diagnosis in a robust epidemiological study based on the Finnish national cancer registry is given in Table 32.2. Overall, this study found an employment rate 9 per cent lower in cancer survivors than in gender- and age-matched controls, 2–3 years after diagnosis.[11]

There is limited evidence on return to work rates in the short term, although a small Dutch study (235 patients diagnosed with primary cancers) found that 24 per cent had returned to work after 6 months and 64 per cent after 12 months.[12] A systematic review of 64 relevant studies, reported a mean duration of absence from work of 151 days in the two-thirds (range 24–94 per cent) of cancer survivors who returned to work.[13]

Table 32.2 Employment rate and relative risk of being employed 2–3 years after diagnosis

Cancer type	Number	% of cancer survivors employed	% of cancer-free controls	Relative risk (95% CI)
Stomach	284	38	54	0.71 (0.59–0.85)
Colon	538	53	59	0.90 (0.81–0.99)
Rectum	331	43	54	0.79 (0.68–0.93)
Cervix uteri	183	58	75	0.77 (0.67–0.90)
Corpus uteri	548	42	51	0.84 (0.74–0.95)
Ovary	534	54	65	0.83 (0.75–0.92)
Prostate	240	30	34	0.87 (0.67–1.13)
Testis	206	72	69	1.02 (0.93–1.19)
Bladder	364	47	57	0.82 (0.72–0.95)
Melanoma of the skin	853	68	66	1.03 (0.97–1.11)
Non-melanoma of the skin	203	56	53	1.06 (0.88–1.26)
Leukaemia	222	45	64	0.70 (0.59–0.84)
Lung	279	19	43	0.45 (0.34–0.59)
Breast	4098	61	65	0.95 (0.92–0.98)

Reprinted from *European Journal of Cancer*, Volume 40, Issue 16, Taskila-Åbrandt et al, The impact of education and occupation on the employment status of cancer survivors, pp. 2488–93, Copyright © 2004, with permission from Elsevier.

Box 32.2 Associations between biopsychosocial factors and return to work

Work may be influenced by the following factors:

- Type of cancer.
- Stage of cancer.
- Whether work is physically demanding.
- Education status of employee.
- Age.
- Treatment type.
- Gender.
- Disease-related factors—fatigue, pain, concentration problems.
- Whether cancer is primary or recurrent.
- Opting for workplace adaptation.
- Workplace interpersonal relationships.
- Perceived workplace support.

A number of associations between biopsychosocial factors and return to work have been reported (Box 32.2). The design and quality of the underlying studies is limited. However, one review looked at studies that took self-reported 'workability' as the outcome measure, defined as '... how able is a worker to do his or her job with respect to the work demands, health and mental resources' rather than the ability to enter or return to employment'.[14] Only studies involving subjects who had continued to work during treatment or returned after treatment were included. This found that workability in cancer survivors (on average, living 2 years after diagnosis) was lower than in non-affected working adults. Workability for a range of common cancers improves over time (usually for at least 18 months), irrespective of age, although the average workability of people with cancer tends to remain lower than in comparison groups and lower than in people with other chronic conditions such as heart disease, stroke, major depression, or panic disorder.[12] Those with lung and gastrointestinal cancers have been reported to have the greatest reduction in workability, patients with testicular cancer to be affected the least. The work productivity of cancer survivors has also been found to be lower and in some reports cancer survivors worked fewer hours. Irrespective of cancer type, chemotherapy has consistently been associated with impaired workability compared to other treatment modalities.

Fatigue, when present, is consistently associated with poor workability, productivity, reduced working hours and absenteeism. Other consequences of disease and treatment, including nausea and vomiting, depressive symptoms, cognitive impairment, and poor sleep have been similarly associated with work limitation. Poor workability is also associated with comorbidities and with cancer recurrence.[12]

In one survey, more than 50 per cent of patients diagnosed with cancer declared their diagnosis to their employer, but fewer than 50 per cent reported any subsequent workplace adaptation or support being put in place, irrespective of cancer type. Those who continued to work during treatment were more likely to report modified work arrangements and paid time off when attending medical appointments. Overall, however, the survey did not provide good evidence of the impact of workplace support or illness disclosure on future workability.[15]

Diagnosis and treatment of cancer: functional prognosis and occupational risk assessment

Adjuvant treatment is a term referring to radio-, chemo-, hormonal, or other pharmacotherapy for cancer. It can be administered prior to (neoadjuvant) or after (adjuvant) primary surgery and given with curative, life-prolonging, or palliative intent. Each treatment has well-recognized acute and long-term side effects that can affect a patient's functional status. Long-term health and functional consequences can also arise directly as a result of surgery for cancer or the nature of the underlying cancer itself. The following section describes some of the common health effects of diagnosis, surgery, and adjuvant treatments, and how these may influence clinical advice on occupational risk assessments relating to employees surviving cancer.

Lymphoedema

Lymphoedema is an accumulation of protein-rich lymph fluid in the interstitial space arising from the interruption of lymph vessel drainage. This may result from various causes including trauma and infection, and also from certain cancers such as uterine, vulval or prostate cancer, melanoma, or lymphoma. The prevalence following gynaecological cancers is estimated at 28–47 per cent.[16]

Lymphoedema caused by breast cancer occurs in 16–28 per cent of patients who have had surgery that has involved dissection of the axillary lymph node (approximately one-third of women at presentation). Of these women, 75 per cent of those who develop lymphoedema will do so within 12 months of surgery, 90 per cent within 3 years,[17] and 1 per cent per year thereafter.[16] Where only sentinel node biopsy is required, 5–7 per cent of women develop lymphoedema. Advice on upper limb exercise after the onset of upper limb lymphoedema can be conflicting, and access to vocational assistance and counselling has been rated highly as an unmet need by women with lymphoedema.[18]

Infection in the limb ipsilateral to the tumour may precipitate lymphoedema.[19] Occupational risk assessment should aim to minimize any risk of trauma to the 'at-risk' limb, and should be discussed with the patient and employer when occupational health advice is provided. Generic advice on good skin care is also available.[20]

Suspicion that exercise of the arm previously subjected to axillary surgery may cause lymphoedema has led to advice to avoid lifting children, heavy bags or other heavy objects with the affected arm. However, a recent major literature review has concluded that non-fatiguing exercise does not increase the risk of upper limb lymphoedema following breast cancer surgery.[16] Moreover, survivors of breast cancer with stable lymphoedema of the arm who continued to lift heavy weights experienced no significant increase in limb swelling. The unrestricted group had fewer exacerbations of lymphoedema, better upper and lower body strength, and reported less severe symptoms from their condition than women advised not to lift. No limit was placed on the non-restricted group as to the limit of resistance exercise they could undertake.[21]

Where upper limb lymphoedema has already developed, consensus holds that a degree of physical activity is beneficial. However, it may be necessary for an individual risk assessment to be undertaken and advice obtained from treating specialists if an employee undertakes repetitive tasks involving isometric exercise or heavy manual handling. In such circumstances, the patient may benefit from advice on recognizing the symptoms of lymphoedema and on a schedule of graded non-fatiguing activity on their return to work.

There is less evidence on how exercise and manual handling affect lower limb lymphoedema. However, specific specialist lymphoedema services provide advice, support, and physical therapies for patients affected by lymphoedema from any cause and are widely available within the UK National Health Service. There are no established pharmacotherapeutic options for the treatment of lymphoedema. Surgical treatment for lymphoedema is rarely performed and limited to severe and refractory cases.[22]

Fatigue

Cancer-related fatigue has been defined as 'a distressing persistent subjective sense of physical, emotional and/or cognitive tiredness or exhaustion related to cancer or cancer treatment that is not proportional to recent activity and interferes with usual functioning'. Fatigue affects some 75–100 per cent of cancer patients at some point[23] and can be functionally debilitating, particularly in combination with the distress of diagnosis, and other symptoms associated with cancer and its treatment. Patients may not disclose that they are affected by fatigue, so it should be asked about and monitored. A number of recognized rating scales can help track symptomatic improvement, particularly after treatment change.

Box 32.3 provides guidance on history taking in cases of cancer-related fatigue. Fatigue often runs a predictable course, arising prior to diagnosis, increasing with treatment, then improving but with a higher baseline thereafter. If fatigue is associated with chemotherapy, symptoms frequently arise a few days after each cycle, although fatigue is often a result of cumulative treatment over a number of months. If associated with fractionated radiotherapy, a cumulative effect can also be seen, with symptoms increasing toward the end of treatment.[24] Cancer survivors report

Box 32.3 Causes of cancer-related fatigue

- Malignancy itself—possibly immune mediated.
- Nausea and vomiting—causes include chemotherapy and radiotherapy, with their associated complications.
- Anaemia—causes include gastrointestinal malignancy with bleeding, nutritional deficiency, myelosuppression from chemotherapy.
- Anorexia.
- Disturbed sleep—causes include pain, anxiety, depression, other emotional problems, not meeting the criteria for formal psychiatric diagnosis.
- Pre-existing comorbidities such as chronic obstructive pulmonary disease.
- Side effects of medication.

fatigue as being more distressing and having a greater functional impact than other cancer-related symptoms, including pain and depression.[25]

Virtually all long-term treatment modalities for cancer, including hormonal treatments and stem cell transplantation, have been associated with fatigue. One survey of breast cancer patients indicated that up to 21 per cent of survivors had persistent fatigue 5–10 years after diagnosis.[26]

Treatment approaches for fatigue include the pacing of activities; overt advice to rest may be inadvisable as it may prolong symptoms. By contrast, there is good evidence suggesting that patients should be encouraged to remain as active as possible.[22] Recent research has suggested possible benefits of high-intensity exercise on physical, functional, and emotional status of patients undergoing chemotherapy, even among those with advanced disease, although research in this area is ongoing.[27]

There is evidence that oncologists may not explore fatigue with patients[23] or consider available evidence-based options for treatment.[28] However, recent guidance from the National Institute for Health and Clinical Excellence has sought to redress this situation by recommending that all patients should have access to an exercise programme if they are experiencing cancer-related fatigue.[20]

Given the subjectivity of fatigue, it is not possible to provide prescriptive advice on whether an employee with cancer is fit to work when experiencing this symptom. However, awareness that a graded return to appropriate work should not prove harmful for those with moderate or mild fatigue, and may prove therapeutic. It can also help to inform clinical assessment and the development of vocational rehabilitation plans with the employee and treating clinicians.

Immunosuppression

Employers may ask for advice from clinicians about the risk of a cancer-affected employee acquiring a work-related infection. There is no definitive evidence available on how specific cancers or work activities may increase susceptibility to a work-related infection. The following section outlines the factors that should be considered when performing a risk assessment.

Chemotherapy

Cytotoxic chemotherapy is widely used in the treatment of many common cancers. Virtually all cytotoxic drugs can lead to immunosuppression, a global term that describes both the quantitative and qualitative effects of chemotherapy on immune function, not all of which can be routinely measured. Leucopenia is easily measurable; the specific type of leucopenia (neutropenia vs. lymphopenia) is noteworthy as the spectrum of infection risk varies.

Neutropenia is a readily identifiable quantitative abnormality, forming a component of overall immunosuppression, during which any infection, especially bacterial, can be life threatening. Neutropenia typically occurs 7–10 days after the administration of chemotherapy in patients who are undergoing cycles of treatment every 3 weeks. The risk of the development of chemotherapy-induced neutropenia (CIN) is reported to be highest during the first cycle of treatment.[29] However, these timings are unpredictable and should not be relied upon in risk assessment. All patients receiving chemotherapy are given guidance on what to do in the event of neutropenic fever.

The incidence of CIN leading to hospital admission has been estimated at 3.4 per cent of cancer patients receiving chemotherapy, with lower rates in non-haematological cancers (2 per cent) compared to haematological cancers (4.3 per cent for all such tumours and 10 per cent in those treated with chemotherapy).[30] In part, this increased risk is secondary to the profound immunosuppressive effects of intensive chemotherapy regimens such as used to combat haematological cancers. In particular, the high chemotherapy doses in the treatment of non-Hodgkin lymphoma have been associated with risk of neutropenia. This can lead to periods of immunocompromise lasting months to years. Such patients may require antibiotic, antifungal, and antiviral prophylaxis over this period.

Febrile neutropenia carries an overall mortality rate of approximately 5 per cent.[31] Fever in a neutropenic patient (usually defined as a neutrophil count of <0.5 cells $\times 10^9/L$, but in some centres up to 1.0 cell $\times 10^9/L$) requires immediate admission for broad-spectrum intravenous antibacterial therapy.[32] Neutropenic sepsis can occur above these levels, but this is likely to be associated with superadded immunocompromise such as arises from concomitant high-dose steroids, hypogammaglobulinaemia (a common accompaniment of the haematological malignancies such as myeloma and chronic lymphocytic leukaemia) or poor marrow reserve due to disease infiltration.

Although evidence is lacking on specific risks in the workplace, those at risk of neutropenia at some point during chemotherapy are generally counselled to reduce their potential exposure to microbes by avoiding work with young children or in roles involving high levels of contact with other people.

Immunomodulatory therapies such as thalidomide, lenalidomide, and the proteasome inhibitor bortezomib, typically used in conjunction with high-dose steroids, can also contribute to immunosuppression and low blood counts.

Monoclonal antibodies, such as the anti-CD20 antibody rituximab, which have an increasing role in cancer therapy, particularly for the haematological cancers, can cause neutropenia months after therapy, rather than in the cyclical way seen with conventional chemotherapy.

Patients receiving chemotherapy or other immunosuppressive treatments are normally considered to be at greater risk of community-acquired infection than average, even with normal neutrophil counts, leading to current UK guidance that those receiving treatment or likely to remain immunosuppressed after treatment ends should receive the seasonal influenza vaccine.[35]

Occupational risk assessment and immunosuppression

It is not possible to make hard and fast recommendations regarding the infective risks in cancer patients who work with varying degrees of immunosuppression across a range of occupations.

However, they should be educated in the avoidance of infection and the steps to take if infection is suspected. The following is a summary of risk management advice provided by medical and charitable bodies in this context, which may inform the occupational physician's guidance regarding microbiological risks at work:

- Avoid large crowds.
- Avoid contact with anyone with a fever, flu, or other infection.
- Wear thick gloves for gardening and wash hands afterwards
- Use moist cleaning wipes to clean surfaces used by other people, such as door handles and keypads.
- Do not wade or swim in ponds, lakes, or rivers.
- Wear shoes at all times.
- Perform prompt first aid for cuts and abrasions to the skin.
- Avoid contact with animal or human faeces (especially the nappies of children who have been recently vaccinated).
- Wash your hands after handling animals, fresh flowers, or pot plants.
- Do not share towels or drinking vessels with others.
- Avoid inorganic dusts (e.g. farms and construction sites).
- Discuss foreign travel with your doctor.

Immunization

The effectiveness of immunization in immunocompromised patients is variable. Live vaccines may be harmful in patients with severe immunosuppression.

Corticosteroids are often used in the treatment of haematological cancers and in end-stage malignant disease. Specialist advice should be sought regarding the appropriateness of live vaccination if patients are receiving 40 mg daily dose equivalents of prednisolone (or lower doses if other immunosuppressive factors are present) for more than 1 week, other immunosuppressive drugs, chemotherapy, or wide-field radiotherapy.

Patients should not receive live vaccines until at least 3 months after they have stopped taking high-dose systemic steroids and at least 6 months after they have discontinued other immunosuppressants or radiotherapy.[35] The *British National Formulary* recommends that there should be at least a 12-month delay before administering live vaccines to a person who has stopped taking immunosuppressants following a stem cell transplant.[32] However, immunosuppression can be severe and prolonged following such procedures. Therefore, it is essential to clarify fitness for live vaccines with the treating specialist.

Inactivated vaccines are safe to administer to immunosuppressed patients, but may elicit a lower immunological response than in immunocompetent individuals. Ideally, where immunization is warranted, this should be administered 2 weeks before commencement of immunosuppressive treatment. The same advice applies to patients who undergo splenectomy. In severely immunosuppressed patents, consideration should be given to repeat immunizations after completion of treatment and recovery. In particular, after stem cell transplantation, patients are likely to lose both natural and immunization-derived antibodies from most vaccine-preventable diseases. Current advice is for such patients to be offered re-immunization, having sought confirmation from the treating physician or an immunologist.[33]

Radiotherapy

Radiotherapy rarely leads to immunosuppression and neutropenia, unless a large volume of active marrow is included in the field. The likelihood of this depends on the total radiation dose and treatment volume, the radiotherapy fractionation schedule, and the body area being irradiated. Severe immunosuppression occurs after total body irradiation, which is used in stem cell transplant settings, but patients typically remain under specialist care until there is an improvement. In most settings, radiotherapy schedules for primary treatment involve 3–8 weeks of daily fractionated doses delivered every weekday at tertiary treatment centres. The incidence of acute side effects is limited by using such schedules and by the localized nature of most treatments. However, depending on the size of the field, inclusion of mucous membranes and number of fractions, many patients do experience significant side effects, including skin or mucous membrane breakdown with resultant pain or nausea and vomiting and significant fatigue. In the event of skin or mucous membrane breakdown, the extent of microbiological exposures in the workplace should be considered. In most cases the intrusiveness of the treatment schedule and ongoing side effects make it impractical to work during treatment.

Hormonal adjuvant treatment

Employees returning to work after a cancer diagnosis may continue on long-term adjuvant treatment, particularly when affected by hormone-driven cancers such as breast and prostate. Adjuvants can lead to side effects or involve treatment schedules that impact on functional capacity and work. The following section outlines some of the most common adjuvant treatments and their effects.

Herceptin®

Herceptin® (Trastuzumab) is a chemotherapeutic agent that specifically targets a subset of 15–20 per cent of breast cancers that have the HER2 receptor. Herceptin® is used in adjuvant and palliative treatment which can last up to a year. Where advised to be the right treatment.[20] Herceptin® is commonly administered for 18 cycles that take place every 3 weeks, at the end of the primary chemotherapy/radiotherapy regimen for breast cancer. The drug is administered by intravenous infusion in an outpatient setting; it takes 30 minutes to complete the infusion. It does not have the immunosuppressive effects of traditional non-targeted chemotherapeutic regimes. Herceptin® is typically well tolerated, the most common side effects being chills and fevers during the course of infusion. Echocardiograms are carried out every 3 months during treatment, as the drug can reduce left ventricular ejection fraction. If this occurs, the drug may need to be discontinued or delayed to allow recovery, so increasing the overall duration of therapy. Once many of the side effects of the drug have begun to abate, patients who have been absent from work during this treatment may contemplate a return to work. At this juncture, occupational health advice should reflect the ongoing demands the treatment will have on an employee's time.

Hormonal treatments

Two-thirds of breast cancers contain receptors for the female hormones oestrogen and progesterone and are termed 'hormone receptor positive'. The treatments for such cancers, Tamoxifen and the aromatase inhibitors, are long-term oral hormone antagonists that are typically well tolerated, although they can cause menopausal symptoms and fatigue. The product characteristics of individual treatments are available from the websites of pharmaceutical manufacturers.

Pain

Pain is estimated to affect up to 50 per cent of patients with cancer and may arise at any stage following diagnosis. Pain can arise from the cancer itself, such as bone or brain metastatic cancer; the long-term effects of treatment, for example, neuropathic pain from chemotherapy (particularly platinum-containing therapies and the proteasome inhibitor, bortezomib); brachial or sacral plexopathy caused by radiotherapy to these areas; or phantom limb pain or post-mastectomy pain after surgery.

The application of the World Health Organization's analgesia three-step 'ladder' has been found to improve pain in 85 per cent of cancer patients, although breakthrough pain still arises in up to 50 per cent. Additionally, the further physical, behavioural, cognitive, emotional, spiritual, and interpersonal effects pain has on a person are well-recognized and have been subject to detailed appraisal.[34] A modern evidence-based approach based on the pathophysiological cause of specific types of pain is desirable.[35]

Where pain affects the workability of employees with cancer, the clinical occupational assessment should consider the adequacy of symptomatic support before commenting on the likely long-term functional impact.

Organ effects

With increasing numbers of cancer survivors returning to work, occupational health doctors need to be aware of the late effects of treatment. Well-recognized effects include:

- Cardiovascular disease, such as premature coronary artery disease or cardiomyopathy (may result from radiotherapy to the mediastinum or anthracycline use).
- Respiratory disease (may be caused by radiotherapy to the chest, or certain agents such as bleomycin).
- Osteoporosis (can be induced by gonadotropin-releasing hormone analogues for prostate cancer, aromatase inhibitors for breast cancers, and prolonged steroid usage).
- Endocrine effects such as hypothyroidism (may occur following radiotherapy to the neck, or hypogonadism) and infertility (due to intensive chemotherapy).
- Increased risk of secondary or subsequent malignancies.

Pelvic radiotherapy has been estimated to lead to later bowel and/or bladder dysfunction in up to 50 per cent of patients. For 50 per cent of these people, the effects are severe, including diarrhoea and incontinence. In one study, 19 per cent of patients undergoing radiotherapy for rectal cancer reported having to toilet more than eight times a day. Patients affected in this way may not say so when asked.[36]

Musculoskeletal

Upper limb function can be impaired in the long term as a result of surgery and/or radiotherapy for breast cancer. However, while upper limb symptoms are common in patients treated for breast cancer, long-term symptoms do not appear to have a major impact on quality of life provided that disease is early does not involve axillary node clearance or axillary radiotherapy.

Even in the absence of lymphoedema, patients who have undergone axillary node clearance or axillary radiotherapy are at risk of long-term upper limb morbidity. The impact on shoulder function can range from minor to substantial and is thought to arise from surgical and radiotherapy-induced fibrosis. One study found that the impact of radiotherapy on upper limb function can manifest over 4 years after treatment has ended.[37,38]

Psychological impact of cancer

A diagnosis of cancer usually has a significant psychological impact on a patient, and can act to undermine self-image and self-confidence; lead to persistent intrusive thoughts of recurrence years after successful treatment; and lead to symptoms of fear, anxiety, and anger.

Although symptoms such as these may not fulfil the criteria of a formal psychiatric diagnosis, they may significantly impair well-being and functioning. The psychosocial impact of a diagnosis may change over the course of a patient's treatment and recovery and into the longer term, possibly requiring a re-evaluation of the support required over time.

When addressing the workability and potential to return to work of an employee with psychological distress, a clinical assessment approach adopting illness representation theory may help to elicit the nature of any barriers to work.[39] This approach may also inform what practical support is needed within the workplace.

Studies have reported significant psychosocial distress in up to 50 per cent of cancer patients, with up to 25 per cent developing major depression.[40] Significant anxiety and/or depression has been found in approximately 50 per cent of breast cancer patients in the first year after diagnosis, 25 per cent in the second to fourth years, and 15 per cent in the fifth year.[41] Long-term psychological symptoms were associated with pre-cancer psychological treatment, younger age, and experience of severe non-cancer related life stressors. However, anxiety and depression were not related to any clinical factors.[41]

Health professionals commonly underestimate the psychological impact of cancer and significant psychiatric morbidity is underdiagnosed.[42] There is some evidence that psychological support can ease the distress arising from a breast cancer diagnosis, and access to such services is recommended in UK clinical management guidelines.[20]

The role of psychological stressors in the onset of primary and recurrent breast cancer has been a topic of research. However, a meta-analysis of the few well-designed studies in this area reported no reliable evidence of such a link,[43] and a more recent prospective cohort study which followed women under 60 for the 5 years following primary breast cancer diagnosis, found no increase in incidence of stressful life events in those who developed a relapse.[44] A link between psychosocial stress and prostate cancer has also been proposed but evidence on this is inconclusive.

Vocational rehabilitation

For cancer survivors, survey data suggests that work ranks only behind their personal health and the well-being of their families in order of importance.[45,46] Work can be a significant part of the individual's identity and a source of self-esteem. Many people who return to work do so without medical or rehabilitation advice. A survey of patients by Cancerbackup revealed that less than half of cancer patients were advised by their doctors about the impact of treatment on their work.[47] Few services are available specifically to support individuals remaining in or returning to work.[13,48]

The experiences of cancer survivors in the workplace are recorded only in small cross-sectional surveys, with little control for confounding factors. Within these limits, patient surveys suggest that timely support in relation to work is desired and appreciated by many, while poor employer understanding of the significance and implications of the diagnosis in relation to work continue to be reported.[49]

Survey results suggest that 73 per cent of UK employers have no formal policy on managing employees with cancer.[49] Support from employers is thus variable, with 50 per cent of employees stating that their employers did not inform them of their statutory rights. Less than half were offered flexible working arrangements.[15] There is evidence to suggest that for a vocational rehabilitation service to be effective, it should intervene early and ensure that good communication takes place between the key players.[50] However, a survey of occupational physicians in the UK revealed that 48 per cent felt the referral of employees with cancer happened too late after the onset of sick leave to allow optimal intervention. Occupational physicians recognized the need to learn more about advising on cancer at work and improving their care plans.[51,52]

Quantitative studies looking at the psychosocial work environment and workability are few and inconclusive. The few qualitative studies in this area have consistently reported a failure by employers to recognize the persisting psychological effects of a cancer diagnosis and its treatment and to introduce appropriate adjustments. Equally, there are reports of unwanted changes to work patterns being imposed by employers, for example, demotion.

The employment provisions of the Equalities Act in 2010 apply to all cancer patients from the point of diagnosis. The Act gives people living with cancer protection from discrimination in a range of areas, including employment and education. However, one survey found that 80 per cent employers were unaware that employees with cancer fell within the provisions of the Disability Discrimination Act (the predecessor of the Equalities Act 2010).[51] It is worth noting that in the USA, cancer survivors are more likely to claim against their employers for discrimination under the Americans with Disabilities Act. Although these claims only comprise 2.9 per cent of all discrimination claims, 27 per cent were successful, compared to an overall success rate of 5 per cent.[53]

There are a wide range of options for work adjustments to support cancer patients to join or remain in the labour market (Box 32.4). These changes to employee working conditions can be temporary or permanent and may have an impact on their terms of employment. In view of this,

Box 32.4 Possible short- and longer-term approaches to vocational rehabilitation after cancer diagnosis and treatment

◆ Changes to and/or flexibility in working hours/days.

◆ Changes to shift working arrangements.

◆ Provision of additional breaks during the working day.

◆ Changes to start/finish times to reduce travel during the busiest times.

◆ Help with travel, e.g. designated parking space or taxi through Access to Work.

◆ Home working to reduce travel demands.

◆ Changes to work duties, e.g. redistribution of duties to/from colleagues.

◆ Consideration of an alternative job role.

◆ Physical adaptations or reorganization of the working environment.

◆ Additional equipment, aids, and adaptations, e.g. communication aids/software.

◆ Advice on specific symptom management, e.g. fatigue management.

◆ Advice on the use of coping strategies, e.g. for cognitive impairment.

◆ Job coaching/support worker in the workplace.

> **Box 32.4 Possible short- and longer-term approaches to vocational rehabilitation after cancer diagnosis and treatment** *(continued)*
>
> ◆ Additional training, supervision and/or support, e.g. mentoring, advocacy, etc.
>
> ◆ Education for supervisor, manager, and colleagues about the condition and its effects.
>
> ◆ Advice/support for supervisor, manager, and colleagues.
>
> ◆ Regular reviews between the employee and supervisor/manager to plan and prioritize future work.
>
> ◆ Additional support from colleagues in the workplace.
>
> ◆ Support from outside of work, e.g. from a rehabilitation service or vocational practitioner.
>
> ◆ Flexibility for employees to attend outpatient appointments if they fall within working hours.
>
> Source: Data from T Carter (2006), Fitness to drive: A guide for health professionals, RSM Press Ltd, London and Skills for Health, Skills for Care, Common core principles to support self care, available at: <http://www.dh.gov.uk/prod_consum_dh/groups/dh_digitalassets/@dh/@en/documents/digitalasset/dh_084506.pdf>.

the occupational physician should ensure that recommendations are made as to the duration of adaptations to produce clarity on this issue before substantial changes are agreed. There is only limited evidence for the effectiveness of the suggested workplace support options in promoting job retention, absence minimization, or enabling cancer survivors to rejoin the workforce; further study of the effectiveness of these interventions is required.[54-56] Moderate quality evidence to support a multidisciplinary rehabilitation approach for cancer survivors, which includes physical, psychological, and vocational components, was found by one systematic review, but again the need for further robust studies of different rehabilitation models was noted.[5]

Fitness to drive

For all tumours, fitness to drive depends in large part upon intracranial (primary or secondary) involvement and subsequent risk of a seizure or visual impairment. If a person has been affected in this way, a decision on their fitness to drive would be made by the Driving and Vehicle Licensing Agency (DVLA).

Because lung cancer most commonly metastasizes to the brain, the fitness to drive of people diagnosed with the illness should be considered. For Group 1 (people with an ordinary licence) the DVLA does not need to be notified about the person's lung cancer unless they have cerebral metastases or are affected by other significant complications. For Group 2 (people who hold a heavy goods vehicle (HSV) or public service vehicle (PSV) licence) the DVLA should be notified about a person's lung cancer. Non-small cell lung cancer classified as T1N0M0 may be considered on an individual basis. Otherwise, driving must cease until 2 years has elapsed from the time of definitive treatment. However, driving may resume if brain scans show no evidence of secondaries.[57]

Where there is no intracerebral involvement, there is no consistent evidence that a cancer diagnosis affects a person's fitness to drive. However, a risk assessment should consider relevant clinical factors (Box 32.5).[58] An increasingly relevant potential impediment to driving capacity is the onset of peripheral nerve damage due to treatments such as bortezomib which are increasingly being used to treat haematological malignancies such as myeloma and lymphoma.

Box 32.5 Factors in assessing fitness to drive[59,60]

- Specific limb impairment, e.g. from primary or secondary bone cancer or surgery.
- A person's general state of health (including the impact of treatment such as chemotherapy or radiotherapy).
- Advanced malignancies causing symptoms such as general weakness or cachexia to such an extent that safe driving would be compromised is not acceptable for safe driving.
- The impact of strong analgesics on cognitive functioning. The use of the World Health Organization's analgesic three-step 'ladder' and adjuvant analgesia involves the use of many drugs with potential cognitive side effects.

Data from Carter T. *Fitness to drive: A guide for health professionals*. London: RSM Press Ltd, 2006 and Skills for Health, Skills for Care. *Common core principles to support self-care*, (http://www.dh.gov.uk/prod_consum_dh/groups/dh_digitalassets/@dh/@en/documents/digitalasset/dh_084506.pdf)

If patients confirm symptoms suggestive of peripheral neuropathy, an assessment of the effect of this on capacity to drive should be undertaken.

Follow-up

Traditionally, follow-up has been designed to screen individuals for signs of recurrent cancer at regular intervals after the completion of treatment, as well as to identify late side effects of treatment.

Currently, the traditional pattern of follow-up care is not effective in managing the immediate after-effects of cancer treatment, where symptoms such as fatigue can persist for many months. It also fails to provide adequate support to individuals who have experienced recurrent cancer or had to repeat treatment over several years.

Engaging patients so that they are interested in their health and, in particular, self-management is widely recognized as crucial to the improvement in care and outcomes for people with long-term conditions.[59] This approach has encouraged a move towards personalized care plans, supported by a 'survivorship information prescription' tailored to individual needs. It is a shift towards information and support, to make patients aware of the signs of recurrent or progressive illness and what they should do if they believe they are affected in this way.

In the context of occupational health, clinical screening is usually not relevant and any follow-up is likely to take place during or immediately after vocational rehabilitation. Following this, arrangements for review in the event of occupational difficulties may be most appropriate, whilst ensuring the employee is aware of the range of support services available.

Health promotion

There is emerging evidence that lifestyle factors including physical activity and diet can influence the rate of cancer progression, improve quality of life, reduce side effects during treatment, reduce the incidence of relapse, and improve overall survival.[60,61] Recent studies have shown that around 2–3 hours of moderate exercise a week after a cancer diagnosis is associated with a 40–50 per cent lower risk of breast cancer death. A similar amount of physical activity after colon cancer has been associated with around a 60 per cent lower risk of cancer death.[62,63]

Epidemiology of cancer

Cancer Research UK[64] provides details on the latest cancer incidence, mortality, and survival statistics in the UK, as well as information on the causes, diagnosis, treatment, screening, and molecular biology and genetics of cancer. A number of validated indices for the common cancers are available, such as the Nottingham Prognostic Index for breast cancer and Gleason grading system for prostate cancer.

Within the context of work, it is important that an employee diagnosed with advanced cancer has access to the benefits they are entitled through their occupational pension scheme.

References

1 Health and Safety Executive. *The burden of occupational cancer in Great Britain.* [Online] (<http://www.hse.gov.uk/research/rrhtm/rr595.htm>)

2 Cancer Research UK. *Cancer incidence by age—UK statistics.* [Online] (<http://info.cancerresearchuk.org/cancerstats/incidence/age/index.htm>)

3 Stiller C. *Childhood cancer in Britain—incidence, survival, mortality.* Oxford: Oxford University Press, 2007.

4 Maddams J, Brewster D, Gavin A, *et al.* Cancer prevalence in the United Kingdom: estimates for 2008. *Br J Cancer* 2009; **101**: 541–7.

5 de Boer AGEM, Taskila T, Ojajarvi A, *et al.* Cancer survivors and unemployment: a meta-analysis and meta regression. *JAMA* 2009; **301**(7): 753–62.

6 Health and Safety Executive. *Occupational Health Advisory Committee report and recommendations on improving access to occupational health support.* [Online] (<http://www.hse.gov.uk/aboutus/meetings/iacs/ohac/access.htm>)

7 Macmillan Cancer Support. *Living with the long term effects of cancer.* [Online] (<http://www.macmillan.org.uk/Documents/GetInvolved/Campaigns/Campaigns/itsnolife.pdf>)

8 Armes J, Crowe M, Colbourne L, *et al.* Patients' supportive care needs beyond the end of cancer treatment: a prospective, longitudinal survey. *J Clin Oncol* 2009; **27**(36): 6172–9.

9 Oeffinger K, Martens A, Sklar C. Chronic health conditions in adult survivors of childhood cancer. *N Eng J Med* 2006; **355**: 1572–82.

10 Macmillan Cancer Support. *Macmillan study of the health and well-being of cancer survivors—follow-up survey of awareness of late effects and use of health services for ongoing health problems.* London: Macmillan Cancer Support, 2008.

11 Taskila-Brandt T, Martikainen R, Virtanen SV, *et al.* The impact of education and occupation on the employment status of cancer survivors. *Eur J Cancer* 2004; **40**: 2488–93.

12 Spelten ER, Verbeek JH, Uitterhoeve AL, *et al.* Cancer, fatigue and return to work of patients to work—a prospective cohort study. *Eur J Cancer* 2003; **39**: 1562–7.

13 Mehnert A. Employment and work-related issues in cancer survivors. *Crit Rev Oncol Hematol* 2011; **77**(2): 109–30.

14 Munir F, Yarker J, McDermott H. Employment and the common cancers: correlates of work ability during or following cancer treatment. *Occup Med* 2009; **40**: 381–9.

15 Pryce J, Munir F, Haslam C. Cancer survivorship and work: symptoms, supervisor response, co-worker disclosure and work adjustment. *J Occup Rehab* 2007; **17**: 83–92.

16 National Cancer Institute. *Lymphedema (PDQ®).* [Online] <http://www.cancer.gov/cancertopics/pdq/supportivecare/lymphedema/healthprofessional>)

17 Mortimer PS, Bates DO, Brassington HD, *et al.* The prevalence of arm oedema following treatment for breast cancer. *Quar J Med* 1996; **89**: 377–80.

18 Girgis A, Stacey F, Lee T, *et al.* Priorities for women with lymphoedema after treatment for breast cancer: population based cohort study. *BMJ* 2011; **342**: d3442.

19 National Institute for Clinical Excellence. *Guidelines for early and locally advanced breast cancer: full guideline.* London: National Institute for Clinical Excellence, 2009. (<http://guidance.nice.org.uk/CG80/Guidance/pdf/English>)

20 Macmillan Cancer Support. *Skin care and lymphoedema.* [Online] <http://www.macmillan.org.uk/Cancerinformation/Livingwithandaftercancer/Symptomssideeffects/Lymphoedema/Skincare.aspx>)

21 Schmitz KH, Ahmed RL, Troxel AB, *et al.* Weight lifting in women with breast-cancer-related lymphedema. *N Engl J Med* 2009; **361**: 664–73.

22 Pain SJ, Purushotham AD. Lymphoedema following surgery for breast cancer. *Br J Surg* 2000; **87**(9): 1128–41.

23 Ahlberg K, Ekman T, Gaston-Johansson F, *et al.* Assessment and management of cancer-related fatigue in adults. *Lancet* 2003; **362**(9384): 640–50.

24 Portenoy RK, Itri LM. Cancer-related fatigue: guidelines for evaluation and management. *Oncologist* 1999; **4**(1): 1–10.

25 Morrow GR. Cancer-related fatigue: causes, consequences, and management. *Oncologist* 2007; **12**(Suppl 1): 1–3.

26 Hofman M, Ryan JL, Figueroa-Moseley CD, *et al.* Cancer-related fatigue: the scale of the problem. *Oncologist* 2007; **12**(suppl 1): 4–10.

27 Adamsen L, Quist M, Andersen C, *et al.* Effect of a multimodal high intensity exercise intervention in cancer patients undergoing chemotherapy: randomised controlled trial. *BMJ* 2009; **339**: b3410.

28 Stone P, Ream E, Richardson A, *et al.* Cancer-related fatigue—a difference of opinion? Results of a multicentre survey of healthcare professionals, patients and caregivers. *Eur J Cancer Care (Engl)* 2003; **12**(1): 20–7.

29 Dale DC. Advances in the treatment of neutropenia. *Curr Opin Support Palliat Care* 2009; **3**(3): 207–12.

30 Caggiano V, Weiss RV, Rickert TS, *et al.* Incidence, cost, and mortality of neutropenia hospitalisation associated with chemotherapy. *Cancer* 2005; **103**; 1916–24.

31 Naik JD, Sathiyaseelan SR, Vasudev NS. Febrile neutropenia. *BMJ* 2010; **341**: c6981.

32 British Medical Association/Royal Pharmaceutical Society of Great Britain. *British National Formulary,* 57th edn. London: BMJ Group, 2009.

33 CDC, the Infectious Disease Society of America, and the American Society of Blood and Marrow Transplantation. *Guidelines for Preventing Opportunistic Infections Among Hematopoietic Stem Cell Transplant Recipients Recommendations of Transplantation.* [Online] (<http://mmserver.cjp.com/gems/bbmt/7-83.pdf>)

34 NHS Quality Improvement Scotland. *The management of pain in patients with cancer. Best practice statement.* Edinburgh: NHS Quality Improvement Scotland, 2009.

35 The British Pain Society. *Cancer pain management—a perspective from the British Pain Society, supported by the Association for Palliative Medicine and the Royal College of General Practitioners.* [Online] (<http://britishpainsociety.org/book_cancer_pain.pdf>)

36 Bruheim K, Guren MG, Skovlund E, *et al.* Late side effects and quality of life after radiotherapy for rectal cancer. *Int J Radiat Oncol Biol Phys* 2010; **76**(4): 1005–11.

37 Levangie PK, Droin J. Magnitude of late effects of breast cancer treatments on shoulder function: a systematic review. *Breast Cancer Res Treat* 2009; **116**(1): 1–15.

38 Lee TS, Kilbreath SL, Refshauge KM, *et al.* Prognosis of the upper limb following surgery and radiation for breast cancer. *Breast Cancer Res Treat* 2008; **110**: 19–37.

39 National Cancer Institute. *Illness representations.* [Online] (<http://www.cancercontrol.cancer.gov/brp/constructs/illness_representations/index.html>)

40 National Comprehensive Cancer Network. *Distress management.* [Online] (<http://www.nccn.org/professionals/physician_gls/pdf/distress.pdf>)

41 Burgess C, Cornelius V, Love S, *et al.* Depression and anxiety in women with early breast cancer: five year observational cohort study. *BMJ* 2005; **330**: 702–5.

42 Fallowfield L, Ratcliffe D, Jenkins V, *et al*. Psychiatric morbidity and its recognition by doctors in patients with cancer. *Br J Cancer* 2001; **84**(8): 1011–15.

43 Petticrew A, Fraser J, Regan M. Adverse life-events and risk of breast cancer: a meta analysis. *Br J Health Psychol* 1999; **4**: 1–17.

44 Graham J, Ramirez A, Love S, *et al*. Stressful life experiences and risk of relapse of breast cancer: observational cohort study. *BMJ* 2002; **324**: 1420.

45 Spelten E, Spragers M, Verbeek J. Factors reported to influence the return to work of cancer survivors: a literature review. *Psycho-Oncology* 2002; **11**: 124–31.

46 Amir Z, Neary D, Luker K. Cancer survivors' views of work 3 years post diagnosis—a UK perspective. *Eur J Oncol Nurs* 2008; **12**: 190–7.

47 CancerBACUP. *Work and cancer: how cancer affects working lives*. London: CancerBACUP, 2005.

48 Pryce J, Munir F, Haslam C. Cancer survivorship and work. *J Occup Rehabil* 2007; **17**: 83–92.

49 Simm C, Aston J, Williams C, *et al*. *Organisations' responses to the Disability Discrimination Act*. Research Report 410. London: Department of Work and Pensions, 2007.

50 Waddell G, Burton AK, Kendall NAS. *Vocational Rehabilitation what works, for whom and when?* Commissioned by the Vocational Rehabilitation Group in association with the Industrial Injuries Advisory Council (report). London: TSO, 2008.

51 Amir Z, Wynn P, Whitaker S, *et al*. Cancer survivorship and return to work: UK occupational physician experience. *Occup Med* 2009; **59**: 390–6.

52 Verbeek J, Spelten E, Kammeijer M, *et al*. Return to work of cancer survivors: a prospective cohort study into the quality of rehabilitation by occupational physicians. *Occup Environ Med* 2003; **60**: 352–7.

53 Amir Z, Brocky J. Employment and the common cancers: epidemiology. *Occup Med* 2009; **59**: 373–7.

54 Nieuwenhuijsen K, Bos-Ransdorp B, Uitterhoeve LL, *et al*. Enhanced provider communication and patient education regarding return to work in cancer survivors following curative treatment: a pilot study. *J Occup Rehabil* 2006; **16**: 647–57.

55 de Boer AGEM, Fring-Dresen MHW. Employment and the common cancers: return to work of cancer survivors *Occup Med* 2009; **59**: 378–80.

56 Tamminga SJ, de Boer AG, Verbeek JH, *et al*. Return-to-work interventions integrated into cancer care: a systematic review. *Occup Environ Med* 2010; **67**: 639–48.

57 Driver and Vehicle Licensing Agency. *At a glance guide to the current medical standards of fitness to drive*. [Online] (<http://www.dvla.gov.uk/at_a_glance/>)

58 Carter T. *Fitness to drive: A guide for health professionals*. London: RSM Press Ltd, 2006.

59 Skills for Health, Skills for Care. *Common core principles to support self care*. [Online] <http://www.dh.gov.uk/prod_consum_dh/groups/dh_digitalassets/@dh/@en/documents/digitalasset/dh_084506.pdf>)

60 Irwin ML, Smith AW, McTiernan A, *et al*. Influence of pre and post diagnosis physical activity on mortality in breast cancer survivors: the health, eating, activity and lifestyle study. *J Clin Oncol* 2008; **24**: 3958–64.

61 Thomas R, Davies N. Lifestyle during and after cancer treatment. *J Clin Oncol* 2007; **19**; 616–27.

62 Holmes MD, Chen WY, Feskanich D, *et al*. Physical activity and survival after breast cancer. *JAMA* 2005; **293**: 2479–86.

63 Meyerhardt JA, Heseltine D, Niedzwiecki D, *et al*. Impact of physical activity on cancer recurrence and survival in patients with stage III colon cancer; findings from CALGB 89803. *J Clin Oncol* 2006; **24**: 3535–41.

64 Cancer Research UK. *CancerStats—cancer statistics for the UK*. [Online] (<http://info.cancerresearchuk.org/cancerstats/>)

Further reading

Wynn P. In-depth review: Cancer and employment. *Occup Med* 2009; **59**: 369–72.

<http://www.macmillan.org.uk/GetInvolved/Campaigns/WorkingThroughCancer/ WorkingThroughCancer.aspx> The Working Through Cancer resources for employers.

<http://www.medicine.ox.ac.uk/bandolier/booth/booths/cancer.html> Systematic reviews on cancer related subjects, including risk factors, screening, and treatments.

<http://www.ncsi.org.uk/> NCSI website.

Appendix 1

Civil aviation

Stuart J. Mitchell

Introduction

The civil aviation industry has a well-developed and tested system of regulatory medical standards for workers in safety-critical roles that is regularly scrutinized and reviewed to preserve the safety of the travelling public. In the first instance this is addressed by the national authority responsible for air safety. In the UK this is the Civil Aviation Authority (CAA), which is concerned to ensure that a licence holder can function effectively, and is not likely to suffer sudden or subtle incapacitation during the period (6 months to 1 year) for which their medical certificate is valid. An employer takes a more long-term view, seeking not only to satisfy the safety requirement, but also to recruit an employee who will remain fit throughout a full career and give regular and efficient service. This is particularly important when the high cost of training a professional pilot or air traffic controller is considered. An individual with a progressive disability might be given a medical certificate subject to regular reviews and may even gain a licence, but might not be trained and/or employed by a major airline.

Risk

Risk management is the main principle of aviation medical certification. It is not possible, nor is it policy, to seek a zero-risk environment. The best airlines operating the best aircraft now achieve a fatal accident rate close to or even better than the CAA safety target of one fatal accident in ten million flights. Many factors contribute to accident causation: the flight crew may be considered to be one of the 'systems' on the aircraft, so the safety target for accidents from medical incapacitation is now less than one in 1000 million flights. This risk target can be achieved in larger aircraft by having two or more pilots, who have been exposed to incapacitation scenarios during routine simulator training, and by only certificating pilots with medical conditions that carry an incapacitation risk of 1 per cent per year or less. This has become known as the '1 per cent rule'. With the development of ever more sophisticated aircraft and improved training, it may be that this figure can be reviewed, as having the 1 per cent standard results in a number of very experienced pilots being grounded, and a balance has to be struck between managing a very small medical risk and the loss of highly experienced pilots (see 'Further reading').

Passenger aircraft smaller than 5700 kg (air-taxi size) usually carry only one pilot, whose incapacitation would inevitably result in an accident. Therefore health standards are higher and, since 1999, these harmonized European standards also apply to pilots engaged in flying instruction and non-passenger-carrying activities, such as banner towing.

Local UK interpretation of operational limitations allows some flexibility within an envelope of acceptable overall risk.

'Acceptable risk' mismatch

One issue of regular concern for occupational physicians practising aviation medicine is that patients' own doctors often advise applicants that the complications of a particular condition or treatment do not affect their fitness to hold a medical certificate. This misconception may arise from a lack of understanding of the aviation environment and a wish to reassure an individual over what is perceived as a low risk in terms of everyday life and work. This mismatch becomes manifest when an individual with a very small risk of developing some medical complication discovers that they fall outside the aviation risk criteria and is, therefore, denied a medical certificate. Dealing with such a situation demands experience, skill, and a degree of tact towards both the individual and their doctors. An individual's career may be interrupted, albeit temporarily, for a reason that is self-evident to the aviation physician but is difficult for the patient to understand.

A similar problem may arise when individuals present for examination to renew their medical certificates and an abnormality is found that has not caused any symptoms (electrocardiogram changes). Individuals in this situation often do not understand that such an abnormality may give rise to a risk of incapacitation in the future. Again, an occupational physician experienced in aviation medicine will be familiar with this scenario and will explain and discuss the situation with understanding and care. Similarly, where there is a mismatch between the aviation regulations and normal practice, physicians must take care not to endorse medical treatment purely for certificatory purposes, although there may be significant financial pressure on an affected pilot who insists on this.

Medical standards

The medical standards for pilots, flight engineers, and air traffic control officers are internationally agreed and are contained in Annex 1 to the Convention on International Civil Aviation. A few, such as the visual requirements, are specific, but many are couched in general terms such as 'cases of metabolic, nutritional or endocrine disorders likely to interfere with the safe exercise of the applicant's licence privileges shall be assessed as unfit'. There is also a waiver clause known as 'accredited medical conclusion', which allows a national authority to issue a medical certificate, if the standards are not fully met, if it believes it is safe to do so. The International Civil Aviation Organization (ICAO), a United Nations (UN) organization, issues a manual of guidance material on the interpretation of the standards.

Since the 1990s there has been a process of harmonization that covers all aspects of civil aviation in Europe. Licensing and medical certification are covered by this process and, since 1999, the European states known as the Joint Aviation Authorities (JAA) have been required to apply common licensing and medical standards (known as Joint Aviation Requirements—Flight Crew Licensing Part 3 (Medical)). This allowed the states to accept each other's licences without further test or expense. The European Aviation Safety Agency (EASA) has been created with responsibility for setting these common standards, which are implemented in each state by the National Aviation Authorities.

In Europe, the initial medical examinations of professional pilots, flight engineers, and air traffic control officers are conducted in an Aeromedical Centre approved by the CAA. Airline transport pilots and commercial pilots below the age of 40 years are then examined annually and 6-monthly above the age of 40, the renewal examinations being undertaken by aeromedical examiners who have had postgraduate training in aviation medicine and who are authorized by the CAA.

Pilots

In terms of medical standards, possible exposure to a hostile environment, notably hypoxia, and sudden changes of pressure and temperature, require very good cardiorespiratory function and freedom from conditions likely to be aggravated by sudden changes in pressure and volume, such as middle ear and sinus disorders, lung bullae, and bowel herniation.

The special senses, especially vision, are clearly important. Uncorrected or corrected vision should be 6/9 (20/30) or better, and there are near (N5) and intermediate (N14) visual requirements. Correction of refractive error and/or astigmatism by the use of spectacles or contact lenses is allowed within certain limits. Normal trichromatic colour vision is not necessary and various screening tests are available to ensure that candidates are 'colour safe'. The latest tests measure colour thresholds using calibrated screens, whilst many states still accept colour lantern tests.

Pilots with static disabilities resulting from orthopaedic or neurological conditions are given a practical test in each aircraft type they wish to fly, which may require approved modifications, such as hand-rudder controllers.

The lifestyle of a professional pilot is necessarily irregular and this can cause significant problems to applicants with gastrointestinal and metabolic disorders. Applicants with diabetes treated with insulin are accepted in a few states, and, as monitoring technologies improve, wider acceptance seems likely provided that the risks of hypoglycaemia and complications are managed. Diabetes controlled by oral therapy is less contentious and does not preclude flying in trained professional pilots subject to regular follow-up, and may be acceptable for initial fitness for private pilots.

Because the continual exercise of judgement and self-discipline are so vital to the pilot's task, significant mental and personality disorders are unacceptable. A history of established psychosis is permanently disqualifying. Neurotic illness is assessed on the probability of recurrence, as is alcohol and drug abuse. Antidepressant medication is fairly common and well tolerated in general and pilot populations, and this has meant that some states accept the use of such medications under controlled conditions in operational aircrew.

A pilot's licence is temporarily suspended on presumption of pregnancy but flying in a two-pilot commercial aircraft is usually possible in the middle trimester provided the pregnancy is progressing normally. Many airlines, however, ground pilots on declaration of pregnancy to minimize any potential exposure of the foetus to solar radiation.

Some commonly used therapeutic agents are unacceptable because of their potential or actual side effects. Performance testing in a flight simulator may be carried out, if necessary, to assess this. In many cases the disorder requiring the therapy will be disqualifying, at least temporarily. For example, the majority of antihypertensive agents are acceptable subject to satisfactory blood pressure control in the absence of side effects. Short-acting hypnotics may be acceptable for short-term use depending on the indication. An aviation medicine specialist should assess such cases individually.

Flight engineers

Some older types of aircraft have a flight engineer as part of the flight crew. They play an important part in monitoring the actions of the pilots as well as controlling the systems on the aircraft, e.g. fuel management. The required medical standards for these crew members are therefore essentially similar to those of pilots, but because they do not physically handle the flying controls at critical stages of flight, their sudden incapacitation does not present the same threat to safety as it would for pilots, and medical standards for incapacity are more lenient.

Cabin crew

Cabin crew do not hold licences and formal medical standards have not previously been regulated. The Joint Aviation Regulations merely required airlines to ensure by 'medical examination or assessment' that cabin crew were fit to carry out their assigned duties. However, EASA has produced new medical requirements for cabin crew which are still to be implemented at the time of writing. These will require periodic examination and/or assessment by either an aeromedical examiner or occupational physician and will be implemented shortly. Airline employers screen for good cardiorespiratory function and freedom from conditions aggravated by pressure changes. The effects of irregular working and worldwide travel are also important in determining whether a health condition is likely to cause problems at work or down-route. Airlines have minimum crewing requirements that could be affected by cabin crew with conditions that cause frequent incapacitation.

Air traffic control officers

Air traffic control officer (ATCO) medical standards are derived from those applied to commercial pilots. However, the working environment and tasks performed by ATCOs vary significantly from those performed by pilots. Although ATCOs follow a common training programme, they usually work in either tower units or large operational area control centres. The working environment of ATCOs in such control centres varies depending on the type of unit. In the UK, those working in 'Area Control' work in pairs, one ATCO directing the traffic whilst the other ATCO performs planning and liaison duties. Other centre-based ATCOs work in 'Terminal Control', supervised by a coordinator shared between several control areas. Visual controllers work in the control towers at airports and direct traffic manoeuvring on the ground and give clearances to take-off and landing aircraft. The sudden incapacitation of an ATCO can pose a risk to flight safety which varies according to the speed of onset and seriousness of the illness event, the speed of reaction of colleagues and supervisors, and the duration and circumstances of incomplete surveillance of the airspace. Research in the UK into risks and consequences of incapacitation suggests that fitness standards should vary between the differing ATCO roles.

In the early to mid 2000s, the standards for ATCOs were harmonized under the direction of Eurocontrol (an agency of the UN responsible for harmonization of regulations and air traffic flow management across Europe). EASA is now the competent authority for air traffic management regulations.

Other legislation

The Equality Act 2010 does not apply to matters of disability employment on board a ship, aircraft, or hovercraft. Civil aviation legislation (The Civil Aviation Act 1982 and the Air Navigation Order 2010) specifies the requirements instead for licensed jobs.

Further reading

Bennett G. Pilot incapacitation and aircraft accidents. *Eur Heart J* 1988; **9**(Suppl. G): 21–4.
Bennett G. Medical-cause accidents in commercial aviation. *Eur Heart J* 1992; **13**(Suppl. H): 13–5.
Chaplin JC. In perspective—the safety of aircraft pilots and their hearts. *Eur Heart J* 1988; **9**(Suppl. G): 17–20.
European Aviation Safety Agency (EASA). *Flight standards*. [Online] (<http://www.easa.europa.eu/flightstandards>)

Evans ADB. International regulation of medical standards. In: Rainford DR, Gradwell DP (eds), *Ernstings Aviation Medicine*, 4th edn, pp. 547–66. London: Arnold, 2006.

International Civil Aviation Organization. *Manual of civil aviation medicine*, 2nd edn. Montreal: International Civil Aviation Organization, 1985.

International Civil Aviation Organization. *Annex 1 to the Convention on International Civil Aviation*, 9th edn. Montreal: International Civil Aviation Organization, 2001.

Mitchell SJ, Evans ADB. Flight safety and medical incapacitation risk of airline pilots. *Aviat Space Environ Med* 2004; **75**: 260–8.

Tunstall Pedoe H. Acceptable cardiovascular risk in aircrew. *Eur Heart J* 1988; **9**(Suppl. G): 9–11.

Appendix 2

Seafarer fitness

Tim Carter

Seafaring is a job and a way of life. As a job it has both risks and performance requirements. As a way of life the consequences of being at sea in terms of diet, exercise, social interactions, distance from healthcare facilities, and, in some cases worldwide travel, are all important. The sector has complex international patterns of staffing, ownership of vessels, and employment contracts, which mean that any maritime country has limited freedom to set its own policies and standards.

Work demands vary widely. Service may be worldwide, inshore, or on inland waterways. Vessel types include bulk carriers, container ships, cruise liners, ferries, commercial yachts, and canal boats. Responsibilities differ between officers and ratings, while the risks and performance requirements on the bridge, in the engine room, and while catering or serving passengers have little in common. In an emergency, physically and psychologically demanding tasks have to be undertaken, such as fire-fighting in restricted spaces, launching and manning lifeboats, or rescuing casualties from the sea.

Several major international organizations have a role in standard setting:

- The International Labour Organization (ILO) has a series of maritime labour conventions and recommendations that cover food, accommodation, medical standards, and care and welfare. These have recently been consolidated into a single Maritime Labour Convention 2006, which will be ratified in August 2013.[1]

- The International Maritime Organization (IMO) is concerned with vessel safety and the contribution of human performance to this. Its recently amended convention on standards for training, competence, and watchkeeping includes requirements from 2012 for medical fitness in safety critical jobs.[2]

- The World Health Organization is important in relation to infection control, port health agreements and emergency care of seafarers[3] WHO and ILO published joint guidance on medical fitness standards in 1997,[4] which is now being revised. These guidelines take account of duties at sea and the widely different patterns of disease and healthcare arrangements in different countries.

- The European Union (EU) regulates working hours[5] and emergency medical supplies carried on EU vessels.[6]

- There is also a wide range of internationally integrated employer,[7] trade union,[8,9] and professional bodies.[10]

Within each country a 'maritime authority' implements these standards and may also be concerned with their enforcement. In the UK, the responsibility for this lies with the Maritime and Coastguard Agency (MCA), an agency of the Department for Transport. Medical standards for determining the fitness of seafarers are produced and regularly updated by the MCA.[11] These standards align with international requirements. Seafarers serving on UK flagged ships must have a medical certificate, issued within the last 2 years, confirming that they meet these standards. Certificates of certain other countries are accepted as equivalent.[12]

The rationale of the fitness criteria for each condition is specified and is increasingly based on validated risk-based evidence. There are two patterns of medical assessment against the standards, one for the majority of merchant seafarers who need to comply with international requirements[13] and another for the masters of small commercial craft such as yachts, work-boats, and passenger vessels in inland and estuarial waters.[14]

Merchant seafarer medicals are undertaken by doctors approved by the Agency, and approval is based on local need. There are about 240 approved doctors in UK and overseas. Most are available to any seafarer but a few are approved only in relation to a single company or a range of companies.[15] Approved doctors are guided by a procedural manual and have access to MCA administrative and medical staff for advice.[16] Standards of work are monitored and most doctors have relevant occupational medical or maritime experience.

Some 50 000 merchant seafarer medicals are performed each year. Of these about 2000 lead to some restriction on service or to failure. Seafarers have the right of appeal to a medical referee and about 80 request a review each year.

Those who work on local commercial boats and yachts may alternatively go to any doctor registered in UK, but normally use their general practitioner, who will complete a medical screening form (ML5). If there are no positive findings, an MCA marine office or the Royal Yacht Association will, subject to other tests of knowledge and competency, issue a Boatmaster's licence or commercial endorsement. If a possibly relevant medical condition is identified, an MCA appointed medical assessor will review the medical information. They may fail the applicant or issue a full or restricted ML5 certificate, which can then be used to support the licence application.

For some conditions fitness criteria are straightforward. Thus, in an environment where navigation lights are red, green, and white, anyone who cannot distinguish these colours cannot undertake lookout duties. Others may be complex. Someone who has had a cardiac event may have continuing impairment of physical performance which could affect their ability to undertake routine or emergency duties. They may also have an increased risk of recurrence and sudden incapacity—critical if they are navigating the ship or working alone. This may pose a particular risk to them and others if evacuation is needed at sea, as well as operational problems if other crew members need to care for them or the ship has to be diverted. Fitness decisions will depend on the person's duties and where the ship is operating.

As seafarers live in close quarters and food is prepared on board, infection risks need to be identified, both in food handlers and in those who may spread infections. Formal standards are contentious where they concern risk factors rather than disease; for instance those concerned with future cardiac risk such as hypertension and obesity—two of the commonest reasons for restriction. Related lifestyle interventions concerned with diet and smoking may be difficult for the individual to implement at sea unless there is commitment from owners and masters.

Most standards depend on the job of the seafarer and on the part of the world in which the vessel sails.[17] Like other statutory measures affecting employment and livelihood the assessment system has to be demonstrably fair and credible, applied uniformly, and subject to independent review.

Some maritime employers have additional fitness criteria but they may not go below the statutory minimum. Seafarers sometimes fail to disclose health problems or seek to avoid treatment of conditions that require medications, such as insulin or warfarin, which can be a bar to work at sea.

A wide range of health professionals can be involved in the care of seafarers. In such situations there are a number of considerations:

1 Young people who want work at sea must understand that they have to meet certain medical standards. Issues that commonly cause work limitation relate to colour vision, asthma (usually better at sea but dangerous in the event of a sudden exacerbation), congenital heart and limb conditions, seizures, and diabetes.

2 Immunizations and antimalarial prophylaxis may be needed.[18]

3 Seafarers requiring elective surgery may need to seek priority to ensure that they can comply with medical standards and return to work.[19]

4 After diagnosis of a significant illness, such as heart disease, diabetes, or epilepsy, the seafarer will need to obtain a new medical certificate but may have to wait until the condition has stabilized and may find that they are restricted or found unfit.

5 When continuing medication is needed, the acceptability of the person for sea service will need to be reassessed. In some cases the medication itself will be the reason for restricting duties or finding the person unfit.

6 If cardiac risk factors are poorly controlled, especially weight and blood pressure, the patient will need to be reminded that failure to achieve control may lead to their career at sea being terminated, even in the absence of a cardiac event.

References

1 International Labour Organization. *Maritime Labour Convention 2006*. (<http://www.ilo.org>)

2 International Maritime Organization. *International Convention on Standards of Training, Certification and Watchkeeping for Seafarers (STCW Convention) 1978*, as amended. (<http://www.imo.org>)

3 World Health Organization. *International medical guide for ships*, 3rd edn. Geneva: World Health Organization, 2007

4 World Health Organization/ILO. *Guidelines for conducting pre-sea and periodic medical fitness examinations for seafarers*. Geneva: World Health Organization /ILO, 1997. (<http://www.ilo.org/public/english/standards/relm/gb/docs/gb271/stm-5a.htm>)

5 The Maritime Working Time Directive (1999/63/EC). (<http://www.europa.eu.int/eurlex/en/index.html>)

6 Maritime and Coastguard Agency. *Merchant Shipping Notice MSN 1768 (M + F). Ships' medical stores*. Southampton: Maritime and Coastguard Agency, 2003.*

7 International Shipping Federation: <http://www.marisec.org>

8 International Transport Workers' Federation: <http://www.itf.org.uk>

9 Nautilus International (the officers trade union): <http://www.nautilusint.org>

10 International Maritime Health Association: <http://www.imha.net>

11 Maritime and Coastguard Agency. *Merchant Shipping Notice MSN 1822 (M). Seafarer medical examination system and medical and eyesight standards*. Southampton: Maritime and Coastguard Agency, 2002.*

12 Maritime and Coastguard Agency. *Merchant Shipping Notice MSN 1822 (M). Seafarer medical examination system and medical and eyesight standards*, p. 8. Southampton: Maritime and Coastguard Agency, 2002. [List kept live on MCA website: <http://www.mcga.gov.uk/seafarer information/health and safety/>.]

13 Maritime and Coastguard Agency. *Marine Guidance Note MGN 219(M). Seafarer medical examinations: guidelines for maritime employers and manning agencies*. Southampton: Maritime and Coastguard Agency, 2002.*

14 Maritime and Coastguard Agency. *Seafarer Medical Report Form (ML5) and ML5 Certificate*. MSF 4112/rev 0810, 2010. [See MCA web site.*]

15 Maritime and Coastguard Agency. *Merchant Shipping Notice MSN 1821 (M). List of approved medical practitioners (approved doctors).* Southampton: Maritime and Coastguard Agency2009. [Also see MCA web site for up-to-date names.*]

16 Maritime and Coastguard Agency. *Approved doctor's manual: seafarer medical examinations.* Southampton: Maritime and Coastguard Agency. [Controlled document periodic updates—current version on Agency website.*]

17 Carter T. The evidence base for maritime medical standards. *Int Maritime Health* 2002; **53**: 1–4.

18 Maritime and Coastguard Agency. *Marine Guidance Note MGN 257 (M). Prevention of infectious disease at sea by immunisations and anti-malaria medication (prophylaxis).* Southampton: Maritime and Coastguard Agency, 2003.*

19 Dreadnought Unit, Guy's and St Thomas' Hospital. [A service providing treatment for seafarers.]: <http://www.seabal.co.uk/dreadnought.htm>

Note

* Maritime and Coastguard Agency (MCA) publications are regularly updated and subject to change. Access to current versions relevant to seafarer medicals can be obtained from the MCAs website: http://www.dft.gov.uk/mca/mcga07-home/workingatsea/mcga-healthandsafety.htm.

Appendix 3

Offshore workers

Mike Doig

Introduction

Offshore oil and gas production is a major, safety critical, global industry with increasing public visibility, found in almost all the oceans of the world (shallow and deep water, arctic and tropical). The quest is to find and extract this finite resource through further exploration and development. The activity is encouraged by higher oil prices and new technology, and many mature fields are being given a new lease of life because of enhanced recovery techniques. The UK still ranks in the top 20 of the world's oil producers[1]—total production of oil and gas peaked in 1999, but was still 2.35 million barrels of oil equivalent per day in 2010. The industry still provides employment for 330 000 people, with 32 000 directly employed by oil and gas companies and 49 960 personnel visiting UK offshore platforms (Figure A3.1).

Offshore installations

There are currently 290 mobile drilling and accommodation rigs (150 manned, 140 unmanned) in the North Sea. These range in size from small exploration and drilling semisubmersibles to massive semi-permanent oil production and export installations (Figure A3.2). The latter represent a complex engineering feat, piecing together all the plant required to safely receive the pressurized hot crude oil, process it, and export it under pressure through an undersea pipeline to an adjacent holding and discharge vessel. Production installations are usually fixed-leg platforms, but sometimes they are floating moored facilities. They are connected to the seabed and hence the oilfields by large-bore risers that carry the hot oil from the deep subterranean reservoirs to the processing plant on the platform.

The offshore working environment

These complex, compact facilities pose a challenging working environment for the offshore workforce. Each offshore installation is a self-sufficient community in which people work and sleep for the duration of their offshore tour (normally 2 or 3 weeks). Logistic support is provided by helicopters and supply vessels, transferring personnel and delivering food and equipment. Shift work is the norm and typically involves rotating 12-hour shifts. Living quarters offshore are necessarily modest but comfortable and usually shared, with two bunks per cabin. Food is of good quality and abundant at mealtimes, but no alcohol is allowed. There are recreational facilities, normally including lounges with papers, magazines, and satellite television, a gym, and often a cinema. Constraints on manning and accommodation mean that anyone who falls sick for more than a brief length of time will have to return onshore and be replaced by another worker. Emergency medical evacuations can be expensive for the company and can be required in inclement weather.

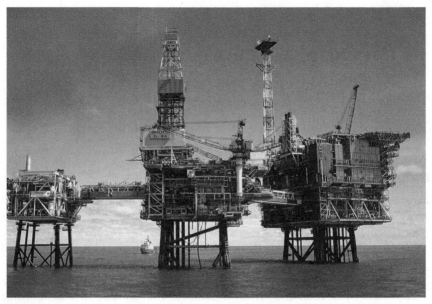

Figure A3.1 Picture of oil rigs. Reproduced with permission from BP Exploration Operating Company Ltd.

Communication with the mainland can be fragile—links are normally by radio or satellite and subject to interference in bad weather conditions. Depending on geographical location, there may be periods in which travel by helicopter is impossible for several days, owing to high winds and heavy seas in the winter or fog in the summer. Visits by supply vessels can also be disrupted by the weather, interfering with the supply of engineering tools, service supplies, and fresh food and water from the mainland.

Range of functions

Typically, a core crew of 50–250 mans each installation, undertaking a wide range of duties associated with running, maintaining, and supporting a complex heavy engineering and oil production operation. Many of the tasks are physically arduous and require a lot of heavy lifting; many valves are still manually operated. Equipment needs regular maintenance and repair, often in a confined working space. Along with the physically demanding roles of the operators, mechanical technicians, instrument technicians, drillers, and roustabouts (labourers) there are specialized functions such as control room operators, chemists to test the oil and drill cuttings, health and safety professionals, caterers, geologists, and importantly an offshore medic (see 'Health legislation'). Each installation falls under the authority of the offshore installation manager (OIM) who is deemed for legislative purposes to be the person in charge.

Health legislation

The Continental Shelf Act of 1964[2] extended petroleum exploration licensing arrangements to the offshore environment with provision for the safety, health, and welfare of persons employed on operations undertaken under licence authority. The Management of Health and Safety at Work

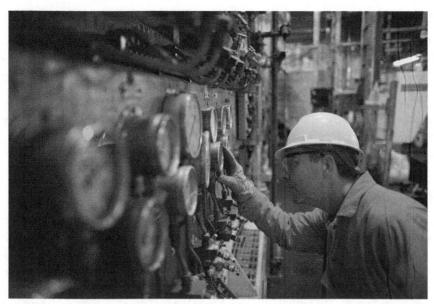

Figure A3.2 Picture of worker looking at dials. Reproduced with permission from BP Exploration Operating Company Ltd.

Act, Control of Substances Hazardous to Health (COSHH), and Working Time Directives have all been extended to cover the offshore workforce.

The offshore regime is based around the Safety Case Regulations (2005)[3] which requires operators to have a safety case for fixed and mobile installations accepted by the Health and Safety Executive (HSE). These regulations are amplified by other rules such as the Offshore Installations and Pipeworks (Management and Administration) Regulations 1995,[4] which require provision of health surveillance, food and drinking water.

The Offshore Installations and Pipeline Works (First Aid) Regulations 1989[5] set out the requirements to provide healthcare facilities on offshore installations and the responsibilities of the dedicated on-site medical provider (the offshore medic).

The Offshore Installations (Prevention of Fire and Explosion, and Emergency Response) Regulations 1995 (PFEER)[6] set out requirements to plan an effective emergency response, including that of the medical team, in the event of serious incidents on an offshore installation.

The provisions of the National Health Service do not extend offshore, so private health providers deliver the health services mandated by legislation, industry standards, and best practice.

Industry guidance

Guidelines on health and fitness standards in the oil industry are developed and published by the Energy Institute (EI) through the Health Technical Committee (HTC) and the Occupational Health and Hygiene Committee. They include the Physical Fitness Standards for the Oil Industry,[7,8] the Medical Standards of fitness to wear Respiratory Protective Equipment,[9] and Medical Aspects of Work for the Onshore Oil industry.[10] Oil & Gas UK (OGUK) publishes guidance for physicians examining offshore workers,[11] again using the EI HTC for expert input.

Offshore survival training

Transport to offshore installations is usually by helicopter. In a major emergency evacuation is likely to be by lifeboat into the sea. Every employee offshore must hold a valid Certificate of Offshore Survival Training, approved by the Offshore Petroleum Industry Training Organization (OPITO) which is valid for 4 years.

This physically demanding Basic Offshore Safety Induction and Emergency Training course[12] involves significant physical stressors such as water immersion, embarking a life raft from the water, and helicopter underwater escape training. Successful completion of the course requires a significant level of fitness and mobility (as does real emergency evacuation) (Figure A3.3). Refresher courses are required every 4 years.

Offshore health facilities

All offshore installations must have a fully equipped medical clinic under the supervision of an offshore medic. These dedicated facilities usually comprise an examination area, a small one- or two-bedded ward, and the wherewithal to treat hypothermia. Sickbay medical equipment is usually very comprehensive, and the basic items defined in the industry first-aid and medical equipment guidelines[13] are often supplemented by more sophisticated medical response and emergency equipment. The facility will stock a wide range of drugs to cover most routine treatment and common emergencies.

The offshore medic

The offshore medics are usually trained nurses or armed services medical attendants who have all passed the specific HSE-approved medic training course as defined in the First Aid Regulations.[5] This 4-week intensive course equips the medic with the extra skills the role demands. They must

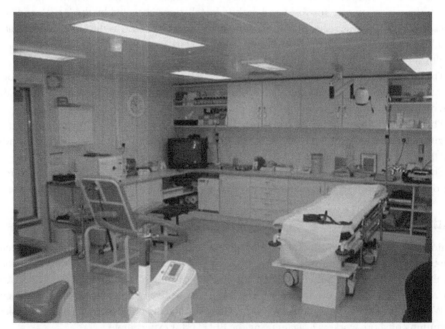

Figure A3.3 Photo of sickbay. Reproduced with permission from Chevron North Sea Limited.

be able to initiate a wide range of medical interventions with no expectation of immediate medical back-up, relying only on the advice of the on-call physician, and perhaps in extremis with help from the first aid team.

The medic has an essential role on the offshore installation, bearing primary responsibility for the treatment of all on-site illness or injury in the workforce and visitors. Their duties include the provision of medical and primary care to personnel, developing the medical plan for emergency response, conducting local medical surveillance for occupationally-related exposures, advising on hygiene, and offering health promotion. Normally a platform has only one medic who is always on call 24 hours per day for any advice or treatment.

A consulting onshore physician ('the topside doctor') provides 24-hour on-call advice to the offshore medic on the diagnosis and clinical management of difficult cases, medical evacuation, and the use of non-standard treatments.

Medical screening

Physicians need to appreciate the greater fitness standards demanded by this remote and special-ized workplace, and the hazard posed by even common medical conditions whose treatment will be delayed in the event of an emergency. The examining physician should assess the physical and mental health of offshore employees in order to:

+ Anticipate and prevent illness which by its nature could place the individual, colleagues, or the emergency rescue services at undue risk.
+ Ensure so far as is reasonably practicable, that offshore personnel are medically and physically fit for their designated work duties.

An individual's fitness for work offshore will be predicated on the following:

+ Diagnosis, aetiology, and prognosis of any medical conditions that are present.
+ The impact of current or planned treatment.
+ The risk of relapse, including acute exacerbations that could require urgent medical intervention.
+ The risk of any adverse effects which could be precipitated or exacerbated by the offshore environment.
+ Restrictions in the availability of specialized medical support, facilities, and supplies.
+ The match between their fitness and the essential tasks in their job.

Assessment of fitness to work offshore must be made by an examining physician approved by UKOG as fulfilling minimum criteria related to clinical evaluation, experience, knowledge, and understanding of the offshore environment. The UKOG medical examination is now a biannual examination with more frequent reviews for workers with significant pathology that requires ongoing surveillance.

Workers for the Norwegian and Dutch sectors have separate certification to their country-specific standards OLF and NOGEPA respectively. Norway (OLF) requires that physicians are approved and listed whereas the Dutch authorities accept OGUK medical certificates.

Increasingly, functional capacity evaluations (FCEs) are being employed by oil operators to confirm physical fitness of their offshore workforce. These include tests of muscular strength, stamina, aerobic capacity, and functional task simulation related to the essential job functions for the employee. These may be defined by the operating company and separately the EI has defined industry guidelines for the UK offshore workforce.

Emergency response team

Offshore installations must have arrangements in place to provide an effective response in the event of an offshore emergency.[14] One element of the response is a specially trained emergency response team (ERT) with various specialized roles including rescue of casualties and firefighting. ERT members have other full-time duties while on board and so the emergency response duty is invariably additional, rather than a full-time responsibility. The EI has published evidence-based guidelines for oil and gas workers both offshore and onshore, including ERT members, developed by Portsmouth University.[7,8] The OGUK Medical Guidelines[11] stipulate task-related physical fitness guidelines for ERT members. They must undergo specific training, again at an OPITO-approved facility. This in itself will involve physical activity and require commensurate fitness to participate in the training. Tasks may include: use of multiple cylinder breathing apparatus, repeated or sustained lifting and carrying (e.g. of casualties), firefighting, search and rescue in smoke filled/hot environments, rescue of casualties from platform legs or vessel holds, running out fire hoses, and moving foam barrels.

Medical fitness and disability

The Equality Act 2010[15,16] applies offshore and to offshore workers, but the demanding nature of the offshore environment means that it may be justified, on safety grounds, to exclude persons with significant disability which might reduce mobility in an emergency or impede the egress of others, including escape from a ditched helicopter. The final decision on the fitness of anyone with a significant disability should always be made by an occupational physician who has a thorough knowledge of the offshore environment—usually with reference to the medical advisor of the operating oil company.

Obesity

In the absence of resulting disease, obesity is now dealt with offshore primarily as a safety issue related to transport and evacuation in an emergency. Standards are currently being proposed so that where an individual is found to have an absolute body weight of more than 115 kg, they should undergo assessment related to seat-belt use and egress from the escape hatch of the helicopters in which they may travel, and other safety parameters related to the specific offshore installation(s) they will be working on (Table A3.1).

Occupational health

The offshore workforce is potentially exposed to the panoply of occupational exposures arising from heavy engineering, petrochemical processing, drilling, and exposed environments. The confined spaces in which people work may aggravate the situation.

A range of potential hazards and toxic exposures need to be considered. These include the following factors:

- Chemical: toxic, corrosive, irritant, sensitizing, and potentially carcinogenic agents.
- Physical: noise, vibration, radiation, and extremes of temperature.
- Biological: risk of food poisoning and legionella.
- Ergonomic: heavy manual handling.
- Psychosocial: work overload, shiftwork, tour patterns, work relationships, travel, isolation from home and family.

Table A3.1 OH hazards chart: example of a risk matrix used to rank safety and environmental issues on offshore installations

	Health/ safety risk	Threat to environment	Cost of threat to plant and equipment	1 Improbable/ remote	2 Occasional	3 Probable	4 Frequent
1	Slightly harmful/ minor	Negligible	<£10 000	L	L	M	M
2	Harmful/ serious	Minor	£10 000– £200 000	L	M	M	H
3	Very harmful/ major	Moderate	£200 000– £1 million	M	M	H	H
4	Extremely harmful/ fatality	Major	>£1 million	M	H	H	H

L: Acceptable but additional controls should be considered if cost effective.

M: Should only proceed with management authorization after additional controls are implemented.

H: Task must not proceed—must be redefined/further control measures put in place to reduce risk. The controls should be reassessed prior to the task commencing.

Reproduced with permission of Chervon North Sea Limited.

A robust strategy is needed to identify, assess, control, and monitor these factors. It is important in calculating exposure limits in the offshore environment to allow for the 12-hour shift pattern. It is also an environment where multiple exposures may be present with potential interaction and potentiation. Health surveillance should be initiated where there is a known adverse health effect and a means of delivering it. This duty is required by health law. EI publish a comprehensive guidance on health surveillance applicable to the oil industry.[17]

Catering

Food safety is critical on offshore installations. Each installation has a single catering facility for the whole workforce which must observe the highest standards of food hygiene and comply with the Offshore Environmental Health Guidelines.[18] A significant episode of food poisoning offshore could be catastrophic, both for the crew and the safe production of oil (Figure A3.4).

Drilling

Drilling, whether exploratory or on established fields, is a high-risk activity with physical and chemical hazards. Heavy drill pipes are manhandled and fabricated into drill-stings many kilometres in length as they descend through the rock formation into the oil-retaining sands. Although now highly mechanized, this part of the offshore operation continues to be one of the most hazardous in terms of manual handling and risk of musculoskeletal injury. Noise is also a constant hazard. Drilling muds may contain toxic chemicals that need to be handled with care.

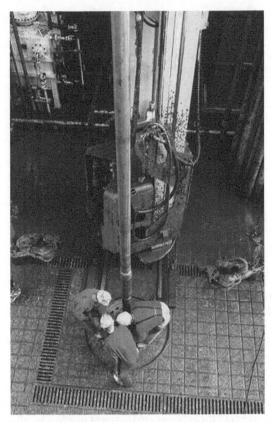

Figure A3.4 Picture of drill floor. Reproduced with permission from Chevron North Sea Limited.

Drugs and alcohol

Offshore oil and gas production facilities are extremely hazardous, safety-sensitive environments, not least because of the large-scale industrial processing of flammable and explosive hydrocarbons under pressure. Alcohol and drugs that interfere with performance cannot be tolerated at any time (emergency evacuation may require an immediate and disciplined response from everyone on board, even if off duty). Normally, therefore, operating companies have strictly enforced mandatory drug and alcohol policies, monitored by random testing and searches at the heliport prior to travel and sometimes offshore. Searches may be made of personal effects, sniffer dogs used to scan the offshore accommodation and living quarters, and urine testing used post incident or for random personal screening.

Infectious diseases

The close, intimate community of an offshore oil installation is a perfect environment for spread of infectious diseases.

The recent impact of SARS (severe acute respiratory syndrome), the H5N1 pandemic, the continuing threat of avian influenza, and the possible use of biological agents by terrorists has led to the realization that offshore installations are potentially vulnerable. The industry has infectious disease protocols that define processes the companies will implement to minimize the risk of the transfer of an infectious agent in an infectious disease or pandemic situation.

Mental well-being

The demands of this working environment, including shift work, isolation, and separation from family and friends for 2–3 weeks at a time, may threaten mental well-being. The spouse or partner who is expected to run the household while the worker is away may also be under considerable pressure. Because of this, many operating and contracting companies have 'stress awareness' programmes for the benefit of offshore workers and their families. Employee Assistance Programmes (EAPs) are now also often provided by the major oil operators. These provide information on a broad range of domestic, personal, financial, and work-related issues. Additionally, these services provide focused support to business organizations managing the stressful consequences of reorganization or redundancy and traumatic incidents such as major accidents or workplace deaths.

Shift work

The 24-hour operation of an offshore installation requires that many employees work shifts. Unmanaged circadian desynchrony can threaten safety through reduced alertness and a fall in reaction times. Following a shift change, it takes several days for circadian-chronological synchrony to occur, so workers on the new nightshift may not be at optimal performance for the first few nights. Some studies suggest that in some cases synchrony may not take place at all during the period of a nightshift, and this can lead to potential sleep disturbance, fatigue, and performance decrement.[19] There is HSE guidance setting out specific advice related to working practices for managing shiftwork and fatigue offshore.[20] These include recognizing the importance of the following factors:

- Providing appropriate staff where and when they are required.
- Minimizing the physiological and psychological penalties associated with adjustment to shifts.
- Promotion of alertness over the working period.
- Minimization of tiredness and fatigue.
- Recognition of individual variability.
- Control of occupational exposure.
- Avoidance of an increase in travel hazards above those for day workers.

It also lists the known hazards of shift-working offshore which include:

- Early shifts before 6am.
- Overtime beyond the 12-hour shift.
- Off-duty call outs.
- Being too long offshore without breaks.
- Long periods of attention.
- Failure to provide back-ups for no shows.
- Tasks with low error tolerance combined with high consequences.
- Long journey times prior to travel offshore and commencing shift on arrival at the installation.

The ageing workforce

The offshore workforce shows a bimodal demographic distribution with the first peak at around 30 years of age, reflecting recent initiatives to attract new entrants to the industry. The mean and median of the population remains at 41 years with a gentle tail off into the late 60s. There has been an increase in personnel in the 50–54, 55–59, 60–64, and 65+ age groups.[21] There are no age limits to working in the offshore environment and the workers are subject to the same factors of any aging workforce—decreasing physical capacity, decrements in coordination and balance, psychological changes, and an increase in pathological conditions that may affect performance. Initiatives to combat these issues include programmes to optimize health and physical fitness, optimized workplace design, better control of job content and allocation of tasks, and, importantly, functional capacity evaluation to ensure individual capability matches task requirements.

Human factors: behavioural-based safety

Safety continues to be of great concern to the offshore industry, with constant efforts to minimize work-related illness and injury. There is greater focus on human factors and behavioural-based safety (BBS), considering safety-critical situations in which individuals can make mistakes through error or violation and how best to maintain a safe working environment. BBS sets out to change safety consciousness through the creation of a culture of modified health and safety sensitive behaviours.

In considering the interface of the individual, the job, and the organization, five main factors play a role: fatigue, communication, risk perception, risk-taking behaviour, and the health and safety culture of the organization. The EI has a useful website which covers this subject in some detail: <http://www.energyinst.org.uk/humanfactors>.

Acknowledgement

Thank you to the following corporations for providing the photographs in this appendix: BP and Chevron North Sea Limited.

References

1 Oil & Gas UK. *Economic report 2010*. London: United Kingdom Offshore Oil and Gas Industry Association Limited trading as Oil & Gas UK, 2010.

2 United Kingdom Continental Shelf Act 1964.

3 *The Offshore Installations (Safety Case) Regulations SI 2005/311*. London: The Stationery Office, 2005.

4 *Offshore Installations and Pipeline Works (Management and Administration) Regulations 1995*. London: The Stationery Office, 1995.

5 *Offshore Installations and Pipeline Works (First-Aid) Regulations 1989 SI 1989/1671*. London: The Stationery Office, 1989.

6 *The Offshore Installations (Prevention of Fire and Explosion, and Emergency Response) Regulations 1995*. Approved Code of Practice and Guidance L65. London: HSE Books, 1995.

7 Energy Institute. *A recommended fitness standard for the oil and gas industry*. London: Energy Institute, 2010.

8 Energy Institute. *Fitness assessment manual*. London: Energy Institute, 2011.

9 Energy Institute. *Medical standards for fitness to wear respiratory protective equipment*. London: Energy Institute, 2011.

10 Energy Institute. *Guidelines for the medical aspects of work for the onshore oil industry*. London: Energy Institute, 2011.

11 Oil & Gas UK. *Guidelines for medical aspects of fitness for offshore workers*, Issue 6. London: Oil & Gas UK, 2008.

12 *Basic offshore safety induction and emergency training and further offshore emergency training*. Aberdeen: Offshore Petroleum Industry Training Organisation, 2003.

13 UK Offshore Operators Association. *Industry guidelines for first aid and medical equipment on offshore installations*. London: UK Offshore Operators Association, 2000.

14 UK Offshore Operators Association. *The management of competence and training in emergency response for offshore installations*. London: UK Offshore Operators Association, 2004.

15 *Equality Act 2010*. London: HMSO, 2010.

16 *Equality Act (Offshore Work) Order 2010*. London: HMSO, 2010.

17 Energy Institute. *Guidance on Health Surveillance*. London: Energy Institute, 2010.

18 UK Offshore Operators Association. *Environmental health guidelines for offshore installations*, Issue 3. London: UK Offshore Operators Association, 1996.

19 Gibbs M, Hampton S, Morgan L, *et al. Effect of shift schedule on offshore shiftworkers' circadian rhythms and health*. Research Report 318. London: Health and Safety Executive, 2005.

20 Health and Safety Executive. *Guidance for managing shiftwork and fatigue offshore*. Offshore Information Sheet 7/2008. London: Health and Safety Executive, 2008.

21 Oil & Gas UK. *2011 UKCS workforce demographics report*. London: United Kingdom Offshore Oil and Gas Industry Association Limited trading as Oil & Gas UK, October 2011.

Appendix 4

The medical assessment of working divers

Robbert Hermanns and Phil Bryson

Introduction

Commercial diving in the UK, including the UK continental shelf, is regulated by the Diving at Work Regulations 1997 (DWR),[1] which are enforced by the Health and Safety Executive (HSE).

Diving is considered commercial under the DWR when it is carried out for employment or reward. (The exact definition and exemptions are given in the regulations.) This chapter only considers health risks in relation to traditional diving in water,[2] matters relating to working in an atmosphere of an ambient pressure greater than 100 millibar or short term use of self-rescue equipment for escape from aircraft are not considered.

Commercial diving covers a large number of activities, ranging from shallow police diving, training of recreational divers, cleaning of aquariums, to scientific, media, and construction diving. Diving techniques range from the use of self-contained underwater breathing apparatus (SCUBA) to surface supply diving, where the diver is supplied from the surface through a hose (umbilical), and saturation diving at depths of several hundred metres.

In the commercial world, diving is just the way a diver 'commutes' to work. Specialist work activities in the workplace include non-destructive testing, inspection, construction or welding, use of power tools and cutting equipment, media or scientific work. The HSE publishes the approved dive qualifications and five approved codes of practice[3] (ACoPs) applicable to different sectors of diving.

These ACoPs cover:

+ Commercial diving projects offshore.
+ Commercial diving projects inland/inshore.
+ Media diving projects.
+ Recreational diving projects.
+ Scientific and archaeological diving projects.

Occupational health aspects of commercial diving

The fitness to dive of any individual diver influences the risks to the entire dive team, making diving a safety critical activity. HSE Approved Medical Examiners of Divers (AMEDs) therefore need to have a detailed appreciation of the diving environment and the relevant workplace risks in order to perform an appropriate medical examination, correctly interpret the information gathered, and form a sound judgement as to a diver's physical and mental fitness to dive. For further information on different diving techniques we refer to the relevant literature and/or Internet media.

The regulations do not stipulate a minimum age for commercial divers. However, the safety critical nature of diving requires an adult attitude to learning and risk appreciation. In practice, training organizations and/or employers will only recruit people of 18 years or older, and working offshore is only permitted at this age threshold.[4]

This brief introduction to diving medicine cannot cover every diving activity. However, the example of saturation diving may help the reader to appreciate some of the challenges of diving and in assessing the medical fitness of divers.

During saturation, divers are kept at working depth pressure during the entire dive project. They live in steel chambers onboard specialized diving support vessels (see Figure A4.1). They 'travel' to work by transferring from their living habitat into a small diving bell in which they are lowered into the water to reach their working depth, where they leave the bell to travel short distances to their work site.

Saturation diving allows for up to 4–8 hours of work under water per shift. After a shift divers will return to their pressurized living habitat without experiencing any significant change in pressure. The UK DWR allows up to a maximum of 28 days in saturation, but elsewhere in the world this limit is sometimes significantly exceeded. Depending on the working depth pressure, the gas pressure in human tissue reaches equilibrium with the gas pressure in the living environment within hours to a few days. Consequently, decompression at the end of a work period can take up to 4–5 days of slowly reducing the gas pressure in the habitat, in order to prevent decompression illness.

The breathing gas in the habitat is depth dependant and usually consists of variable gas mixtures of oxygen and helium. Helium has a much greater ability to conduct heat than air. Consequently, the habitat temperature has to be kept at much higher temperatures (28–32°C) to maintain core body temperature than in air. Environmental humidity can also be high. These conditions create ideal circumstances for bacterial contamination, with a raised risk of infections despite best efforts to control all relevant habitat parameters. Up to six people live together in a chamber for extended periods of time, relatively isolated from the outside world. In large diving vessels several of these chambers can be connected so that the largest diving systems can now hold up to

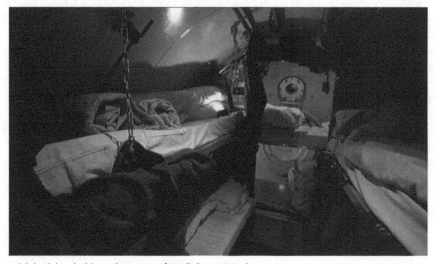

Figure A4.1 Living habitat. Courtesy of Well Ops UK Ltd.

24 divers at a time. While it is possible to introduce small medical instruments, equipment, and medication into the habitat with ease, the provision of advanced medical care within a diving habitat is severely limited, not least because medical personnel will usually need to be transported to the site by helicopter.

AMEDs should therefore always consider in their assessments the 'safety critical' nature and isolation of saturation diving, which to a degree can apply to all commercial diving.

Diving medical examination and training of medical practitioners

Before medical practitioners can apply to the HSE for approval to conduct commercial diving medical examinations they must attend a dedicated training course. This initial 5-day training course covers basic diving physics, physiology, and diving medicine. Once approved, an AMED should participate in at least 2 days of refresher training for every 5 years of practice. AMEDs should also aim to conduct a minimum of 10 examinations per year in order to maintain their competency and ongoing approval.

HSE has implemented a moratorium on new approvals since September 2010 (status February 2012),[5] leading to concern about the future viability of centres of diving medical excellence to advise the industry.

In comparison to the current situation in the UK, the European Diving Technology Committee (EDTC) and other international groups have proposed that commercial divers should only be examined by physicians with a minimum level of training and/or qualification in occupational medicine. However, it is recognized that many specialists outside the field of occupational medicine will also need to play a role in assessing the health of divers.

Examination and diver fitness certification mechanism

Advice for AMEDs regarding 'the medical examination and assessment of divers (MA1)' is available from HSE's website. The latest edition, published in December 2011,[6] is substantially similar to that published in 2005. The MA1 provides administrative advice and a framework for the fitness assessment. AMEDs need at all times to maintain detailed documentation, justifying their judgements and decisions.

On initial approval the AMED will receive a number of carbon copy medical examination documentation forms (MA2 forms). The first two pages of the form record the diver's and the doctor's details and the outcome of the fitness assessment. They need to be returned to the HSE's diving section within 7 days of finalizing the examination. The AMED can also issue a temporarily unfit or otherwise restricted certificate, for instance, to allow further investigations to take place. The standard rules for informed consent for disclosure of medical information to the HSE will apply.

A detailed examination is important, with particular emphasis on the cardiopulmonary, nervous, and musculoskeletal systems. The diver should receive a completed copy of the HSE MA2 and should bring this to their next diving medical examination, failing which an AMED should refuse to examine the diver. Continuity of information is essential.

A certificate of fitness to dive is valid for a maximum of 12 months. It is strongly recommended that the AMED retains in the medical file, a copy of the previous MA2 presented to them by the diver.

International context and reciprocity of medical certificates within Europe

The medical subcommittee of EDTC, an international forum of diving interested medical practitioners, has published guidelines for medical assessment of working divers.[7] The Diving Medical Advisory Committee (DMAC), under the secretarial umbrella of the International Marine Contractors Association (IMCA), is a voluntary group of international medical practitioners which produces advice aimed at the diving industry.[8] In 2009, the DMAC produced a position statement in collaboration with the EDTC regarding the required fitness expectations and suitable exercise framework for commercial divers.[9]

The HSE accepts reciprocity of dive certificates with some European countries as issued by 'approved' classes of medical practitioners.[5] Commercial diving is an international business in which MA2 fitness to dive certificates, as issued by UK-based AMEDs, are accepted by many employers worldwide.

Examination—process considerations

The first examination of an aspiring diver is critically important in setting the right mindset in relation to the medical and fitness requirements. At this exam the diver must confirm their previous medical history with a general practitioner (GP)-signed health questionnaire. An example of the minimum dataset is provided at the end of the HSE MA1 guidance.

The MA1 guidance does not separately differentiate the physical requirements and levels of fitness of male and female divers. Particularly in relation to the physical fitness test and percentage body fat measurements, this is unrealistic and could potentially discriminate against female divers. In practice this does not appear to cause a major problem considering that saturation, offshore, and inshore civil/construction diving are almost exclusively male domains, whereas in scientific, media, aquarium, shellfish/clam, or police/fire and rescue diving more female divers can be found.

Where an AMED is in doubt whether or not full ability for all possible diving activities is present, they are able to issue a dive certificate that is restricted to a particular category of diving.

The MA1 details a diver's right of appeal. Missing clinical information or expert medical opinion must be obtained; however, this should be sorted at the AMED examination stage and at cost to the diver rather than through an appeal to the HSE. For peer support and informal expert opinion and advice AMEDs can consult the UK Sport Diving Medical Committee and join its discussion forum: 'the UK Diving Medical Community' (UKDMC).[10] This is a voluntary affiliation of medical practitioners with an interest in recreational and/or commercial diving medicine.

Medical examination

The medical examination of divers follows the same template as any other medical examination. Given the safety critical nature of diving and the fact that working under water can affect many organ systems, the examination has to be thorough and detailed. This should be appropriately reflected in the health questionnaire, the clinical examination, communication with other health professionals, the regular calibration of instruments, and in the auditable way in which the AMED reaches a judgement.

Investigations that are required as a minimum are detailed in the MA1. At follow-up examination a full blood count is not required and the need for a resting electroencephalogram (ECG) may be determined by clinical indication. As a minimum, however, ECG recording should start again at age 40 in at least 5-yearly intervals. Appropriate investigations can be performed outside of these minimum requirements as clinically indicated.

Routine radiology of the lungs and/or long bones has not proven to be of value and should only be undertaken when a clear clinical indication can be identified.

Obesity

Obesity is increasingly common and strongly associated with poor physical fitness and poor general health. It is also thought to moderately increase the risk of decompression illness (DCI), largely on the theoretical basis, that more body fat could store more inert gas and therefore cause a higher gas load in the body at depth and a higher bubble load during decompression.

Therefore, and because of its general link to poor physical fitness, obesity should be viewed critically when assessing fitness to dive. However, body mass index (BMI) (weight in kg/height in m²) alone is a poor descriptor of body morphology and adiposity, and use of BMI in HSE's MA1 guidance came under intense international criticism at a diving conference in 2011.[11] It was recommended that an individual's BMI measurement should be supplemented by waist circumference or skin calliper measurements, to identify more precisely which divers are overweight or obese with a given BMI value. A fuller discussion can be found in the relevant National Institute for Health and Clinical Excellence guidelines.[12]

Where doubt about continued fitness arises, the issuing of time-restricted certificates of less than 12 months, detailed advice to the diver, and/or referral to their GP for further input and support may be appropriate.

Background to the physical fitness requirements of divers and other safety critical work

Diving is an inherently dangerous activity where the margins for error are small. For example, at a recent diving conference, an HSE inspector reported eight fatal incidents under investigation, five of which were in commercial divers. The fitness assessment of commercial divers aims to ascertain whether or not a diver has sufficient physical and mental reserves to deal with emergency situations. An American study of fire and rescue workers showed that 45 per cent of fatalities on duty were caused by cardiovascular events, mainly coronary heart disease, rather than from smoke inhalation.[13]

The HSE MA1 requirement for an aerobic capacity of 13 metabolic equivalents (METs) or 45 mL/kg/min of oxygen consumption for young and fit divers appears to have been derived from early Navy research. Although 45 mL/kg/min VO₂max still seems a reasonable requirement at the start of a diving career, it is clear that as divers age, many will have difficulty meeting this standard.

Various other high metabolically demanding and/or safety critical occupations such as the Emergency Response Team function in the offshore industry and in the fire and rescue services in the UK[14] also support specific physical fitness requirements.

The question is where should one draw the line for the still permissible fitness performance for commercial divers, taking into account any diving restrictions?

Controversy surrounding exercise testing

Differences of opinion exist within the different specialist groups involved in the medical assessment of divers. Discussions centre on the wisdom of exercise testing by AMEDs, to what level, and by what method. Some advocate that these tests are performed in the working setting. However, most commercial divers are self-employed and there is at present no system that could be used to run these tests in an appropriate real-life setting.

Exercise testing is also associated with potentially serious and even fatal health risks. Difference of opinion exists as to how these risks should best be managed in occupational health practice. Pre-exercise risk screening questionnaires have been criticized, given the obvious possibility of biased reporting when continued work depends on receiving a fitness certificate. Indeed the best predictor for conducting a safe exercise capacity test is ongoing regular exercise.[15,16] A very large study reported 17 deaths and 96 severe complications during or subsequent to exercise testing among 700 000 patients but no incidents from exercise testing among a group of 350 000 sports people.[17]

We are firmly of the opinion that robust aerobic fitness capacity of divers contributes significantly to the in-water safety of the whole dive team. In our opinion it is appropriate to include a robust, safe, and repeatable exercise capacity test in the fitness to dive medical examination. In view of the UK-agreed reciprocity with several other European countries, the question is, how best to integrate this requirement into the UK setting?

HSE's recommended practice for exercise testing

The last substantive revision of the MA1 occurred in 2005, after the HSE conducted an expert workshop on exercise testing in 2004.[17] Now the MA1 states that an 'appropriate protocol for testing and calculation of VO_2max must be followed in a standardized manner'. This should have moved all AMEDs away from less consistent and less reliable step tests that would not report in VO_2max. In his 02/2007 AMED newsletter,[18] the HSE diving medical advisor further expanded on this point and proposed to use ' . . . the Chester step test or other tests that are incremental, and allow pulse and/or ECG measurements during the exercise, and which measure VO_2max indirectly' as the recommended minimum protocol to determine aerobic capacity.

The Chester step test is a specific example of a graded (incremental) exercise step test protocol that is widely used in the UK. It is thought to be substantially safer and more accurate than constant speed step test protocols that rely on post-recovery heart rate measurement. These have a poor correlation with true VO_2max.

Although the absolute accuracy of the Chester step test has a standard error estimated to be 12–15 per cent,[19] the intrapersonal repeatability appears to be acceptable. Detecting changes in fitness over a diving career as measured with the same screening test by all AMEDs may be of greater benefit than the absolute accuracy of the result. For an overview of exercise and step test physiology see the relevant literature.[20-22]

Recommended benchmarks for aerobic capacity testing in divers

The current MA1 guidance of an exercise level equivalent to 13 METS or 45 mL/kg/min (lean body mass) oxygen consumption is thought to be unrealistically high in aging and/or overweight divers. At an international conference, the alternative safety limit of at least 12 METS or approximately 42 mL/kg/min was proposed. Byrne et al. have shown that the accepted conversion of MET in VO_2 (1 MET = 3.5 mL/kg/min O_2 consumption) may overestimate the actual resting VO_2 on average by 35 per cent and that the greatest variance occurs in people with a high percentage of body fat.[23] Consequently, the use of the MET system could overestimate energy expenditure in individuals with a high BMI due to adiposity.

HSE's audit experience of AMEDs (R.H., personal communication) suggests that confusion and inconsistencies exist over what to do when divers perform below this benchmark. For established divers it would seem prudent to start issuing time- and/or dive activity-restricted certificates at an exercise capacity result equal or lower than 42 mL/kg/min VO$_2$max, as measured with an appropriate exercise test. Alternatively, a direct VO$_2$max determination in a physiology laboratory under closely monitored conditions could investigate an unexpected low performance with a step test. Where doubt remains, divers should be excluded from diving until their aerobic capacity has improved sufficiently.

Safeguards for aerobic capacity testing

The MA1 has revised the safety precautions needed to support safe aerobic capacity testing. The testing is estimated to cause 1 in 2500 to 1 in 10 000 cases of myocardial infarction or death in patients with coronary artery disease.[24] The residual risk in apparent asymptomatic divers requires AMEDs to conduct a specific risk assessment for their particular circumstances. This risk assessment should include their practice location, accessibility, and egress in case of emergency and their access to qualified emergency personnel and relevant equipment. AMEDs should note the guidance from the Resuscitation Council UK regarding cardiopulmonary resuscitation.[25]

Exercise testing with a step test in the occupational practice is rarely monitored with an ECG. To exclude post-exercise arrhythmias, AMEDs should consider repeating the ECG after the exercise test or capture a single lead rhythm ECG afterwards. This is the recommended approach in the Norwegian guidelines.[26]

Introduction to organ-specific observations

Fundamental to the understanding the effects of gas and water pressure on the different organ systems and the body is an appreciation of the gas laws and the physiological changes caused by hydrostatic pressure and gas pressures. These are part of the training of AMEDs and are explained in detail in relevant textbooks. Suffice it to say that barotrauma effects can occur during descent and ascent, and that hydrostatic pressure causes significant fluid shifts from the periphery into the body core with associated rise in blood pressure and cardiac stroke volume. The gas laws (Boyle's inverse relationship between volume and absolute pressure) dictate that the most significant changes in gas expansion occur during the first and last 10 metres of descending and surfacing respectively.

The following sections should be read in conjunction with the HSE MA1 and other texts such as the EDTC *Fitness to Dive Standards*.[7] The purpose here is to cover only the most frequently encountered issues. Where indicated, the AMED must communicate clearly with the consultant to whom he refers the diver. Most specialists do not work in the field of diving medicine and will not necessarily understand all the nuances.

Communicable diseases

The medical examiner should be satisfied that the diver is not suffering from an infectious disease. Where there is doubt whether a person is infectious, then further assessment and referral should be made to a medical microbiologist or specialist in infectious diseases. Ongoing communicable diseases would probably bar a worker from diving until resolution because good hygiene practices are more difficult in a diving environment.

Psychiatric assessment

Evidence of psychological states that might affect the safety of the diver or others in the water must be sought. Diving itself will impose a specific stress, depending upon the type of work, its location, and the operational risks involved. Living and working for significant periods of time (up to a month in the UK) in a saturation chamber system will also bring its own psychological stresses. Divers should be free from psychiatric illness or impairment of cognitive function.

Alcohol or drug dependence would normally be a bar from diving unless there has been a period of abstinence of at least 1 year for alcohol and 3 years for drugs, off medication and without relapse while under continuous monitoring by a competent health professional. Detailed evidence from treatment facilities, current psychological and/or psychiatric assessment, including ongoing drug screening, may be required before a return to commercial diving can be allowed.

A detailed referral for an opinion from a psychiatrist should be obtained in cases of doubt. This referral must explain the nature of the work involved.

Respiratory system

The integrity of the respiratory system is vital for diving. The British Thoracic Society has produced guidelines for the examination of fitness to dive.

Any condition that might compromise gas exchange, or exercise response must be sought. Any abnormality that may cause air trapping and could lead to barotrauma on ascent from depth should be investigated. Pulmonary barotrauma represents escape of air from the lung/alveoli into various other anatomical structures and can lead to pneumothorax, pneumomediastinum or arterial gas embolism or any combination of these. Right-to-left shunting in the lung circulation, for instance, from arterio-venous malformations, can circumvent the normal filter function of the lung with the potential for increased risk of bubbles crossing from the right to the left circulation with an increased risk of decompression illness.

Clinical assessment of the chest and pulmonary function testing should also be normal. When variations from normal are found, AMEDs should, where necessary, clarify these with peers or arrange appropriate referral. However, the routine taking of chest X-rays seldom contributes to the detection of relevant pathology and should only be undertaken if there is a clear clinical indication and specialist support.

Approach to assessment of lung function

Routine spirometry is required. The target should be a forced expiratory volume in 1 second (FEV_1) of greater than 80 per cent of predicted and greater than 70 per cent of predicted FEV_1/forced vital capacity (FVC) ratio. An exercise test should not cause a drop of more than 15 per cent of predicted FEV_1 after exercise. Post-exercise peak flow measurements are required according to the MA2 examination form and may assist in identifying exercise-induced asthma. Where required, the AMED should also consider more formal exercise testing, which may include testing in a cold environment to exclude cold-induced asthma.

Asthma

Safety to dive in those with asthma is controversial. There is no convincing evidence that asthma is a significant cause of pulmonary barotraumas, but careful initial assessment is necessary in a new candidate. Those with asthma induced by cold, exercise, or emotion are barred from diving. Diving may be permitted for asthmatics who are at either step 1 or step 2 of the BTS Asthma

Guidelines. GPs have recently started to implement step 3 of the British Thoracic Society's guidance, involving combination therapy of long-acting β_2-agonists and anti-inflammatory medication, at a much earlier point in the patient's treatment. In this situation if diving is still thought to be possible, it is recommended that AMEDs only take such a decision in consultation with the diver's GP and possibly a respiratory specialist with an interest in diving.

Cardiovascular system

This organ system is the one which is the most complex and which stimulates the most debate. The basic rules are outlined within the MA1, but the UKDMC forum is a useful place to debate the nuances of interpretation and to discuss each case individually.

A history, or finding on examination, of any type of heart disease including septal defects, cardiomyopathies, ischaemic heart disease, valvular disease, shunts, and dysrhythmias, except for sinus arrhythmia and infrequent ventricular extrasystoles not related to exercise, should lead to certification of unfitness for diving and the individual should be referred for a cardiological opinion assuming they wish to pursue diving. The cardiologist should have knowledge of diving medicine.

Patent foramen ovale and other causes of right-to-left shunting

Patent foramen ovale (PFO) is a common condition, affecting an estimated 25 per cent of the population to some degree. Most lesions are small and appear not to introduce a significant risk of right-to-left shunting, relevant for paradoxical embolism and hence also for cross-over of bubbles during decompression in diving. The gold standard for detecting PFO is by transthoracic echocardiography, provided the correct protocol is followed by a well-trained investigator.

Screening for PFO is not routinely conducted in either the preliminary or annual medical assessments. However, where there is a history of unexplained neurological, cardiorespiratory or cutaneous decompression illness (DCI), particularly if there is also a history of migraine with aura, then transthoracic echo bubble testing should be performed under supervision of a cardiologist experienced in the procedure. The PFO can now be effectively repaired through a percutaneous approach, thereby reducing the risk of bubble transfer from the right to left circulation. This procedure carries a 1–2 per cent risk of life-threatening complications, even in experienced hands. Other conditions that permit intracardiac shunting from right to left, such as atrial septal defects, are contraindications to diving until repaired and deemed safe.

Blood pressure

Twenty-four-hour readings during daily activities or blood pressure measurements under exercise load may need to be considered to exclude significant hypertension in certain situations. Hypertension and/or left ventricular diastolic dysfunction may constitute a risk factor for developing pulmonary oedema when diving and has in rare cases been reported along with other physical activities. If in any doubt, the advice of a cardiologist with an interest in diving medicine should be sought.

The central nervous system

Assessment of the central nervous system is extremely important initially and at subsequent intervals. AMEDs should consider documenting the detail of the diver's neurological examination. The documentation on the MA2 dive certificate is not detailed enough to form the basis for future comparison of any change or as the basis for incident investigations. A diver must have no functional disturbance of motor power and sensation, coordination, level of consciousness or cognition, special senses and balance, bowel, or bladder.

Neurological symptoms of acute DCI may present with loss or alteration of sensation, or with muscular weakness. Thus, any neurological condition with these symptoms may mimic DCI and if present in a diver may greatly complicate its management.

Where there is doubt an opinion must be sought from an appropriate specialist with an interest in diving.

Ear, nose, and throat system

A history of surgery of the ear is usually a contraindication to commercial diving, and individual advice should be sought from a specialist. Stapedectomy has previously been an absolute contraindication to diving; however, recent evidence indicates that this may be too strict and that each case should be judged individually.

Visual system

Any condition that leads to reduced vision or surgical procedure or injury that could lead to secondary infection may pose a hazard in diving.

Effect of immersion on vision

As the diver goes deeper, progressively less light from the surface arrives at depth. Only 20 per cent of available surface light is perceived when at 10 metres of sea water (msw) and this can be made worse by backscatter from suspended silt and particles. Colour vision is also progressively lost; reds disappear at 10 msw and at 30 msw only blues and greens remain. Most commercial diving for inspection or construction purposes will, however, use artificial light to compensate for darkness at depth. The full-face mask or helmet reduces the visual field considerably and the air/mask interface causes distortion, such that objects appear about one-quarter nearer and magnified by about one-third.

Corneal corrective surgery

Myopic correction may now be accomplished in a number of surgical ways. As these procedures are increasingly used, more is known about the effects of this type of surgery in terms of success rates, healing times and complication rates. Communication between the AMED and treatment facility should clarify these details. The Divers Alert Network provides some relevant information.

Dental

Dental care is important. Scuba divers need to be able to retain a mouthpiece. Dental caries and periodontal disease need to be treated. Unattached dentures should be removed during diving. Changes in pressure can cause pain in teeth or exploding fillings, due to small pockets of air or gas being trapped within the tooth. It is therefore recommended that divers see a dentist every 6 months to maintain a high standard of dental health. Ideally they should be able to (and encouraged to) produce evidence of these consultations at each diving medical. If in doubt, the AMED should issue a temporary unfit dive certificate until a certificate of dental fitness is obtained.

Endocrine system

Most endocrine conditions are contraindications to professional diving. However, well-controlled hypothyroidism is acceptable. It is sensible to obtain evidence of this control and to ensure there are no secondary organ complications.

Diabetes mellitus of any type and controlled by any means has until recently been a contraindication to diving. Since the last substantive revision of the MA1 in 2005, there are possibilities for people with diabetes to gain work within the diving industry.

Diving under close supervision in a pool, aquarium, very sheltered inland waters, or even as a sport diving instructor (for example) may be acceptable in some cases. The AMED should discuss each potential case with an appropriate Diving Medical Specialist with a specific interest in this area. Consultation with the diver's treating physician is required to ascertain the facts of each case. It is clearly appropriate to ensure that the potential diver's diabetic control and level of fitness have been good for some time and that there is no end-organ damage. Should the diver be passed fit with restrictions, his level of care and control must be monitored regularly. Ongoing consultation should regularly occur between the AMED, the diver's treating physician, and the Diving Medical Specialist.

Gastrointestinal system

Active peptic ulceration is not compatible with diving, but the relapse rate after a course of *triple therapy* is sufficiently low to allow return to air diving. However, objective evidence of ulcer healing and symptom resolution is required. Saturation diving, given its long periods of isolation and potentially stressful environment, is unlikely to be appropriate.

Asymptomatic cholelithiasis may not be problematic. However, saturation diving would be unsuitable and the same may apply to all types of diving depending on the remoteness of the location. Chronic hepatic disease requires specialist assessment.

Stomas need to be individually assessed and free draining ones are compatible with diving. 'Continent' ones requiring a catheter to relieve pressure are not compatible with diving. However, stomas may not be suitable for saturation diving for social reasons, rather than medical ones, associated with living in confined spaces with other divers.

Dermatological system

Integrity of the skin is important for the diver. Immersion, use of diving suits and equipment, and raised temperature and humidity of saturation diving chambers can lead to skin damage and risk of secondary infection. Professional divers are at increased risk of infections of hands, ear canals, facial skin, and the most prevalent infection in saturation diving, *Pseudomonas aeruginosa*. The confined and easily contaminated living space, high temperature, high humidity, and a hyperoxic atmosphere significantly contribute to the risk of bacterial skin contamination. Fungal infections of the skin are not uncommon and may require repeated treatment.

Haematological system

Blood dyscrasias, even in remission, will usually be cause for rejection and polycythaemia will increase the risk of acute DCI. Coagulation disorders are incompatible with diving. Divers who have had splenectomy are at an increased risk of overwhelming infection from *Pseudomonas* and are not fit for saturation diving.

Malignancy

After conclusion of treatment, cases of malignancy should be individually assessed for factors affecting in-water safety and fitness to dive. If involved in saturation diving then suitability for an extended stay in an isolated environment needs to be assessed. Ongoing or intermittent chemotherapy, liable to compromise the immune system, would bar patients from working in saturation diving and possibly other types of diving. Fitness certificates and any restriction need to be carefully considered and documented. Regular and frequent reviews of the diver's fitness are required. Full involvement of the diver's treating physician is appropriate.

The disabled diver

The question of a disabled diver requiring an MA2 AMED examination is mostly raised within the context of recreational instruction diving, or after a return to work diving medical following a previous accident. In most instances divers with obvious impairments would find it very difficult to gain employment in the wider dive industry. Although it is sometimes suggested that the Equality Act 2010 should also be considered, it seems unlikely that an employer would be able to make a 'reasonable adjustment' for an impairment of a diver if that could lead to an increase in risk for the rest of the dive team. In practice, the employer and the dive team will have to be able to compensate for any diminished work capacity of a disabled diver, including emergency egress. It is important to assess individuals in conjunction with their proposed work as divers. The assessment should include the individual's ability to look after themselves and others in the water and should also consider the overall safety of the dive team. Full details of the restriction regarding the type of diving and other safety considerations should be recorded on the diving medical certificate. Peer discussions before issuing a certificate of fitness to dive may be required.

Return to diving after acute decompression illness

This is well documented within the MA1 and is discussed in DMAC guidance. It is recommended that all cases of DCI in a diver are reviewed by the AMED and/or a diving medical specialist to consider the need to further assess the diver for potential predisposing causes.

Long-term health effects

There has been much consideration of long-term effects but so far the only proven and potentially disabling condition is dysbaric osteonecrosis. This can, in most cases, be prevented through safe diving practice in the now standard procedures for regulated professional diving. Magnetic resonance imaging scanning is the most sensitive method of investigation

Aberdeen University has conducted a study called the Examination of Long Term Health Impact of diving (ELTHI). Overall, the ELTHI study did not identify any long-term health effects associated with professional diving that amounted to clinical abnormality compared to matched off-shore workers, although the complaint of 'forgetfulness or loss of concentration' was associated with significant impairment of health-related quality of life. The only factor that appeared to unexpectedly amplify any symptoms experienced by divers was the occupation of welding, albeit that the number of welders in the group was too small to draw definitive conclusions.

Hyperbaric chamber workers

The DWR covers the use of hyperbaric chambers within diving projects. People who may be routinely subjected to hyperbaric conditions need to have the same level of medical fitness. Hyperbaric chambers in hospitals are not covered by the DWR but the British Hyperbaric Association recommends that medical attendants working in such chambers undergo medical examinations and that the standards are similar to those for professional divers. As a general rule, employers should not examine their own staff for fitness to enter into the chamber. This could likely be taken as a potential conflict of interest and could introduce bias on behalf of both parties.

Summary

The statutory diving medical examination is designed to exclude factors that might affect the diver's ability to work safely under water. In addition the examination has a strong emphasis on the need to avoid danger to others, which clearly defines diving as a safety critical activity. Finally, the long-term health effects on divers should be monitored by comparing the results of each year's examination.

Divers have a legal obligation to declare any factor, of which they are aware, that might affect their own personal safety prior to every dive and the employer or diving contractor has the responsibility for ensuring that a diving operation is carried out in as safe a manner as is reasonably practicable.

The HSE rightly continues to require safe diving practices, the appropriate training of HSE AMEDs, and a high quality of medical assessment of commercial divers.

One of the main reasons HSE called for an expert workshop on exercise testing for divers in 2004 was the realization that 'significant variation existed between AMEDs in the way that they carry out and interpret the results of exercise tests for the diving medical'. This situation seems to have continued.

It is beyond the scope of this chapter to arbitrate over the optimal screening test for aerobic capacity testing in general AMED practice and whether it should only be performed within the AMED framework for certifying fitness to dive. This debate is likely to continue for some time. In the meantime the AMED community as a group should seek and agree the best current practice and attempt to implement this for the benefit of the diver and the diving industry as a whole.

Acknowledgement

We thank D. Bracher and N. K. I. McIver who prepared the chapter in the previous edition.

References

1 The Diving at Work Regulations 1997, SI 1997/2776.

2 Health and Safety Executive. *Diving in benign conditions, and in pools, tanks, aquariums and helicopter underwater escape training.* HSE Information sheet No 8. [Online] (<http://www.hse.gov.uk/pubns/dvis8.pdf>)

3 Health and Safety Executive. Approved codes of practice for the Diving at Work Regulations 1997: <http://www.hse.gov.uk/diving/acop.htm>

4 Opito training requirements for worksite placements (industry standards): <http://www.opito.com/uk/entry-requirements.html>.

5 Health and Safety Executive. Diving pages: (<http://www.hse.gov.uk/diving/index.htm>)

6   Health and Safety Executive. *The medical examination and assessment of divers (MA1)*. [Online] (<http://www.hse.gov.uk/diving/ma1.pdf>)

7   The European Diving Technology Committee. *Fitness to dive standards. Guidelines for medical assessment of working divers*. [Online] (<http://www.edtc.org/Fitness%20to%20dive.htm>)

8   Diving Medical Advisory Committee: <http://www.dmac-diving.org/>

9   The Diving Medical Advisory Committee. *DMAC statement on exercise testing in medical assessment of commercial divers*, October 2009. [Online] (<http://www.dmac-diving.org/guidance/DMAC-Statement-200910.pdf>)

10 UK Sports Diving Medical Committee. Discussion forum for recreational examiners and AMEDs. Available via the secretariat for registered medical practitioner members only: <http://www.uksdmc.co.uk/>

11 UKSDMC Diving Medicine Conference, 18–19 November 2011, Bristol Royal Infirmary.

12 National Institute for Health and Clinical Excellence. *Quick reference guide 2 for the NHS*, 2006. [Online] (<http://www.nice.org.uk/nicemedia/live/11000/30364/30364.pdf>)

13 Kales SN, Soteriades ES, Christophi CA, *et al.* Emergency duties and deaths from heart disease among firefighters in the United States. *New Engl J Med* 2007; **356**: 1207–15.

14 FireFit Steering committee. *Testing physical capability in the UK Fire & Rescue Service. Review and recommendations.* [Online] (<http://www.firefitsteeringgroup.co.uk/richard.pdf>)

15 Kokkinos P, Myers J, Peter J, *et al.* Exercise capacity and mortality in black and white men. *Circulation* 2008; **117**: 614–22.

16 Peterson P, Magid D, Ross C, *et al.* Association of exercise capacity on treadmill with future cardiac events in patients referred for exercise testing. *Arch Intern Med* 2008; **168**: 174–9.

17 Smith JS, Evans G. *HSE workshop on exercise testing for divers, 19 April 2004*. Sheffield: Health & Safety Laboratory, 2004. (<http://www.hse.gov.uk/research/hsl_pdf/2004/hsl0410.pdf>)

18 AMED newsletters. Available from the HSE Corporate Medical Unit at HQ in Bootle at amed@hse.gov.uk

19 Syres K. *The Chester aerobic fitness tests: assist physiological measurement resource manual*. Wrexham: Fitness Assist, 2005. (<http://www.fitnessassist.co.uk>)

20 Katch V, McArdle W, Katch F. *Essentials of exercise physiology*, 4th edn. Philadelphia, PA: Lippincott Williams and Wilkins, 2010.

21 American Heart Association. Exercise standards for testing and training: a statement for healthcare professionals from the American Heart Association. *Circulation* 2001; 104; 1694–740. (<http://www.circ.ahajournals.org>)

22 American Heart Association. Exercise standards—a statement for healthcare professionals. *Circulation* 1995; **91**: 580. (<http://www.circ.ahajournals.org>)

23 Byrne NM, Hills AP, Hunter GR, *et al.* Metabolic equivalent: one size does not fit all. *J Appl Physiol* 2005; **99**: 1112–19.

24 Glen S. Exercise testing for divers. Presentation at UK SDMC conference, Shrewsbury, 23–4 March, 2006.

25 Resuscitation Council (UK) guidelines: <http://www.resus.org.uk/SiteIndx.htm>

26 Statens Helsetilsyn. [The Norwegian Board of Health]. *Norwegian guidelines for medical examination of occupational divers*. Oslo: Statens Helsetilsyn. (<http://www.helsetilsynet.no/upload/Publikasjoner/veiledningsserien/guideline_examination_divers_ik-2708.pdf>)

Further reading

Bove AA (ed.). *Bove and Davis' diving medicine*, 4th edn. Philadelphia, PA: WB Saunders, 2005.

Brubakk AO, Neuman TS (eds). *Bennett and Elliott's physiology and medicine of diving*, 5th edn. London: Saunders, Elsevier Science Ltd, 2003.

Edmonds C, Lowry C, Pennefather J, *et al.* (eds). *Diving and subaquatic medicine*, 4th edn. London: Arnold, 2002.

Fife C, St. Leger Dowse M (eds). *Women and pressure. Diving and altitude*. Flagstaff, AZ: Best Publishing 2010.

General aspects of fitness for work overseas

Dipti Patel

Introduction

Overseas travel is a common feature of employment. An estimated 12 per cent of UK residents travel for business and professional purposes annually and some reside overseas in the longer term.[1] The various approaches to preparation and support for an overseas assignment can be as diverse as workers' occupational backgrounds. Organizations that send employees overseas owe them a legal and moral duty of care regardless of where in the world they work. Additionally, employers have a vested interest in supporting their employees, ensuring that they are fit and adequately prepared for their overseas assignment, and that appropriate procedures are in place to take care of them if they become ill or injured. The financial costs of healthcare overseas, sickness absence, and, in extreme cases, of repatriation, can be considerable.

Epidemiology of travel-related health problems

Those travelling overseas have a higher and well-recognized risk of illness and injury. They are exposed to a variety of new cultural, psychological, physical, physiological, environmental, and microbiological challenges. Their ability to adapt and cope with these challenges is affected by many variables including their pre-existing physical, psychological, immunological, and medical health, and their personality, experience, and behaviour while overseas.

Numerous studies have considered the health of travellers. A consistent and coherent body of data in large study populations has made it possible to obtain consensus on the type of illnesses and risks experienced by different groups of travellers. These studies show that a high proportion of travellers (regardless of their reason for travel) experience health problems, with illness attack rates per trip ranging from 36 per cent to 75 per cent. Diarrhoea, upper respiratory infections, and skin disorders are the most commonly reported illnesses. Most conditions tend to be minor and self-limiting, but up to 30 per cent of affected individuals are confined to bed, 19 per cent will need to consult a doctor, and 2 per cent of cases result in hospital admission, medical repatriation, or death. Deaths are rare, the main causes being cardiovascular disease, accidents, and injuries.[2]

Research on business travellers has produced similar results, although illness rates tend to be higher and psychological problems more prominent than in holidaymakers.[3] In expatriates, in particular, illnesses, hospital admissions, injuries, violent episodes, and psychological problems are reported with higher frequency as a result of their longer stay overseas and cumulative exposure to country-related hazards.[3]

Role of occupational health departments

Occupational health (OH) departments have a key role in supporting overseas workers. The degree of involvement will vary depending on the potential hazards associated with the overseas assignment and the organization's approach to international health and safety. The approach adopted should be based on a suitable risk assessment; for example, the risks relevant to a charity sending staff to work on a long-term aid project in Latin America will differ from those for a financial service organization sending executives on short-term trips to Central Asia.

At a strategic level, OH can help ensure that clear processes and policies are in place to meet the OH needs of overseas workers, and the global nature of the organization. These could, for example, include assistance in developing a global health and safety policy, advice on disability-related adjustments, advice on healthcare and repatriation arrangements, and assistance with contingency planning for major disasters overseas (e.g. pandemics, earthquakes, tsunamis, civil unrest). At an individual level, OH input should focus on pre-travel preparation, support while overseas, and support on return home.

Pre-travel preparation

Risk assessment is a fundamental component of pre-travel preparation, and helps guide any advice and interventions offered. The risk assessment should focus on individual, occupational, and destination-related factors. Preparation should include a medical assessment of an individual's fitness to work abroad, provision of preventive advice and measures such as immunizations, malaria prophylaxis, or medical kits, and a process for managing problems identified before travel or whilst abroad.

Fitness to travel and work abroad

OH departments have a role in ensuring that an individual is fit to work overseas without risk to themselves or others. There are few data in the literature that provide evidence-based guidance on pre-travel fitness assessments for overseas workers, so individual risk assessment is important. Use can be made of a general traveller's assessment and health questionnaires, telephone enquiry, face-to-face consultation, and medical examination. The assessment should be conducted by healthcare professionals who have an understanding of occupational health in an overseas context and designed and performed in a way that allows identification of actual or potential health problems that may be problematic during the overseas assignment. It is essential that the assessment occurs well in advance of the departure date so that there is sufficient time for identified health problems to be appropriately managed. Owing to the different demands of overseas work, many employees who are considered fit to work in the UK may not be fit to do the same work overseas.

While there should be no absolute health contraindication to work overseas, certain groups of travellers are at higher risk than others of developing illness or injury whilst overseas, including those at the extremes of age, pregnant women, workers with pre-existing medical conditions, and those who are immunocompromised. In these groups, decisions should be made on a case-by-case basis, with a thorough evaluation of the risks and tailored preparation and advice.

Where pre-existing health concerns are identified, not only must the stability of the condition and any impact it has on functional ability be considered, but also the efficacy of preventive measures, the impact of travel, the overseas environment, the adequacy of local medical facilities, and in some cases the availability of medication/medical equipment. An easily managed illness in the UK can be a major challenge overseas. For example, an individual at higher risk of deep vein thrombosis may require heparin prophylaxis during long-haul air travel; someone with diabetes on insulin may find that their glucose control is affected by hot climates (due to quicker insulin absorption in warm temperatures); a pregnant woman may be limited in terms of immunizations and malaria prophylaxis; and an individual with chronic liver disease on a long-term posting may find that specialist liver facilities are not available in the host country. Therefore, for employees with pre-existing medical problems, preparation for an overseas assignment requires careful planning and informed decision-making, which may include liaison with treating doctors and, in some instances, doctors overseas.

Relevant disability or employment legislation must always be considered, but practicability and financial costs may preclude adjustments that would have been feasible in the UK.[4] The final decision on fitness for work overseas may have to be balanced against organizational needs. An organization's working policy may require individuals with particular and unique skills to travel to areas where the risk to their health is higher than would ordinarily be accepted.

Some countries impose entry restrictions (e.g. those infected with human immunodeficiency virus may be barred from working in some countries).[5]

Psychological fitness

One of the most difficult areas to assess is psychological risk, particularly for long-term or expatriate assignments. Expatriates have been shown to have a consistently higher incidence of affective and adjustment disorders, and mental health problems are one of the principal causes of premature departure and repatriation from overseas assignments.[3] Risk factors include a previous history of psychological problems, depressed mood, family history of mental ill-health, home country anxieties, physical ill health, occupational anxiety, and work stressors. In the case of work stressors, more than 40 per cent of International Red Cross expatriates reported that their mission had been more stressful than expected, mostly due to the working environment.[6] In British diplomats, the risk of ill-health was significantly higher than that in their partners, suggesting that work demands could be a contributory factor to ill health overseas.[7]

Research in the 1960s suggested that overseas performance could be predicted if in-depth psychological assessment was carried out by experienced psychiatrists or interviewers familiar with the placement environment.[8] More recent research indicates that future mental health problems are associated with a number of identifiable risk factors such as a personal or close family history of psychosis, attempted suicide, personality disorder or neurosis, one or more attendances at a psychiatric outpatient department, consultation with a general practitioner for psychological reasons, or evidence of depressed mood at assessment.[9] Consequently, a more pragmatic approach for assessing psychological risk may involve screening questionnaires, with further medical assessment and onward referral to a psychiatrist where concerns are raised.

Occupational health hazards

Conventional OH hazards also need to be considered. These may pose a challenge as such exposures may be less well controlled overseas and opportunities for, and the quality of, health surveillance may be more limited. In some cases, hazards that are no longer routinely experienced in developed countries (e.g. asbestos, benzene) may be prevalent. Patterns of work on an overseas assignment—longer working hours, isolation, and leave arrangements—may create additional health risks or aggravate pre-existing ones.

Assessment of dependants

In the case of expatriates there may also be a requirement to assess the fitness of partners and dependant children. Successful expatriate assignment often rests importantly on good family support, communication and adjustment.[10] The problems that relocation may bring for the non-working partner must be considered, particularly if they abandon a career in their home country with no overseas job in prospect. However, the perception that partners are more susceptible to decreased well-being has not been confirmed in prospective expatriate studies.[11]

Children tend to adapt well to living overseas, but may have medical or developmental conditions or educational requirements that prove more difficult to manage overseas. In many countries facilities for medical care of children are even less adequate than those for adults, and the threshold for seeking medical advice or repatriation may be correspondingly lower. Fitness considerations may pose a particular challenge both for children with pre-existing health problems and for healthy children who cannot access a suitable standard of medical care. In consequence, the organizational policy may occasionally preclude the overseas posting of children.

Travel health

Pre-travel preparation includes provision of immunizations, malaria prophylaxis, and other preventive health advice, and should be started after an individual (and if relevant, their family) is considered fit for their overseas assignment. Employees should be encouraged to organize immunizations at least 4–6 weeks in advance of their departure date to allow for completion of courses, monitoring for adverse reactions, and time to mount an adequate immune response to vaccine preventable diseases. For example, a full rabies course is given over 1 month (at 0, 7, and 21–28 days); for the Japanese encephalitis vaccine, the course should ideally be completed at least 10 days prior to departure in case of possible delayed allergic reactions; and for the typhoid vaccines immunity usually takes 2–3 weeks to develop from injection.

Detailed advice on immunizations, malaria prophylaxis, and other travel-related disease risks (e.g. traveller's diarrhoea, dengue fever) is beyond the scope of this appendix. Destination-specific requirements for travel health advice must be obtained from computerized databases. These provide the most up-to-date and valid information on the global distribution of infectious diseases and other health risks, the changing patterns of infection and drug-resistant organisms, advances in preventive measures, and the health regulations in different countries.[12,13] This information will help determine the additional immunizations needed, as a requirement of entry into a country (e.g. yellow fever vaccine), or recommended to counter endemic infections at the destination (e.g. hepatitis A vaccine). Similarly, it will help inform malaria prevention choices and advice on other protective measures.

Support while overseas

The cost of healthcare overseas can be high. For example, the cost of an air ambulance from the East coast of the USA can be up to £45 000, air-ambulance evacuation from the Canary Islands can cost up to £16 000, and repatriation on a scheduled flight, on a stretcher with a doctor escort from Australia, can cost up to £20 000 at the time of writing.[14] Additionally, the medical (and dental) facilities in some parts of the world can be basic. It is vital, therefore, to ensure that adequate arrangements (including medical insurance cover) are in place to deal with medical and dental emergencies, which may extend to repatriation. Such arrangements must include the mechanism by which the costs of local care can be met, as in most countries medical care has to be purchased and, in many places payment, or guarantee of payment, is required before admission to hospital can be arranged or treatment commenced.

For expatriates or long-term assignees, arrangements should also include access to routine non-urgent medical care, including cover for pre-existing medical conditions. Additional considera-tion needs to be given to the provision of OH support and employee assistance programmes for this group. If dependants accompany the employee, then their medical needs will also need to be addressed.

Importantly, employees must be familiar with medical cover arrangements and medical evacu-ation processes, regardless of whether they are travelling on a brief business trip or are on long-term assignment. The emergency evacuation of a sick employee is often a hazardous experience for the patient and an expensive, worrying, and time-consuming exercise for those organizing repatriation.

Return to the UK

The overseas worker should be advised of the possible need for follow-up after travel. This may arise in the context of an acute illness, screening of asymptomatic travellers, and OH support.

The ill returned traveller

Prompt and effective treatment of travel-related illnesses reduces morbidity and mortality, and (for infectious diseases) reduces the risk of transmission to the community. OH departments do not generally manage acute illness, but are a point of contact for returned employees and can signpost them to sources of further medical care. Frequently the first port of call will be the indi-vidual's general practitioner and a number of algorithms are available to support decision-making when dealing with the common illnesses in returned travellers.[15] In some situations (e.g. febrile travellers returning from the tropics), referral to an infectious/tropical disease hospital will be a more suitable option.

Screening of asymptomatic travellers

Post-travel screening remains a contentious area, but in a UK study of a cohort of travellers who had been in the tropics or subtropics for at least 3 months, it was found that potentially serious asymptomatic infection was common (e.g. schistosomiasis).[16] A number of algorithms are avail-able to assist healthcare professionals assessing the asymptomatic traveller.[15]

Occupational health follow-up

OH follow-up may be required as part of a return-to-work plan for those who have significant ill-ness, injury, or exposure (physical or psychological) while overseas. Long-term assignees require specific attention as, for some individuals, readjustment to home life can be difficult. In a study of aid workers, 75 per cent reported difficulty in readjusting, 33 per cent felt disorientated, and 73 per cent felt inadequately supported on their return.[17] In another study, of returned aid workers, 46 per cent reported psychological difficulties. Of these, 87 per cent had depression, 7 per cent chronic fatigue, and 4 per cent post-traumatic stress disorder.[18]

Conclusion

Travel-related health problems are common, but adequate preparation and support can reduce the risk of illness and injury in overseas workers. Careful risk assessment, appropriate and effective risk management, clear risk communication, and health education are essential.

Medical preparation for overseas working is an essential precursor that should be completed well in advance of departure and, in the case of expatriates, should include every member of the family who is travelling. The cost of such a procedure is small compared with the costs of potentially avoidable medical repatriation.

Finally, it must be remembered that many people are working abroad, often in hostile areas, without any support from well-organized parent organizations. In these circumstances, the principles in this appendix still apply, but appropriate arrangements for the provision of medical care in the event of illness become even more important.

Acknowledgements

This chapter is based in part on two articles written for *Occupational Health [at Work]* (Patel D. Workers abroad—part 1: the epidemiology of travel related illness. *Occup Health [at Work]* 2008; **5**(3): 22–6 and Patel D. Workers abroad—part 2: the role of occupational health. *Occup Health [at Work]* 2008; **5**(4): 26–30).

Useful websites

<http://www.cdc.gov/travel> Travel health advice from the US Centers for Disease Control and Prevention.

<http://www.dh.gov.uk> Official health advice including that for travel and updated chapters of the 'Green Book'.

<http://www.hpa.org.uk> Information on communicable disease and other health hazards in the UK.

<http://www.iamat.org> Access to a searchable database of English-speaking doctors throughout the world who have an interest in travel medicine and have committed to assist travellers in need of medical care.

<http://www.nathnac.org/pro/index.htm> UK travel health information for health professionals and the public.

<http://www.who.int/en> A large international database covering all aspects of travel health including the weekly epidemiological record (WER) and outbreak news.

References

1 Barnes W, Smith R. *Travel trends 2010*. London: Office for National Statistics, 2010.

2 Reid D, Keystone, JS, Cossar JH. Health abroad; general considerations. In: DuPont HL, Steffen R (eds), *Textbook of travel medicine and health*, 2nd edn, pp. 3–10. Ontario: BC Decker Inc, 2001.

3 Patel D. Occupational travel. *Occup Med* 2011; **61**: 6–183.

4 *Cordell* v. *Foreign and Commonwealth office*. UKEAT/0016/11/SM.

5 The Global Database on HIV related travel restrictions: <http://hivtravel.org/>

6 Dahlgren AL, Deroo L, Avril J, *et al.* Health risks and risk-taking behaviors among International Committee of the Red Cross (ICRC) expatriates returning from humanitarian missions. *J Travel Med* 2009; **16**(6): 382–90.

7 Patel D, Easmon C, Seed P, *et al.* Morbidity in expatriates—a prospective cohort study. *Occup Med* 2006; **56**(5): 345–52.

8 Gamble K, Lovell D, Lankester T, *et al.* Aid workers, expatriates and travel. In: Zuckerman J (ed), *Principles and practice of travel medicine*, pp. 449–50. Chicester: Wiley, 2001.

9 Foyle M. Expatriate mental health. *Acta Psychiatr Scand* 1998; **97**: 278–83.

10 Caliguri PM, Hyland MM, Joshi A, *et al.* Testing a theoretical model for examining the relationship between family adjustment and expatriates' work adjustment. *J Appl Psychol* 1998; **83**: 598–614.

11 Anderzen I. *The internationalization of work. Psychophysiological, predictors of adjustment to foreign assignment.* Stockholm: Karolinska Institute 1998.

12 Leggat PA. Risk assessment in travel medicine. *Travel Med Infect Dis* 2006; **4**(3–4): 127–34.

13 Keystone JS, Kozarsky PE, Freedman DO. Internet and computer-based resources for travel medicine practitioners. *Clin Infect Dis* 2001; **32**: 757–65.

14 Foreign and Commonwealth Office. *Travel insurance advice.* [Online] (<http://www.fco.gov.uk/en/travelling-and-living-overseas/staying-safe/travel-insurance/>)

15 Field VF, Ford L, Hill DR (eds). *Health information for overseas travel.* London: National Travel health Network and Centre, London, 2010.

16 Whitty CJM, Carroll B, Armstrong M, *et al.* Utility of history, examination and laboratory tests in screening those returning to Europe from the tropics for parasitic infection. *Trop Med Int Health* 2000; **5**(11): 818–23.

17 Macnair R. *Room for improvement: the engagement and support of relief and development workers.* London: Overseas Development Institute, 1995.

18 Lovell DM. *Psychological adjustment amotjeng returned overseas aid workers.* DClinPsy Thesis, University of Wales, 1997.

Further reading

Centers for Disease Control and Prevention (CDC). *CDC health information for international travel.* New York: Oxford University Press, 2012. (<http://www.cdc.gov/yellowbook>)

Chiodini P, Hill D, Lalloo D, *et al. Guidelines for malaria prevention in travellers from the United Kingdom.* London: Health Protection Agency, 2007. (<http://www.hpa.org.uk/infections/topics_az/malaria/guidelines.htm>)

Department of Health (Joint Committee on Vaccination and Immunisation). *Immunisation against infectious diseases.* London: HMSO, 2006.

Field V, Ford L, Hill DR. *Health Information for overseas travel.* London: National Travel Health Network and Centre, 2010.

World Health Organization (WHO). *International travel and health.* Geneva: WHO, 2012. (<www.who.int/ith/en>)

Appendix 6

Workers exposed to hand-transmitted vibration

Ian Lawson and Roger Cooke

Introduction and background

Occupational health professionals are often asked to give advice on establishing health surveillance programmes for workers exposed to hand-transmitted vibration (HTV). This appendix covers the clinical features, case assessment, and management of cases to assist in providing such advice. Prior to giving advice on health surveillance, it is imperative that the employer draws up a policy covering worker information on HTV hazards, identification and assessment of exposure, management of cases, and control measures. It is also advisable to include consultation with the company legal advisers and employee union representatives. Those advising multinational enterprises should be aware of significant differences in regional legislation and approaches to health surveillance outside the UK, touched on only briefly in this appendix.

The term hand–arm vibration syndrome (HAVS) is used to describe the constellation of symptoms resulting from exposure to HTV. The syndrome consists of three components: the sensorineural, the vascular (previously known as vibration-white finger (VWF)), and musculoskeletal effects. The diagnosis of each of these is largely dependent upon the history presented by the individual, supported by findings of clinical examination; in some cases there may be more objective evidence, such as witnessing an attack of whiteness, or more subjective evidence from sensorineural test results, demonstrating a loss of sensory perception.

The diagnosis of HAVS is primarily based upon the following:

♦ A history of relevant exposure to HTV.

♦ The presence of symptoms compatible with such a diagnosis.

♦ Exclusion of other causes of such symptoms.

A survey in Great Britain for the Health and Safety Executive (HSE) estimated that approximately 4.9 million workers were exposed to HTV. Similar European surveys in Sweden and Germany, estimated 350 000 and 6.7 million workers exposed respectively.[1,2] There are many potential sources of HTV, the common feature being tools and equipment that are capable of transmitting an external source of vibrational energy to the hand–arm system. Contrary to information provided on some websites, sources without this characteristic—such as keyboards or pianos—will not produce HAVS. The main industries with exposure involve construction and heavy engineering, but significant exposures can arise in many trades, such as construction workers, metal-working and maintenance fitters, welders, miners, foresters, shipbuilders, foundry workers, utility service workers, and gardeners.[3,4]

Relevant exposure to hand–arm vibration

Although a detailed understanding of vibration assessment techniques is not required of the occupational health professional, a rudimentary knowledge of nomenclature and the interpretation of risk assessment is necessary. Vibration magnitude is measured in terms of its acceleration, averaged by the root-mean square method. Mounted accelerometers are used to measure frequency-weighted values (a_{hw}) in three axes relative to the tool handle and these are summated to produce the 'vibration total value', as defined in ISO standard 5349-1, 2001.[5] Injury is assumed to relate to the total energy entering the hand, with a specific relation between time and vibration magnitude. Akin to the approach for noise, the dose or 'daily vibration exposure' or 'A(8)' can then be re-expressed in terms of the equivalent acceleration that would impart the same energy over an 8-hour reference period:

$$A(8) = a_{hw}\sqrt{(t/T_0)} \ (ms^{-2})$$

where:

$A(8)$ = the daily vibration exposure (8-hour energy-equivalent vibration total value or a $hw(eq(8))$).

a_{hw} = the frequency-weighted vibration total value.

t = duration of exposure in a day to the vibration a_{hw}.

T_0 = 8 hours (in the same units as t).

There is no 'safe' level of hand–arm vibration exposure, since there is considerable variation in individual susceptibility to vibration, although a daily A(8) level of 1 m/sec^2 is regarded as posing negligible risk (ISO 5349, Annex C). In the UK, the HSE uses an A(8) level of 2.5 m/sec^2 as an action level (exposure action value (EAV)), above which employers are required to introduce risk reduction measures, and introduce health surveillance.[6] This value is based on the ISO 5349 standard which refers to this magnitude of vibration producing symptoms of finger blanching in 10 per cent of exposed people after a 10-year period. By contrast, the daily A(8) which predicts the likelihood of onset of sensorineural symptoms of HAVS is uncertain.

It is generally accepted that lifetime cumulative hand–arm vibration exposure is the major determinant of onset. Both occupational and non-occupational exposures must be considered as contributory to this lifetime exposure.

When taking a history of vibration exposure, it should be noted that operators tend to overestimate the usage time of vibratory tools. It is the tool or equipment contact or 'trigger' time that is important to estimate. Workers tend to overestimate this time, which in reality is typically 50–70 per cent of their estimate. For some tools overestimation may be as high as 90 per cent.[7]

A lot of information can be obtained on possible vibration exposure from tool supplier data and formal assessments are not always necessary. Partial doses from several tools can be summed to an equivalent daily dose. Sources of data on vibration magnitudes can be found in equipment handbooks or suppliers' information sheets. Along with an estimate of hand-tool contact times these will help assess putative daily exposures. Tools may be conveniently grouped as 'high-', 'medium-', or 'low-' risk (see <http://www.hse.gov.uk/pubns/indg175. pdf>). HSE provides an exposure ready-reckoner, to estimate A(8) from exposure time and vibration magnitude (<http://www.hse.gov.uk/vibration/hav/readyreckoner.htm>), and an exposure calculator to facilitate the summation of doses from several tools (<http://www.hse. gov.uk/vibration/hav/hav.xls>).

Clinical features of HAVS and differential diagnosis

Onset of symptoms

Symptoms of HAVS develop after the exposure has begun, and usually after a number of years. The interval between first exposure and onset of symptoms, referred to as the latent interval, is primarily determined by magnitude and duration of exposure, but also influenced by individual susceptibility. This interval can range from several months to 20 or more years.

It is accepted that in some people symptoms may begin after cessation of exposure, although this may reflect change in cold exposure rather than initial development of the condition. A workshop in Stockholm[8] and the HSE guidance, *Control of Vibration at Work Regulations 2005*, took a 1-year interval as an appropriate maximum, although a national scheme that compensated mineworkers in the UK accepted symptoms developing up to 2 years after exposure had ceased.[9]

Vascular symptoms

The vascular effect of hand–arm vibration is manifest as Raynaud's phenomenon, which is episodic digital vasospasm. Although individuals may vary in their ability to report a classical triphasic history (whiteness, followed by blueness, followed by redness), the diagnosis of Raynaud's phenomenon ideally requires the following features:

- Discrete episodes, typically lasting around 20–30 minutes, with a range of a few minutes up to about an hour or so, perhaps up to 2 hours.
- An initial tingling or coldness followed by:
  - Numbness and clearly demarcated whiteness (blanching) that is uniform over the affected area, and normally extends around the circumference of the finger.
  - Whiteness that develops distally (at the tips) and spreads proximally at the start of an attack. The end of an attack is marked by return of normal colour beginning proximally. During this phase the affected area may take on a blue hue, resulting from the flow into the skin capillaries of de-oxygenated blood, probably from the venules. This blueness is described by some individuals as the only noticeable feature.
  - Return of blood to the affected area, typically with tingling, pain, sensation of swelling ('hot aches'), and a bright red discolouration (reactive hyperaemia) before the normal circulation and colour returns.

Raynaud's phenomenon also occurs naturally in some people, when it is known as primary Raynaud's phenomenon, Raynaud's syndrome, or Raynaud's disease. In the UK, about 5 per cent of males and 15 per cent or more of females are affected, but rates in other countries vary, depending on ambient climate. It is important to differentiate a history of true vasospasm, as described in the list, from simple physiological vasoconstriction as occurs with cold exposure. Some people describe a general cold sensitivity for several months before the onset of finger blanching.

Where a cause is identified it is known as secondary Raynaud's phenomenon. Hence vibration is one of the causes of secondary Raynaud's phenomenon. Other causes of Raynaud's phenomenon include: connective tissue diseases (such as scleroderma, systemic lupus erythematosus, rheumatoid arthritis), trauma following injury, frost bite, thoracic outlet syndrome, Buerger's disease and toxins, including medications (such as beta-blockers, and some cytotoxics) and chemicals at work. Raynaud's phenomenon associated with these other secondary causes is usually more severe and affects all four limbs. Primary Raynaud's affects fingers only in approximately 50 percent of cases. Recent research has shown vasospasm can also occur in the feet of those exposed to hand–arm vibration (albeit only when hands are affected), suggesting that this point of difference is not absolutely diagnostic.

The mechanism by which HTV produces Raynaud's phenomenon is not known, but it is thought to be multifactorial, with contributions from neural control, vascular wall changes, and intravascular abnormalities.

There is increasing recognition that hypothenar hammer syndrome (damage to the ulnar artery as it courses round the hamate bone) may be associated with heavy manual work, and possibly with HTV. This can be distinguished from HAVS by careful clinical assessment, including Allen's test and Doppler ultrasonography.[10]

Features suggesting that Raynaud's phenomenon may be due to HTV include:

♦ Onset and deterioration of symptoms after commencement of exposure to HTV and before 12 months after cessation of that exposure.

♦ The initial distribution of colour changes. Typically, the initial changes arising from hand–arm vibration exposure show a distribution over the hands and fingers most exposed to vibration.

♦ Stabilization or improvement of symptoms after cessation of exposure, if the condition is at an early stage.

Sensory symptoms

The neurological damage due to hand–arm vibration is thought to represent a combination of damage to mechanoreceptor nerve endings,[11] demyelinating neuropathy,[12] an increase in intra- and extra-neural connective tissue collagen, and epineural oedema. It may manifest as a peripheral digital neuropathy or a regional neuropathy, of which the commonest example is median nerve damage. The separate roles of vibration, repetitive movements, grip and push forces, non-neutral postures, and other ergonomic stressors can be difficult to distinguish when neurological symptoms appear to result from work with vibratory tools. Such disorders may be more appropriately identified as being caused by the work than by exposure to HTV per se. The effects are described separately here, although in practice they can be co-morbid and present a challenge to diagnosis as they share some common features.

Sensorineural HAVS

The damage caused to neurological structures typically causes a 'diffuse neurosensory deficit in the fingers with symptoms of numbness and/or tingling, also loss of tactile sensitivity, manual dexterity, and grip strength'.[13] In progressing to such damage, the sensorineural component of HAVS develops through a number of phases, which are identified in workers exposed to hand–arm vibration.

1 In phase one there is exposure to HTV but no symptoms (the latent interval).

2 In phase two, exposure to HTV produces symptoms of tingling and or numbness associated with vibration exposure and shortly thereafter.

3 In phase three symptoms become more protracted and constitute the sensorineural component of HAVS.

It is generally accepted that pathological damage is present in the third of these phases, but prior to the development of pathological changes, the symptoms reflect a normal physiological response to vibration. It is widely thought that symptoms of tingling and numbness lasting 20 minutes or more after tool use mark the change from a normal physiological response to development of the pathological changes that are referred to as the sensorineural component of HAVS. However, this threshold is arbitrary and based on consensus, rather than scientific knowledge on the development of pathology.

The differential diagnosis will include consideration of factors such as systemic disease, medication, and neurotoxins, although in the UK the key potential alternative diagnoses will be cervical spondylosis, when tingling and numbness of the finger is the second most common symptom (50 per cent),[14] thoracic outlet syndrome, and peripheral neuropathy due to alcohol or diabetes.

The 2005 HSE guidance[6] notes that 'numbness occurring separately from blanching is of prime interest as this may indicate the neurological component of HAVS'. The possibility of alternative causes will be raised by a history of dermatomal or peripheral nerve distribution of the neurological symptoms. Pain, tingling or numbness associated with cold exposure, or an episode of Raynaud's phenomenon suggests those symptoms have a vascular basis. Pain per se is generally not a feature of sensorineural HAVS. There remains the diagnostic problem of those presenting with intermittent tingling or numbness, not associated with colour changes, and occurring in approximately 20 per cent of presentations.

Carpal tunnel syndrome

Carpal tunnel syndrome (CTS) is the commonest of the nerve compression syndromes. It is usually regarded as arising from elevated pressure within the carpal tunnel, which has a direct effect and also interferes with capillary circulation to the median nerve leading to conduction block. If sustained, these effects may lead to demyelination and axonolysis. Additionally, it has been suggested that ischaemia of the median nerve, resulting from strain to and relative stretching of the nerve itself, causes a relatively diffuse nerve ischaemia. The pathological process in CTS associated with hand–arm vibration is less well established.

CTS is characterized by pain or paraesthesiae, or sensory loss in the median nerve distribution, and one or more of the following: Tinel's test positive, Phalen's test positive, nocturnal exacerbation of symptoms, motor loss with wasting of abductor pollicis brevis, and abnormal nerve conduction time.[15] Additional features that might support the diagnosis are absence of signs in the little finger and on the dorsum of the hand, and a history of successful surgery or steroid injection.

While the classical sensory distribution of the median nerve is the thumb, index, and middle fingers and lateral side of the ring fingers, along with a corresponding area over the palm, some patients find that all digits are affected—perhaps through a communication with the ulnar nerve in the palm or concomitant compression of the ulnar nerve in the Guyon tunnel.

There are a number of reports of an association between primary Raynaud's phenomenon and idiopathic CTS.[16] Causes of CTS include tenosynovitis, over-use injuries, pregnancy (due to water retention), old distal radius fractures, diabetes mellitus, hypothyroidism, acromegaly, amyloidosis, mycobacterial infections, and tumours within the carpal tunnel space. Well-established risk factors include: being a woman of menopausal age, obesity, diabetes or having a family history of diabetes, osteoarthritis of the carpometacarpal joint of the thumb, smoking, and lifetime alcohol intake. It is a widely held view that symptoms of CTS may be caused or aggravated by fast repetitive or sustained forceful wrist activity, particularly with the wrist in a position of flexion or extension. Hand–arm vibration is associated with a neuropathy of the median nerve that may present in the same way as CTS, although it is thought that the pathological background may differ from that of classical CTS. A recent evidence-based review by the Faculty of Occupational Medicine[13] referred to a paper which concluded that 'the evidence supported a positive association with CTS and the use of vibrating tools, but the evidence was stronger for a positive association between exposure to a combination of risk factors such as repetitive and forceful work, awkward postures and vibration'.[17] Although it has generally been accepted that there is no dose–response relationship between vibration exposure and CTS, the same review concluded that there is 'limited evidence that suggests a dose–response relationship between vibration exposure and the prevalence of CTS'.

Musculoskeletal effects and Dupuytren's contracture

Weakness of grip has been reported in workers with HAVS, and is thought to be associated with dysfunction in the intrinsic muscles of the hands.[18–20] Although the pathological process and aetiology is unclear, a measure of grip strength should form part of the overall clinical assessment. Bone and joint disorders are recognized for state compensation in some countries, but it is difficult to differentiate these from the effects of heavy manual work. Similarly, studies on the association of hand–arm vibration and Dupuytren's contracture have produced conflicting findings, with some in favour and others against an association.[21,22]

Clinical assessment and standardized tests

Following a detailed history to elicit the features described earlier, a clinical assessment primarily to assess other causes should be undertaken and should include:

- The overall condition, temperature, colour of hands, presence of scars, Dupuyten's nodules or fibrosis.
- Bilateral measurement of blood pressure, radial and ulnar pulses, Allen's test, Adson's or Roos tests, auscultation for subclavian bruits.
- An assessment of sensory perception using Semmes Weinstein or West monofilament fibres, and of tactile discrimination (moving two-point discrimination) and manipulative dexterity (Purdue pegboard). The distribution of abnormalities of sensation should be recorded.
- If appropriate, assessment of cervical spine, vascular and neurological assessment of lower limbs.
- Phalen's and Tinel's tests for CTS.

It should be noted that many of these tests are of low discriminatory value for HAVS. Additional standardized tests and investigations may include:

- Thermal aesthesiometry and vibro-tactile threshold assessment, which are likely to have particular value in distinguishing early from late-stage 2SN cases.
- Doppler ultrasound, which may be useful in identifying hypothenar hammer syndrome.
- Nerve conduction studies, which are of value in diagnosing CTS that occurs in manual workers as well as those exposed to HTV.

Cold provocation (rewarm) testing is no longer regarded as providing additional useful evidence (Figure A6.1).[6,23]

Grading

The vascular and neurological components are graded separately according to two scales that were developed by a workshop in Stockholm and published in 1987 (Table A6.1).[24,25] These scales have international currency and have been modified recently in order to assist with the management of cases.[6]

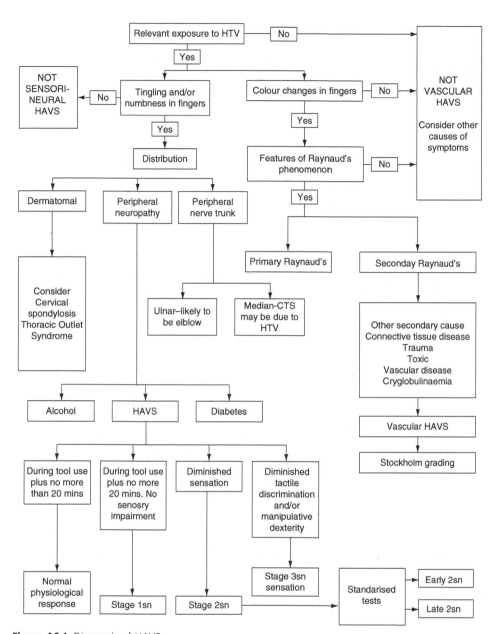

Figure A6.1 Diagnosis of HAVS.

Health surveillance and management of cases

The main elements of a health surveillance programme for HAVS comprise: (1) a system of symptom reporting; (2) periodic health inquiry and examination; (3) the formal clinical assessment of suspected cases; (4) the management of affected individuals; and (5) statutory record keeping.

In practice, the process begins with education and the encouragement of workers to report relevant symptoms to a responsible authority (doctor, nurse, line manager, or designated responsible

Table A6.1 The Stockholm Workshop Scale for the classification of the hand–arm vibration syndrome

Vascular component

Stage	Grade	Description
0		No attacks
1V	Mild	Occasional attacks affecting only the tips of one or more fingers
2V	Moderate	Occasional attacks affecting distal and middle (rarely also proximal) phalanges of one or more fingers
3V	Severe	Frequent attacks affecting all phalanges of most fingers
4V	Very severe	As in Stage 3, with trophic changes in the fingertips

Reprinted with permission from Gemne G et al., The Stockholm Workshop scale for the classification of cold induced Raynaud's phenomenon in the hand-arm vibration syndrome (revision of the Taylor Pelmear scale). *Scandinavian Journal of Work, Environment and Health* 1987; 13: 275–8, Copyright © 1987.

Sensorineural component

Stage	Description
0SN	Vibration-exposed but no symptoms
1SN	Intermittent numbness with or without tingling
2SN	Intermittent or persistent numbness, reduced sensory perception
3SN	Intermittent or persistent numbness, reduced tactile discrimination and/or manipulative dexterity

Note: The staging is made separately for each hand. The grade of the disorder is indicated by the stage and number of affected fingers on both hands, e.g. stage/hand/number of digits.

Reprinted with permission from Brammer AJ et al., Sensorineural stages of the hand arm vibration syndrome. *Scandinavian Journal of Work, Environment and Health* 1987; 13: 279–83, Copyright © 1987.

person). In addition, for those exposed above the EAV a screening questionnaire is completed at regular intervals, at, say, the pre-placement stage and then annually (with a check over the first 6 months to identify early and unusual susceptibility). Direct inquires are made about cold-induced finger blanching, sensorineural symptoms, problems of grip and dexterity, and sometimes other health effects.

The HSE suggests a tiered approach, as this is sparing of limited medical resource.[6] Evaluation by an appropriately trained and experienced clinician (having undergone a Faculty of Occupational Medicine approved training programme) is needed for those with symptoms—to confirm the nature, pattern, and history of complaints, to perform a clinical examination, and to consider differential diagnoses and the need for further tests and care.

At pre-employment assessment, consideration will be required of those who have pre-existing Raynaud's phenomenon. It would be appropriate to treat those with known HAVS in the same way as existing employees. Those who present at pre-employment with Raynaud's phenomenon due to another cause should be advised of a possible increased risk when exposed to HTV. This should not be considered an automatic bar to employment but workers in this position should certainly be kept under more regular surveillance. Also, it will be impossible to determine whether any progression is due to the pre-existing disease or to the effects of HTV. Similar arguments may be applied to pre-existing peripheral neuropathy. With careful assessment, symptoms due to cervical spondylosis or thoracic outlet syndrome may be distinguishable from a peripheral neuropathy, and hence need not influence decisions regarding exposure to HTV.

Those with CTS in emission—whether through treatment or not—can use vibratory tools, although recurrence of symptoms will raise the question of whether that is due to vibration or the pre-existing condition. There is no evidence that HTV leads to exacerbation of pre-existing compressive CTS, although much work with vibratory tools also includes other risk factors for CTS; it is advisable to inform both employee and employer of the potential increased risks. This is true also of those returning to work after CTS surgery and each case should be considered individually.

Attacks of cold-induced blanching are a source of discomfort, and work and leisure-time interference, but do not appear to cause much loss of working time and have little effect on long-term function. Sensory impairment is a much more important cause of functional disability.

It is now accepted that vascular symptoms can improve on withdrawal from exposure, albeit slowly over several years, and with the likelihood of recovery being influenced by the age of the worker, severity of the disease, and duration of post-symptomatic exposure. In contrast, the neurological effects of HAVS do not seem to improve. Against that background, the principle of management should be avoidance of progression to the more severe stage, which will increase the likelihood of improvement in symptoms as well as avoiding severe functional impairment which is likely to affect social and domestic activities as well as working ability. It is for this reason that a distinction has been drawn between early and late stage 2. The shift from early stage 2 to late stage 2 will indicate the need to avoid further exposure to HTV. However, other factors will also need consideration, including the speed of development of the symptoms (which may reflect individual susceptibility) and the age of the employee. Hence a 62-year-old worker with late stage 2SN who has shown no progression for 10 years might continue work without restriction, while a 35-year-old worker who has progressed from asymptomatic to stage 2 in a few years should certainly be advised to avoid further HTV exposure.

In affected workers, both categories of disease tend to progress if the degree of exposure continues unchecked. However, the rate of progression varies between individuals, and is not entirely predictable. It depends on many factors, including vibration magnitude, operator technique, and (probably) personal susceptibility.

Regardless of the decision on fitness for work, employers should receive a written record confirming that surveillance has taken place and the outcome. These 'health records' need to be retained by the employer. Group anonymized results of the health surveillance should be offered to the employer with a review of control measures if required (Figure A6.2).

Industrial Injuries Benefit

In the UK, HAVS (A11) is prescribed for Industrial Injuries Benefit in employed earners for both vascular and sensorineural components if they have worked in a listed occupation (<http://iiac. independent.gov.uk/pdf/command_papers/Cm6098.pdf>).

This state benefit may be claimed irrespective of fault and without a requirement for the individual to cease their job. Vibration-associated CTS (A12) is also prescribed. There are similar benefits in some European countries, some of which additionally compensate joint and bone disorders.

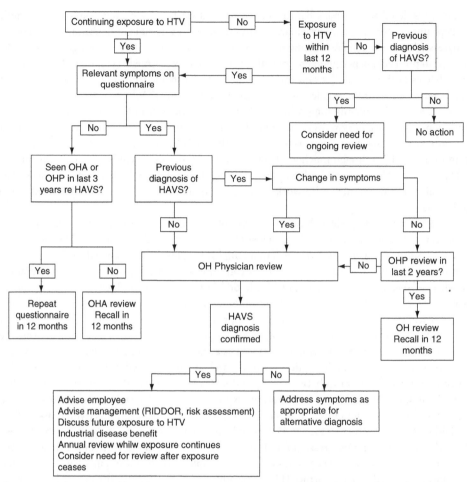

Figure A6.2 Occupational health management of cases. OHA, occupational health adviser; OHP, occupational health physician.

Reporting of Injuries, Diseases, and Dangerous Occurrences Regulations (RIDDOR)

Under separate legal provisions (the RIDDOR Regulations), employers have a statutory duty to notify cases of HAVS to the appropriate enforcing authority (HSE or local authority), once they become aware that a diagnosis has been made by a medical practitioner, irrespective of the severity (grade) of the symptoms.

The occupational health professional may be called upon to give advice on primary prevention and control measures. The usual hierarchy of control should be used: avoidance (can the requirement be designed out?), substitution (of tool or material worked), interruption of the vibration transmission pathway (by isolation or vibration-damping), and safer systems of work.

Regular tool maintenance programmes are often offered by tool suppliers, routinely replacing worn out tool parts. Training on tool usage, avoiding excessive grip and push forces, and the proper selection of tools for the tasks is also important. Sometimes tools and processes can be redesigned to avoid the need to come into contact with vibrating parts. Rest breaks and rotation of tasks that limit exposure time where practicable should be implemented. Although anti-vibration gloves are recommended in some countries, this is not presently the case in the UK.

References

1 Health and Safety Executive. *Regulatory impact assessment of the draft Control of Vibration at Work Regulations 2005 as they relate to hand-arm vibration.* Sudbury: HSE Books, 2004.

2 Bovenzi M, Peretti A, Nataletti P, *et al.* (eds). Workshop; 'Application of 2002/44/EC Directive in Europe'. In: *Proceedings of the 11th International Conference on Hand-Arm Vibration*, Bologna, Italy, 2007.

3 Griffin MJ. *Handbook of human vibration.* London: Academic Press, 1990.

4 Palmer KT, Griffin MJ, Syddall H, *et al.* Risk of hand-arm vibration syndrome according to occupation and sources of exposure to hand-transmitted vibration: a national survey. *Am J Ind Med* 2001; **39**: 389–96.

5 International Organization for Standardization (ISO). *Mechanical vibration – Measurement and evaluation of human exposure to hand-transmitted vibration. Part 1: General requirements.* ISO 5349-1. Geneva: ISO, 2001.

6 Health and Safety Executive. *Hand-arm vibration. The Control of Vibration at Work Regulations 2005. Guidance on regulations*, p. 71. L140. Sudbury: HSE Books, 2005.

7 Palmer KT, Haward B, Griffin MJ, *et al.* Validity of self-reported occupational exposures to hand-transmitted and whole-body vibration. *Occup Environ Med* 2000; 57: 237–41.

8 Gemne G, Brammer AJ, Hagberg M, *et al.* (eds). *Proceedings of the Stockholm workshop 94. Hand-arm vibration syndrome: Diagnostics and quantitative relationships to exposure.* Solna, Sweden: NIOH/Arbete Och Halsa, 1995.

9 Lawson IJ, McGeoch KL. HAVS assessment process for a large volume of medico-legal compensation cases. *Occup Med* 2003; 53: 302–8.

10 Cooke R, Lawson I. Use of Doppler in the diagnosis of hypothenar hammer syndrome. *Occup Med* 2009; 59: 185–90.

11 Ekenvall L, Nilsson BY, Gustavsson P. Temperature and vibration thresholds in vibration. *Br J Ind Med* 1986; 43: 825–9.

12 Takeuchi T, Imanischi H. Histopathological observations in finger biopsy from thirty patients with Raynaud's phenomenon of occupational origin. *J Kumanato Med Soc* 1984; 58: 56–70.

13 Mason H, Poole K. *Clinical testing and management of individuals exposed to hand-transmitted vibration: an evidence review.* London: Faculty of Occupational Medicine, 2004.

14 Ahmed Z, Khan M, Islam N. Cervical spondylosis. *Asian Med J* 1982; 25: 275–7.

15 Harrington JM, Carter JT, Birrell L, *et al.* Surveillance case definitions for work related upper limb pain syndromes. *Occup Env Med* 1998; 55: 264–71.

16 Hartmann P, Mohokum M, Schlattmann P. The association of Raynaud's syndrome with carpal tunnel syndrome. *Rheumatol Int* 2012; 32: 569–74.

17 Lozano-Calderón S, Anthony S, Ring D. The quality and strength of evidence for aetiology: example of carpal tunnel syndrome. *J Hand Surg* 2008; 33A: 525–38.

18 McGeoch KL, Gilmour WH. Cross sectional study of a workforce exposed to hand-arm vibration: with objective tests and the Stockholm workshop scales. *Occup Environ Med* 2000; 57: 35–42.

19 Necking LE, Lundstrom R, Lundborg G, *et al.* Hand muscle pathology after long term vibration exposure. *J Hand Surg* 2004; **29B**: 431–7.

20 Lawson IJ, Burke FD, Proud G, *et al.* Grip strength in miners with hand-arm vibration syndrome. *Occup Environ Med* 2006; **114**: 28–9.

21 Burke FD, Proud G, Lawson IJ, *et al.* An assessment of the effects to vibration, smoking, alcohol and diabetes on the prevalence of Dupuytren's disease in 97,537 miners. *J Hand Surg* 2007; **32E**: 400–6.

22 Descatha A, Jauffret P, Chastang JF, *et al.* Should we consider Dupuytren's contracture as work-related? A review and meta-analysis of an old debate. *BMC Musculoskelet Disord* 2011; 12: 96.

23 Proud G, Burke F, Lawson IJ, *et al.* Cold provocation testing and hand-arm vibration syndrome-an audit of the results of the Department of Trade and Industry scheme for the evaluation of miners. *Br J Surg* 2003; 90; 1076–9.

24 Gemne G, Pyykkö I, Taylor W, *et al.* The Stockholm Workshop scale for the classification of cold-induced Raynaud's phenomenon in the hand–arm vibration syndrome (revision of the Taylor Pelmear scale). *Scand J Work Environ Health* 1987; **13**: 275–8.

25 Brammer AJ, Taylor W, Lundborg G. Sensorineural stages of the hand–arm vibration syndrome. *Scand J Work Environ Health* 1987; **13**: 279–83.

Index